Frontiers in Neurosurgery

(Volume 4)

(Craniopharyngiomas - Classification and Surgical Treatment)

Editor

Songtao Qi

Department of Neurosurgery, Nanfang Neurosurgery Research Institution, Nanfang Hospital, Southern Medical University, 1838 North Guangzhou Avenue, 510515 Guangzhou, China

Associate Editors

Jun Pan and Yuntao Lu

Department of Neurosurgery, Nanfang Neurosurgery Research Institution, Nanfang Hospital, Southern Medical University, 1838 North Guangzhou Avenue, 510515 Guangzhou, China

Frontiers in Neurosurgery

Volume # 4

Craniopharyngiomas - Classification and Surgical Treatment

Editor: Songtao Qi

Associate Editors: Jun Pan and Yuntao Lu

ISSN (Online): 2405-741X

ISSN (Print): 2405-7401

ISBN (Online): 978-1-68108-532-6

ISBN (Print): 978-1-68108-533-3

General:

1. Any dispute or claim arising out of or in connection with this License Agreement or the Work (including non-contractual disputes or claims) will be governed by and construed in accordance with the laws of the U.A.E. as applied in the Emirate of Dubai. Each party agrees that the courts of the Emirate of Dubai shall have exclusive jurisdiction to settle any dispute or claim arising out of or in connection with this License Agreement or the Work (including non-contractual disputes or claims).
2. Your rights under this License Agreement will automatically terminate without notice and without the need for a court order if at any point you breach any terms of this License Agreement. In no event will any delay or failure by Bentham Science Publishers in enforcing your compliance with this License Agreement constitute a waiver of any of its rights.
3. You acknowledge that you have read this License Agreement, and agree to be bound by its terms and conditions. To the extent that any other terms and conditions presented on any website of Bentham Science Publishers conflict with, or are inconsistent with, the terms and conditions set out in this License Agreement, you acknowledge that the terms and conditions set out in this License Agreement shall prevail.

Bentham Science Publishers Ltd.
Executive Suite Y - 2
PO Box 7917, Saif Zone
Sharjah, U.A.E.
Email: subscriptions@benthamscience.org

BENTHAM SCIENCE

CONTENTS

PREFACE

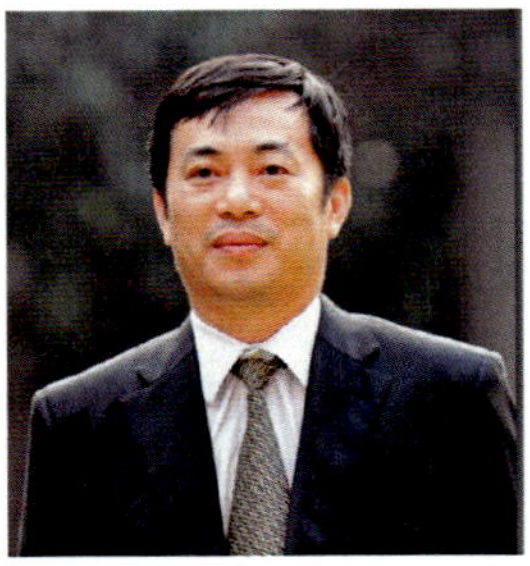

Chief Editor: Song-tao Qi

In the 30th years of last century, Dr. Harvey Cushing, the great master of neurosurgery, stated that "craniopharyngioma (CP) is the most buffering problem to the neurosurgeon". Although a century has since passed, this famous comment has been used frequently until now, indicating that the refractoriness of CP continues to challenge both patients and doctors.

During the past 10 years, epidemiological data regarding brain tumors have revealed that CP accounts for 6–9% of all intracranial tumors and 54% of pediatric tumors in the sellar region. Furthermore, the annual prevalence of CP within a given population was 1.3/million. The above data confirm that CP is not a rare type of tumor, but rather is a common intracranial tumor in pediatric patients.

Histopathologically, CP originates from residual embryonic Rathke's cyst cells, which are associated with a benign tumor. However, given the extreme difficulty associated with surgical treatment, various treatments for malignant cancers, such as conventional radiotherapy, stereotactic radiosurgery, internal radiation therapy, and chemotherapy, have been accepted by many neurosurgery centers in different countries worldwide. Despite this acceptance, the high rate of recurrence, low quality of life, and low tumor-free survival rate associated with CP unfortunately have not been significantly altered. Taken together, these findings suggest that this benign tumor exhibits malignant biological behaviors.

Undoubtedly, surgery is the optimal treatment method for CP. In other words, CP is a strictly surgical disease, and thus surgery might be the only curative method. In light of the advanced development and applications of microsurgical techniques in the most recent half-century, radical surgical CP removal has become increasingly accepted by high-level skull base neurosurgeons, and several publications have reported gross total CP removal rates exceeding 80%. However, given the deep location of CPs in close proximity to vital structures, the high levels of difficulty associated with surgical removal and risk during the perioperative period remain major problems associated with surgical treatment. Regarding reasonable surgical treatment methods for CP, several masters of neurosurgery, including Pascau, Yasargil, and Kassam, summarized large numbers of clinical cases and published several important papers in which they used their experiences to propose methods for selecting the appropriate surgical approach and best intraoperative techniques. These authors also proposed several widely influential clinical classifications of CP, which remain in current usage. Invariably, those classifications accounted for the relationship between the tumor and the third ventricle, and described the anatomical occupation as a purely radiological classification. It is difficult for an inexperienced neurosurgeon to completely understand the true origin of CP, particularly the true relationship of the tumor with the hypothalamic structures. Terminology such as intra-extra-ventricular CP and non-strictly or strictly intra-ventricular CP led to tremendous confusion regarding whether the surgical treatment of CP would inevitably injure the hypothalamic structures. As a result, the concept of unresectable CP was proposed and is considered the primary reason for the wide acceptance of radiotherapeutic and chemotherapeutic treatment of CP.

Since 1998, our group has accumulated experience in the surgical treatment of CP, based on the principle of radical gross total removal, in more than 500 cases. First, we paid more attention to the anatomical location of the tumor, and subsequently we shifted our focus to the various origins of CP and the relationships between tumors and surrounding vital structures during the development of the various types of CP. Interestingly, the clinical outcome improved dramatically. As a result, we proposed a new classification for CP, according to the stratification of anatomical features and based on the tumor origin.

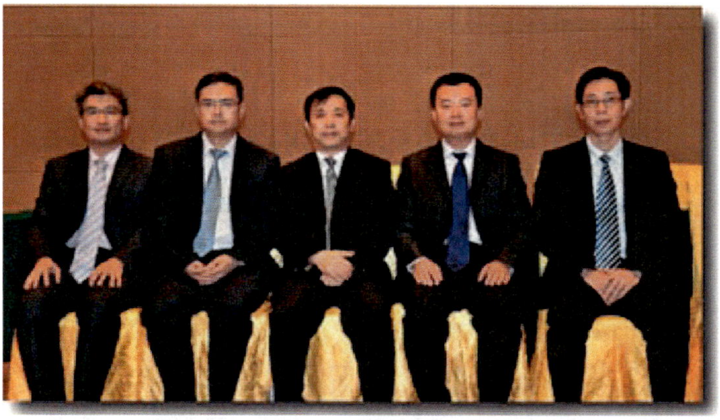

Major Contributing editors (Left to right): Lu Yuntao, Pan Jun, Qi Songtao, Zhang Xi-an, Fan Jun.

A restored understanding of the anatomical details of CP and their applications resulted in the advanced development of surgical techniques and clinical treatments. Our histological and anatomical studies of the hypophyseal gland, pituitary stalk and third ventricular floor provided a foundation for our clinical applications with regard to sellar region surgery, and comprise a highlighted feature of this book. Of course, a book containing such important clinical and experimental data could not have been completed only by the named authors. We therefore offer our appreciation for all students and observers who have ever studied at our clinical center, all technicians in our laboratory, and the secretaries in my office.

An understanding of CP, as well as difficulties of perioperative treatment and long-term hormone substitution, are likely to become strictly required for relevant workers, along with increased patience, thanksgiving and compassion. It is encouraging to note that this attitude has been accepted, inherited, and forwarded by all members of our team. I believe that this quality will not only benefit patients, but will also fill our own lives like a sunny and inspiring breeze.

I dedicate this book to all patients and their families for placing their trust in us. In addition, we offer the greatest appreciation to our unsung families for their tremendous and uncomplaining dedication.

Songtao Qi
Department of Neurosurgery
Nanfang Neurosurgery Research Institution
Nanfang Hospital, Southern Medical University
1838 North Guangzhou Avenue
510515 Guangzhou
China

List of Contributors

Chun-ling Ye	College of Pharmacy, Ji'nan University, 601 Western Huangpu Avenue, Guangzhou, China
Guang-long Huang	Department of Neurosurgery, Nanfang Neurosurgery Research Institution, Nanfang Hospital, Southern medical university, 1838 North Guangzhou avenue, Guangzhou, China
Jie Zhou	Department of Neurosurgery, The First Affiliated Hospital of Sichuan Medical University, 25 Taiping Road, Luzhou, China
Jun Fan	Department of Neurosurgery, Nanfang Neurosurgery Research Institution, Nanfang Hospital, Southern medical university, 1838 North Guangzhou avenue, Guangzhou, China
Jun Pan	Department of Neurosurgery, Nanfang Neurosurgery Research Institution, Nanfang Hospital, Southern medical university, 1838 North Guangzhou avenue, Guangzhou, China
Jun-xiang Peng	Department of Neurosurgery, Nanfang Neurosurgery Research Institution, Nanfang Hospital, Southern medical university, 1838 North Guangzhou avenue, Guangzhou, China
Songtao Qi	Department of Neurosurgery, Nanfang Neurosurgery Research Institution, Nanfang Hospital, Southern medical university, 1838 North Guangzhou avenue, Guangzhou, China
Xi-an Zhang	Department of Neurosurgery, Nanfang Neurosurgery Research Institution, Nanfang Hospital, Southern medical university, 1838 North Guangzhou avenue, Guangzhou, China
Xiao-rong Yan	Department of Neurosurgery, The First Affiliated Hospital of Fujian Medical University, 20 Chazhong Road, Fuzhou, China
Yi Liu	Department of Neurosurgery, Nanfang Neurosurgery Research Institution, Nanfang Hospital, Southern medical university, 1838 North Guangzhou avenue, Guangzhou, China
Yuntao Lu	Department of Neurosurgery, Nanfang Neurosurgery Research Institution, Nanfang Hospital, Southern medical university, 1838 North Guangzhou avenue, Guangzhou, China

CHAPTER 1

History and Epidemiology of Craniopharyngioma

Yuntao Lu*

Department of Neurosurgery, Nanfang Neurosurgery Research Institution, Nanfang Hospital, Southern Medical University, 1838 North Guangzhou Avenue, Guangzhou, China

Abstract: In this chapter, we firstly briefed reviewed the history and the terminology of craniopharyngioma (CP). Then with summarizing our own data based on 10 top hospitals in China and previous publications, we focused on description of the Epidemiology of craniopharyngioma (CP). And correspondingly, clinical manifestation of CP patients was depicted as well.

Keywords: Craniopharyngioma, Epidemioloty, History, Neurosurgery, Sellar region.

HISTORY AND TERMINOLOGY

In 1857, Zenker first described a mass composed of squamous epithelial cells along the pars distalis and pars tuberalis of the pituitary [1]. In 1860, Luschka [2] extensively researched adenohypophyseal squamous cells; however, his study was overlooked during the next several decades [3]. Therefore, the origin and terminology of such masses comprising squamous epithelial-like cells remained unclear at that time. In 1902, however, Saxer [4] reported tumors comprising the same type of squamous cells and two years later, after conducting systematic studies of adeno-hypophyseal squamous epithelial cells, Erdheim [5] reported in 1904 that these cells only existed in the pituitary glands of adult patients. Further details regarding location revealed that these cells were usually found on the anterior surface of the infundibulum and were distributed in islets or groups of variable size, shape, and number. Moreover, at that time, several masses comprising these squamous epithelial cells were found to contain various small cysts that were similar to an unnamed type of tumor that originated from the pituitary gland; therefore, the term "hypophyseal duct neoplasms" was used to describe those lesions.

* **Corresponding author Yuntao Lu:** Department of Neurosurgery, Nanfang Neurosurgery Research Institution, Nanfang Hospital, Southern Medical University, 1838 North Guangzhou Avenue, Guangzhou, China; Tel/Fax: +8620-61641806; E-mail: lllu2000yun@gmail.com

Songtao Qi (Ed.)

More interestingly, Erdheim found no residual cells along the regressed craniopharyngeal duct, in contrast to a proposal by Von Mihalkovitcs who postulated that during development, the pituitary gland would undergo an upward and forward rotation accompanied by intracranial insertion. It is possible that in terms of the route of development, some residual craniobuccal cyst cells remain. Subsequently, Hirsch O., Duffy, Kiyono, and Carmichael *et al.* reported similar theories [6]. Along with the development of embryonic pituitary gland studies, several terms were used in later years to describe this type of tumor, including hypophyseal duct tumor, craniopharyngeal duct tumor, Rathke's pouch tumor, interpeduncular and suprasellar tumors, craniobuccal cysts, suprasellar epithelioma, and adamantinoma. In 1932, Cushing initially proposed the name "craniopharyngioma" to define this type of tumor. Cushing explained this term as follows: "This admittedly somewhat cumbersome term has been employed for want of something more brief to include the kaleidoscopic tumors, solid and cystic, which take their origin from epithelial rests ascribable to an imperfect closure of the hypophyseal or craniopharyngeal duct" [7]. In the same year, Susman observed squamous epithelial cells in the pituitary glands of pediatric patients [8].

EPIDEMIOLOGY AND DEMOGRAPHY

Craniopharyngioma, which originates from residual Rathke's pouch cells, is a type of common benign sellar lesion that accounts for 2-5% of all intracranial tumors [9]. This is also the most common type pituitary mass in children, accounting for 6-13% of all childhood brain tumors and approximately 50% of childhood sellar tumors [10 - 12]. The Childhood Cancer Registry of Piedmont, Italy, has estimated an annual incidence of 1.4 cases per million children [13]. Similar data (*e.g.*, 0.11–0.13 cases per 100,000 people per year) have been reported by other registries in Western countries [14], thus constituting Class III evidence. According to Bunin [14], an annual incidence of 1.3 cases per million people (135 cases of craniopharyngioma) was reported in the USA during the period from 1990 to 1993 (Fig. **1**). Among pediatric populations, the incidence is slightly higher. For example, among children aged 5-14 years, the annual incidence is 1.8-2.0 cases per million children (Table **1**) [15]. There are no data to support a genetic or environmental basis for this disease. Similar result was also reported by CBTRUS (Central Brain Tumor Registry of the United States) and GDVPTR (Greater Delaware Valley Pediatric Tumor Registry) based on 300 newly diagnosed cases of craniopharyngioma in the USA, irrespective of race.

Pediatric cancer registries systematically include intracranial tumors with benign or unspecified behaviors, a category that includes craniopharyngioma [15, 16].

Table 1. The incidence of craniopharyngioma among various races and sexes in the US population.

<table>
<tr><th colspan="3">CBTRUS (1990–1993)</th><th colspan="4">Brain tumor registry of Los Angeles (LAC, 1972–1995)</th></tr>
<tr><th></th><th>Cases</th><th>Incidence*</th><th colspan="2"></th><th>Cases</th><th>Incidence*</th></tr>
<tr><td>Total</td><td>135</td><td>0.13</td><td colspan="2">Total</td><td>221</td><td></td></tr>
<tr><td>Male</td><td>68</td><td>0.13</td><td colspan="2">Male</td><td>118</td><td>0.13</td></tr>
<tr><td>Female</td><td>67</td><td>0.12</td><td colspan="2">Female</td><td>103</td><td>0.11</td></tr>
<tr><td>Caucasian</td><td>109</td><td>0.12</td><td rowspan="2">Male</td><td>Caucasian</td><td>62</td><td>0.14</td></tr>
<tr><td>African-American</td><td>11</td><td>0.13</td><td>African-American</td><td>12</td><td>0.12</td></tr>
<tr><td colspan="3" rowspan="2"></td><td rowspan="2">Female</td><td>Caucasian</td><td>59</td><td>0.11</td></tr>
<tr><td>African-American</td><td>11</td><td>0.10</td></tr>
</table>

*Incidence per million people (The descriptive epidemiology of craniopharyngioma, Neurosurgical Focus, 3(6): Article 1, 1997). CBTRUS, Central Brain Tumor Registry of the United States; LAC, Los Angeles County

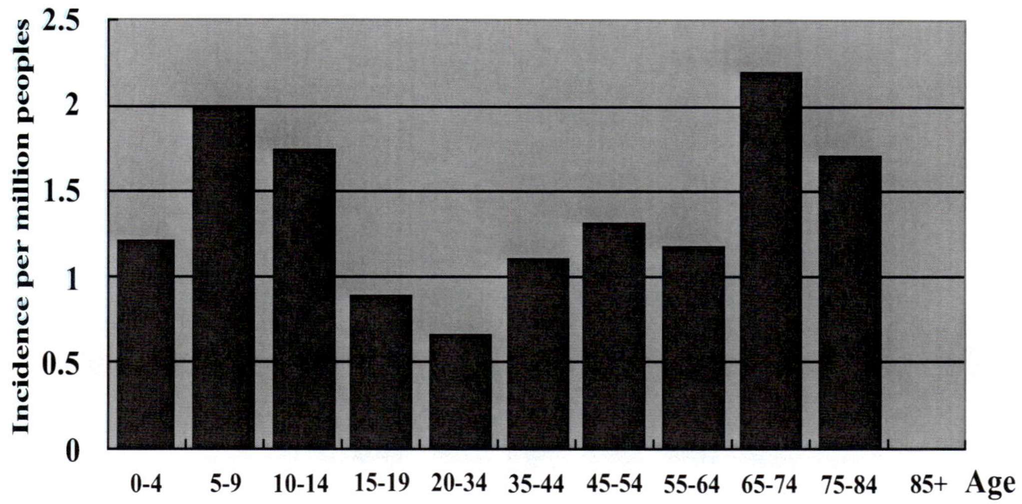

Fig. (1). Incidence of craniopharyngioma during the period from 1990 to 1993 as reported by the Central Brain Tumor Registry of the United States (CBTRUS) [15] (The descriptive epidemiology of craniopharyngioma, Neurosurgical Focus, 3(6): Article 1, 1997).

Although this disease can be detected at any age, even in prenatal and neonatal periods [17, 18], it exhibits a bimodal age distribution with the first peak in children between 5 and 14 years of age and the second in adults older than 65 years [14]. There is Class III evidence of clinical presentation usually in children aged 5–14 years, but there is a second peak in craniopharyngioma incidence in adults older than 75 years [19]. No gender-based differences have been observed in population-based studies from the USA and Finland [14, 20, 21] (Table **3**).

Craniopharyngioma is often associated with an enigmatic and unpredictable growth pattern. Despite the benign histological appearance of this tumor, its frequent tendency to infiltrate critical parasellar structures and aggressive behavior, even after apparently successful therapy, can lead to significant morbidity and mortality, thus posing a considerable medical and social problem. Rutka stated, "There is perhaps no other primary brain tumor that evokes more passion, emotion, and as a result, controversy than does the craniopharyngioma" [21]. Craniopharyngioma is classified as a tumor of the sellar region but may present elsewhere in the central nervous system (CNS) or nasopharynx. Predisposing risk factors (*e.g.*, genetic, environmental) are unknown [11]. Multiple craniopharyngioma cases have been reported within 2 families [22, 23], but there is no data to support a genetic or environmental basis for this disease.

Although limited, reports from Asia and Africa indicate a higher incidence of craniopharyngioma relative to Western countries (8). Among 2587 Chinese patients with craniopharyngioma, 586 were aged 0–10 years (22.7%) and 778 were aged 11–20 years (30.1%). Prenatal and neonatal craniopharyngiomas have also been described in multiple reports (2, 9, 11–13, 19, 23). According to our data, which were collected from January 1, 2000 to December 31, 2012, there were 248 cases of craniopharyngioma (age range, 0–72 years) in our department; these accounted for 3.8% of the 6487 total cases of CNS tumors and 18% of the 1365 cases involving sellar region tumors. Regarding pediatric patients, 85 patients presented with craniopharyngioma during childhood (<15 years), accounting for 64.9% of all pediatric sellar region tumors (131 cases); 54 and 31 of these cases were observed in boys and girls, respectively, for a male/female ratio of 1.74:1. Among adult patients (≥15 years), the incidence of craniopharyngioma was 13.2% among all cases involving sellar region tumors. Of these, 103 cases and 60 cases occurred in men and women, respectively, for a male/female ratio of 1.72:1. The prevalence of craniopharyngioma at various ages is summarized in (Fig. **2**).

Data representing a total of 538 craniopharyngioma cases (patient age range, 0–86 years) were collected from 10 of the top Chinese hospitals between January 1, 2006 and December 31, 2011. These hospitals included 1) Nanfang hospital, Southern medical university; 2) Xuanwu hospital, Capital Medical University; 3) Tangdu hospital, The fourth military medical university; 4) The first affiliate hospital of Harbin medical university; 5) Qilu hospital of Shandong university; 6) West China Hospital of Sichuan University; 7) Tianjin medical university general hospital; 8) The first Affiliated Hospital of China Medical University; 9) The first teaching hospital of Xinjiang medical university; 10) The first affiliated hospital of Fujian medical university. Among these patients, 120 (22.3%) were pediatric: 71 boys and 49 girls. The male/female ratio was 1.45:1. The total number of adult cases was 418 (77.7%), including 243 men and 175 women for a male/female ratio of 1.39:1. Similar craniopharyngioma prevalence rates were observed in various age groups based on these data from multiple Chinese neurosurgery centers (Fig. **3**). The incidence among men was also higher than that among women within various age groups. Craniopharyngioma occurrence remained most common during the period from 0 to 10 years of age (20.4%).

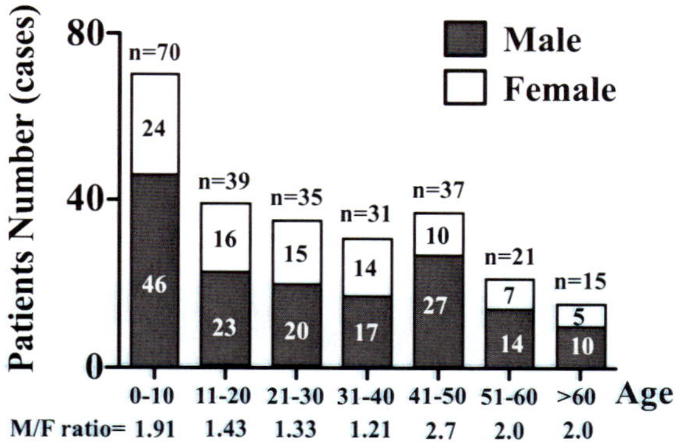

Fig. (2). The prevalence of craniopharyngioma at various ages. The 0–10 year age group accounted for 70 of 248 cases (28.2%), representing the most predominant period of occurrence; 39 (15.7%), 35 (14.1%), 31 (12.5%), 37 (14.9%), 21 (8.5%), and 15 cases (6.1%) occurred in the 11–20, 21–30, 31–40, 41–50, 51–60, and >60-year age groups, respectively. Our data showed significant gender bias; specifically, the prevalence among male patients was significantly higher than that among female patients. The male/female ratios within different age groups ranged from 1.21 to 2.7.

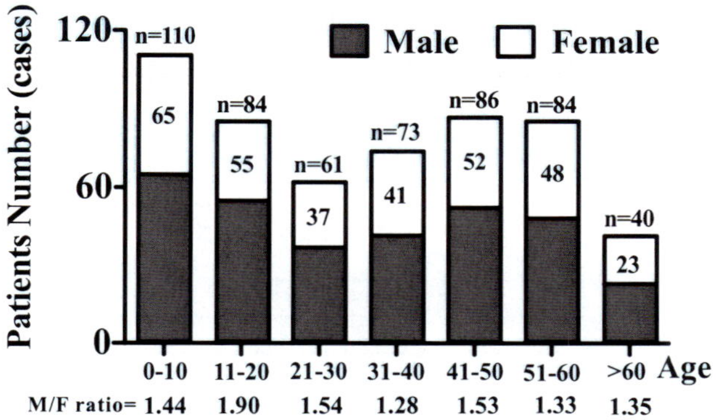

Fig. (3). Data from craniopharyngioma cases at the 10 top hospitals in China; the prevalence of cases at various ages is presented. The predominant period of occurrence was age 0–10 years (110 of 538 cases [20.4%]); in 84 (15.6%), 61 (11.3%), 73 (13.6%), 86 (16.0%), 84 (15.6%), and 40 (7.4%) cases, craniopharyngioma occurred in the 11–20, 21–30, 31–40, 41–50, 51–60, and >60 year age groups, respectively. Our data demonstrated significant gender bias; specifically, the prevalence was significantly higher among men than among women. The male/female ratios in different age groups ranged from 1.28 to 1.9.

CLINICAL MANIFESTATION

The clinical symptoms of craniopharyngioma are due to pressure exerted by the tumor on the surrounding vital structures of the sellar region, including the optical pathway, hypothalamus, pituitary stalk, ventricular system, and pituitary gland. Manifestation severity is closely related to tumor location, size, and potential growth [24 - 27]. Several publications have reported average periods from the presentation of symptoms to diagnosis ranging from 1 week to 372 months [28 - 31]. The most common presenting manifestations are headache, nausea/vomiting, visual disturbance, growth retardation (in children), and hypogonadism (in adults). Other manifestations are listed in (Table **2A, 2B**) [21]. Visual field defects, which usually manifest as bitemporal hemianopsia, are among the most common symptom presentations with an incidence as high as 49% [26, 28, 29]. Notably, this symptom can occasionally be relieved temporarily following cyst rupture and fluid drainage to the ventricles [32]. Other less common features include motor disorders such as hemi- or monoparesis [24, 33 - 35]; seizures [24]; psychiatric symptoms such as emotional lability, hallucinations, paranoid delusions [24, 28, 33, 35]; autonomic disturbances [24]; precocious puberty [29, 35]; inappropriate antidiuretic hormone secretion [36]; chemical meningitis due to spontaneous cyst rupture [37]; hearing loss [38]; anosmia [24]; nasal obstruction [39]; epistaxis [40]; photophobia [41]; emaciation [42, 43]; Weber's syndrome (ipsilateral III cranial nerve palsy with contralateral hemiplegia consequent to midbrain infarction) [44]; and Wallenberg's syndrome (consequent to occlusion of the posterior inferior cerebellar artery).

Table 2A. Most common presenting clinical manifestations of craniopharyngioma in children and adults (Craniopharyngioma. *Endocrine Reviews*, 2006, 27(4): 375) [21].

Ref.	No.	Age (yr)	Headache (%)	Nausea/ vomiting(%)	Papilloedema (%)	Cranial nerves palsy(%)	Ataxia/ Unsteadiness (%)	Cognitive dysfunction (%)[a]	Decreased consciousness /coma(%)	Optic atrophy (%)	Visual Field defects(%)
[45]	57	All<16	81	68	53						58
[46]	67	All<16	66	37	31	6		3b	7	20	35
[47]	241		78	34	25			36			71c
[48]	74	38<18	50								72
[49]	61	All<21	77	43	29	20	18		3		59d
[50]	56	26<19	7 adults,					20 adults,			60 adults,
			15 children	21		8 children		8 children			54 children
[51]	121	32≤16	74		10	2		10	29	15	62
[52]	122	29<16	53	49	16	3		13	8	40	79
[53]	75	All<16.4	65		32	15	17		16	40	44
[54]	119	41<16	56 adults,	26 adults,	6 adults,	9 adults,	3 adults,	17 adults,	4 adults,	14 adults,	60 adults,
			78 children	54 children	29 children	27 children	7 children	10 children	10 children	5 children	46 children

(Table 2A) contd.....

Ref.	No.	Age (yr)	Headache (%)	Nausea/ vomiting(%)	Papilloedema (%)	Cranial nerves palsy(%)	Ataxia/ Unsteadiness (%)	Cognitive dysfunction (%)[a]	Decreased consciousness /coma(%)	Optic atrophy (%)	Visual Field defects(%)
Range			7-81	21-68	6-53	2-27	3-18	3-36	3-29	5-40	35-79

[a] Memory loss, confusion, disorientation [b] Reported as 'slow mentality' [c] Reported as 'visual difficulties'
[d] Patients with decreased visual acuity are also included

Table 2B. Most common presenting clinical manifestations of craniopharyngioma in children and adults (Craniopharyngioma. *Endocrine Reviews*, 2006, 27(4): 375) [21].

Ref.	No.	Age(yr)	Decreased visual acuity or visual deterioration (%)	Growth failure[a] (%)	Failure of sexual development[a] (%)	Hypogonadism (adults) (%)	Poor energy (%)	Somnolence (%)	Anorexia/poor weight gain or weight loss (%)	Obesity or weight gain (%)	Polyuria/ polydipsia (%)
[45]	57	All<16	58	39							9
[46]	67	All<16		7 (42% with retarded bone age)	20 (of pubertal children)			9			12
[47]	241							20			6
[48]	74	38<18		93		85					23
[49]	61	All<21		25							13
[50]	56	26<19	47 adults,	8	4	10					3 adults
			50 children							4 children	
[51]	121	32≤16	62	17	14		23			8	12
[52]	122	29<16	80	45		40					18
[53]	75	All<16.4	47	33	5			20	31	15	28
[54]	119	41<16	40 adults,	32	24	28	32 adults,	10 adults,	8 adults,	13 adults,	15 adults,
			39 children				22 children	5 children	20 children	5 children	15 children
Range			39-80	7-93	4-24	10-85	22-32	5-20	8-31	4-15	3-28

[a] children

Endocrinological evaluation is indispensable for craniopharyngioma patients. At presentation, the hypothalamic–pituitary function has likely undergone severe destruction. Following the experimental detection of 122 patients with craniopharyngioma, Effenterre and Boch [34] observed that 85% had single-axis or multiple-axis hormone deficits. Despite the use of different endocrinological evaluation methods and criteria, a summary of multiple research results revealed that 35–95% of patients presented with growth hormone (GH) deficiency, 38–82% with follicle stimulating hormone/luteinizing hormone deficiency, 21–62% with adrenocorticotropic hormone deficiency, 21–42% with thyroid-stimulating hormone deficiency, and 6–38% with diabetes insipidus [21] (Table **3**). However, Karavitaki thought that the incidence of GH deficiency might have been overestimated and that the real incidence was not as high as the reports because of selection bias among patients who underwent testing (particularly adults), as these more likely represented symptomatic cases.

Table 3. Pituitary hormone deficits and hyperprolactinemia at presentation in children and adults with craniopharyngioma (Craniopharyngioma. *Endocrine Reviews*, 2006, 27(4): 375) [21].

Ref	No.	Age(yr)	GH deficiency	FSH/LH deficiency[a]	ACTH deficiency	TSH deficiency	Hyper-prolactinemia	DI
[55]	42	All≤17.2	13/18(72)	3/8(38)	4/17(24)	7/29(24)		4/24(17)
[48]	74	38<18			18/74(24)	31/74(42)		8/74(12)
[56]	61	All<21	12/34(35)		7/34(21)	7/34(21)		8/34(23)
[57]	35	13<19	27/35(77)	27/33(82)	12/35(34)	13/35(37)	7/29(24)	13/35(38)
[58]	75	All<16.3	13/15(87)	3/6(50)	16/50(32)	20/62(32)	12/37(32)	22/75(29)
[59]	143	30<16	59/82, 17/23 in children(74)	96/143(77), 10/11 in children(91)	45/143(32), 8/30 in children(27)	35/143(25), 6/30 in children(20)	59/143(41), 5/30 in children(17)	23/143(16), 3/30 in children(10)
[60]	18	No age range reported	7/18(39)	10/18(56)	9/18(50)	7/18(39)	6/18(33)	1/18(6)
[54]	121	42<16	21/22(95) 15/15 in children(100)	40/54(74)[b]	40/65(62), 15/22 in children(68)	29/81(36), 7/28 in children(25)	24/44(55)[b]	19/104(18), 7/32 in children(22)
Range			35-100	38-91	21-68	20-42	17-55	6-38

The use of different tests and diagnostic criteria for establishing the compromised pituitary function in the various series should be taken into account. Data are presented as the number of patients with the defect/total number of patients tested (relevant percentages). [a] Prepubertal children were excluded from the evaluations. [b] Only adults were included in the evaluations. Note: GH, growth hormone; FSH, follicle stimulating hormone; LH, luteinizing hormone; ACTH, adrenocorticotrophic hormone; TSH, thyroid-stimulating hormone; DI, diabetes insipidus

Some of the previous literature reports have described particular manifestations as restricted to various age groups. For example, in such reports, increased intra-cranial pressure always occurred in pediatric patients; sexual immaturity, in adolescents; visual deficits and hypopituitarism, in young and middle-aged adults (preferentially); and mental dysfunction, in elderly patients. A series investigation that compared pediatric and adult patients found that headache, nausea/vomiting, papilloedema, and cranial nerve palsy were more frequent among children; this is likely associated with the higher rates of hydrocephalus among young patients. However, regarding clinical manifestations, no significant differences were found between children and adults with respect to symptom duration and endocrinological dysfunction. Karavitaki *et al.* also stressed a more cautious interpretation of clinical manifestation data because these data were extracted from several retrospective studies rather than specific systematic questionnaires.

The detailed clinical information collected from 144 patients at our own hospital between January 1, 1996 and December 31, 2010 was respectively reviewed. Regarding clinical manifestations, diabetes insipidus occurred more frequently among all patients (68.8%) than visual disturbances (66%) and headache (46.8%). Other symptoms such as sexual disturbances (17.7%), epilepsy (2.1%), mental disorders (3.5%), lethargy (9.2%), and emaciation (2.8%) were also presented. As indicated in Fig. (**4**), headache was the most common presenting symptom in pediatric patients (65.4%), followed by diabetes insipidus (63.5%) and visual disturbances (59.6%). Moreover, growth retardation is usually a pediatric presentation (30.8%). However, mental disorders and emaciation were not observed in young patients.

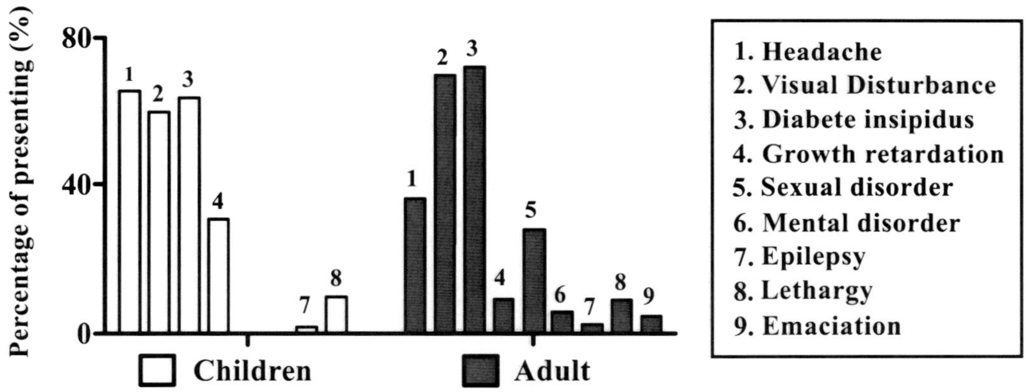

Fig. (4). The percentage of various craniopharyngioma symptoms upon presentation in Children and adult patients.

Regarding endocrinological function, 83% of all patients exhibited either single-axis dysfunction (58%) or panhypopituitarism (25%). Notably, this rate was even higher among pediatric patients. Among the 58 pediatric cases, 98% suffered from endocrine deficiency, including 53.8% with single-axis and 44.2% with multiple deficits. Most adult patients exhibited single hypothalamic-pituitary axis dysfunction (62.5%), whereas only 4.2% exhibited panhypopituitarism. Additionally, 6.7% of adult patients exhibited amenorrhea.

An analysis of craniopharyngioma data from multiple centers in China (top 10 hospitals nationwide) yielded similar results with respect to clinical manifestation. The most frequent symptoms included the visual acuity deficits (69.8%), headache (69.1%), diabetes insipidus (58.9%), and visual field defects (45.9%). Other presentations such as amenorrhea (10.2%), lethargy (9.4%), and memory deficit (2.4%) were also observed. Similar to our data, the most common symptom among pediatric patients was headache (84.1%), followed by visual acuity deficits (55.3%), visual field defects (43.6%), and diabetes insipidus (35.9%). Growth retardation was observed in 13.8% of patients. However, in adults, decreased visual acuity was the most common symptom (72.4%), followed by headache (65.7%) and visual field defects (46.4%). Both the data from our department and from multiple centers in China revealed some differences between pediatric and adult patients.

CONFLICT OF INTEREST

The author (editor) declares no conflict of interest, financial or otherwise.

ACKNOWLEDGEMENTS

Declared none.

REFERENCES

[1] Raimondi AJ, Rougerie J. A critical review of personal experiences with craniopharyngioma: clinical history, surgical technique and operative results. 1983. Pediatr Neurosurg 1994; 21(2): 134-50. [http://dx.doi.org/10.1159/000120827] [PMID: 7986744]

[2] Luschka H. Der Gehirnhang und die Steissdruese des Menschen. Berlin: G. Reimer 1860.

[3] Hirsch O. Hypophyseal duct tumors (craniopharyngiomas) versus adamantinomas. J Neuropathol Exp Neurol 1958; 17(2): 305-14. [http://dx.doi.org/10.1097/00005072-195804000-00013] [PMID: 13525990]

[4] Saxer F. Ein Beitrag zur Kenntniss der Dermoide und Teratome. Ziegler's Beitr 1902.

[5] Erdheim J. Über hypophysengangsgeschwulste und hirmcholesteatome. Sitzungsb Kais Akad Wissen Math Naturw Klin 1904; 113: 537-726.

[6] Hirsch O. Hypophyseal duct tumors (craniopharyngiomas) versus adamantinomas. J Neuropathol Exp Neurol 1958; 17(2): 305-14. [http://dx.doi.org/10.1097/00005072-195804000-00013] [PMID: 13525990]

[7] Cushing H. The craniopharyngioma Intralcranial tumors. London: Bailliere, Tindal and Cox 1932; pp. 93-8.

[8] Susman W. Embryonic epithelial rests in the pituitary. Br J Surg 1932; 19(76): 571-6. [http://dx.doi.org/10.1002/bjs.1800197607]

[9] Parisi JE. Mena H., Nonglial tumors.Principles and practice of neuropathology. 1st ed. St. Louis, MO: Mosby 1993; pp. 203-66.

[10] Matson DD, Crigler JF Jr. Management of craniopharyngioma in childhood. J Neurosurg 1969; 30(4): 377-90. [http://dx.doi.org/10.3171/jns.1969.30.4.0377] [PMID: 4308176]

[11] Schoenberg BS, Schoenberg DG, Christine BW, Gomez MR. The epidemiology of primary intracranial neoplasms of childhood. A population study. Mayo Clin Proc 1976; 51(1): 51-6. [PMID: 1249998]

[12] Kuratsu J, Ushio Y. Epidemiological study of primary intracranial tumors in childhood. A population-based survey in Kumamoto Prefecture, Japan. Pediatr Neurosurg 1996; 25(5): 240-6.

[http://dx.doi.org/10.1159/000121132] [PMID: 9309787]

[13] Haupt R, Magnani C, Pavanello M, Caruso S, Dama E, Garrè ML. Epidemiological aspects of craniopharyngioma. J Pediatr Endocrinol Metab 2006; 19 (Suppl. 1): 289-93. [PMID: 16700303]

[14] Bunin GR, Surawicz TS, Witman PA, Preston-Martin S, Davis F, Bruner JM. The descriptive epidemiology of craniopharyngioma. J Neurosurg 1998; 89(4): 547-51. [http://dx.doi.org/10.3171/jns.1998.89.4.0547] [PMID: 9761047]

[15] Bunin GR, Surawicz TS, Witman PA, Preston-Martin S, Davis F, Bruner JM. The descriptive epidemiology of craniopharyngioma. Neurosurg Focus 1997; 3(6): e1. [http://dx.doi.org/10.3171/foc.1997.3.6.4] [PMID: 17206775]

[16] Haupt R, Magnani C, Pavanello M, Caruso S, Dama E, Garrè ML. Epidemiological aspects of craniopharyngioma. J Pediatr Endocrinol Metab 2006; 19 (Suppl. 1): 289-93. [PMID: 16700303]

[17] Bailey W, Freidenberg GR, James HE, Hesselink JR, Jones KL. Prenatal diagnosis of a craniopharyngioma using ultrasonography and magnetic resonance imaging. Prenat Diagn 1990; 10(10): 623-9. [http://dx.doi.org/10.1002/pd.1970101002] [PMID: 2274487]

[18] Müller-Scholden J, Lehrnbecher T, Müller HL, *et al.* Radical surgery in a neonate with craniopharyngioma. report of a case. Pediatr Neurosurg 2000; 33(5): 265-9. [http://dx.doi.org/10.1159/000055967] [PMID: 11155065]

[19] Surawicz TS, McCarthy BJ, Kupelian V, Jukich PJ, Bruner JM, Davis FG. Descriptive epidemiology of primary brain and CNS tumors: results from the Central Brain Tumor Registry of the United States, 1990-1994. Neuro-oncol 1999; 1(1): 14-25. [PMID: 11554386]

[20] Sorva R, Heiskanen O. Craniopharyngioma in Finland. A study of 123 cases. Acta Neurochir (Wien) 1986; 81(3-4): 85-9. [http://dx.doi.org/10.1007/BF01401226] [PMID: 3489356]

[21] Rutka JT. Craniopharyngioma. J Neurosurg 2002; 97(1): 1-2. [http://dx.doi.org/10.3171/jns.2002.97.1.0001] [PMID: 12134898]

[22] Boch AL, van Effenterre R, Kujas M. Craniopharyngiomas in two consanguineous siblings: case report. Neurosurgery 1997; 41(5): 1185-7. [http://dx.doi.org/10.1097/00006123-199711000-00031] [PMID: 9361074]

[23] Green AL, Yeh JS, Dias PS. Craniopharyngioma in a mother and daughter. Acta Neurochir (Wien) 2002; 144(4): 403-4. [http://dx.doi.org/10.1007/s007010200058] [PMID: 12021891]

[24] Petito CK, DeGirolami U, Earle KM. Craniopharyngiomas: a clinical and pathological review. Cancer 1976; 37(4): 1944-52. [http://dx.doi.org/10.1002/1097-0142(197604)37:4<1944::AID-CNCR2820370446>3.0.CO;2-#] [PMID: 1260697]

[25] Weiner HL, Wisoff JH, Rosenberg ME, *et al.* Craniopharyngiomas: a clinicopathological analysis of factors predictive of recurrence and functional outcome. Neurosurgery 1994; 35(6): 1001-10. [http://dx.doi.org/10.1227/00006123-199412000-00001] [PMID: 7885544]

[26] Baskin DS, Wilson CB. Surgical management of craniopharyngiomas. A review of 74 cases. J Neurosurg 1986; 65(1): 22-7. [http://dx.doi.org/10.3171/jns.1986.65.1.0022] [PMID: 3712025]

[27] Paja M, Lucas T, García-Uría J, Salamé F, Barceló B, Estrada J. Hypothalamic-pituitary dysfunction in patients with craniopharyngioma. Clin Endocrinol (Oxf) 1995; 42(5): 467-73. [http://dx.doi.org/10.1111/j.1365-2265.1995.tb02664.x] [PMID: 7621564]

[28] Duff J, Meyer FB, Ilstrup DM, Laws ER Jr, Schleck CD, Scheithauer BW. Long-term outcomes for surgically resected craniopharyngiomas. Neurosurgery 2000; 46(2): 291-302. [http://dx.doi.org/10.1097/00006123-200002000-00007] [PMID: 10690718]

[29] Hoffman HJ, De Silva M, Humphreys RP, Drake JM, Smith ML, Blaser SI. Aggressive surgical management of craniopharyngiomas in children. J Neurosurg 1992; 76(1): 47-52. [http://dx.doi.org/10.3171/jns.1992.76.1.0047] [PMID: 1727168]

[30] Graham PH, Gattamaneni HR, Birch JM. Paediatric craniopharyngiomas: a regional review. Br J Neurosurg 1992; 6(3): 187-93. [http://dx.doi.org/10.3109/02688699209002926] [PMID: 1632917]

[31] Love JG, Marshall TM. Craniopharyngiomas. Surg Gynecol Obstet 1950; 90(5): 591-601. [PMID: 15418429]

[32] Chen C, Okera S, Davies PE, Selva D, Crompton JL. Craniopharyngioma: a review of long-term visual outcome. Clin Experiment Ophthalmol 2003; 31(3): 220-8. [http://dx.doi.org/10.1046/j.1442-9071.2003.00648.x] [PMID: 12786772]

[33] Karavitaki N, Brufani C, Warner JT, *et al.* Craniopharyngiomas in children and adults: systematic analysis of 121 cases with long-term follow-up. Clin Endocrinol (Oxf) 2005; 62(4): 397-409. [http://dx.doi.org/10.1111/j.1365-2265.2005.02231.x] [PMID: 15807869]

[34] Van Effenterre R, Boch AL. Craniopharyngioma in adults and children: a study of 122 surgical cases. J Neurosurg 2002; 97(1): 3-11. [http://dx.doi.org/10.3171/jns.2002.97.1.0003] [PMID: 12134929]

[35] Banna M, Hoare RD, Stanley P, Till K. Craniopharyngioma in children. J Pediatr 1973; 83(5): 781-5. [http://dx.doi.org/10.1016/S0022-3476(73)80369-5] [PMID: 4742571]

[36] Gonzales-Portillo G, Tomita T. The syndrome of inappropriate secretion of antidiuretic hormone: an unusual presentation for childhood craniopharyngioma: report of three cases. Neurosurgery 1998; 42(4): 917-21. [http://dx.doi.org/10.1097/00006123-199804000-00131] [PMID: 9574658]

[37] Patrick BS, Smith RR, Bailey TO. Aseptic meningitis due to spontaneous rupture of craniopharyngioma cyst. Case report. J Neurosurg 1974; 41(3): 387-90. [http://dx.doi.org/10.3171/jns.1974.41.3.0387] [PMID: 4412094]

[38] Honegger J, Buchfelder M, Fahlbusch R. Surgical treatment of craniopharyngiomas: endocrinological results. J Neurosurg 1999; 90(2): 251-7. [http://dx.doi.org/10.3171/jns.1999.90.2.0251] [PMID: 9950495]

[39] Kanungo N, Just N, Black M, Mohr G, Glikstein R, Rochon L. Nasopharyngeal craniopharyngioma in an unusual location. AJNR Am J Neuroradiol 1995; 16(6): 1372-4. [PMID: 7677045]

[40] Ahsan F, Rashid H, Chapman A, Ah-See KW. Infrasellar craniopharyngioma presenting as epistaxis, excised via Denker's medial maxillectomy approach. J Laryngol Otol 2004; 118(11): 895-8. [http://dx.doi.org/10.1258/0022215042703688] [PMID: 15638981]

[41] Kawasaki A, Purvin VA. Photophobia as the presenting visual symptom of chiasmal compression. J Neuroophthalmol 2002; 22(1): 3-8. [http://dx.doi.org/10.1097/00041327-200203000-00002] [PMID: 11937897]

[42] Svolos DG. Craniopharyngiomas. A study based on 108 verified cases. Acta Chir Scand Suppl 1969; 403: 1-44. [PMID: 5280972]

[43] Miyoshi Y, Yunoki M, Yano A, Nishimoto K. Diencephalic syndrome of emaciation in an adult associated with a third ventricle intrinsic craniopharyngioma: case report. Neurosurgery 2003; 52(1): 224-7.

[PMID: 12493122]

[44] Waga S, Handa H. Radiation-induced meningioma: with review of literature. Surg Neurol 1976; 5(4): 215-9.
[PMID: 817405]

[45] Matson DD, Crigler JF Jr. Management of craniopharyngioma in childhood. J Neurosurg 1969; 30(4): 377-90.
[http://dx.doi.org/10.3171/jns.1969.30.4.0377] [PMID: 4308176]

[46] Banna M, Hoare RD, Stanley P, Till K. Craniopharyngioma in children. J Pediatr 1973; 83(5): 781-5.
[http://dx.doi.org/10.1016/S0022-3476(73)80369-5] [PMID: 4742571]

[47] Petito CK, DeGirolami U, Earle KM. Craniopharyngiomas: a clinical and pathological review. Cancer 1976; 37(4): 1944-52.
[http://dx.doi.org/10.1002/1097-0142(197604)37:4<1944::AID-CNCR2820370446>3.0.CO;2-#]
[PMID: 1260697]

[48] Baskin DS, Wilson CB. Surgical management of craniopharyngiomas. A review of 74 cases. J Neurosurg 1986; 65(1): 22-7.
[http://dx.doi.org/10.3171/jns.1986.65.1.0022] [PMID: 3712025]

[49] Hetelekidis S, Barnes PD, Tao ML, *et al.* 20-year experience in childhood craniopharyngioma. Int J Radiat Oncol Biol Phys 1993; 27(2): 189-95.
[http://dx.doi.org/10.1016/0360-3016(93)90227-M] [PMID: 8407391]

[50] Weiner HL, Wisoff JH, Rosenberg ME, *et al.* Craniopharyngiomas: a clinicopathological analysis of factors predictive of recurrence and functional outcome. Neurosurgery 1994; 35(6): 1001-10.
[http://dx.doi.org/10.1227/00006123-199412000-00001] [PMID: 7885544]

[51] Duff J, Meyer FB, Ilstrup DM, Laws ER Jr, Schleck CD, Scheithauer BW. Long-term outcomes for surgically resected craniopharyngiomas. Neurosurgery 2000; 46(2): 291-302.
[http://dx.doi.org/10.1097/00006123-200002000-00007] [PMID: 10690718]

[52] Van Effenterre R. Boch AL2002 Craniopharyngioma in adults and children. J Neurosurg •••; 97: 3-11.
[http://dx.doi.org/10.3171/jns.2002.97.1.0003] [PMID: 12134929]

[53] DeVile CJ. Craniopharyngioma.Oxford textbook of endocrinology and diabetes. 1st ed. Oxford, UK: Oxford University Press 2002; pp. 218-25.

[54] Karavitaki N, Brufani C, Warner JT, *et al.* Craniopharyngiomas in children and adults: systematic analysis of 121 cases with long-term follow-up. Clin Endocrinol (Oxf) 2005; 62(4): 397-409.
[http://dx.doi.org/10.1111/j.1365-2265.2005.02231.x] [PMID: 15807869]

[55] Thomsett MJ, Conte FA, Kaplan SL, Grumbach MM. Endocrine and neurologic outcome in childhood craniopharyngioma: Review of effect of treatment in 42 patients. J Pediatr 1980; 97(5): 728-35.
[http://dx.doi.org/10.1016/S0022-3476(80)80254-X] [PMID: 7431164]

[56] Baskin DS, Wilson CB. Surgical management of craniopharyngiomas. A review of 74 cases. J Neurosurg 1986; 65(1): 22-7.
[http://dx.doi.org/10.3171/jns.1986.65.1.0022] [PMID: 3712025]

[57] Paja M, Lucas T, García-Uría J, Salamé F, Barceló B, Estrada J. Hypothalamic-pituitary dysfunction in patients with craniopharyngioma. Clin Endocrinol (Oxf) 1995; 42(5): 467-73.
[http://dx.doi.org/10.1111/j.1365-2265.1995.tb02664.x] [PMID: 7621564]

[58] DeVile CJ, Grant DB, Hayward RD, Stanhope R. Growth and endocrine sequelae of craniopharyngioma. Arch Dis Child 1996; 75(2): 108-14.
[http://dx.doi.org/10.1136/adc.75.2.108] [PMID: 8869189]

[59] Honegger J, Buchfelder M, Fahlbusch R. Surgical treatment of craniopharyngiomas: endocrinological results. J Neurosurg 1999; 90(2): 251-7.
[http://dx.doi.org/10.3171/jns.1999.90.2.0251] [PMID: 9950495]

[60] Shin JL, Asa SL, Woodhouse LJ, Smyth HS, Ezzat S. Cystic lesions of the pituitary: clinicopathological features distinguishing craniopharyngioma, Rathke's cleft cyst, and arachnoid cyst. J Clin Endocrinol Metab 1999; 84(11): 3972-82.
[PMID: 10566636]

CHAPTER 2

The Pituitary Gland and Etiology of Craniopharyngioma

Yuntao Lu*

Department of Neurosurgery, Nanfang Neurosurgery Research Institution, Nanfang Hospital, Southern Medical University, 1838 North Guangzhou Avenue, Guangzhou, China

Abstract: As histological benign tumor with malignant cellular characteristic, craniophayrngyioma (CP) caused big trouble not only for surgery but also for the postsurgical management. So, it is important to emphase the understanding of the pituitary gland and also it's connected structures, such as pituitary stalk, hypothalamus, and so on. In this chapter, we described the anatomical and cytological constructors of pituitary gland. As with combined the etiology of CP, we depicted the embryonic development of gland and its accessory structures. On the other hand, several hypotheses about the origin of CP were also analysed and described.

Keywords: Craniopharyngioma, Embryonic development, Histology, Pituitary gland.

INTRODUCTION

Despite its benign pathological and cellular features, the clinical prognosis of craniopharyngioma remains unsatisfactory. The current consensus regarding the reasons for this poor prognosis includes the close relationships formed between the tumor and several vital neurovascular structures such as the hypophysis, pituitary stalk, hypothalamus, and some important perforating branches of the internal carotid artery (ICA), anterior cerebral artery (ACA), or anterior communicating artery (AcoA). In clinical studies, the closest adherence is always observed at the originating site of the craniopharyngioma. In this context, neurosurgeons worldwide have attempted to determine the exact etiologies of craniopharyngiomas with various types of growth patterns in order to reveal this elusive information.

However, great controversies regarding the etiology of craniopharyngioma, a type

* **Corresponding author Yuntao Lu:** Department of Neurosurgery, Nanfang Neurosurgery Research Institution, Nanfang Hospital, Southern Medical University, 1838 North Guangzhou Avenue, Guangzhou, China; Tel/Fax: +8620-61641806; E-mail: lllu2000yun@gmail.com

Songtao Qi (Ed.)

of sellar tumor with a widely varied and non-uniform morphology, have remained for several decades. Despite the above-mentioned disputes, several hypotheses based on normal anatomy and embryonic pituitary gland development is currently accepted. Therefore, to describe the etiologies of craniopharyngiomas, the morphology, cytology, and developmental process of the normal pituitary gland should first be understood.

MORPHOLOGY AND CYTOLOGY OF THE PITUITARY GLAND

Anatomical Conceptions

In the sellar region, the pituitary gland is located within the pituitary fossa, which connected to the hypothalamus *via* the pituitary stalk. The pituitary gland is oval-shaped with an approximate length of 1 cm, width of 1-1.5 cm, and height of 0.5 cm. The weight of the neonatal pituitary gland is approximately 0.1 g; this, however, increases significantly with age, reaching weights of 0.5-0.7 g in adult men and even heavier weights in women. During pregnancy, the pituitary gland volume enlarges significantly, and the weight can reach 1.5 g in multiparous women. Despite its small volume, the pituitary gland is among the most important endocrinological organs; this organ not only secretes various hormones that target other organs, but also connects to the high-grade endocrinological center through the hypothalamic–pituitary axis. Therefore, the pituitary gland plays pivotal roles within the endocrine and nervous regulatory control systems.

Classic textbooks divide the pituitary gland into the anterior (adenohypophysis) and posterior lobes (neurohypophysis). The adenohypophysis occupies the anterior three quarters of the gland and can be further divided into the pars distalis, pars tuberalis, and pars intermedia. The normal human pars distalis, which constitutes the major part of the gland, is kidney-shaped and golden-yellow and is located in the anterior extremity. The pars distalis contains glandular endothelial cells and capillaries and can secrete various types of hormones.

The neurohypophysis occupies the posterior quarter of the gland and comprises the pars neuralis, infundibulum or median eminence, and infundibular stem. Between the posterior margin of the optic chiasm and mammillary body, the holly-shaped infundibulum or median eminence extents downwards from the tuber cinereum and contains the infundibular recess of the third ventricular cavity. Previous literature reports have claimed that approximately 20% of the infundibular recess reaches the lower half of the pituitary stalk. Under the hydrocephalus, this recess enlarges and inflates significantly; this is commonly observed in craniopharyngiomas of the third ventricular floor (3rd VF). The median eminence is another important vascular connection between the hypothalamus and pituitary gland. The supraoptic nucleus and paraventricular nucleus secretes arginine vasopressin (AVP) and oxytocin, respectively, which are transferred to and stored within the pars neuralis.

The pituitary stalk comprises the pars tuberalis of the adenohypophysis and infundibulum or median eminence of the neurohypophysis, as well as the infundibular stem. The eminence separates the stalk from the hypothalamus (Fig. **1**). No particular or detailed descriptions regarding conceptions of the pituitary stalk were found in anatomical textbooks. In fact, the stalk is not an independent organ but is a part of the gland. Moreover, the conception of the pituitary stalk has been widely described in clinical works. The infra-diaphragmatic and supra-diaphragmatic hypophysis are generally called the pituitary gland and pituitary stalk, respectively. In living humans, the stalk is carmine-colored with numerous longitudinal stria vascularis.

Classical textbooks have divided the pars intermedia into anterior and posterior lobes; however, some authoritative texts such as Gray's Anatomy do not indicate a clear division. Some scholars have even thought that the pars intermedia lacks function and, therefore, considered the division into anterior or posterior lobes to be meaningless. In our opinion, which considers the cellular origin, morphological features, and endocrine function, the pars intermedia are similar to the adenohypophysis. In addition, this tissue is a residual component of Rathke's pouch and likely contains residual cells. The pars intermedia should therefore be included in the anterior lobe of the pituitary gland.

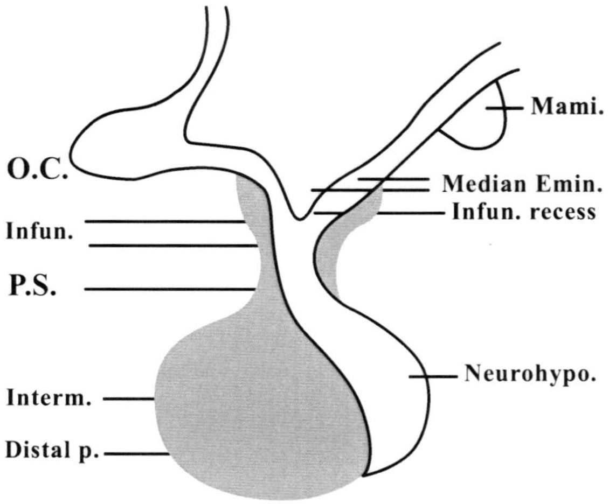

Fig. (1). Normal pituitary anatomy(O.C., Optical chiasm; Mami., Mamillary body; Emin., Eminence; Infun., Infundibulum; P.S., Pituitary stalk; Interm., Intermedian).

Cytology of the Pituitary Gland

Adenohypophysis Fig. (2)

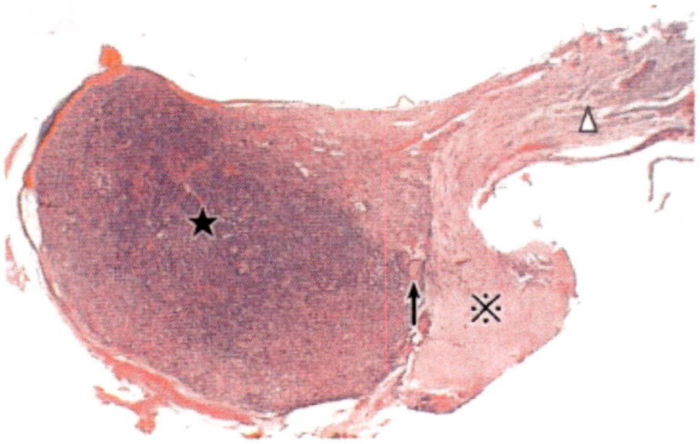

Fig. (2). Pituitary stalk (Human); hematoxylin/eosin (H.E.) staining, 2.5× magnification (★ Pars distalis; △ Pituitary stalk; ↑: Pars intermedia; ※ Pars neuralis).

The origins of adenohypophyseal cytological research can be traced to the early 20th century. The cytology of the pituitary gland has been clearly defined during the three eras of light microscopy, electron microscopy, and immunohistochemistry. Most recent studies have indicated that various types of adenohypophyseal cells originate from the same multipotent stem cells and harbor the potential of bidirectional differentiation to acidophilic and basophilic cells that could further differentiate into various types of endocrine cells. These mature cells, however, are unable to undergo cellular cleavage. Following the aging and death of these cells, stem cells again proliferate and differentiate to compensate for the cellular loss. This hypothesis is closely related to the development of lesions in the sellar region.

The pars distalis constitutes the largest portion of the adenohypophysis. Generally, glandular cells are distributed within the pars distalis as cords or clumps of cells that are closely associated with blood vessels and often include large perivascular spaces (Fig. **3**). The quantities and percentages of secretory cells in the pars distalis differ according to age and physiological status. The secretory cells present in this tissue include acidophilic cells, basophilic cells, chromophobe cells, and follicular cells. Acidophilic cells can be further divided according to size and immunohistochemical detection of secretory granules into growth hormone (GH), somatotropin (STH), prolactin (PRL), or lactogenic hormone (LTH) secreting cells. Similarly basophilic cells can be further divided into thyroid stimulating hormone (TSH), adrenocorticotrophic hormone (ACTH), follicle-stimulating hormone (FSH), and luteinizing hormone (LH) secreting cells.

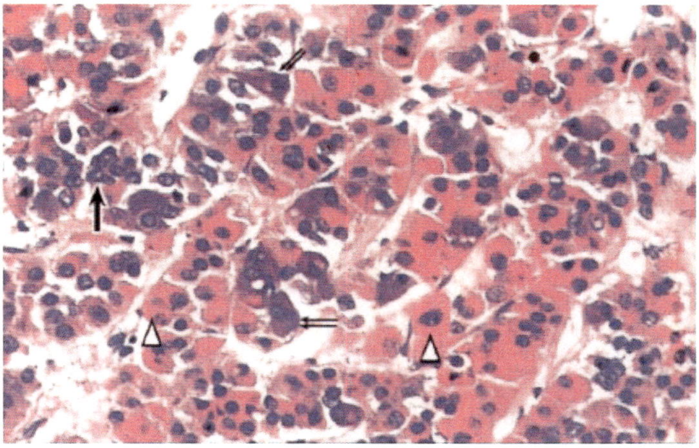

Fig. (3). Pars distalis (human); H.E. staining, 40× magnification (↑: chromophobe cell; ↑↑: basophilic cell; △ acidophilic cell).

Recently, some scholars thought that a subset of secretory cells might produce only one type of hormone, whereas other cells might secrete multiple hormones. Many studies have indicated close relationships and interactions within and between the various endocrinological cell compartments with respect to aspects of development, differentiation, and other physiological functions. In addition, various secretory cells are distributed within the preferential zone (Fig. **4**). PRL- and GH-secreting cells are located in the bilateral wings, TSH-, FSH-, and LH-secreting cells in the middle third, and ACTH-secreting cells in the posteromedial section. This distribution pattern also coincides with the site-related predilections of various types of pituitary adenomas.

Chromophobe cells comprise the largest population and conglobate within the pars distalis (Fig. **3**). In recent years, only a few chromophil cells have been observed to lack secretory granules; the overwhelming majority of these cells contain at least one type of granule as well as Golgi complexes similar to those observed in basophilic cells. Currently, chromophil cells are divided into different groups. Previous hypotheses have suggested that chromophil cells can differentiate bidirectionally into acidophilic or basophilic cells. In addition, scholars have hinted that chromophil cells are in fact adenohypophyseal stem cells. Within the chromophil cell compartment, the few undifferentiated cells that lack secretory granules are progenitor cells; these cells can differentiate in a multidirectional manner. Correlations between these progenitor cells and adenoma tumorigenesis as well as the repair functions of these cells following hypopituitarism are worthy of further study.

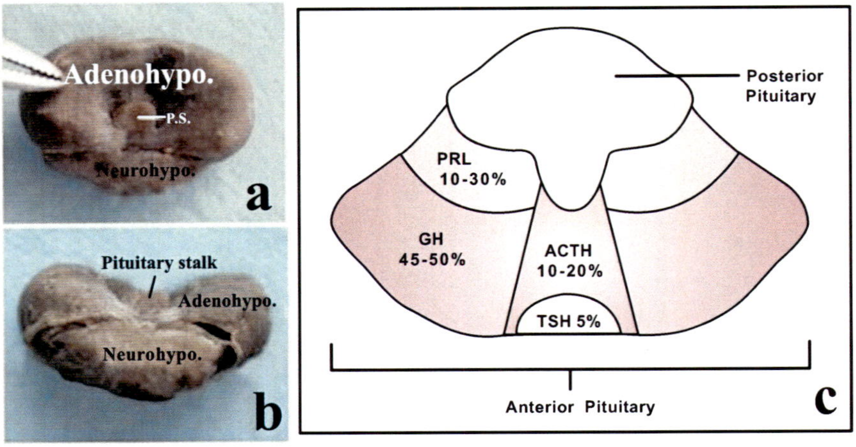

Fig. (4). The preferential locations of various types of secretory cells. Adenohypo., adenohypophysis; P.S., Pituitary stalk; Neurohypo., neurohypophysis.

Pars Tuberalis

The pars tuberalis is contiguous with the main adenohypophyseal tissue mass, with an extension around the stalk and on the inferior hypothalamic surface. The thickest anterior part of the pars tuberalis is currently thought to envelope the entire infundibular stem. However, the posterior part is relatively thinner and may even be congenitally absent. The hypothalamic–hypophyseal portal vein passes through the pars tuberalis to ultimately enter the pars distalis; as a result, the pars tuberalis is highly vascularized and in the living body, is carmine-colored with numerous longitudinal stria vascularis. The cells in this tissue are generally described as chromophobic and although granular cells resembling those of the pars tuberalis may be present, the majority of cells are apparently of the former type. These cells are aligned longitudinally between the vessels and include many undifferentiated cells with few basophilic and acidophilic cells. Large amounts of granules, lipid droplets, and glycogen are observed in the cellular cytoplasm. Furthermore, the pars tuberalis cells are the only type of pituitary cells to contain large amounts of glycogen. Some islets of squamous epithelial cells have also been identified in this tissue. Commonly, vessels within the pars tuberalis comprise a transport pathway between the hypothalamus and pars distalis. However, the cytological function of the pars tuberalis remains unknown. Some previously published evidence suggests that, at any rate, some pars tuberalis cells may contain (and hence possibly secrete) and provide some regulation and supplementation to the secretory products of the pars distalis.

The pars tuberalis is mentioned as playing an important role in cranio-pharyngioma etiological hypotheses. These details will be described in subsequent chapters. Regarding the cytological features, the cells in this tissue are thought to be active because of the large quantity of glycogen and many undifferentiated cells, which might form the cellular basement described in the metaplastic hypothesis of craniopharyngioma pathogenesis. On the other hand, although both the pars tuberalis and distalis develop from the anterior wall of Rathke's pouch, there are significant differences with respect to cellular morphology and constitution. Therefore, some scholars have proposed that the pars tuberalis provides cellular storage for the pars distalis. When secretory cells within the pars distalis are injured, cells of the pars tuberalis might differentiate directionally with respect to these cells and thus play a compensatory role. The above-mentioned issue is important to an understanding of the true etiology of craniopharyngioma and the compensatory endocrinological mechanism during surgical pituitary stalk dissection.

Pars Intermedia

The pars intermedia of the pituitary gland varies considerably and often comprises only a thin lamina of cells that are more or less co-extensive with the posterior aspect of the pars distalis and separated from the pars distalis by the intraglandular cleft. The pars intermedia may extend further over the infundibular process and either may maintain the same type of relationship with the pars distalis or, as in the rodent, may be congenitally absent. The human pars intermedia is composed of variably sized, colloid-filled cysts surrounded by chromophobic and basophilic cells (Fig. **5**). These cysts comprise of either cuboid or stylolitic ciliated cells and are filled with colloids of different viscosities. However, the function of these cysts remains unknown. Significant degeneration of the pars intermedia can be observed during human development. The pars is obviously identifiable in the embryonic and infancy periods but disappears with age.

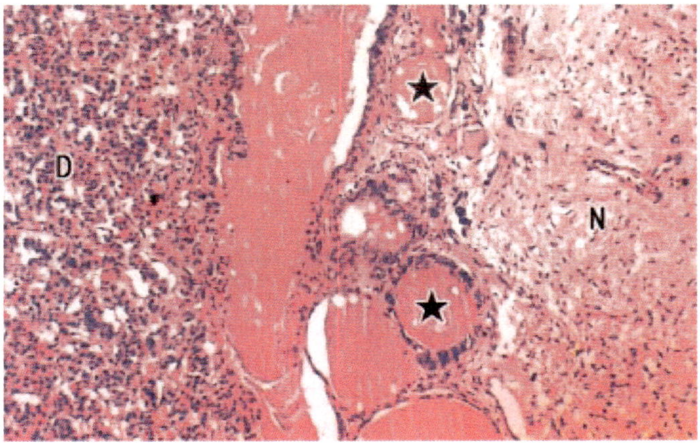

Fig. (5). Pars intermedia (human); H.E. staining, 10× magnification (**D:** Pars distalis; **N:** Pars neuralis; ★: Colloid-containing follicle in the pars intermedia).

The basophilic cells of the pars intermedia include melanophore-stimulating hormone (MSH)-secreting cells with some cells similar to the ACTH-secreting cells found in the pars distalis. The secretory function of MSH cells has been proven in amphibians. Specifically, frogs from which the pars intermedia was dissected developed darker skin color. Another example occurs in pregnant humans, in whom colored spots on the skin are caused by increased MSH secretion.

Neurohypophysis

The neurohypophysis develops from the basal part of the diencephalon, which connects directly to the hypothalamus. The neurohypophysis comprises numerous nonmyelinated nerve fibers and gliocytes (pituicytes) (Fig. **6**). These fibers originate from the hypothalamic–pituitary axis, which contains approximately 50,000 hypothalamic large cell neuronal axons. Most of these nervous fibers were experimentally proven to originate from the supraoptic nucleus and paraventricular nucleus. Secretory granules containing hormones such as antidiuretic hormone (ADH) and various kinds of stimulants are transmitted from hypothalamic neurons to the pars neuralis through these axons and are stored within varicosities. Accordingly, the neurohypophysis is actually an organ that serves to accumulate and release these hormones.

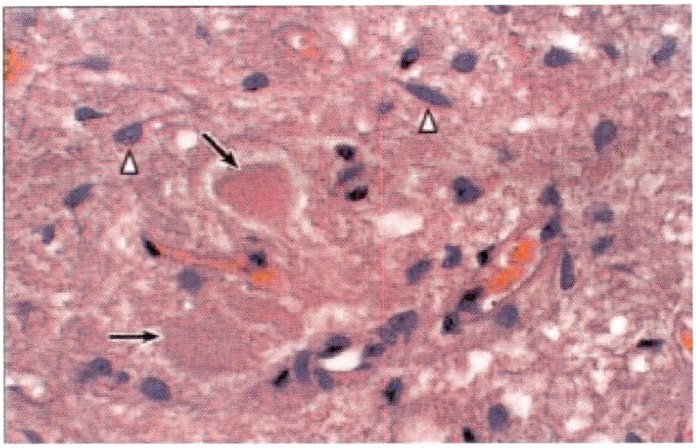

Fig. (6). Pars neuralis of the pituitary gland (human); H.E. staining, 40× magnification (↑: Herring body; Δ Pituicyte).

Numerous nervous fibers and some acidophilic masses of unequal size, known as Herring bodies, can be observed *via* light microscopy. Under careful electron microscopic observation, these nonmyelinated nerve fibers are of unequal thickness, and longitudinal microtubules, scattered neurofilaments, a few mitochondria, and secretory granules can be identified within the axons. Some intumescent axons form string-of-beads-like shapes or varicosities. The varicosities and axon terminals are filled with dense granules that are also revealed to be Herring bodies under light microscopy.

The neurohypophysis has neuroendocrine functions that are predominantly represented by the storage and release of oxytocin (OT) and AVP/ ADH. Therefore, this organ plays indispensable roles in water–electrolyte balance maintenance and blood pressure stabilization, the details of which will be described in a later chapter. Besides the above-mentioned hormones, a small quantity of peptidergic nerve fibers have also been identified within the neurohypophysis, and these control chemicals such as substance P, enkephalins, endorphins, and dynorphins as well as hormones such as LH-releasing hormone (LHRH), thyrotropin-releasing hormone (TRH), cholecystokinin (CCK), and somatostatin (SOM/SRIF). There are also other nerve fibers that control amines and amino acids such as catecholamine (CA), norepinephrine (NT), dopamine (DA) and gamma-aminobutyric acid (γ-GABA). The presence of these nerve fibers indicates that the neurohypophysis can internally regulate anterior pituitary hormone secretion. Moreover, some previous studies have illustrated that regulation is conferred not only by the above nerve fibers, but also through the fibers themselves through inter-synapses or nerve-pituicyte interactions.

Pituicytes are the primary cellular constituents of the neurohypophysis, and their role remains unknown. These cells essentially appear to be modified glial cells and are distributed between the nerve fibers. Using electron microscopy [26], some scholars have shown that pituicytes always contain several dendrons that connect to different cells and thus form a network. Additionally, nerve fibers are intimately associated with these dendrons. The pituicytes may act as sheath cells for the fibers, similar to neuroglia in the central nervous system (CNS). However, current, widely accepted findings indicate that pituicytes are not simply inert supporting elements but can also phagocytose degenerating neuronal material. Furthermore, some scholars believe that pituicytes may also release an active substance that promotes the growth of new nerve fibers and induces regeneration. These cells might also produce and secrete GABA and other chemicals to regulate the nerve fiber activity and hormone secretion.

In a study of the relationship between craniopharyngiomas and the hypothalamus, Songtao *et al.* [43] identified significant phagocyte zone reactions and gliosis in some cases; these reactions formed a stratified alignment at the posteroinferior or lateral area where the tumor closely adhered to the pituitary stalk or pars neuralis (Fig. 7). In rare cases, isolated tumoral islets can also be found within the gliosis zone. As pituicytes play the same role as gliocytes in the CNS, the gliosis between the tumor and infundibular stem (nerve fibers) is formed by pituicytes. Regarding craniopharyngioma, whether pituicytes continue to provide supportive, protective, and phagocytic functions merits further study.

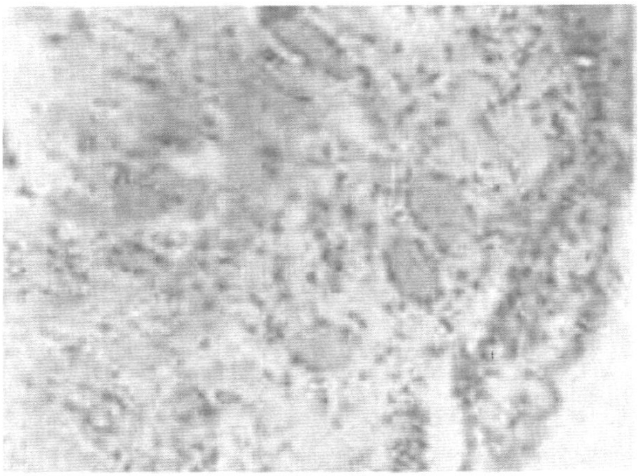

Fig. (7). The gliosis zone around the craniopharyngioma.

Pathological Influence of Pituitary Stalk Dissection

Following amputation of the hypothalamic–pituitary axis, the Herring bodies in the distal axon disappear and a significant accumulation of secretory granules occurs in the proximal axon. In the context of hormone exhaustion, Herring bodies in the neurohypophysis also disappear. Simultaneously, retrograde degeneration occurs in the supraoptic nucleus and periventricular nucleus of the hypothalamus. Transport and accumulation of existing secretory granules to the extremities continues. Qi *et al* [42] summarized the triphasic clinical features of diabetes insipidus following pituitary stalk dissection as the acute phase, mesophase, and persistent phase.

(1) During the acute stage, secretory granules accumulate at the distal nerve fibers because ADH secreted by the supraoptic and periventricular nuclei cannot be transported to the pars neuralis through the normal hypothalamic–pituitary axis. Diabetes insipidus occurs during the early stage as a result of decreased ADH levels in the blood. **(2)** However, within the mesophase, accumulated secretory granules are released into the blood because of the retrograde nuclear degeneration and neuronal apoptosis/necrosis. As a result, the urine volume may be temporarily maintained within a normal range. **(3)** During the persistent phase, further progression occurs in the absence of new ADH granule production, and continuous and persistent insipidus finally occurs.

Pharyngeal Hypophysis

The pharyngeal hypophysis is located in the submucosal layer of the posterior margin of the nasal septum and top of the pharynx and develops from the residual Rathke's pouch. This tissue was first named by Erdherim in 1904 and is thought to maintain a constant presence in the human body, despite its rare observance in other animals. Pharyngeal craniopharyngiomas are occasionally observed in clinical studies. Furthermore, most scholars believe that the residual Rathke's pouch is an important site of craniopharyngiomal origin. Carlos *et al.* reported that the pharyngeal hypophysis has a width of $\leq$1 mm and length of 3.5-7 mm. Additionally, as proven *via* immunohistochemistry, the pharyngeal hypophysis secretes both GH and PRL; as a result, some scholars believe it to be an accessory gland of the adenohypophysis. At particular ages, this gland might have limited endocrinological regulatory functions.

EMBRYONIC DEVELOPMENT OF THE PITUITARY GLAND AND ITS ACCESSORY STRUCTURES

The following points have been clarified: the pituitary gland is derived from the ectoderm, and it is always composed of two structurally distinct parts. The anterior lobe is derived from the buccal epithelium, or somatic ectoderm, whereas the posterior lobe is derived from the ectodermal neural tube. As depicted in several literature reports, including ours [34], this gland is enveloped in a connective tissue membrane (pituitary capsule) and lamina propria. An understanding of the origin and clinical, pathological, and iconographic features of craniopharyngioma is inseparable from an understanding of the closely related embryonic development of the pituitary gland and its accessory structures.

Embryonic Development: Pituitary Gland

Although the adenohypophyseal and neurohypophyseal parts connect to form the pituitary gland, the different development processes of the two lobes are widely accepted. In accordance with this description, we will illustrate separately the development of the anterior and posterior lobes (Fig. **8**).

The adenohypophyseal nomenclature is derived from directly from the ectoderm of the primitive stomodeum. At embryonic development day 24, the entire epithelial portion of this gland first develops as Rathke's pouch, a pocket of the buccal ectoderm. This pouch associates closely with the neural down-growth and at approximately 7–8 weeks of development, the petiole part of the pouch, which is connected to the oral epithelium, begins to degenerate and seal the corridor to the primitive oral cavity. Finally, a rudimentary and residual structure, the craniopharyngeal canal, is formed; this will later degenerate and disappear in the normal human body. Cytogenesis varies considerably in different areas of Rathke's pouch. The cells in the posterior pouch wall grow slowly and persistently, such that a cleft (Rathke's cleft) separates the lamina of cells that lay opposite to the neural down-growth; this is the pars intermedia. Meanwhile, two lateral outgrowths of the upper part of the pouch grow forward and toward the midline; these usually join and become attached near the tuber cinereum, thus forming the pars tuberalis. The anterior wall of the pouch develops into the pars distalis, which constitutes the major epithelial part of the gland.

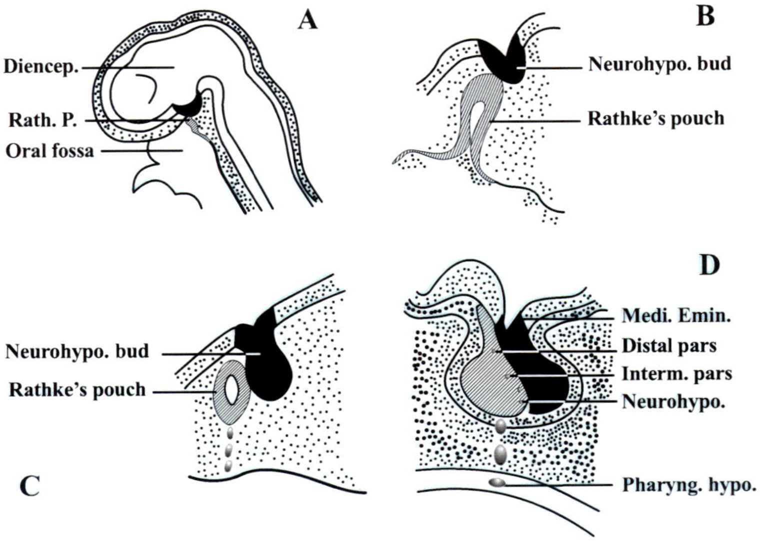

Fig. (8). Schematic diagram of pituitary gland development in the embryonic human (Reference from Sartoretti-Schefer [32]). **A:** 24 days; **B:** 6 weeks; **C:** 8 weeks; **D:** Later stages. Diencep., diencephalon; Rath. P., Rathke's pouch; Neurohypo., neurohypophysis; Medi. Emin., median eminence; Interm., Intermedian; Pharyng. Hypo., Pharyngeal hypophysis.

The neurohypophysis arises as a down-growth from the basal part of diencephalon (also called the neurohypophyseal bud) towards the oral cavity, which later forms the hypothalamus and retains a connection with this part of the brain through a nerve fiber stalk. At 10-11 weeks of embryonic development, the distal part of the neurohypophyseal bud extends sharply downwards and develops into the pars neuralis while connecting with the posterior wall of Rathke's pouch. The neuroepithelial cells in the bud proliferate and differentiate into pituicytes. However, the proximal part, along with the consecutive part of the hypothalamic pars neuralis, forms the median eminence and infundibular stem. Subsequently, the axons arising from the hypothalamic secretory nervous nucleus grow within the pars neuralis through the infundibulum.

Embryonic Development: Pituitary Capsule

To date, great controversies remain regarding the embryonic development of the pituitary capsule; however, its mesodermal origin is widely accepted. Generally [16, 18, 32, 38, 43], it is believed that mesodermic mesenchymal cells surround the adenohypophysis, which is derived from the primitive stomodeal ectoderm. At weeks 7–8 of embryonic development Fig. (**9**), the mesenchymal cells mature, leading to an increased collagen filament component and decreased cellular component and thus marking the formation of the pituitary capsule foundation. At weeks 9–10 of embryonic development, in addition to the accelerated cartilaginification of the skull base, pituitary growth is restricted by the clival and osteochondral sphenoid. Furthermore, the center part of the gland has descended into the pituitary fossa and the primitive capsule, comprising a few fibrous layers, has already formed. This capsule separates the gland from the bilateral primitive cavernous sinus (CS). At week 12, ossification of skull base is basically completed, and additional matrix cells surround the primitive capsule in an irregular manner. Furthermore, the pituitary capsule protrudes bilaterally and significantly. Moreover, at weeks 14-16, the capsule develops further and increases in thickness while exhibiting a more regular fibrous alignment. The capsular component of the proximal pituitary, which surrounds the pituitary stalk, formed the sellae diaphragm ultimately by fusing with the meningeal dura. Some vessels also invade the pituitary capsule and perichondrium. At week 17, additional stromal cells accumulate around the pituitary gland and connect loosely with capsule, which thickens along with increasing embryonic age. Finally, an intact pituitary capsule is formed.

Studies of early embryonic stages indicated that along with enveloping of the adenohypophysis, the capsule also encloses the neurohypophysis. However, because neurohypophyseal development occurs later than adenohypophyseal development, the posterior part of the capsule is relatively thinner than the anterior part. In fact, all of the above descriptions demonstrate that the pituitary capsule comprises dense connective tissue that is independent of the sellar region pia mater.

However, several previous researchers have reported the origins of the pituitary capsule and dura and arachnoid mater during embryonic development, and different authors have supported different theories [9 - 11, 14, 15, 35]. Wisloki [14, 15] and Ciric [10], respectively, proposed that the capsule derives from the dura and pia arachnoid, whereas Chi and Lee studied 21 human embryos and 35 fetuses by a histological analysis [9] and suggested that it derives from Rathke's pouch [13, 28, 30, 38, 41], which grows from the distal stomodeal ectoderm to connect and finally fuse with the neurohypophysis; the mesenchymal cells around the pituitary gland then develop and differentiate to form a prominent pituitary capsule.

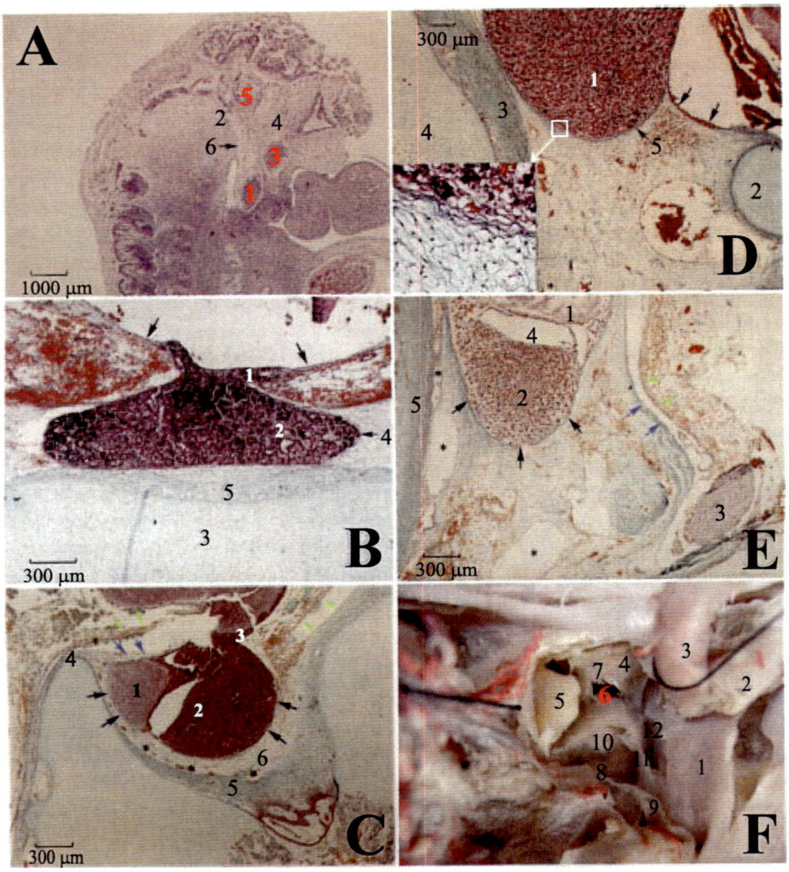

Fig. (9). (Reference from Ding *et al.* [44]). Embryonic development of the pituitary capsule. **A:** Sagittal section from a 6-week embryo (H.E staining). 1, Adenohypophyseal primordium; 2, Neurohypophyseal primordium; 3, Trigeminal ganglion; 4, Trigeminal root; 5, Primitive cephalic vein; 6, Rathke's pouch. **B:** Coronal section from a 12-week embryo (Masson staining). 1, Pituitary stalk; 2, Adenohypophysis; 3, Sphenoid cartilage; 4, Pituitary capsule; 5, Sphenoidal perichondrium; ↑: Meningeal primordium. **C:** Sagittal section from a 15-week embryo (Masson staining). 1, Neurohypophysis; 2, Adenohypophysis; 3, Pituitary stalk; 4, Clival perichondrium; 5, Sphenoidal perichondrium; 6, Bone matrix; Green arrows, Arachnoid mater; Blue arrows, Diaphragm; Dark arrows, Pituitary capsule; Asterisk, Venous plexus. **D:** Coronal section from a 16-week embryo (Masson staining). 1, Adenohypophysis; 2, Reduced wing cartilage; 3, Sphenoidal periosteum; 4, Sphenoidal cartilage; 5, Pituitary capsule; ↑: Primodium of diaphragm; Asterisk, Vein; Lower left, magnification displays the connective fibers of the pituitary capsule (200× magnification). **E:** Coronal section from a 25-week embryo (Masson staining). 1, Neurohypophysis; 2, Adenohypophysis; 3, Oculomotor nerve; 4, Intermedia cleft; 5, Sphenoidal periosteum; Green arrow, Arachnoid mater; Blue arrows, Diaphragm; Dark arrows, Pituitary capsule; Asterisk, Vein. **F:** Microanatomy of an adult pituitary capsule. 1, Dura mater of the tuberculum sellae; 2, Optic nerve; 3, Clinoid process segment of the ICA; 4, Horizontal segment of the ICA; 5, Posterior clinoid process; 6, Medial space; 7, Connective fibers between the ICA and pituitary capsule; 8, Pituitary stalk; 9, Arachnoid mater; 10, Pituitary gland; 11, Diaphragm; 12, Anterior intercavernous sinus.

In clinical studies, two types of congenital disease have also indicated the pituitary capsule origin. For example, in anencephalic fetuses, a single adenohypophysis is completely enclosed within the fibrous capsule. In contrast, in a case involving the congenital absence of an adenohypophysis, reported by Brewer *et al.* [6], the remaining neurohypophysis in the sella turcica was entirely surrounded by a pia arachnoid membrane derived from the suprasellar arachnoid. However, no clear capsule was identified. All of the above evidence not only suggests that adenohypophyseal development is closely related to Rathke's pouch, but also that rotated pouch development induces a diaphragm that extends to the center of the sellar region. The adherence between the capsule and diaphragm obstructs protrusion of the suprasellar arachnoid into the pituitary fossa. Abnormal development at any stage will cause corresponding clinical issues, such as congenital empty sella turcica. Meanwhile, this development also plays an indispensable role in craniopharyngioma origins and growth patterns.

ORIGIN OF CRANIOPHARYNGIOMA

Since the discovery of craniopharyngioma more than a century earlier, more than 10 nomenclatures have been used for this lesion, including Erdheim tumor, Hypophyseal duct tumor, Craniopharyngeal duct tumor, Rathke's pouch tumor, Epidermoma, Adamantinoma, pituitary stalk tumor, and Medullary carcinoma. The above-listed changes in nomenclatures reflect the understanding of this type of lesion. Although the pathogenesis of craniopharyngioma is not yet completely understood, it can be explained by the following three hypotheses.

Residual Cells of Craniopharyngeal Duct [4, 22, 31, 32, 37]

As described above, at an early stage of embryonic development, the stomodeum epithelium near the dental plate invaginates to form Rathke's pouch and further developing to the adenohypophysis. Subsequently, a sealed cavity is formed and connects to the stomodeum through a degenerated craniopharyngeal duct. Because of diverse growth velocity, the anterior cells grow more rapidly and exhibit an upward and rotated growth pattern, directing the residual cells of the craniopharyngeal duct to the intra- or supra-sellar region or even the anterior part of the 3rd VF. This hypothesis assumes that the craniopharyngioma derives from these residual cells (Fig. **10**). In our clinical works, especially for the surgery of the infra-diaphragmatic CP (type Q, see Chapter 10 of this book), a hole located in the floor of pituitary fossa was always observed after the tumor was removed Fig. (**11**), which was the best evidence for supporting the origination of CP from the residual cells of craniopharyngeal duct.

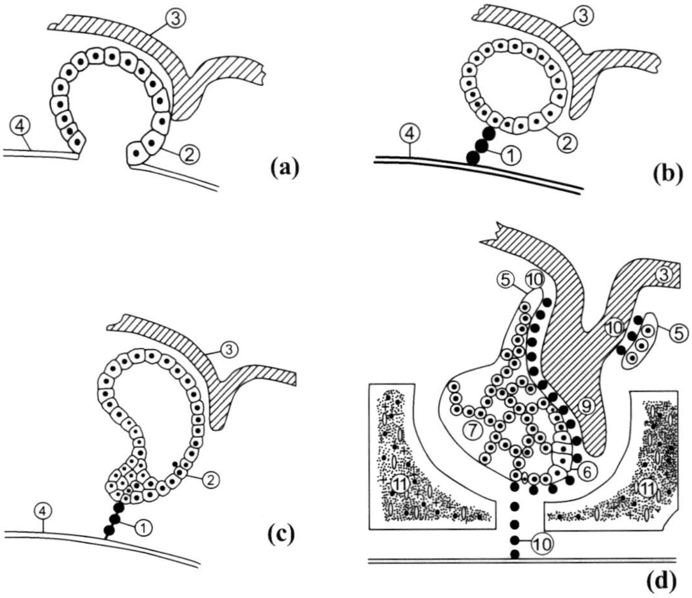

Fig. (10). (Adapted from Sartoretti-Schefer *et al* [32]. This schematic depicts the origin of a craniopharyngioma according to Theory One). (a) At an early stage of embryonic development, the stomodeum epithelium invaginates and forms Rathke's pouch; (b) A further invagination of Rathke's pouch reveals the formation and connection of a sealed pouch cavity to the stomodeum ectoderm *via* the craniopharyngeal duct; (c) During anterior lobe development, which arises from Rathke's pouch, the anteroinferior cells proliferate more rapidly, resulting in a rotated growth pattern through which the ventral cells ultimately comprise the pars tuberalis; (d) Along with this rotated development, some residual craniopharyngeal duct cells are brought to the intra- and suprasellar region and are possibly the origin of craniopharyngioma.① Craniopharyngeal duct cells; ② Rathke's pouch cells; ③Diencephalon;④ Dental lamina;⑤ Pars tuberalis;⑥ Pars intermedia; ⑦ Pars distalis;⑧ Infundibular stem;⑨ Pars neuralis;⑩ Residual craniopharyngeal duct cells; (11) Sella turcica. (Reference from Sartoretti-Schefer *et al.* [8], with modified).

According to the previously depicted pituitary development Fig. (**8**), it is not difficult to understand how residual craniopharyngeal cells might exist in any location from the pharynx oralis to the 3rd VF [1, 5, 8, 12, 19, 20, 29, 33]. Therefore, this theory also explains the presentations of craniopharyngioma of the pharynx nasalis and tumors within the sphenoid bone [21, 25, 39]. Meanwhile, this theory believes that a close relationship exists between tumors and the prenatal stomodeum and dental plate, which will ultimately form the dental enamel. As a result, this theory can also explain why similar histological findings are observed among dental enamel carcinomas, keratinization, classified dental cysts, and adamantinomatous craniopharyngioma [7]. Moreover, some literature reports have described finding teeth within craniopharyngiomas [2, 18, 24].

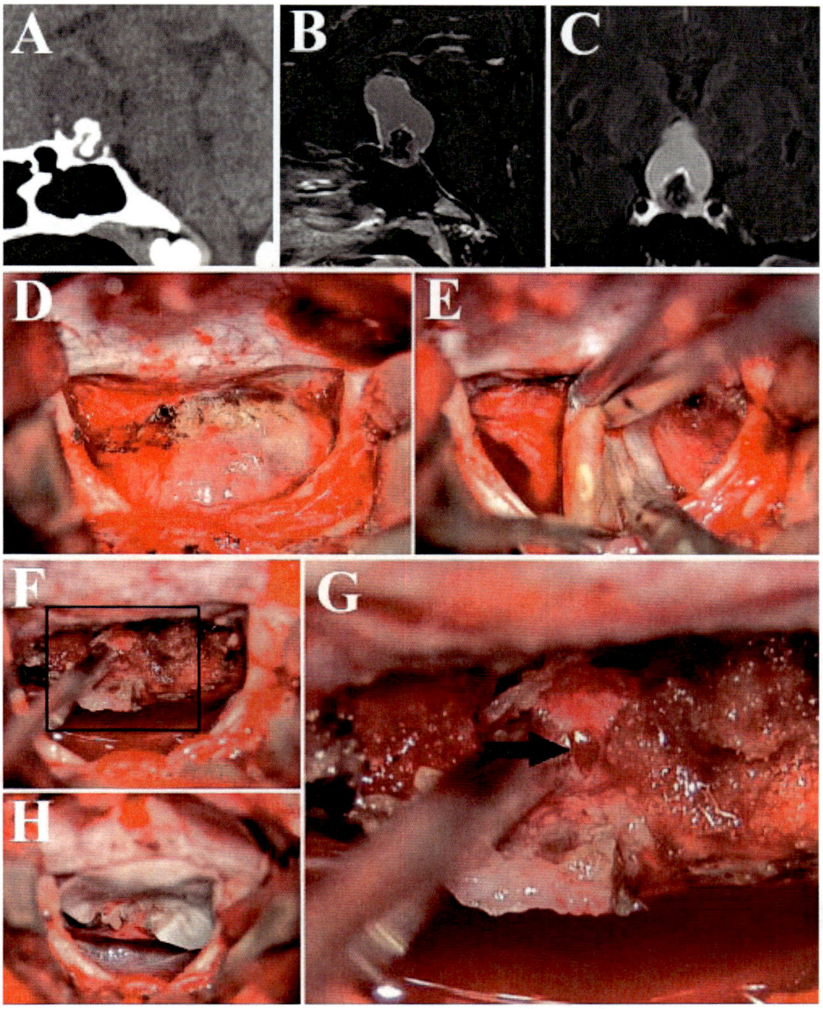

Fig. (11). The clinical case indicated the origination of the Id-CP. **A~C.** CT and MRI scan of a 22 years old female indicated the intra-sellar and supra-seller cystic predominant tumor with a mass of calcification inside the pituitary fossa. **D~E.** The frontobasal interhemispheric approach was selected to remove the tumor. **F.** After the tumor removal, a hole (Black arrow) was observed in the floor of the pituitary fossa, which was magnified in the Fig. (**G**). The hole might indicate the origination of the Id-CP. H. After the tumor total removal, an artificial dura mater was used to cover the pituitary fossa.

Residual Rathke's Pouch Cells

Following neonatal pituitary gland studies conducted by Goldberg and Eshbaugh [16], squamous epithelial cell nests were observed in the pars tuberalis of four cases involving the gland. The researchers thought that these cells were residual Rathke's pouch cells. Following the differentiation of Rathke's pouch, no such cell nests should be identified within the majority of the neonatal hypophysis. Other studies [3, 17, 27] have supported this theory in which craniopharyngioma arises from residual squamous cells of Rathke's pouch. Furthermore, it has been widely accepted that these residual cells are most frequently present in the pars tuberalis.

In addition, this theory also believes that the tumor is located near the location of embryonic sellar region development (Fig. **12**). A previous article described the pia mater as originating from mesodermal inserts between Rathke's pouch and encephalic vesicles prior to the rotation of the pars tuberalis during week 5 of embryonic. Therefore, it would impossible for residual Rathke's pouch cells to exist underneath the pia mater. Moreover, the pia meter ultimately induces a thin connective tissue septation between the anterior and posterior lobes. In contrast, a delay in the formation of this connective layer during development would lead to direct contact between Rathke's pouch and the encephalic vesicles. In this situation, some Rathke's pouch cells might be transplanted in the encephalic vesicles, which are very likely the pathogenetic origin of intraventricular craniopharyngioma (IVC).

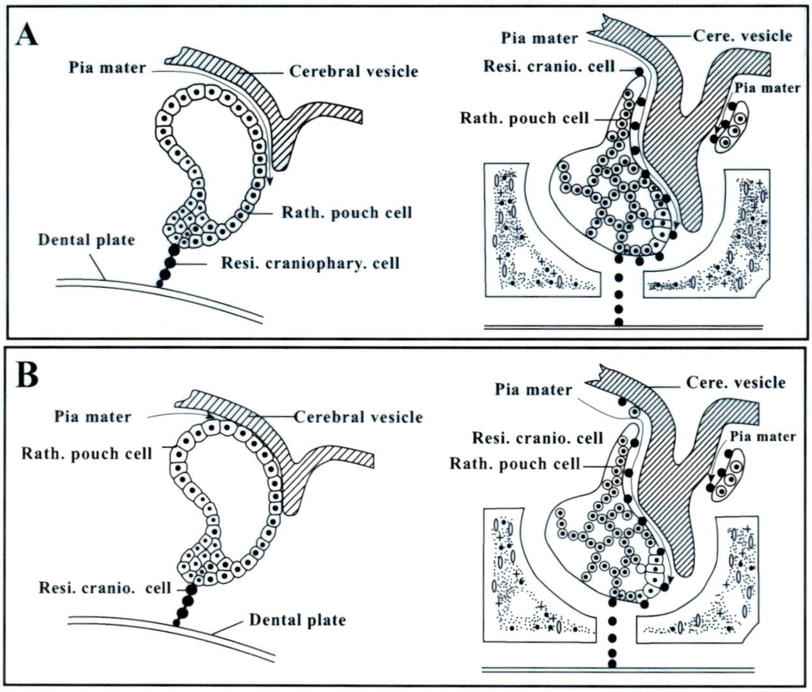

Fig. (12). This schematic depicts the origin of a craniopharyngioma according to Theory Two. During embryonic development, delayed development of the pia mater causes differences in the locations of craniopharyngiomas (Reference from Ciri IS [25], with modified). **A:** The pia mater inserts between Rathke's pouch and the encephalic vesicles, resulting in normal development without residual primitive cells beneath the pia mater; **B:** Delayed development of the pia mater leads to the localization of residual craniopharyngeal duct and Rathke's pouch cells beneath the pia mater.

For centuries, there have been many controversies regarding the occurrence of intrinsic IVC, without credible evidence to support the existence of IVC. According to the above schematic diagram, it appears that residual epithelial cells can be transplanted to the neuroectodermal diencephalon. However, given our understanding of the features of embryonic development, it would be impossible for these residual cells to penetrate the neuroectodermal layer and localize within the third ventricle cavity. Most likely, IVC might localize within the various walls of the third ventricle, beneath the pia mater (see also the chapter concerning the IVC).

Some scholars [23] have studied secretion from the craniopharyngioma lining epithelium and found that the secretory component is similar to that of the tunica mucosa oris and pharyngis. These findings hint at a close relationship between the tumor and Rathke's pouch. Moreover, Tachibana *et al.* [37] found that the pars tuberalis, Rathke's pouch, and craniopharyngioma can all produce P-glycoprotein, thus providing a potential clue regarding a common ectodermal origin of this disease.

Cellular Metaplastic Theory

As in our above description, Rathke's pouch develops and forms various parts of the adenohypophysis. In the context of the histological pituitary gland studies, many scholars have identified squamous epithelial cells in the pars tuberalis. These squamous epithelial nests are observed frequently, particularly in adults, and increase with age. Furthermore, these squamous cells harbor secretory granules that contain gonadotrophins and ACTH [36]. Therefore, a hypothesis was proposed in which these squamous cells derived from the metaplastic secretory cells of the anterior lobe. Moreover, craniopharyngioma, especially the squamous-papillary type, likely originates from these metaplastic squamous epithelial cells [27]. Goldberg and Eshbaugh [16] reviewed 1364 cases of adenohypophysis but did not identify any significant squamous epithelial cell nests among 78 patients younger than 10 years of age. Therefore, the researchers concluded that these squamous cells did not arise from the residual Rathke's pouch but rather from metaplastic normal gland cells. The researchers also observed rare squamous epithelial nests in patients younger than 20 years.

Using immunohistochemical and electron microscopy detection, Songtao Qi [42] studied the hormone secretion from craniopharyngiomas and found that these tumors can secret a range of adenohypophyseal hormones. In addition, the anterior lobe, pituitary adenoma, and craniopharyngioma can all produce human chorionic gonadotropin (HCG), providing further support to the metaplastic theory.

Given a deeper understanding of craniopharyngioma and of the considerable diversity among tumors with different growth patterns and those observed in children and adults, many scholars have proposed a pluralistic theory. As we know, craniopharyngiomas adhere to two incidence peaks that occur in children (5–10 years) and adults (40–60 years). In pediatric cases, adamantinous-type tumors are more frequently observed; these are predominantly cystic and are always accompanied by calcification. On the other hand, in adult patients, squamous-papillary type tumors are more frequently observed, and calcification and cysts occur infrequently [3, 16]. As a result, some scholars believe that pediatric craniopharyngioma might originate from residual cells of the craniopharyngeal duct or Rathke's pouch, whereas adult tumors predominantly arise from metaplastic squamous epithelial cells.

CONFLICT OF INTEREST

The author (editor) declares no conflict of interest, financial or otherwise.

ACKNOWLEDGEMENTS

We should acknowledge Mr. Piao Ying-jie, Department of Histology and Embryology, Southern medical university, China, who provided several elegant histological pictures.

REFERENCES

[1] Akimura T, Kameda H, Abiko S, Aoki H, Kido T. Infrasellar craniopharyngioma. Neuroradiology 1989; 31(2): 180-3.
[http://dx.doi.org/10.1007/BF00698851] [PMID: 2747897]

[2] Alvarez-Garijo JA, Froufé A, Taboada D, Vila M. Successful surgical treatment of an odontogenic ossified craniopharyngioma. Case report. J Neurosurg 1981; 55(5): 832-5.
[http://dx.doi.org/10.3171/jns.1981.55.5.0832] [PMID: 6796660]

[3] Asa SL, Kovacs K, Bilbao JM. The pars tuberalis of the human pituitary. A histologic, immunohistochemical, ultrastructural and immunoelectron microscopic analysis. Virchows Arch A Pathol Anat Histopathol 1983; 399(1): 49-59.
[http://dx.doi.org/10.1007/BF00666218] [PMID: 6299000]

[4] Banna M. Craniopharyngioma: based on 160 cases. Br J Radiol 1976; 49(579): 206-23.
[http://dx.doi.org/10.1259/0007-1285-49-579-206] [PMID: 776317]

[5] Benitez WI, Sartor KJ, Angtuaco EJ. Craniopharyngioma presenting as a nasopharyngeal mass: CT and MR findings. J Comput Assist Tomogr 1988; 12(6): 1068-72.
[http://dx.doi.org/10.1097/00004728-198811000-00034] [PMID: 3183117]

[6] Brewer DB. Congenital absence of the pituitary gland and its consequences. J Pathol Bacteriol 1957; •••: 59-67.
[http://dx.doi.org/10.1002/path.1700730109]

[7] Burger PC, Fuller GN. Pathology--trends and pitfalls in histologic diagnosis, immunopathology, and applications of oncogene research. Neurol Clin 1991; 9(2): 249-71.
[PMID: 1682793]

[8] Byrne MN, Sessions DG. Nasopharyngeal craniopharyngioma. Case report and literature review. Ann Otol Rhinol Laryngol 1990; 99(8): 633-9. [http://dx.doi.org/10.1177/000348949009900809] [PMID: 2200325]

[9] Chi JG, Lee MH. Anatomical observations of the development of the pituitary capsule. J Neurosurg 1980; 52(5): 667-70. [http://dx.doi.org/10.3171/jns.1980.52.5.0667] [PMID: 7373394]

[10] Ciric I. On the origin and nature of the pituitary gland capsule. J Neurosurg 1977; 46(5): 596-600. [http://dx.doi.org/10.3171/jns.1977.46.5.0596] [PMID: 845648]

[11] Conklin JL. The development of the human fetal adenohypophysis. Anat Rec 1968; 160(1): 79-91. [http://dx.doi.org/10.1002/ar.1091600108] [PMID: 4172831]

[12] Cooper PR, Ransohoff J. Craniopharyngioma originating in the sphenoid bone. Case report. J Neurosurg 1972; 36(1): 102-6. [http://dx.doi.org/10.3171/jns.1972.36.1.0102] [PMID: 5007266]

[13] Dietemann JL, Kehrli P, Maillot C, *et al.* Is there a dural wall between the cavernous sinus and the pituitary fossa? Anatomical and MRI findings. Neuroradiology 1998; 40(10): 627-30. [http://dx.doi.org/10.1007/s002340050653] [PMID: 9833890]

[14] GB W. The meningeal relations of the hypophysis cerebi: PartI-The relations in adult mammals. Anat Rec 1937; 273-9.

[15] GB W. The meningeal relations of the hypophysis cerebri: PartII-An embryological study of the meniges and blood vessels of the human hypophysis. Am J Anat 1937; 95-130.

[16] Goldberg GM, Eshbaugh DE. Squamous cell nests of the pituitary gland as related to the origin of craniopharyngiomas. A study of their presence in the newborn and infants up to age four. Arch Pathol 1960; 70: 293-9. [PMID: 13850582]

[17] Goldberg GM, Eshbaugh DE. Squamous cell nests of the pituitary gland as related to the origin of craniopharyngiomas. A study of their presence in the newborn and infants up to age four. Arch Pathol 1960; 70: 293-9. [PMID: 13850582]

[18] Gorlin RJ, Pindborg JJ, Redman RS, Williamson JJ, Hansen LS. PINDBORG JJ, REDMAN RS, WILLIAMSON JJ, HANSEN LS: The calcifying odontogenic cyst. a new entity and possible analogue of the cutaneous calcifying epithelioma of malherbe. Cancer 1964; 17: 723-9. [http://dx.doi.org/10.1002/1097-0142(196406)17:6<723::AID-CNCR2820170606>3.0.CO;2-A] [PMID: 14172078]

[19] Graziani N, Donnet A, Bugha TN, Dufour H, Figarella-Branger D, Grisoli F. Ectopic basisphenoidal craniopharyngioma: case report and review of the literature. Neurosurgery 1994; 34: 346-9.

[20] Hillman TH, Peyster RG, Hoover ED, Nair S, Finkelstein SD. Infrasellar craniopharyngioma: CT and MR studies. J Comput Assist Tomogr 1988; 12(4): 702-4. [http://dx.doi.org/10.1097/00004728-198807000-00044] [PMID: 3392286]

[21] Iwasaki K, Kondo A, Takahashi JB, Yamanobe K. Intraventricular craniopharyngioma: report of two cases and review of the literature. Surg Neurol 1992; 38(4): 294-301. [http://dx.doi.org/10.1016/0090-3019(92)90045-O] [PMID: 1440221]

[22] Julow J, Lanyi F, Hajda M, Szeifert G, Simkovits M, Pasztor E. Intracystic instillation of yttrium 90 silicate colloid in cystic craniopharyngioma Orv Hetil 1989; 130(1367-1368): 1371-5.

[23] Kalnins V. Calcification and amelogenesis in craniopharyngiomas. Oral Surg Oral Med Oral Pathol 1971; 31(3): 366-79. [http://dx.doi.org/10.1016/0030-4220(71)90159-9] [PMID: 5277389]

[24] Kanungo N, Just N, Black M, Mohr G, Glikstein R, Rochon L. Nasopharyngeal craniopharyngioma in

an unusual location. AJNR Am J Neuroradiol 1995; 16(6): 1372-4. [PMID: 7677045]

[25] Krsulovic J, Brückner G. Morphological characteristics of pituicytes in different functional stages. Light- and electronmicroscopy of the neurohypophysis of the albino rat. Z Zellforsch Mikrosk Anat 1969; 99(2): 210-20. [http://dx.doi.org/10.1007/BF00342222] [PMID: 5354169]

[26] Luse SA, Kernohan JW. Squamous-cell nests of the pituitary gland. Cancer 1955; 8(3): 623-8. [http://dx.doi.org/10.1002/1097-0142(1955)8:3<623::AID-CNCR2820080328>3.0.CO;2-D] [PMID: 14379152]

[27] Mastronardi L, Guiducci A. Are nonfunctioning pituitary adenomas extending into the cavernous sinus aggressive and/or invasive? Neurosurgery 2002; 51: 521-2.

[28] Mukada K, Mori S, Matsumura S, Uozumi T, Goishi J. Infrasellar craniopharyngioma. Surg Neurol 1984; 21(6): 565-71. [http://dx.doi.org/10.1016/0090-3019(84)90271-4] [PMID: 6719329]

[29] Parkinson D. Surgical anatomy of the lateral sellar compartment (cavernous sinus). Clin Neurosurg 1990; 36: 219-39. [PMID: 2403883]

[30] Petito CK. Craniopharyngioma: prognostic importance of histologic features. AJNR Am J Neuroradiol 1996; 17(8): 1441-2. [PMID: 8883638]

[31] Sartoretti-Schefer S, Wichmann W, Aguzzi A, Valavanis A. MR differentiation of adamantinous and squamous-papillary craniopharyngiomas. AJNR Am J Neuroradiol 1997; 18(1): 77-87. [PMID: 9010523]

[32] Sener RN. Giant craniopharyngioma extending to the anterior cranial fossa and nasopharynx. AJR Am J Roentgenol 1994; 162(2): 441-2. [http://dx.doi.org/10.2214/ajr.162.2.8310943] [PMID: 8310943]

[33] Songtao Q, Yuntao L, Jun P, Chuanping H, Xiaofeng S. Membranous layers of the pituitary gland: histological anatomic study and related clinical issues Neurosurgery 2009; 64: s1-s10.

[34] Sunderland S. The meningeal relations of the human hypophysis cerebri. J Anat 1945; 79(Pt 1): 33-7. [PMID: 17104964]

[35] Szeifert GT, Pásztor E. Could craniopharyngiomas produce pituitary hormones? Neurol Res 1993; 15(1): 68-9. [http://dx.doi.org/10.1080/01616412.1993.11740111] [PMID: 8098858]

[36] Tachibana O, Yamashima T, Yamashita J, Takabatake Y. Immunohistochemical expression of human chorionic gonadotropin and P-glycoprotein in human pituitary glands and craniopharyngiomas. J Neurosurg 1994; 80(1): 79-84. [http://dx.doi.org/10.3171/jns.1994.80.1.0079] [PMID: 7903692]

[37] Taptas JN. The so-called cavernous sinus: a review of the controversy and its implications for neurosurgeons. Neurosurgery 1982; 11(5): 712-7. [http://dx.doi.org/10.1227/00006123-198211000-00019] [PMID: 7155338]

[38] Teramoto A, Hirakawa K, Sanno N, Osamura Y. Incidental pituitary lesions in 1,000 unselected autopsy specimens. Radiology 1994; 193(1): 161-4. [http://dx.doi.org/10.1148/radiology.193.1.8090885] [PMID: 8090885]

[39] Wang Y, Zhao C, Wang Z, *et al.* Apoptosis of supraoptic AVP neurons is involved in the development of central diabetes insipidus after hypophysectomy in rats. BMC Neurosci 2008; 9: 54. [http://dx.doi.org/10.1186/1471-2202-9-54] [PMID: 18578860]

[40] Yokoyama S, Hirano H, Moroki K, Goto M, Imamura S, Kuratsu JI. Are nonfunctioning pituitary

adenomas extending into the cavernous sinus aggressive and/or invasive? Neurosurgery 2001; 49: 857-63.

[41] Huang C, Tao Q. craniopharyngioma and growth hormone deficiency. Foreign Medical Neurology Neurosurgery 2003; 30: 359-62.

[42] Liu Baoguo, Qi Songtao, Pan Jun, Zhang Xi'an, Peng Yuping, Fang Luxiong. Study and significance of inflammation of craniopharyngioma tissue. Guangdong Medical Journal. 2006; 27: pp. 61-3.

[43] Yong-qian WA, Mei-xiu DI, Duo-sheng TA, Bing-yu WA. Embryonic development and microscopic anatomy of pituitary sacs. Chinese Journal of Clinical Anatomy 2005; 23: 137-41.

CHAPTER 3

Pathological Classification of Craniopharyngioma and its Molecular Aspects

Xiao-rong Yan* and **Yi Liu**

Department of Neurosurgery, Nanfang Neurosurgery Research Institution, Nanfang Hospital, Southern Medical University, 1838 North Guangzhou Avenue, Guangzhou, China

Abstract: Craniopharyngioma is a type of epithelial neoplasm that develops in the sellar region, a feature that distinguishes these tumors from other glial or neuronal lesions in the same location. Although the etiology of craniopharyngioma has not yet been confirmed, this type of tumor is generally thought to derive from the epithelial remnants of the craniopharyngeal duct that eventually forms part of the adenohypophysis. In this chapter, we address the pathological classification of craniopharyngioma and its molecular aspects. craniopharyngiomas can be divided into two subtypes: adamantinomatous craniopharyngioma (ACP) and squamous papillary craniopharyngioma (SPCP). ACP is more common (90% of all craniopharyngiomas), particularly among children. ACP features various types of epithelial characteristics such as peripheral palisades, stellate reticulum, whorl-like array cells, wet keratin, and cholesterol clefts. SPCP tumors are found almost exclusively in adults and generally present as solid masses comprised histologically of sheets of well-differentiated squamous epithelial cells, with prominent papillae composed of squamous epithelial cells that grow around fibrovascular cores. ACp contain mutations in CTNNB1, encoding β-catenin: a component of the adherens junction and mediator of Wnt signalling. reported frequency of CTNNB1 mutations varies widely (16–100%). Recently, it was reported that pCps contain BRAF p.V600e mutations in 95% of cases and that CTNNB1 and BRAF mutations are mutually exclusive and specific to tumour subtype.

Keywords: Beta-catenin, BRAF p.V600e, Craniopharyngioma, Molecular mechanism, Pathway, WNT.

Craniopharyngioma is a type of epithelial neoplasm that develops in the sellar region, a feature that distinguishes these tumors from other glial or neuronal lesions in the same location. Although the etiology of craniopharyngioma has not

* **Corresponding author Xiao-rong Yan**: Department of Neurosurgery, Nanfang Neurosurgery Research Institution, Nanfang Hospital, Southern Medical University, 1838 North Guangzhou Avenue, Guangzhou, China; Tel/Fax: +8620-61641806; E-mail: 178603351@qq.com

Songtao Qi (Ed.)

yet been confirmed, this type of tumor is generally thought to derive from the epithelial remnants of the craniopharyngeal duct that eventually forms part of the adenohypophysis (Fig. **1**).

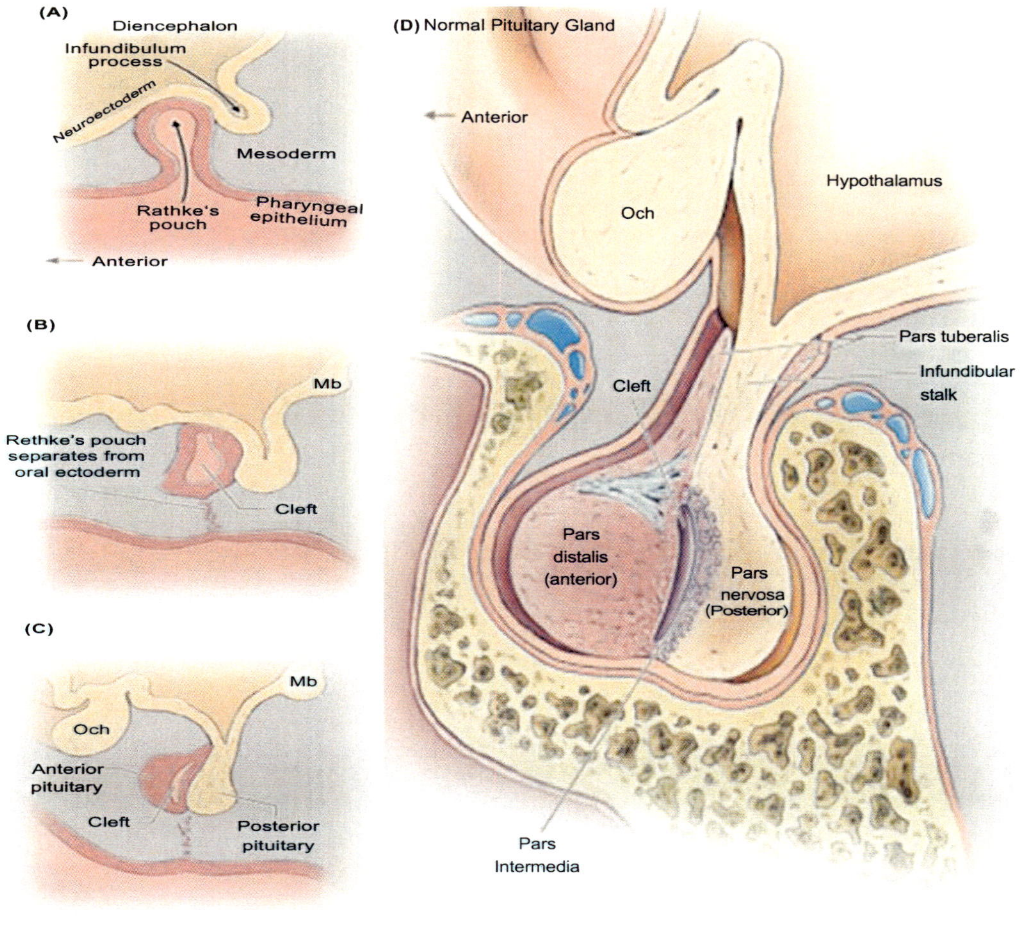

Fig. (1). Development of the hypophysis. (From Seunggu *et al.*).

PATHOLOGICAL TYPES

Histologically, craniopharyngiomas can be divided into two subtypes: adamantinomatous craniopharyngioma (ACP) and squamous papillary craniopharyngioma (SPCP). The incidence of ACP exhibits a bimodal age distribution, with peaks in children aged 5–14 years and adults aged 50–74 years [1]. This subtype is more common (90% of all craniopharyngiomas), particularly among children (nearly 100% of pediatric craniopharyngiomas), and often presents as a lobulated solid or cystic mass with a spongy quality resulting from a variable cystic component. These cystic spaces contain a dark, opaque, brown-green fluid with an appearance that some have compared to motor oil. This fluid contains lipids and polarizable cholesterol crystals (Fig. **2**).

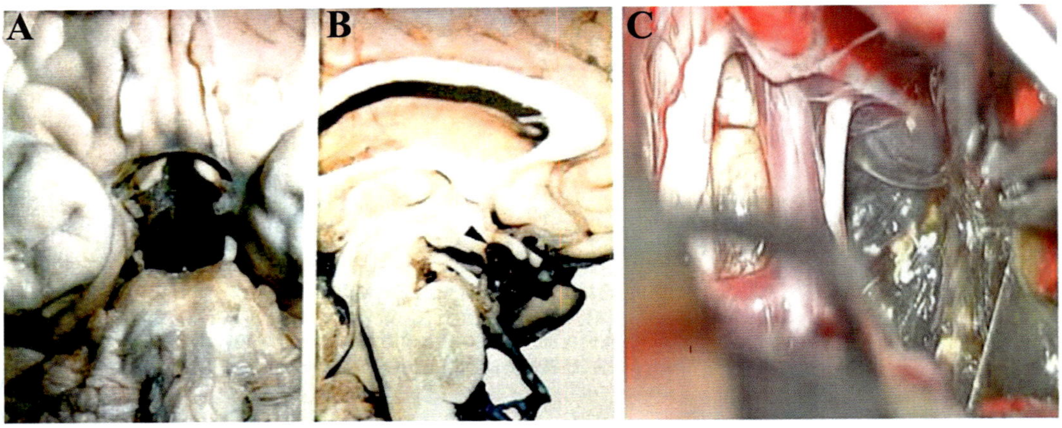

Fig. (2). Gross anatomy of craniopharyngioma.

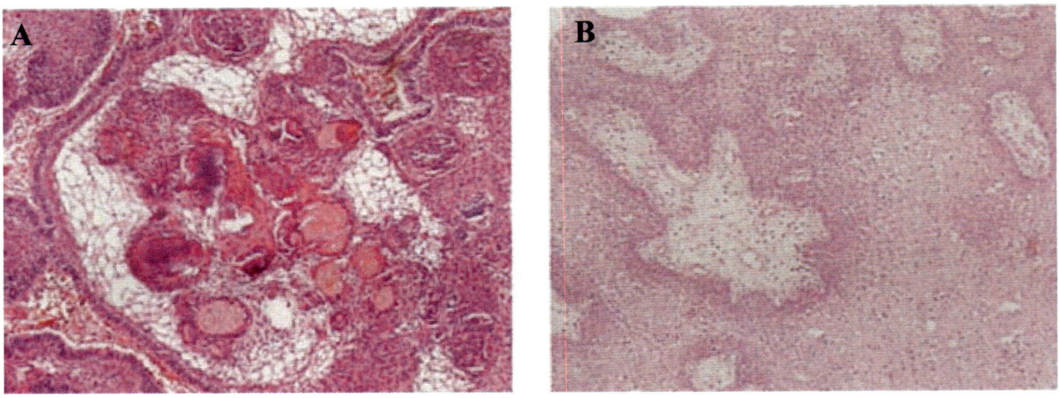

Fig. (3). Hematoxylin/eosin (H.E.) staining of ACP and SPCP. A, ACP: Loosely arranged stellate reticulum, whorl-like array cells, wet keratin, and calcification are surrounded by peripheral palisades; B, SPCP: Well-differentiated squamous epithelial cells contribute to the papillae surrounding fibrovascular cores.

Under the microscope, ACP features various types of epithelial characteristics such as peripheral palisades, stellate reticulum, whorl-like array cells, wet keratin, and cholesterol clefts, none of which are observed in SPCP (Fig. **3**). Peripheral palisades (columnar epithelium) arrange along the leading edge of the mass, within which the stellate reticulum, whorl-like array cells, and wet keratin are contained. The whorl-like array cells are composed of squamous epithelial cells and are thought to arise from the stellate reticulum. The wet keratin, also known as ghost cell structure, derives from degenerative whorl-like array cell nests and is considered the fundamental structure of calcification [2]. Piloid gliosis with distinct accumulations of Rosenthal fibers is often seen at the interface between the tumor and adjacent brain tissue.

In contrast to ACP, SPCP tumors are found almost exclusively in adults and generally present as solid masses comprised histologically of sheets of well-differentiated squamous epithelial cells, with prominent papillae composed of squamous epithelial cells that grow around fibrovascular cores. The palisades, wet keratin, stellate reticulum, calcification, and cholesterol clefts present in ACP are absent in SPCP.

The differences in histological characteristics between ACP and SPCP may be explained by the theory that ACP arises from epithelial remnants of the craniopharyngeal duct or Rathke's pouch, which in turn were derived from parts of the stomadeum epithelium destined to form primitive teeth, and that SPCP develops from residues of the stomadeum epithelium that contribute to development of the buccal mucosa [3, 4]. Similar to other epithelial tumors, both ACP and SPCP express cytokeratin and epithelial membrane antigen.

Recently, both pathological and genetic differences were revealed between ACP and SPCP. Mutation of the Wnt pathway, which induces the translocation of β-catenin into nuclei, appears to play an important role in ACP tumorigenesis.

β-catenin is a submembranous component of the adherens junction and functions as a transcriptional activator of the Wnt signaling pathway. Wnt signaling stabilizes cytoplasmic β-catenin, allowing its translocation to the nucleus and the formation of active transcription complexes with T cell factor-1/lymphoi--enhancing factor-1 (TCF/LEF1). Mutations in β-catenin that affect glycogen synthase kinase-3β (GSK-3β) dependent phosphorylation sites have been reported in various tumors [5]. These mutations stabilize β-catenin by inhibiting proteosomal degradation and thus promote constitutive activation of TCF/LEF1-dependent transcription [6].

In research conducted by Sekine *et al.*, nuclear and cytoplasmic β-catenin accumulation was found in all ACP but not in all SPCP. However, β-catenin expression was observed exclusively in the membrane and was generally observed in nonneoplastic epithelial ACP cells and all SPCP cells Fig. (**4**) [7]. This finding suggests that the constitutive activation of TCF/LEF-dependent transcription might be deeply involved in the craniopharyngioma tumorigenesis. β-catenin gene mutation and overexpression are specific to ACP, indicating a potential genetic difference between ACP and SPCP.

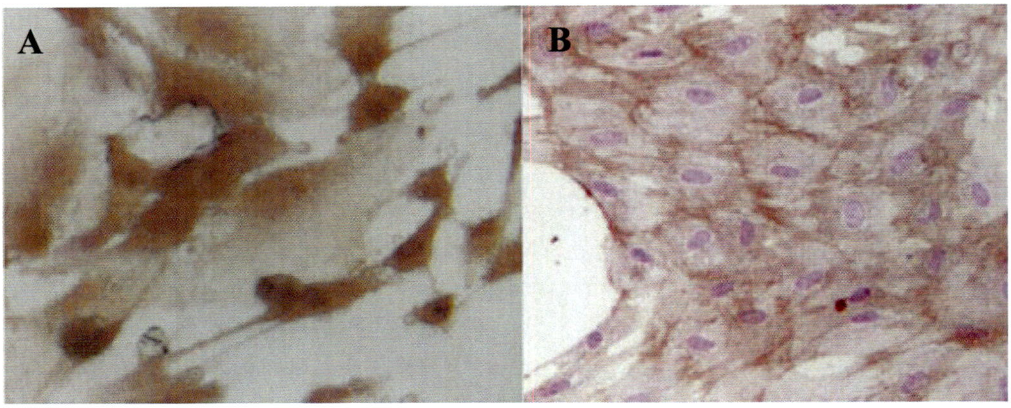

Fig. (4). β-catenin localization patterns differ between ACP and SPCP. Shown are images from immunohistochemical (IHC) β-catenin staining. A, in ACP, β-catenin localizes to the nucleus; B, in SPCP, β-catenin localizes to the cell membrane in SPCP. (From Priscilla *et al.* [7]).

IMAGING FEATURES OF CRANIOPHARYNGIOMA

The variability and diverse histological features of craniopharyngioma are typically evident *via* imaging (magnetic resonance [MR] and computed tomography [CT]). Craniopharyngioma is typically described as a calcified, solid-cystic lesion with a lobular shape. Distinct calcification is present in more than 60% of all cases and is more usual in pediatric patients [8, 9]. The solid component of ACP is usually isointense or hypointense on T1-weighted MR images and inhomogeneously hyperintense on T2-weighted images. The use of Gd-contrast enhancement often yields heterogeneous MR signals in craniopharyngiomas [10, 11]. The cystic elements of ACP typically exhibit hyperintensity on T1-weighted images, hyper- or mixed intensity on T2-weighted images, and cyst wall enhancement was common. The majority of SPCP tumors are predominantly solid tumors with a more regular shape and usually exhibit hypointensity on T1-weighted images, hyperintensity on T2-weighted images, and Gd contrast enhancement of the solid area or cyst wall [11, 12]. In SPCP lesions, the MR imaging appearance of solid regions is frequently similar to that of ACP.

DIFFERENTIAL DIAGNOSIS

Histologically, xanthogranuloma of the sellar region comprises cholesterol clefts, macrophages (xanthoma cells), chronic inflammatory cellular reactions, necrotic debris, and hemosiderin deposits (Fig. **5**). Although this entity is not yet fully defined and transitional cases are known to occur, xanthogranuloma of the sellar region is clinicopathologically distinct from ACP with respect to location, tumor size, age distribution, symptoms, and prognosis. Non-adamantinomatous squamous or cuboidal epithelium, as well as small tubules, may be focally present, whereas typical adamantinomatous epithelium is usually absent or accounts for less than 10% of the tissue. In contrast to ACP, the epithelial cells encountered in xanthogranulomas do not exhibit nuclear β-catenin accumulation.

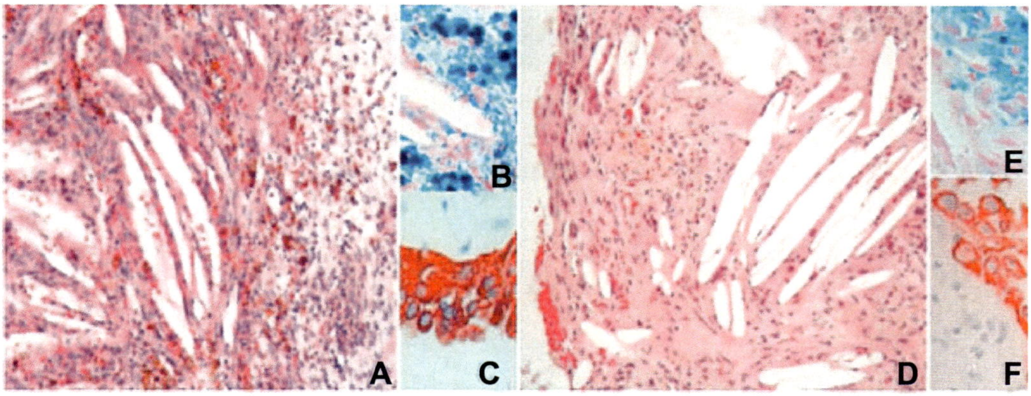

Fig. (5). Histopathological presentation of xanthogranuloma of the sellar region. H.E. staining (A, D) reveals macrophages, cholesterol clefts, and chronic inflammatory cells. Hemosiderin deposits are visualized *via* Prussian blue staining (B, E). Immunohistochemistry with a pan-epithelial antibody (LU5) reveals few epithelial cells (C, F). (H.E., 200× magnification; all others, 400×) (From Jung *et al.*).

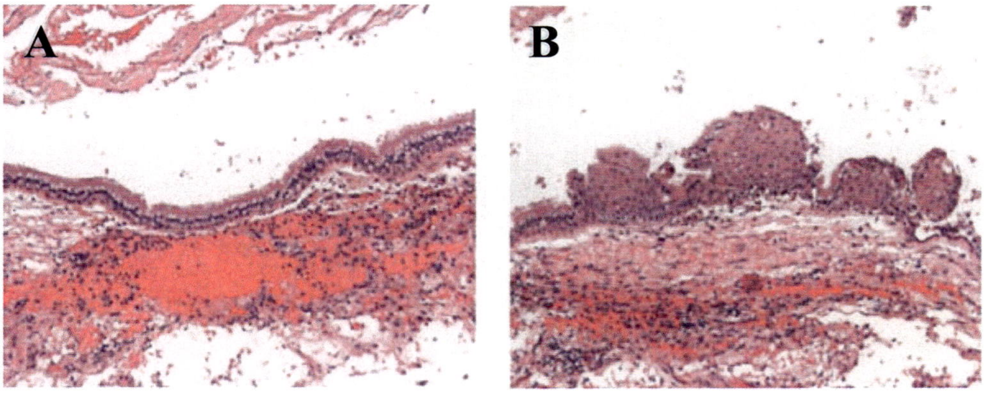

Fig. (6). A, Histological appearance of a Rathke's cleft cyst: a thin layer of supporting mesenchymal tissue lined with a single layer of ciliated columnar epithelium. B. Small clusters of metaplastic squamous epithelium can be found in Rathke's cleft cysts.

Although ACP has a characteristic histological appearance, epidermoid and Rathke's cleft cysts are sometimes suggested in the differential diagnosis. Both entities are reliably and feasibly distinctive; the former is characterized as a uniloculated cyst lined with squamous epithelium and filled with flaky dry keratin. Rathke's cleft cysts rarely pose a significant challenge and are only included in the differential diagnosis when they exhibit extensive squamous metaplasia (Fig. **6b**). More commonly, Rathke's cleft cysts comprise a single layer of either flattened or ciliated epithelium (Fig. **6a**).

HARD STRUCTURES IN CRANIOPHARYNGIOMA (CALCIFICATION, OSSIFICATION AND DENTAL TISSUE)

The etiology of craniopharyngioma remains controversial. Craniopharyngeal duct remnants, squamous metaplasia of anterior hypophysis cells, and enamel organ tissue migration have all been implicated [13 - 15]. The findings of bone and dental tissues in craniopharyngiomas have supported an odontogenic origin of these tumors. Alvarez-Garijo reported a case of highly calcified craniopharyngioma that contained ossified structures and, in particular, some well-developed teeth (Fig. **7**). In that report, a histological study revealed the presence of a typical craniopharyngioma structure, including peripheral palisades, stellate reticulum, wet keratin, and calcification, as well as tooth structure, including pulp, dentine, enamel, and roots [16].

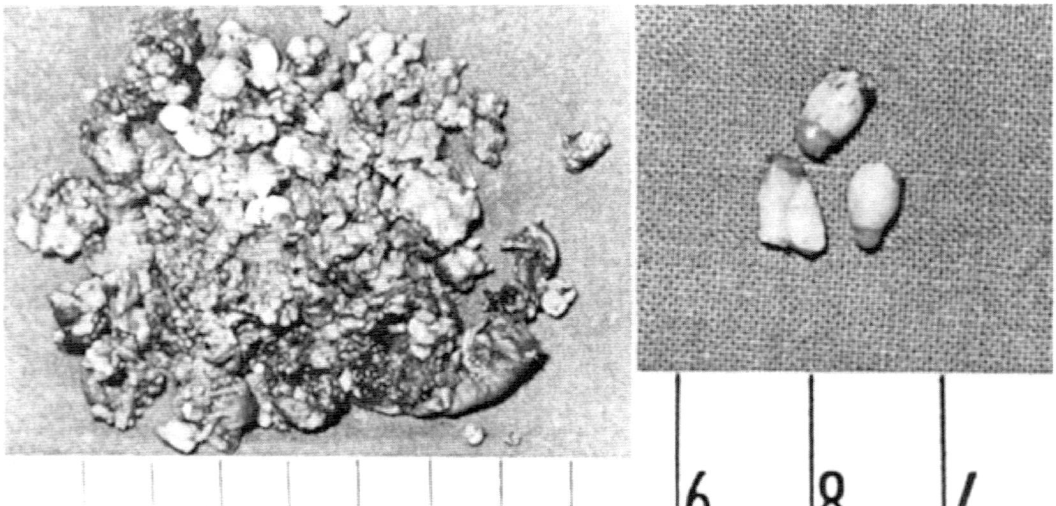

Fig. (7). Left: An operative specimen containing teeth was excised in a piecemeal manner. Observe the formed teeth, complete with roots. Right: Close-up view (From Alvarez-Garijo *et al.* [16]).

In some cases of craniopharyngioma with hard calcification or even ossification, single or clusters of osteoblast-like mesenchymal cells were encountered along the peripheral rim of the wet keratin, which directly contacted the fibrous connective tissue [17].

These finding suggest a relationship between craniopharyngiomal calcification and bone tissue.

Actually, ossified structures are not unusual in craniopharyngiomas; in these tumors, cortical bone lamellae, bone lacuna, and woven bone trabecula are often found to surround wet keratin. Electron microscopy revealed that the wet keratin, which contains numerous cytoplasmic tonofibrils, made directly contact with the fibrous connective tissue. Mesenchymal cells surrounded by collagen fibrils and amorphous ground matrices were occasionally observed alongside the keratinized cells. These mesenchymal cells, which contain numerous glycogen granules, free ribosomes, and vesicles, were morphologically similar to osteoblasts. The spaces created by the mesenchymal cells contained membrane-bound vesicles that often harbored needle-shaped crystals (hydroxyapatite crystals). These vesicles frequently contacted the neighboring collagen fibrils that surrounded the mesenchymal cells. Further hydroxyapatite deposits along the collagen fibrils led to the formation of a larger mineralized mass and, eventually, ossification [17].

The membrane-bound vesicle is an important structure in the process of calcium deposition. These vesicles can be considered as matrix vesicles, matrix giant bodies, or mitochondria, which are generally recognized as the initial mineralization foci in both physiological and pathological calcified tissue [2, 13, 18]. Hydroxyapatite crystals accumulate in the vesicles and can be pooled to form small bone trabecula. Subsequently, collagen fibrils orient this accumulation and promote the formation of thick bone trabecula [13, 18, 19]. The membrane vesicles exist not only around but also within the wet keratin and undergo calcium deposition to form calcified lesions and ossification.

Although calcification is an important feature of ACP, no calcified tissues are found in SPCP. As visualized *via* CT or surgical observation, the calcification patterns in ACP vary from no calcification to solid lumps, popcorn-like foci or, less commonly, an eggshell pattern that lines the cyst wall [20] (Figs. **8**, **9**). Nevertheless, all of these patterns appear as a purple mass under the microscope. The calcified lesions in ACP are substantially composed of hydroxyapatite crystals. These hydroxyapatite crystals deposit in some vesicles, where they increasingly collect to form mineral nodules. Wet keratin is thought to be the basement structure for the formation of calcified lesions.

The findings of bone tissue and teeth led to a theory in which calcification in craniopharyngiomas resemble odontogenesis/osteogenesis. Craniopharyngioma shares an origin with dental tissue, and the histological profile of craniopharyngioma is highly analogous to that of odontogenic tumors. Enamel proteins that are expressed exclusively in teeth have also been found in ACP.

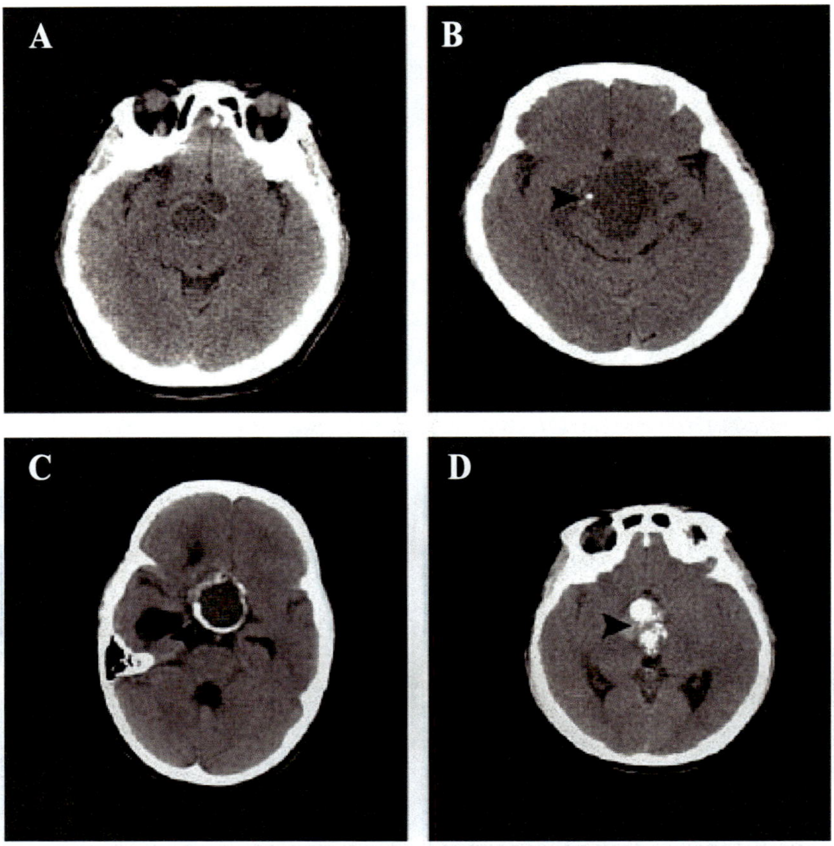

Fig. (8). A representative presurgical brain CT scan reveals a suprasellar cystic lesion (arrowhead). All was ACP after pathological examination. A, ACP without calcification (-, negative); B, ACP with solid mild calcification (+, mild); C, Cystic CP with eggshell-like calcium deposition in the cyst wall (++, moderate); D, CP with popcorn-like focal calcification (+++, severe).

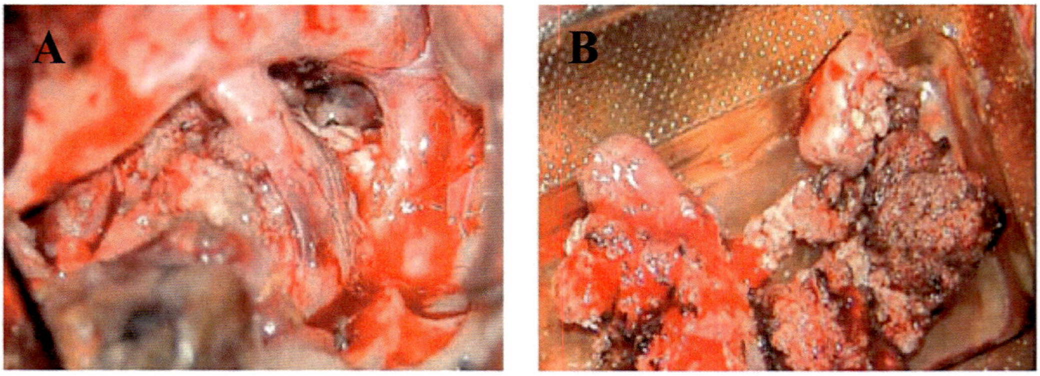

Fig. (9). A, Surgical view of a craniopharyngioma with a calcified lesion that compresses the pituitary stalk. B, the calcified tumor was removed as a single mass.

Our study found that a protein with osteogenic function, osteopontin (OPN), was a core factor in the calcification of craniopharyngioma. OPN is a phosphorylated glycoprotein secreted by activated macrophages, leukocytes, and activated T lymphocytes. It is also presented in numerous human cancers as well as mineralized tissues [21 - 24]. OPN is found to plays an significant role in the mineralization process. Our study demonstrated that both OPN and its receptor CD44v6 was expressed in calcified craniopharyngioma samples. Meanwhile, subcellular localization of OPN was found in craniopharyngioma cells, suggesting that these cells likely synthesize and secrete OPN protein.

As a functional protein secreted by osteoblasts during calcium deposition, OPN may be controlled by osteogenic proteins that induce osteoblast differentiation. Further study revealed that the osteogenic proteins bone morphogenetic protein-2 (BMP2), osterix, and Runx2 might play important roles in the calcification of craniopharyngioma.

BMP2 belongs to the BMP family, which is the largest family of secreted transforming growth factor-beta (TGF-β) superfamily signaling molecules,and was considered as an osteoinductive/odontoinductive protein. BMP2 can promote osteoblast and chondroblast differentiation by inducing new bone formation [25 - 27]. Recent literature has revealed the BMP2's role in teeth development was conducted through the differentiation of odontoblasts and ameloblasts [28 - 30]. Runx2 (also called Cbfal) and osterix (also called Osx) belong to osteoblast-specific transcription factors that are important for osteoblast differentiation. The factors mentioned above are involved in downstream molecules expression, including OPN, bone sialoprotein (BSP), and osteonectin (OCN) [31]. BMP2 can regulate both Runx2 and osterix during osteoblast differentiation [32 - 36].

High levels of BMP2, Runx2, and osterix expression were observed in calcified ACP, and these levels correlated positively with the degree of ACP calcification; however, these proteins were weakly expressed in SPCP. We also detected the expression patterns of these osteogenic proteins. Our results revealed that BMP2 together with Runx2 and osterix were expressed in the stellate reticulum and the whorl-like array cells [4]. Further,both Runx2 and osterix were also found in wet keratin and calcified lesions. Wet keratin, or ghost cell structure, which was considered deriving from degenerating whorl-like array cell nests was thought to be the foundation for calcification [2]. H.E. staining also revealed osteoblast-like cells in calcified lesions of ACP suggesting a similar biological process as osteoblasts differentiation in the bone [37] (Fig. **10**). ALL these findings suggest that osteoblast-like morphology were found in areas of wet keratin and calcification in ACP was a positive process by tumor cells [17]. The factors including BMP2 might play an significant role in calcification.

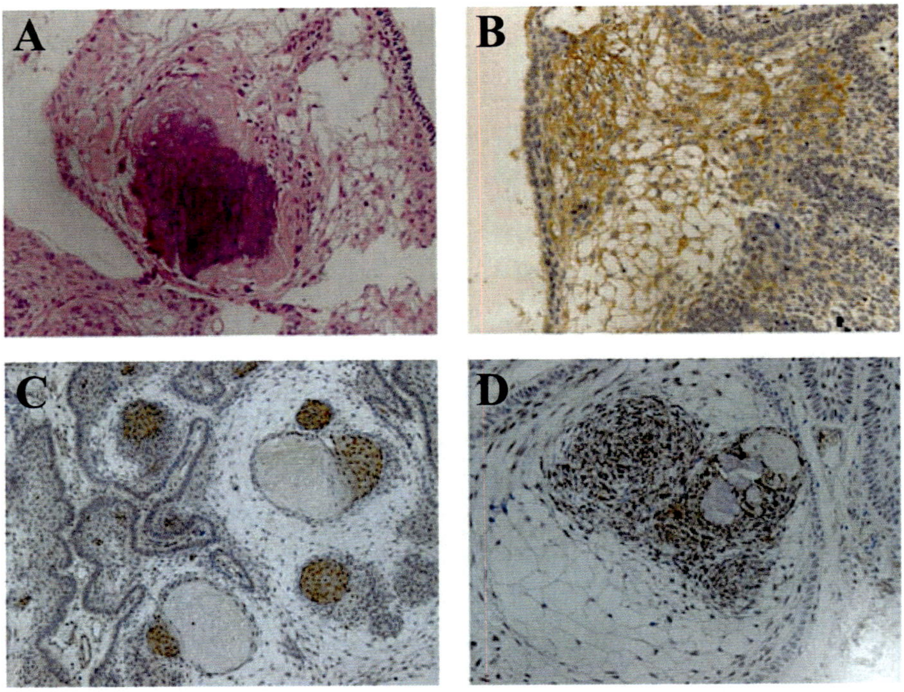

Fig. (10). A, H.E. staining: calcified lesion appears as a purple mass in the wet keratin. B, BMP2 was expressed in the stellate reticulum and whorl-like array cells of ACP. C, Runx2 was mainly found in the whorl-like cells and reticulum. D, Osterix staining was observed in the epithelia surrounding the wet keratin and calcified lesions.

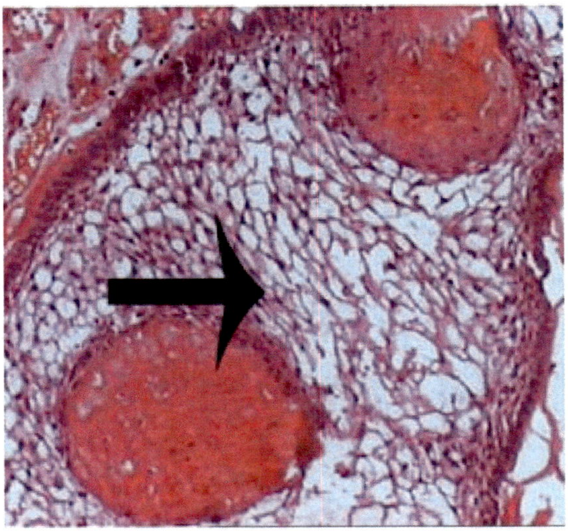

Fig. (11). A calcified lesion that arose from the wet keratin, containing spindle/round-shaped osteoblast-like cells (arrowhead). Inset: magnification of the area indicated by the arrow.

The above-described evidence demonstrates that osteogenic proteins, including BMP2, and the osteoblast differentiation markers Runx2 and osterix were key factors in the craniopharyngiomal calcification and also that some ACP might differentiate into cells exhibiting an osteoblast-like lineage (Fig. **11**).

CONFLICT OF INTEREST

The authors (editor) declares no conflict of interest, financial or otherwise.

ACKNOWLEDGEMENTS

We should acknowledge Dr. Deng Yong-jian for reviewing the pathological sections of craniopharyngioma.

REFERENCES

[1] Bunin GR, Surawicz TS, Witman PA, Preston-Martin S, Davis F, Bruner JM. The descriptive epidemiology of craniopharyngioma. J Neurosurg 1998; 89(4): 547-51. [http://dx.doi.org/10.3171/jns.1998.89.4.0547] [PMID: 9761047]

[2] Sato K, Kubota T, Yamamoto S, Ishikura A. An ultrastructural study of mineralization in craniopharyngiomas. J Neuropathol Exp Neurol 1986; 45(4): 463-70. [http://dx.doi.org/10.1097/00005072-198607000-00007] [PMID: 3723142]

[3] Fernandez-Miranda JC, Gardner PA, Snyderman CH, *et al.* Craniopharyngioma: a pathologic, clinical, and surgical review. Head Neck 2012; 34(7): 1036-44. [http://dx.doi.org/10.1002/hed.21771] [PMID: 21584897]

[4] Kato K, Nakatani Y, Kanno H, *et al.* Possible linkage between specific histological structures and aberrant reactivation of the Wnt pathway in adamantinomatous craniopharyngioma. J Pathol 2004; 203(3): 814-21. [http://dx.doi.org/10.1002/path.1562] [PMID: 15221941]

[5] Polakis P. Wnt signaling and cancer. Genes Dev 2000; 14(15): 1837-51. [PMID: 10921899]

[6] Sekine S, Sato S, Takata T, *et al.* Beta-catenin mutations are frequent in calcifying odontogenic cysts, but rare in ameloblastomas. Am J Pathol 2003; 163(5): 1707-12. [http://dx.doi.org/10.1016/S0002-9440(10)63528-6] [PMID: 14578169]

[7] Sekine S, Shibata T, Kokubu A, *et al.* Craniopharyngiomas of adamantinomatous type harbor beta-catenin gene mutations. Am J Pathol 2002; 161(6): 1997-2001. [http://dx.doi.org/10.1016/S0002-9440(10)64477-X] [PMID: 12466115]

[8] Adamson TE, Wiestler OD, Kleihues P, Yaşargil MG. Correlation of clinical and pathological features in surgically treated craniopharyngiomas. J Neurosurg 1990; 73(1): 12-7. [http://dx.doi.org/10.3171/jns.1990.73.1.0012] [PMID: 2352012]

[9] Karavitaki N, Cudlip S, Adams CB, Wass JA. Craniopharyngiomas. Endocr Rev 2006; 27(4): 371-97. [http://dx.doi.org/10.1210/er.2006-0002] [PMID: 16543382]

[10] Choi SH, Kwon BJ, Na DG, Kim JH, Han MH, Chang KH. Pituitary adenoma, craniopharyngioma, and Rathke cleft cyst involving both intrasellar and suprasellar regions: differentiation using MRI. Clin Radiol 2007; 62(5): 453-62. [http://dx.doi.org/10.1016/j.crad.2006.12.001] [PMID: 17398271]

[11] Sartoretti-Schefer S, Wichmann W, Aguzzi A, Valavanis A. MR differentiation of adamantinous and squamous-papillary craniopharyngiomas. AJNR Am J Neuroradiol 1997; 18(1): 77-87.

[PMID: 9010523]

[12] Crotty TB, Scheithauer BW, Young WF Jr, *et al.* Papillary craniopharyngioma: a clinicopathological study of 48 cases. J Neurosurg 1995; 83(2): 206-14. [http://dx.doi.org/10.3171/jns.1995.83.2.0206] [PMID: 7616262]

[13] Kalnins V, Rossi E. V. and E. ROSSI, ODONTOGENIC CRANIOPHARYNGIOMA: A CASE REPORT. Cancer 1965; 18: 899-906. [http://dx.doi.org/10.1002/1097-0142(196507)18:7<899::AID-CNCR2820180720>3.0.CO;2-L] [PMID: 14308239]

[14] Luse SA, Kernohan JW. Squamous-cell nests of the pituitary gland. Cancer 1955; 8(3): 623-8. [http://dx.doi.org/10.1002/1097-0142(1955)8:3<623::AID-CNCR2820080328>3.0.CO;2-D] [PMID: 14379152]

[15] Russell DS. The Pathology of Intracranial Tumours. Postgrad Med J 1950; 26(293): 109-26. [http://dx.doi.org/10.1136/pgmj.26.293.109] [PMID: 21313511]

[16] Alvarez-Garijo JA, Froufé A, Taboada D, Vila M. Successful surgical treatment of an odontogenic ossified craniopharyngioma. Case report. J Neurosurg 1981; 55(5): 832-5. [http://dx.doi.org/10.3171/jns.1981.55.5.0832] [PMID: 6796660]

[17] Sato K, Kubota T. Fine structure of ossification in craniopharyngiomas. Ultrastruct Pathol 1999; 23(6): 395-9. [http://dx.doi.org/10.1080/019131299281374] [PMID: 10626690]

[18] Anderson HC. Calcification processes. Pathol Annu 1980; 15(Pt 2): 45-75. [PMID: 6256707]

[19] Bernard GW. Ultrastructural observations of initial calcification in dentine and enamel. J Ultrastruct Res 1972; 41(1): 1-17. [http://dx.doi.org/10.1016/S0022-5320(72)90034-2] [PMID: 5075522]

[20] Qi S, Huang G, Pan J, *et al.* Involvement of osteopontin as a core protein in craniopharyngioma calcification formation. J Neurooncol 2010; 98(1): 21-30. [http://dx.doi.org/10.1007/s11060-009-0053-8] [PMID: 19902145]

[21] Diao H, Kon S, Iwabuchi K, *et al.* Osteopontin as a mediator of NKT cell function in T cell-mediated liver diseases. Immunity 2004; 21(4): 539-50. [http://dx.doi.org/10.1016/j.immuni.2004.08.012] [PMID: 15485631]

[22] Furger KA, Menon RK, Tuck AB, Bramwell VH, Chambers AF. The functional and clinical roles of osteopontin in cancer and metastasis. Curr Mol Med 2001; 1(5): 621-32. [http://dx.doi.org/10.2174/1566524013363339] [PMID: 11899236]

[23] Haylock DN, Nilsson SK. Osteopontin: a bridge between bone and blood. Br J Haematol 2006; 134(5): 467-74. [http://dx.doi.org/10.1111/j.1365-2141.2006.06218.x] [PMID: 16848793]

[24] O'Regan A, Berman JS. Osteopontin: a key cytokine in cell-mediated and granulomatous inflammation. Int J Exp Pathol 2000; 81(6): 373-90. [http://dx.doi.org/10.1046/j.1365-2613.2000.00163.x] [PMID: 11298186]

[25] Katagiri T, Yamaguchi A, Ikeda T, *et al.* The non-osteogenic mouse pluripotent cell line, C3H10T1/2, is induced to differentiate into osteoblastic cells by recombinant human bone morphogenetic protein-2. Biochem Biophys Res Commun 1990; 172(1): 295-9. [http://dx.doi.org/10.1016/S0006-291X(05)80208-6] [PMID: 1699539]

[26] Noël D, Gazit D, Bouquet C, *et al.* Short-term BMP-2 expression is sufficient for in vivo osteochondral differentiation of mesenchymal stem cells. Stem Cells 2004; 22(1): 74-85. [http://dx.doi.org/10.1634/stemcells.22-1-74] [PMID: 14688393]

[27] Lecanda F, Avioli LV, Cheng SL. Regulation of bone matrix protein expression and induction of

differentiation of human osteoblasts and human bone marrow stromal cells by bone morphogenetic protein-2. J Cell Biochem 1997; 67(3): 386-96.
[http://dx.doi.org/10.1002/(SICI)1097-4644(19971201)67:3<386::AID-JCB10>3.0.CO;2-B] [PMID: 9361193]

[28] Bègue-Kirn C, Smith AJ, Ruch JV, *et al.* Effects of dentin proteins, transforming growth factor beta 1 (TGF beta 1) and bone morphogenetic protein 2 (BMP2) on the differentiation of odontoblast in vitro. Int J Dev Biol 1992; 36(4): 491-503.
[PMID: 1295560]

[29] Lee HK, Park JT, Cho YS, Bae HS, Cho MI, Park JC. Odontogenic ameloblasts-associated protein (ODAM), via phosphorylation by bone morphogenetic protein receptor type IB (BMPR-IB), is implicated in ameloblast differentiation. J Cell Biochem 2012; 113(5): 1754-65.
[PMID: 22213140]

[30] Coin R, Haïkel Y, Ruch JV. Effects of apatite, transforming growth factor beta-1, bone morphogenetic protein-2 and interleukin-7 on ameloblast differentiation in vitro. Eur J Oral Sci 1999; 107(6): 487-95.
[http://dx.doi.org/10.1046/j.0909-8836.1999.eos107611.x] [PMID: 10625109]

[31] Ducy P, Zhang R, Geoffroy V, Ridall AL, Karsenty G. Osf2/Cbfa1: a transcriptional activator of osteoblast differentiation. Cell 1997; 89(5): 747-54.
[http://dx.doi.org/10.1016/S0092-8674(00)80257-3] [PMID: 9182762]

[32] Nakashima K, Zhou X, Kunkel G, *et al.* The novel zinc finger-containing transcription factor osterix is required for osteoblast differentiation and bone formation. Cell 2002; 108(1): 17-29.
[http://dx.doi.org/10.1016/S0092-8674(01)00622-5] [PMID: 11792318]

[33] Zhang YW, Yasui N, Ito K, *et al.* A RUNX2/PEBP2alpha A/CBFA1 mutation displaying impaired transactivation and Smad interaction in cleidocranial dysplasia. Proc Natl Acad Sci USA 2000; 97(19): 10549-54.
[http://dx.doi.org/10.1073/pnas.180309597] [PMID: 10962029]

[34] Matsubara T, Kida K, Yamaguchi A, *et al.* BMP2 regulates Osterix through Msx2 and Runx2 during osteoblast differentiation. J Biol Chem 2008; 283(43): 29119-25.
[http://dx.doi.org/10.1074/jbc.M801774200] [PMID: 18703512]

[35] Shu B, Zhang M, Xie R, *et al.* BMP2, but not BMP4, is crucial for chondrocyte proliferation and maturation during endochondral bone development. J Cell Sci 2011; 124(Pt 20): 3428-40.
[http://dx.doi.org/10.1242/jcs.083659] [PMID: 21984813]

[36] Celil AB, Campbell PG. BMP-2 and insulin-like growth factor-I mediate Osterix (Osx) expression in human mesenchymal stem cells via the MAPK and protein kinase D signaling pathways. J Biol Chem 2005; 280(36): 31353-9.
[http://dx.doi.org/10.1074/jbc.M503845200] [PMID: 16000303]

[37] Jähn K, Richards RG, Archer CW, Stoddart MJ. Pellet culture model for human primary osteoblasts. Eur Cell Mater 2010; 20: 149-61.
[http://dx.doi.org/10.22203/eCM.v020a13] [PMID: 20818597]

CHAPTER 4

Current Therapeutic Situation

Yi Liu*

Department of Neurosurgery, Nanfang Neurosurgery Research Institution, Nanfang Hospital, Southern Medical University, 1838 North Guangzhou Avenue, Guangzhou, China.

Abstract: Craniopharyngiomas are benign midline tumors that have a propensity for local recurrence and are ideally curable *via* total surgical resection. Many survivors suffer from behavioral, cognitive, endocrine, hypothalamic, and visual disturbances. Optimal management remains highly controversial. In this chapter, we reviewed the therapy strategies for Craniopharyngiomas including surgery, radiotherapy and chemotherapy. Complete resection is even more important in children, especially those younger than 3 years, because of the additional morbidity associated with radiotherapy during early childhood. The aim of radiotherapy is to achieve long-term disease control in patients lacking complete removal or with recurrent tumors. Systemic chemotherapy has rarely been reported in terms of craniopharyngioma management. Local intratumoral chemotherapy for craniopharyngioma was used to treat difficult, recurrent cystic tumors and has subsequently been employed as a strategy to avoid late-term effects of surgery or radiotherapy. The roles of all therapies should be balanced according to factors such as the patient's age, the tumor size and location, and prior treatment.

Keywords: BRAF, Chemotherapy, Craniopharyngiomas, Radiotherapy, Surgery.

MANAGEMENT DURING THE PERIOPERATIVE PERIOD

Craniopharyngiomas are benign midline tumors that have a propensity for local recurrence and are ideally curable *via* total surgical resection. Regardless, their optimal management remains highly controversial, and ongoing debates address both the natural disease history and therapy. Following advances in microsurgical and endoscopic techniques, the complete resection rates have increased from 69% to 90%, with acceptable mortality and morbidity [1, 20, 42, 55, 63, 68, 78, 90, 92, 100, 106, 107, 111, 116, 119, 133, 139, 147, 149, 155, 171, 178, 182 - 185, 207], although some authors might not fully appreciate and underestimate the adverse neuroendocrinological and cognitive effects of surgery in children [18, 22, 47, 54,

* **Corresponding author Yi Liu**: Department of Neurosurgery, Nanfang Neurosurgery Research Institution, Nanfang Hospital, Southern Medical University, 1838 North Guangzhou Avenue, Guangzhou, China; Tel/Fax: +8620-61641806; E-mail: 278679433@qq.com

Songtao Qi (Ed.)

59, 64, 84, 91, 182]. However, complete resection is even more important in children, especially those younger than 3 years, because of the additional morbidity associated with radiotherapy during early childhood [3, 5, 9, 37, 64, 110, 208]. The decision and rationale regarding the optimal microsurgical approach for a craniopharyngioma should be based on an interpretation of the clinical findings and radiological investigations in conjunction with an understanding of the pathological anatomy and embryology of these lesions. Broadly speaking, surgical approaches for these lesions include both craniological and transsphenoidal approaches using endoscopic techniques.

Preoperative Evaluation

The preoperative evaluation includes laboratory, neuroophthalmological, neuroradiological, and neuropsychological evaluations. Laboratory investigations should include a full endocrinological assessment (*e.g.*, growth hormone [GH], thyroid-stimulating hormone [TSH], adrenocorticotropic hormone [ACTH], luteinizing hormone [LH], follicle-stimulating hormone [FSH], and antidiuretic hormone [ADH] levels). Anterior panhypopituitarism should be considered if deficiencies in five anterior pituitary hormones (GH, TSH, ACTH, LH, and FSH) are detected or deficiencies in TSH, ACTH, and GH are observed in a prepubertal child. These assessment methods can be found in Chapter 16 of this book. Hormone deficiencies are common among patients with craniopharyngiomas: hypogonadism occurs in 75–80% of patients, GH deficiency in 80–100%, moderate adrenal insufficiency in 30–60%, hypothyroidism in 20–40%, and diabetes insipidus in 10–20% [15, 63, 69, 84, 87, 103, 134, 140, 152, 163, 166, 186]. Endocrine manifestations are more common in children, in whom short stature and delayed linear growth are detected in 93% of cases [143]. In adult patients, symptoms related to sex hormone imbalances are most common. Decreased libido is reported in 88% of adult male patients and amenorrhea in 82% of adult female patients [60]. Adolescents usually present with delayed or arrested puberty. Diabetes insipidus manifests at presentation in 17% of children and 20% of adolescents [7, 125]. Although rare, adult patients may also present with galactorrhea due to a "stalk effect" that compromises the inhibition of prolactin production. Occasionally, compression of hypothalamus may contribute to precocious puberty due to a lack in the hypothalamic-mediated inhibition of gonadotrophin-releasing hormone (GnRH). However, this condition is not commonly observed because of combined hypopituitarism that balances the effects of increased GnRH. Additionally, 24-hour measurements of fluid intake and output as well as measurements of specific gravity (SG), electrolytes, osmotic pressure, hepatic and renal function, blood coagulation, electrocardiogram (ECG), sternum, and body mass index (BMI) should be evaluated [22, 54, 125, 146].

The neuroophthalmological evaluation should include measurements of visual acuity and perimetry of the visual field as well as an examination of the optic fundus [2, 27, 31, 44, 124, 148]. Combined ophthalmological diseases that cause visual disturbances, such as glaucoma and diabetic retinopathy, should also be evaluated., Appropriate plates for visual acuity test should be used instead for young children. Deterioration should be determined if visual acuity has deteriorated by >0.2 compared to the last test and an additional defect is presented in 1/4 within the visual field. Visual disturbances may manifest as reduced visual acuity, unilateral or bilateral blindness, visual field defects, diplopia, blurred vision, or seesaw nystagmus. As many as 80% of adults present with visual disturbances, whereas only 40% of children complain of similar deficits [2, 27, 31, 44, 124, 148]. The finding that visual deficits are reported in a smaller proportion of children is largely attributed to the notion that children have a higher tolerance of visual loss, compared with adults. This is likely because children have less experience with normal vision and, as a result, are unable to identify abnormalities. Subtle alterations in school performance may be the only presenting feature. For patients harboring craniopharyngiomas who have no visual problems, it is highly likely that their tumors are restricted to the intrasellar region and do not involve the optic apparatus [57].

Neuroradiology evaluations for craniopharyngiomas include a skull X-ray, computed tomography (CT), magnetic resonance imaging (MRI), and Digital Subtraction Angiography(DSA). Historically, calcification associated with craniopharyngioma on a plain skull X-ray has always been an important and virtually pathognomonic feature of suprasellar lesions. However, high-resolution CT with contrast enhancement is very useful when radiologically assessing craniopharyngiomas for both surgical planning and subsequent follow-up. Enhanced CT can reveal both solid and cystic components. Areas of calcification are very clearly demonstrated on fine-cut CT using bone window algorithms. Furthermore, CT can exclude hydrocephalus. Recent advances in CT technology, along with the development of spiral multiple-array combined and advanced software programs, have facilitated high-definition coronal and sagittal reconstructions that were previously exclusive to MRI. Although it is suboptimal for assessments of calcification, the resolution of MRI remains superior to that of CT and is the investigation of choice for craniopharyngiomas, particularly with respect to both sagittal and coronal reconstructions. MRI has the additional advantage of not requiring any radiation; this is beneficial because patients frequently require multiple and sequential scans, which lead to the potential long-term risk of cataract formation, especially in pediatric patients. MRI precisely demonstrates the extent and location of the tumor, including its relationships with important surrounding neurovascular structures. The sizes and consistencies of craniopharyngiomas are also quite variable and are of great importance to the surgical strategy and prognosis: 14–20% of tumors are >4 cm in size, 58–76% are between 2 and 4 cm, and 4–28% are <2 cm. Some 46–64% of cranio-pharyngiomas are purely or predominantly cystic, 18–39% are predominantly solid, and 8–36% are mixed [45, 81, 98, 181]. Perfusion-weighted magnetic resonance imaging (PWI) can provide which provides the differential informations for sellar/parasellar tumors, although is possible to preoperatively differentiate these histological subtypes [14].

It is not uncommon for patients with craniopharyngiomas to present with neuropsychological sequelae. Similar to visual problems, cognitive disturbances are more common in adults than children. This is not surprising, given the comparative difficulty in diagnosing pediatric psychiatric disturbances. Less than 10% of children become affected, whereas approximately 25% of adults experience mental disturbances [57, 85, 86, 140, 144, 162, 169, 188, 191]. In addition to the clinical diagnosis, cognitive disturbances can serve as a predictive factor for treatment outcomes, as prolonged mentation deficits and depression are associated with a worse prognosis. As previously mentioned, craniopharyngiomas can be relatively large at diagnosis. Together with the fact that these tumors usually arise from the sellar region, large craniopharyngiomas can easily disrupt communication between the hypothalamus and various brain regions such as the thalamus, frontal lobe, and temporal lobe, resulting in the evolution of a range of psychological and psychosocial problems. There is a wide spectrum of neuropsychological presentations ranging from mentation deficits, apathy, abulia, and depression to delayed psychomotor responses, hypersomnia, incontinence, and seizures. Complex psychomotor seizures and amnesia have been reported in patients with tumor extension into the temporal lobes or hippocampus. The mechanism behind the manifestation of these symptoms is complex and likely multifactorial. Hydrocephalus and hypothyroidism are thought to be among the many contributing factors.

Preoperative Management

Hydrocephalus and Increased Intracranial Pressure

Many cranio-pharyngiomas will eventually become large enough to impede cerebrospinal fluid (CSF) circulation at the foramina of Munro and cause obstructive hydrocephalus. Hydrocephalus is consequently a common complication that affects a third of patients, regardless of age [21, 49, 72, 168]. Headache and vomiting are typical presentations of an increased intracranial pressure (ICP). Hence, it is not surprising that both symptoms are most common complaints of children with craniopharyngiomas: 80% of affected children present with headache and 60% present with nausea and/or vomiting. Symptoms of increased ICP also occur in adult patients but at a lower incidence: 30% of adult patients present with headache and 20% with nausea and/or vomiting. Upon examination, papilledema is found in 40% of children and 10% of adults [58, 120]. Asymptomatic hydrocephalus may be relieved after tumor resection; however, this can make tumor exposure more difficult during surgery. Preoperative lumbar drainage is helpful, as this can release CSF and reduce brain traction. Patients with symptoms of headache and vomiting and even a loss of consciousness should undergo emergency treatment. The most common and effective treatment is ventricle puncture drainage. The drainage tube should be removed within 72 hours after craniotomy to avoid infection. Hydrocephalus is relieved after tumor resection in most cases. A ventriculoperitoneal shunt may be an option for patients with persistent hydrocephalus.

Hormone Replacement Therapy

Preoperative hormone replacement therapies mainly include corticosteroids and thyroid hormones [103, 189]. 1-desamino-8-d-arginine-vasopressin (DDAVP) treatment for diabetes insipidus should be initiated before surgery. Given the high incidence of post-operative ACTH deficiency, all patients, even those found to have no abnormalities of the adrenal axis, should receive a stress dose of corticosteroids before surgery. Prednisone is usually the first choice in this situation. A total prednisone dose of 7.5 mg can be divided into two or three orally administered subdoses beginning 3 days before surgery. Patients with preoperative hypothyroidism should be treated with euthyrox at a dosage of 20 mg/day for 3 days before surgery. Electrolyte levels, especially Na and K, should be restored to within normal limits.

Postoperative Management

Anti-Epileptic

Phenobarbitol at a dose of 0.1 g should be injected intra-muscularly immediately after surgery and readministered every 12 hours until patients can orally ingest other antiepileptic drugs. Dilantin is the most common orally administered drug. Patients without preoperative epileptic seizures should use this drug for at least 2–3 weeks, whereas those with preoperative or postoperative seizures should be treated routinely with this drug [207]. The risk of epilepsy after 10 years ranges from 12% to 17% [104, 160].

Hormone Replacement Therapy

Corticosteroids should be immediately injected intravenously after surgery. During the first 3 days after surgery, a total hydrocortisone dose of 200–300 mg should be administered with gradual tapering until reaching an oral physiological minimum requirement (*i.e.*, 20–30 mg of hydrocortisone daily). Euthyrox should not be used for 3–5 days after surgery because of the risk of additional cortisol consumption. An initial oral dose of 25 μg/day can be gradually increased to a maintenance dose of 50–100 μg/day [126, 145]. Therapeutic replacement of other hormones, such as GH and sex hormones, is discussed in the endocrine chapters.

Electrolyte Disturbances

Electrolyte disturbances are observed in 80–100% patients with craniopharyngiomas [29] and mainly present as hyperna-tronemia/hyponatremia and hypokalemia. All patients usually should undergo twice-daily serum sodium measurements during the postoperative period. Hypernatronemia is observed immediately after surgery and lasts for 3–5 days because of ADH deficiency. DDAVP should be used to reduce the urine volume, and 5% glucose injections should be administered according to the urine volume and serum sodium concentration [71, 125, 194]. Hypokalemia is common during this period, and K should be supplied either orally or *via* intravenous drip. Hyponatremia will appear in the later postoperative period, usually after 5–7 days, and will persist for 2–4 weeks. Cerebral salt-wasting syndrome (CSWS) and syndrome of inappropriate antidiuretic hormone (SIADH) always contribute to hyponatremia, although the former is more common. It is important for clinicians to differentiate these syndromes because treatments oppose one another. Central venous pressure (CVP) and renal sodium excretion (UNa) are the two most important indicators. CSWS should be treated with sufficient hypertonic saline, whereas fluid restriction is the main treatment for SIADH.

Diabetes Insipidus

Diabetes insipidus is not uncommonafter craniopharyngioma surgery, with previously reported postoperative incidence rates ranging from 70% to 93% [22, 71, 125]. The postoperative diabetes insipidus course may be transient, permanent, or triphasic. It is transient if vasopressinergic neurons regeneration occurs or permanent in the case that most of the neurons in the supraoptic and paraventricular nuclei, or their relationship to the neuro-hypophysis, are damaged or lost. A classic triphasic response was reported while was not common in clinical practice [88]. DDAVP should be administered to reduce the urine volume to 3000–4000 ml/day; however, excessive urine volume control is unwise, as it can cause serious hyponatremia. The most important treatment for diabetes insipidus is maintenance of a balance between fluid intake and loss. Occasionally, and especially in pediatric patients, a slightly higher serum sodium concentration (145–150 mmol/L) may be beneficial [143, 164].

Sudden Disturbance in Consciousness

When patients with craniopharyngioma present with a sudden disturbance in consciousness, a CT scan should be performed to exclude intracranial hematoma or hydrocephalus. Many other factors can result in a disturbance in consciousness disturbance, including an electrolyte disturbance (hyponatremia), acid-base disturbance, serious intracranial infection, and adrenocortical insufficiency [30, 62, 71, 85, 120, 142, 194, 207, 208]. The latter may be observed with dosage reductions or an emerging stress state. Methylprednisolone pulse therapy is particularly effective in this situation.

Other Complications

Other complications include upper gastrointestinal hemorrhage, hyperpyrexia, and infection. Upper gastrointestinal hemorrhage is rare, given the broad use of proton-pump inhibitors (PPI). Hyperpyrexia is caused by abnormal hypothalamus regulation, and physical cooling is the main treatment measure. Occasionally corticosteroids can be administered for a persistent high fever. Intracranial and urinary tract infections are the most common infections in postoperative patients with craniopharyngioma. The drainage tube should not be retained for more than 72 hours, and lumbar puncture should be performed soon after removing the drainage tube. Continuous lumbar cistern drainage, with or without intrathecal antibiotic injection, is effective for most intracranial infection cases; however, cases involving unusual infections such as multi-drug-resistant *Acinetobacter baumannii* always have poor outcomes [102].

Radical surgery is the sole curative measure for patients with craniopharyngioma; however, this procedure carries increased complications and a higher risk. Management during the perioperative period is very important for patients undergoing surgery. Even a perfect operation will precede a poor outcome if good management is not provided during the perioperative period.

SURGICAL TREATMENT FOR CRANIOPHARYNGIOMA

The optimal treatment for craniopharyngioma remains controversial and under debate. It is difficult to find an balance between aggressive therapy and increased complications in both children and adults. At any age, radical resection is usually performed as the primary treatment for craniopharyngioma [1, 42, 68, 78, 90, 92, 106, 107, 111, 116, 119, 133, 139, 147, 149, 155, 171, 182, 184, 185, 207]. The best outcomes can be achieved through radical resection. Nevertheless, the tumor type basing the location, size, and calcifications, frequent involvement of critical neurovascular structures, patient's age at presentation, and the surgeon's experience usually limit resection extent . The risk of significant morbidity in visual, hypothalamic functions, and endocrinological disturbances could be followed by radical resection, which lead to a poor life quality. Moreover, craniopharyngioma can also recur following total resection, despite confirmation *via* negative post-operative brain imaging. For these reasons, many authors prefer a less radical surgical treatment followed by radiation therapy. This section mainly discusses the various surgical modalities for craniopharyngiomas with respect to tumor control rates.

There are two main surgical modalities for craniopharyngiomas: the transcranial and transsphenoidal approaches. For various reasons, the former is more widely applied [43, 54, 99, 129, 196]: first, most craniopharyngiomas are of suprasellar origin and rarely exhibit intrasellar invasion, thus restricting the application of a transsphenoidal approach. Second, a suitable transcranial approach can provide a wide view of the tumor, especially in some critical areas such as the pituitary stalk (PS), optical nerve, anterior cerebral artery (ACA), and the third ventricular floor. Third, only some tumors of entirely intrasellar origin, known as the inferior-diaphragm sellar type, may be completely resected *via* a transsphenoidal approach [1, 54, 94, 130, 200, 205].

Transcranial Approach

The selection and indication of a transcranial approach, such as the fronto-temporal, inter-hemispheric, or subfrontal approach, is beyond the scope of this chapter. The gross-total resection (GTR) and subtotal resection (STR), with or without adjuvant radiotherapy (RT), are the two types of resection currently offered according to the degree of resection. GTR provides improved tumor control when compared with STR alone, whereas adjuvant radiotherapy after STR can provide tumor control rates that are essentially similar to those achieved with GTR during a limited follow-up period [75, 156]. However, radiation-induced hypothalamic pituitary axis dysfunction may occur in up to 80% of patients in a long-term follow-up and is often associated with adverse impacts on growth, skeletal health, fertility, sexual function, and physical and psychological health [46, 75, 114, 117, 138]. Moreover, the residual tumor after adjuvant radiotherapy can induce a recurrence that is more difficult to treat than the primary tumor [36, 132].

Radical surgery has been proposed as curative for selected tumors. The extent of resection depends on many factors, including the tumor classification, hypo-thalamic involvement, presence of hydrocephalus, calcifications, and repeat surgery. The surgeon's experience and attitude also play important roles. GTR is confirmed *via* postoperative brain image in most studies because the neurosurgeon's assessment may not always be accurate during the operative procedure. Indeed, 18–26% of cases were still found remnants in postoperative imaging in in which complete resection was considered by the surgeon [55]. 10-year recurrence rates was from 0% to 62% in those series with radiological confirmation of GTR (Table **1**). These rates are significantly lower than those associated with STR (25–100% at a 10-year follow-up) [75, 156].

Why do the recurrence rates remain high despite radiological confirmation of a GTR? Although craniopharyngioma is histopathologically benign, it can adhere to neighboring tissues such as the hypothalamus *via* inflammatory reactions or other mechanisms [165], thus leading to an unclear resection during surgery.

Table 1. A. Overview of selected craniopharyngioma surgical results from the medical literature.

Publication	Years	Number of cases	GTR (%)	Early mortality (%)	Mean follow-up (months)	Recurrence (%)
Baskin	1986	73	9.5	3	48	14
Yasargil	1990	144	90	9	NA	7
Symon	1991	50	60	4	30	10
Maira	1995	57	75	0	78	0
Fahlbusch	1999	168	49	0.7	65	11
Van Effenterre	2002	122	59	2.5	84	13
Chakrabarti	2005	86	84	0	>60	7
Di Rocco	2006	54	78	3.7	104	7
Shi	2008	306	89.3	3.9	25	17
Gardner	2008	16	60	0	34	NA
Yamada	2010	90	90	2.2	55	7.8
Kim	2011	18	76	0	67.6	5.9
Elliott	2011	2955	60.9	2.6	70	4
Hofmann	2012	73	83.1	0	25.2	17.6

The residual tumor cells in these tissues serve as the origin of recurrence. The other reason for recurrence after radiological confirmation of resection radicality is that most cases are not resected en bloc but rather in a piecemeal manner. Here, we emphasis the use of en bloc resection because, as we know, most cranio-pharyngiomas are cystic with a thin capsule wall. This capsule wall can be easily retained after a piecemeal resection. En bloc resection means that after releasing the cystic fluid, the surgeon carefully dissects the capsule wall from the surrounding tissues. For tumors that have adhered tightly to other tissues, the surgeon should identify another dissecting direction and repeat the above-described steps. Tightly adherent tumor tissue should be resected sharply at the end of surgery (Fig. **1**). The most common place for tightly adherent is PS and the front of the third ventricle floor (3rd VF).

Transsphenoidal Approach

The transsphenoidal approach has been adopted for pituitary adenomas for a long time. However, this approach for supradiaphragmatic has been reported only since the 1980s; this approach was originally described by Weiss as an "extended transsphenoidal approach" [67]. The use of this route allowed the removal of suprasellar lesions involving the 3rd VF, such as craniopharyngiomas, while avoiding the manipulation and/or retraction of any neurovascular structures. Nevertheless, the narrow view and higher rate of CSF leakage limit the widespread application of this technique. The transsphenoidal approach is more difficult in a an enlarged pituitary fossa. Recently, the introduction of the endoscope to this approach awakened renewed interest in this technique [25, 54, 66, 93, 94, 122, 130, 201, 205].

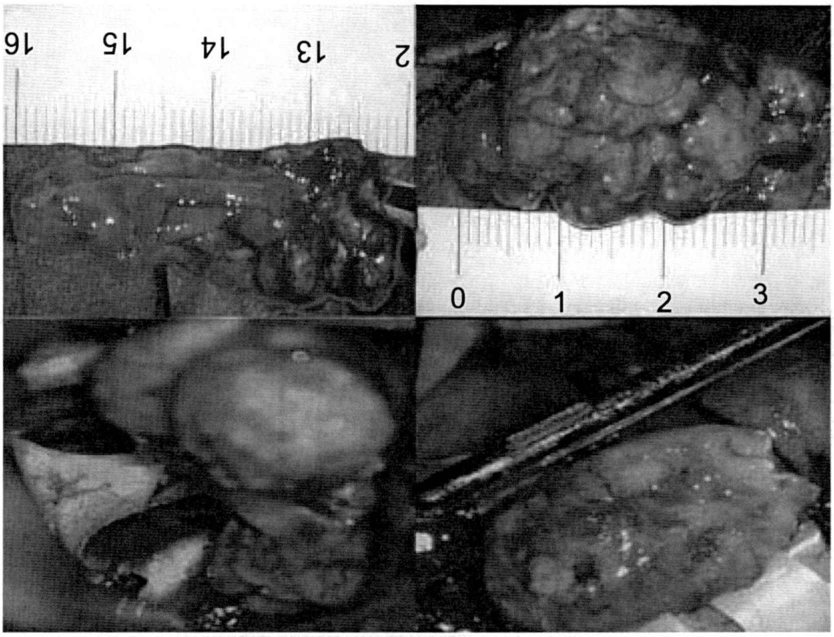

Fig. (1). En bloc resection of craniopharyngiomas.

The endoscopic approach owns the advantages including a direct view of the relevant anatomy and an enlarged working angle for the suprasellar territories as well as the third ventricle. The endoscopic endonasal approach permits visualization of the inferior portion of both the extra- and intraventricular aspects of the third ventricle, which is superior to visualization provided by the conventional transcranial approach.

However, there are some disadvantages of this approach [54]. The first is CSF leakage, which may required a second cranial base repair. Second, the opening of the ventricular cavity creates a direct communication with the sphenoid sinus, which may cause a serious intracranial infection such as ventriculitis[102], for which the mortality rate is as high as 80–100%. Third, arachnoid dissection in the subchiasmatic area could bilaterally disrupt Liliequist's membrane, causing the flow of a large amount of CSF from the basal cisterns and possibly inducing a subdural hematoma. Fourth, given the limited surgery field and instrument restriction, en bloc resection is very difficult. Fifth, many craniopharyngiomas affect the 3rd VF without truly invading the ventricular cavity; in other words, the 3rd VF is pushed upward by the tumor. In such cases, the tumor will be exposed earlier and the 3rd VF obstructed from view by the tumor through a transsphenoidal approach. Unless the tumor is partly resected, the 3rd VF cannot be exposed. During tumor resection, the 3rd VF may be disturbed, and arterial perforating feeders from the internal carotid artery (ICA), medial choroidal artery, posterior communicating arteries, and posterior cerebral arteries may be damaged.

Prognostic Factors for Tumor Recurrence

Craniopharyngiomas are more likely to recur during the first 3 years after primary resection, after which the recurrence incidence plateaus [18, 127, 142, 198]. The presence of tumor remnants after surgery was the strongest predictor of tumor recurrence [42]. The 5-year RFS in patients without residual tumor was 84.9%, *versus* 48.3% in patients with residual tumor [23]. Age was usually not a predictor for recurrence while in those patents less than 5 years old age may become a predictor [202]. Gender was not a predictor for worse prognosis.However,large calcified lesions have been associated with an increased risk of recurrence. 3rd VF involvement is another risk factor for recurrence. Whether the pathological subtype was a predictor of prognosis was remain unknown,future work should include more cases for a longer term follow up [158].

Long-term Outcomes of Craniopharyngioma After Resection

During recent follow-ups, the overall survival rates associated with adult craniopharyngioma in recent years have ranged 89-94% at 5 years and 85%-90% at 10 years [60]. The 5- and 10-year OS rates associated with childhood craniopharyngiomas are 88–94% and 70–92%, respectively, with a 20-year survival rate of 76% [143].

Pereira *et al.* [160] and Karavitaki *et al.* [104] recorded respective visual morbidity rates of 40% and 48% of patients with craniopharyngioma who were treated *via* surgery alone or with chemoradiotherapy (CRT) after 10 years of follow-up. Duff *et al.* [52] recorded outcomes of at least quadrantanopia in 63% of patients treated with surgery alone or combined with CRT and followed up for 10 years. Visual outcomes are adversely affected by the presence and duration of visual symptoms at diagnosis, tumor localization in the prechiasmatic area, and a radiation dose of 2 Gy/day.

The reported rates of post-surgical pituitary hormone deficiencies have increased to 80–100% [84, 87, 103, 166]. In a recent study, the long-term prevalence rate of total anterior pituitary insufficiency was 89%, and the rates for GH-, gonadotropin-, ACTH-, and TSH-deficiency were 91%, 93.5%, 92%, and 86%, respectively [87]. GH deficiency following treatment is observed in approximately 70–92% of patients treated for pediatric craniopharyngioma [77]. Transient postoperative diabetes insipidus has been reported in nearly all patients in some series. The incidence of permanent postoperative diabetes insipidus was found to range from 40% to 93% [17, 40, 87, 151].

Symptoms attributed to hypothalamic dysfunction, including obesity, fatigue, abnormal behavior, sleep irregularities, and thirst regulation imbalances are common during long-term follow-ups. Hypothalamic obesity are the most common complications consequent to hypothalamic damage in pediatric patients with craniopharyngioma. Obesity was found in the first 6–12 months after treatment [39, 79, 136, 143, 153].

In children, the quality of life may be severely affected both directly by the craniopharyngioma and by the treatment received. It was reported that up to 50% of patients experience psychosocial impairment and up to 1/4 patients are not able to work in their previous occupations or fall behind in school [143]. Duff *et al.* [52] reported 40% of cases suffer an impaired life quality after surgery during a 10-year follow-up study. Van Effenterre and colleagues [191] reported that 16% of the adults and 26% of the children did not achieve an independent living status and exhibited unfavorable social integration and work or school performances after a mean observation period of 7 years. In another surgical series,at a 10-year follow-up the cumulative probability of permanent motor deficits was 11%; that of epilepsy, 12%; of psychological disorders requiring treatment, 15%; and of total dependency for daily activities, 9% [157]. Pereira *et al.* [160] found that 47% of patients exhibited long-term psychosocial impairment such as compromised independent living, social integration, professional occupation, and school performance, whereas 49% experienced neurological morbidity.

The best treatment strategy would be tailored to the individual patient and based upon the imaging appearance of the tumor, general clinical condition of the patient, and experience of the treatment team; additionally, and mostly in pediatric cases, the reliability of and resources available to the family and community to provide for needed assistance are also factors. We cannot absolutely apply a specific approach to each case. One issue that we should remember at least is that at any age, radical resection is usually considered the primary treatment of choice for craniopharyngioma.

RADIOTHERAPY FOR CRANIOPHARYNGIOMA

Radiotherapy has been and remains important to craniopharyngioma management. The aim of radiotherapy is to achieve long-term disease control in patients lacking complete removal or with recurrent tumors. Many studies have reported increased morbidity and mortality following radical surgery *versus* conservative surgery [1, 20, 42, 63, 68, 78, 90, 92, 106, 107, 111, 116, 119, 133, 139, 147, 149, 155, 171, 182 - 185, 207]. Patients with residual tumors may avoid or delay needed repeat surgery after radiotherapy, and repeat surgery for craniopharyngiomas has been associated with additional morbidity and mortality [4, 8, 24, 33, 38, 53, 55, 56]. This section reviews the current evidence advocating the use of radiotherapy, particularly in light of technical advances in radiotherapy delivery.

External Beam Irradiation

External beam irradiation is the most common radiotherapeutic approach used in neurosurgery. A number of studies have reported the efficiency of fractionated radiotherapy for craniopharyngioma management [5, 6, 28, 48, 50, 61, 65, 74, 75, 110, 167, 170, 177, 180, 192, 195, 202]. The 10-year recurrence rates after external beam irradiation without surgery range from 0% to 23%. Recurrence-free survival at a 10-years follow-up improved to an average of 80% in patients who underwent STR plus external beam irradiation [159]. In 2002, Varlotto reported a study of 24 patients with craniopharyngioma who had undergone radiotherapy [192]. In that study, the control rates at 10 and 20 years were 89% and 54%, respectively.

For fractionated radiotherapy, the optimal total radiation dose for cranio-pharyngioma is between 50 and 65 Gy [65, 159, 176, 192]. Fractionation into daily doses of 180–200 cGy permits the administration of a larger total radiation dose and is better tolerated by the brain, thus sparing normal tissues within the radiation field [159]. Smaller daily fractions and a larger radiation field may enhance the protective effects on the brain and normal tissues. Complications have been reported in many papers and include radionecrosis, optic neuritis, dementia, hypothalamic-pituitary dysfunction, radiation-induced tumors and decreased IQ [5, 6, 11, 12, 19, 26, 28, 32, 50, 51, 70, 80, 123, 128, 174, 179].

Stereotactic Radiotherapy

Stereotactic radiotherapy, or three-dimensional (3D) conformal external beam radiotherapy, has undergone considerable development in the last 10 years [83, 101, 135]. Currently, stereotactic radiotherapy is a standard treatment for most intracranial lesions, including craniopharyngioma. As both deliver radiation *via* photons with a linear accelerator, the greatest difference between stereotactic radiotherapy and two-dimensional external beam irradiation is use of a radiation field that conforms to the tumor shape. The radiation field requires precise immobilization, accurate tumor localization with the best available imaging, and computerized 3D treatment planning. Radiation field planning requires both high-quality enhanced MRI images and co-registered CT images. The extent of visible residual craniopharyngioma in the images and the presumed microscopic tumor cell extension are delineated to define the gross tumor volume (GTV). The GTV is manually contoured on fused MRI images. However, the target localization, computer planning, and treatment delivery remain somewhat uncertain, and therefore, an additional 3–5 mm 3D margin is usually added to cover the entire lesion; this new volume is defined as the planning target volume (PTV). Different departments set their own additional margin specifications based on departmental measurements. The highest radiation dose is applied to the PTV. Computer planning defines the beam positions to achieve dose homogeneity within the PTV and allows the optimum avoidance of surrounding critical normal structures. These structures, which include the eyes, optic nerves, optic chiasm, and hypothalamus, are also outlined. Patients are treated in a supine position using a Gill–Thomas–Cosman frame (a specially designed and more suitable frame is provided for pediatric patients). A general anesthetic is administered to patients, particularly pediatric patients, who cannot tolerate the frame. Patients subjected to anesthesia should be immobilized using proper equipment to prevent displacement. High-resolution planning CT images (2–3-mm and 5-mm slice thickness and separation throughout and beyond the target area, respectively) are fused with a MRI scan.

The advantage of stereotactic radiotherapy is that it is suitable for lesions >3 cm or those adjacent to important neural structures. One study of 14 children with recurrent craniopharyngioma reported that stereotactic radiotherapy could yield 5-, 10-, and 15-year relapse-free survival rates of 100%, 83%, and 83%, respectively, *versus* 67%, 0%, and 0%, respectively, with surgery alone. The use of the GTV plus an additional margin to generate the PTV possible, along with high-precision stereotactic techniques, reduces the normal brain volume subjected to high radiation doses, and this technique can achieve good tumor control and low toxicity levels similar to those observed following standard-dose conventional radiotherapy.

Proton Beam Therapy

Protons can provide the same biological effects as photons, and therefore these therapies are similar in theory. The greatest advantage of proton beam therapy is the deposition of energy within a defined area, with little radiation escaping to areas beyond.

Compared with the best photon radiotherapy, reductions in whole brain volume have been detected after a dosimetric evaluation of 3D conformal proton therapy in pediatric patients with craniopharyngioma; however, an improved target dose distribution has not been found [12, 16, 76, 118, 121, 137, 197]. Early small-cohort studies have reported that proton therapy can achieve similar results as fractionated external beam irradiation and stereotactic radiotherapy, with 5-year progression-free survival rates exceeding 90% [118, 197]. However, despite administering lower doses to normal tissues beyond the irradiated target, potential advantages such as lower toxicity have not yet been reported. The potential advantage that proton beam therapy provides lower irradiation to normal tissues in young children with craniopharyngiomas may be considered important after a longer follow-up.

Internal Irradiation (Brachytherapy)

One characteristic of craniopharyngiomas is the presence of single or multiple cysts that can account for 80–90% of the total tumor bulk and serve as the anatomical basement of internal craniopharyngiomal irradiation [82]. Internal irradiation was first reported in 1952 by Leksell and Linden. The irradiation, which is mainly produced *via* β-or λ-emission, has a short range of tissue penetrance and even dose distribution, thus supporting its wide clinical application for the treatment of craniopharyngiomas, especially in children. Many β- and λ-emitting isotopes have been used, including yttrium-90, phosphorous-32, rhenium-186, and gold-198, the first of which is most common. Theoretically, internal irradiation may provide higher radiation doses to the cyst lining than external beam radiotherapy, the latter of which is more likely to damage secretory epithelial cells, leading to the elimination of fluid production and, eventually, cyst involution. A frame-based stereotactic needle insertion is used to deliver these isotopes into the cystic cavity [13, 131, 135, 150, 154, 173, 187, 204]; this procedure can also be performed through an Ommaya reservoir after extracting cystic fluid [82, 89, 96, 109, 161, 172, 206]. Both ways have their own characteristics. The former provides the opportunity to target multicystic lesions in a single session, whereas the latter provides repeated access and decompression in monocystic tumors. The target radiation dose to the cyst wall is approximately 200–250 Gy. In a meta-analysis of four studies, Karavitaki and Wass demonstrated complete or partial cyst involution in 71–88% of cases treated with radiation doses of 200–267 Gy during follow-up periods of 3.1–11.9 years [105]. The stabilization and progression rates ranged from 3% to 19% and 5% to 10%, respectively. New cyst formation or an increase in the solid component was observed in 6.5–20% of these cases. Surprisingly, the overall recurrence and survival rates achieved with brachytherapy cannot be compared to those achieved with external beam radiotherapy [127]. There are some disadvantages associated with internal irradiation. As it is difficult to measure the tumor capsule thickness using MRI or other imaging modalities, the radiation doses to adjacent normal tissues such as the visual pathway are unpredictable. The rate of visual impairment or blindness after internal irradiation may be as high as 30% [97].

Stereotactic Radiosurgery

Stereotactic radiosurgery (SRS) delivers multiple convergent ionizing radiation beams that intersect at the target lesion. The surrounding normal tissue is well protected because of the sharp dose fall-off beyond the target area. SRS can be performed with a Gamma Knife or linear accelerator, which is also called an X-ray Knife [95, 108, 114, 175, 199]. The obvious limitations of SRS include the fact that lesions larger than 3 cm or in close proximity to the optic chiasm are not indicated. As mentioned above, SRS is consequently a therapeutic option for small residual or recurrent craniopharyngiomas. According to several studies, the outcome of residual or recurrent craniopharyngioma after SRS is inferior to that after conventional fractionated external beam radiotherapy. In a study of 164 patients, a reduction in tumor size was observed in 58–79% after treatment with radiation doses ranging between 8 and 20 Gy, with a mean tumor margin dose of 10 Gy [112]. To date, the largest series includes 98 consecutive patients [113].In that study, SRS planning indicated tumor treatment with a maximal dose of 21.8 Gy and a tumor margin dose of 11.5 Gy, using a mean 4.5 isocenters. The 5- and 10-year progression-free survival rates were 60.8% and 53.8%, with overall 5- and 10-year survival rates of exceeding 90% (94.1 and 91%, respectively). Reported complications after SRS included both vision and endocrinological function deterioration in 6.1% of the sample. Other studies involving smaller numbers of cases have reported similar results and complications [34, 35, 73, 95, 108, 112 - 115, 123, 141, 175, 190, 203].

The optic chiasm can only tolerate radiation doses of 8–10 Gy, and the associated 25% optic neuropathy incidence is attributed to single radiation doses above 8–10 Gy; this limits the application of this technique to lesions far from the optic chiasm and is the main reason for unsatisfactory tumor control rates [123]. Some studies in which smaller lesions were treated with SRS reported minimal morbidity and a visual impairment rate of 3%. The limitation may directly restrict the application of SRS to small lesions, and some authors have reported worse outcomes with SRS than with other radiotherapies when comparing tumor control rates [10].

Radiation-induced Disturbances in Hypothalamic Pituitary Function

The nature of radiation-induced damage to the hypothalamic pituitary axis is not fully understood. Direct neuronal damage caused by ionizing radiation followed by degeneration and death is the current preferred theory. Radiation-induced h–p dysfunction may occur in about 80% of patients subjected to long-term follow-up and is associated with unfavourable effects on growth, skeletal health, fertility, sexual function, and physical and psychological health [41, 193]. Moreover, stereotacticradiotherapy for pituitary tumors does not appear to reduce the long-term risk of hypopituitarism.

CHEMOTHERAPY FOR CRANIOPHARYNGIOMA

Craniopharyngioma management is complex. Both radical surgery and radiotherapy can result in behavioral, cognitive, endocrine, hypothalamic, and visual dysfunction. This has led to the exploration of local intratumoral chemotherapy for craniopharyngioma management. Initially, this approach was used to treat difficult, recurrent cystic tumors but has subsequently been employed as a strategy to avoid late-term effects of surgery or radiotherapy. Systemic chemotherapy has rarely been reported in terms of craniopharyngioma management.

Intracavitary Chemotherapy

Bleomycin is the most frequently used intracavitary chemotherapeutic agent for cystic craniopharyngioma. Bleomycin is a chemotherapeutic agent that targets epithelial tumors. As that craniopharyngiomas are thought to have an epithelial origin, bleomycin was initially tested against craniopharyngioma tissue cultures in 1974. Its use is indicated in selected cases of predominantly cystic craniopharyngiomas, especially cases of cystic recurrence and cases in young children, in whom radiotherapy is best delayed or avoided. Bleomycin is administered *via* a stereotactically positioned catheter connected to a subcutaneous Ommaya reservoir. Although experience with this approach is limited, the initial results are encouraging. In 1989, Broggi *et al.* reported the involution of craniopharyngioma cysts in 13 of 18 patients treated with stereotactic intracystic bleomycin instillation. During a follow-up period ranging from 3 to 12 years, decreases in the cystic tumor size of at least 50% were observed in 64–86% of treated children. In a study of 24 patients with craniopharyngioma who were treated with intracystic bleomycin, Mottolese and colleagues observed complete tumor resolution in nine patients and decreases in cyst sizes of 50–70% in 15. No recurrences occurred during a median follow-up of 5 years. In 1996, Cavalheiro observed the regression of calcification after bleomycin treatment. More recent experiences with longer follow-up periods have shown that although the initial response rate is high, the regression-free survival rate is poor. Bleomycin therapy is further associated with serious complications related to its toxicity; these include hypothalamic damage following instillation after STR, ischemic attacks, peritumoral edema, cranial nerve palsies, and blindness and death related to leakage into the CSF space.

As an alternative to bleomycin, intracystic interferon (IFN) can also be administered to patients with cystic craniopharyngiomas. The mechanism of action remained unknown, some studies have suggested that IFNs exert antitumoral activity through their anti-proliferative, cytotoxic, and maturational effects, while simultaneously modulating the patient's immune response.

IFNs are glycoprotein members of the cytokine family and are related to transforming growth factor-beta and tumor necrosis factor, which are responsible for regulating cell differentiation and proliferation. The efficacy of IFN-α has been well established with respect to its activity against squamous cell carcinoma of the skin, in which it induces apoptosis. Ikiċ *et al.* were the first to apply IFN-α intratumorally to treat squamous cell carcinoma and demonstrated the reduction and even disappearance of this tumor type. Jakacki *et al.* first used systemic IFN-α to treat recurring craniopharyngiomas and those refractory to conventional treatment. Given that craniopharyngiomas and squamous cell carcinomas have the same embryological origin and that squamous epithelium is found in both the cyst wall and solid component of craniopharyngiomas, a phase II study was conducted with a group of 15 patients aged 4.2–19.8 years of age. Three patients who demon-strated a complete response (defined as the complete radiological disappearance of the tumor) had predominantly cystic tumors. In the study, all patients experienced febrile episodes during the first weeks of treatment, along with muscle cramps and myalgia. Seven patients developed important signs and symptoms of IFN-α toxicity, leading to either treatment interruption or a reduction in administered doses. In 2002, Chamberlain was the first to use an intra-ventricular application of IFN-α to treat neoplastic meningitis. The manifestations of neurotoxicity (described mainly as chronic fatigue syndrome) were easily treated and did not impede the continuation of treatment.

Cavalheiro *et al.* first inserted a catheter into a tumor cyst and then attached this catheter to a subgaleal reservoir to withdraw the cyst fluid; 5 days later, the catheter was used to inject 3 MIU of IFN into the cyst. This process was repeated on alternate days for a total of 12 injections. A second cycle of IFN was possibly indicated after 30 days if no response was radiologically evident. Of the 21 children treated in that study, all of whom had tumors with more than 60% cystic matter, 11 complete responses (>90% reduction), seven partial responses (>70% reduction), and three minor responses were achieved (<70% reduction). Two patients experienced tumor progression and underwent resection. In an empirical study by Dastoli et al., 3,000,000 MIU of IFN-α were administered to the cyst interior thrice weekly for 4 weeks. All patients (100%) experienced significant reductions in tumor volume at the end of treatment. The mean initial volume was 33.50 cm^3, and the mean final volume was 3.10 cm^3. The reduction in tumor volume exceeded 90% in 11 patients (57.89%) and ranged from 81% to 87% in five patients (26.31%); only three patients (15.78%) had lesser reductions in tumor volume, with reduction rates of 60%, 70%, and 72%.

The treatment complications included fatigue, weight loss, anorexia, and behavioral changes. Few patients required treatment interruption, and no hormonal deficits were added to the preexisting deficits. Patients with craniopharyngioma live with a chronic disease and are subject to periods of intensified symptoms or deterioration that can be treated *via* the intratumoral application of IFN-α. Provided that these patients experience improved vision, recover normal hormone levels and growth patterns, attend school, and exhibit adequate cognitive performance and neuropsychomotor development with little or no impairment of the quality of life during this important life stage, the application of additional chemotherapy cycles is considered less aggressive than additional surgical interventions or radiotherapy sessions. However, as this treatment modality is new, a longer follow-up is needed to assess its effectiveness for long-term craniopharyngioma control.

The practicalities of therapy involve the safe insertion of a catheter into the cyst. Although a variety of surgical techniques have been used for catheter placement, a stereotactic approach is generally advocated. Complications can occur because of the cyst wall thickness: too thin, and the cyst wall can tear and allow backflow of the sclerosant bleomycin; too thick, and stereotactic puncture can be difficult. Catheter design should be considered, as bleomycin leakage has been associated with severe adverse effects, including death. A reduction in cyst volume can cause the catheter to become dislodged, and the absence of easy cyst fluid withdrawal should indicate a need for further imaging to demonstrate water-tightness.

Systemic Chemotherapy

Systemic chemotherapy has been used in a limited number of patients, and its value remains to be established. Only four papers have described the use of systemic chemotherapy for craniopharyngioma. Several cases of recurrent tumors were reported to respond to conventional chemotherapy. In one paper, a patient who had refused surgery and radiotherapy upon relapse was treated with eight courses of vincristine, carmustine, and procarbazine administered at 6-week intervals. The patient experienced an unequivocal neurological improvement and a reduction in cyst size as determined by serial CT scans. The toxicity was mild and chiefly hematological.

In another paper, four children with multiple recurrent tumors were treated with chemotherapy, as surgery and radiotherapy were restricted because of prior administration. The regimen consisted of five intravenous ambulatory courses of adriamycin (doxorubicin) plus oral lomustine at 6-week intervals. After completing chemotherapy, the patients experienced no further tumor recurrences after 12, 10, 3, and 3 years. The third patient experienced a cystic relapse after a 3-year remission. In the fourth patient, a complete regression of the cystic part of the tumor was observed. The chemotherapy side effects comprised alopecia and bone marrow depression. Another report documents the case of a 21-year-old woman who developed a malignant tumor that arose from a craniopharyngioma at 14 years after the original diagnosis. This tumor responded remarkably to cisplatin-based chemotherapy, although doubts concerning the tumor histology should be addressed.

The largest drug-treated cohort was used to investigate IFN-α, as squamous cell carcinoma was reported to respond to this agent. Fifteen patients with progressive or recurrent craniopharyngiomas and ages ranging from 4 to 19 years were treated daily with 8 MIU of IFN-α/m^2 for 16 weeks (induction phase), followed by the same dose thrice weekly for an additional 32 weeks. Of the 12 patients who were evaluated through radiological studies, three with predominantly cystic tumors demonstrated responses to treatment; one of these patients also exhibited visual field improvements. The cystic size often increased temporarily during the first several months of therapy. Three patients were found tumor progressive during therapy. The median time to progression was 25 months. Among the IFN-treated patients, in six patients the need for radiation therapy was delayed for 18– 35 months (median, 25 months).

Recent studies showed that nearly all papillary craniopharyngiomas harbor BRAFV600E mutation, and the incidence range is from 81% to 100% in different institutions. Considering the homogeneity of the benign tumor, BRAFV600E mutation gives a great perspective in both diagnosis and treatment. It was reported that pyrosequencing and VE1 stain, a immunohistochemical marker of BRAFV600E, in removal tumor can be a reliable method to differential diagnosis of Rathke's cyst from papillary craniopharyngioma.

BRAFV600E mutation can led to the activate of MAPK pathway continuously and was considered to be key point in the tumorigenesis of papillary cranio-pharyngioma. It was also reported that BRAFV600E mutations are present in cutaneous melanoma, hairy-cell leukemia, thyroid carcinomas and, less commonly, in ovarian, colon, lung, and other malignancies. Fortunately, molecular targeted inhibitor drugs for BRAFV600E or MAPK pathway, such as Vemurafenib, Trametinib, Dabrafenib, were developed and an established treatment protocols has been used for melanoma and colorectal cancer with BRAFV600E mutation. There is a study reported a recrudescent papillary craniopharyngioma case with BRAFV600E mutation. After 3 months' treatment of Vemurafenib (960 mg, orally bid), the MRI showed a marked reduction in the size of the tumor but the regrowth of tumor showed up after drug withdrawal. Another study reported a multiply recurrent papillary cranio-pharyngioma case with confirmed BRAFV600E mutation by whole exome sequencing on the pre- and post-treatment resection samples and peripheral blood, showed significant reduction of tumor volume by the treatment of RAF inhibitor dabrafenib (150 mg, orally bid) and MEK inhibitor trametinib (2 mg, orally bid). Endoscopic transsphenoidal surgery for consolidation tumor resection in the day 38 from the beginning of molecular targeting treatment was preformed and radiation treatment (50.4 Gy in 28 fractions) was followed 3 weeks later. The patient didn't show new symptom 7 month later after comprehensive treatment. It seems that targeted drugs are effective in treatment of papillary cranio-pharyngioma, however, severe inflammatory response caused by drugs creates potential obstacle for operation procedure, therefore, clinic trial is needed to evaluate security and effectiveness of the target therapy.

Although craniopharyngioma is a benign tumor and is potentially curable by surgery alone, its management remains difficult and controversial. Many survivors suffer from behavioral, cognitive, endocrine, hypothalamic, and visual disturbances. Late deaths from endocrine complications reduce overall survival even in apparently cured patients. Both surgery and radiotherapy have been implicated in the etiologies of cognitive, endocrine, and hypothalamic damage, and the roles of both therapies should be balanced according to factors such as the patient's age, the tumor size and location, and prior treatment. Chemotherapy has become an important component of management in children with central nervous system tumors and has allowed the avoidance, delay, or reduction of damaging surgery or radiotherapy.

CONFLICT OF INTEREST

The author (editor) declares no conflict of interest, financial or otherwise.

ACKNOWLEDGEMENT

We should acknowledge Dr. Wang Chao-hu and Zhang Shi-chao for the assistant of article organization and literature reviewing.

REFERENCES

[1] Transsphenoidal surgery of craniopharyngioma: form palliative surgery to radical removal. Zh Vopr Neirokhir Im N N Burdenko 2013; 77: 3-12.

[2] Abrams LS, Repka MX. Visual outcome of craniopharyngioma in children. J Pediatr Ophthalmol Strabismus 1997; 34(4): 223-8.
[PMID: 9253736]

[3] Aggarwal A, Fersht N, Brada M. Radiotherapy for craniopharyngioma. Pituitary 2013; 16(1): 26-33.
[http://dx.doi.org/10.1007/s11102-012-0429-1] [PMID: 22948229]

[4] Alen JF, Boto GR, Lagares A, de la Lama A, Gomez PA, Lobato RD. Intratumoural bleomycin as a treatment for recurrent cystic craniopharyngioma. Case report and review of the literature Neurocirugia (Astur) 2002; 13: 479-85.

[5] Amacher AL. Craniopharyngioma: the controversy regarding radiotherapy. Childs Brain 1980; 6(2): 57-64.
[PMID: 7353444]

[6] Backlund EO. Treatment of craniopharyngiomas: the multimodality approach. Pediatr Neurosurg 1994; 21 (Suppl. 1): 82-9.
[http://dx.doi.org/10.1159/000120867] [PMID: 7841083]

[7] Bajwa SJ, Bajwa SK, Bindra GS. The anesthetic, critical care and surgical challenges in the management of craniopharyngioma. Indian J Endocrinol Metab 2011; 15(2): 123-6.
[http://dx.doi.org/10.4103/2230-8210.81944] [PMID: 21731872]

[8] Barua KK, Ehara K, Kohmura E, Tamaki N. Treatment of recurrent craniopharyngiomas. Kobe J Med Sci 2003; 49(5-6): 123-32.
[PMID: 15141142]

[9] Becker G, Kortmann RD, Skalej M, Bamberg M. The role of radiotherapy in the treatment of craniopharyngioma--indications, results, side effects. Front Radiat Ther Oncol 1999; 33: 100-13.
[http://dx.doi.org/10.1159/000061227] [PMID: 10549481]

[10] Belen D, Er U, Yigitkanli K, Bolay H. Delayed neurotoxic complication of intracavitary bleomycin therapy for craniopharyngioma in a child who had previously undergone radiosurgery. Case report. J Neurosurg 2007; 106(5) (Suppl.): 391-3.
[PMID: 17566208]

[11] Beltran C, Naik M, Merchant TE. Dosimetric effect of target expansion and setup uncertainty during radiation therapy in pediatric craniopharyngioma. Radiother Oncol 2010; 97(3): 399-403.
[http://dx.doi.org/10.1016/j.radonc.2010.10.017] [PMID: 21074883]

[12] Beltran C, Roca M, Merchant TE. On the benefits and risks of proton therapy in pediatric craniopharyngioma. Int J Radiat Oncol Biol Phys 2012; 82(2): e281-7.
[http://dx.doi.org/10.1016/j.ijrobp.2011.01.005] [PMID: 21570209]

[13] Blackburn TP, Doughty D, Plowman PN. Stereotactic intracavitary therapy of recurrent cystic craniopharyngioma by instillation of 90yttrium. Br J Neurosurg 1999; 13(4): 359-65.

[http://dx.doi.org/10.1080/02688699943457] [PMID: 10616561]

[14] Bladowska J, Zimny A, Guziński M, *et al.* Usefulness of perfusion weighted magnetic resonance imaging with signal-intensity curves analysis in the differential diagnosis of sellar and parasellar tumors: preliminary report. Eur J Radiol 2013; 82(8): 1292-8. [http://dx.doi.org/10.1016/j.ejrad.2013.01.033] [PMID: 23466030]

[15] Blethen SL, Weldon VV. Outcome in children with normal growth following removal of a craniopharyngioma. Am J Med Sci 1986; 292(1): 21-4. [http://dx.doi.org/10.1097/00000441-198607000-00004] [PMID: 3717202]

[16] Boehling NS, Grosshans DR, Bluett JB, *et al.* Dosimetric comparison of three-dimensional conformal proton radiotherapy, intensity-modulated proton therapy, and intensity-modulated radiotherapy for treatment of pediatric craniopharyngiomas. Int J Radiat Oncol Biol Phys 2012; 82(2): 643-52. [http://dx.doi.org/10.1016/j.ijrobp.2010.11.027] [PMID: 21277111]

[17] Bohn D, Davids MR, Friedman O, Halperin ML. Acute and fatal hyponatraemia after resection of a craniopharyngioma: a preventable tragedy. QJM 2005; 98(9): 691-703. [http://dx.doi.org/10.1093/qjmed/hci101] [PMID: 16055476]

[18] Bojanowski K, Marchel A. Long-term result of the surgical treatment of craniopharyngiomas Neurol Neurochir Pol 2006; 40: 478-83.

[19] Bonilha L, Borges G, Fernandes YB, Ramina R, Carelli EF, Alvarenga M. Pilocytic astrocytoma following radiotherapy for craniopharyngioma: case report. Arq Neuropsiquiatr 2000; 58(3A): 731-5. [http://dx.doi.org/10.1590/S0004-282X2000000400022] [PMID: 10973118]

[20] Bret P, Beziat JL. [Sphenoido-nasopharyngeal craniopharyngioma. A case with radical excision by Le Fort I-type maxillotomy]. Neurochirurgie 1993; 39(4): 235-40. [Sphenoido-nasopharyngeal craniopharyngioma. A case with radical excision by Le Fort I-type maxillotomy]. [PMID: 8208331]

[21] Brihaye J, Brihaye-van Geertruyden M. Management and surgical outcome of suprasellar meningiomas. Acta Neurochir Suppl (Wien) 1988; 42: 124-9. [PMID: 3189002]

[22] Bucci MN, Chin LS, Hoff JT. Perioperative morbidity associated with operative resection of craniopharyngioma: a review of ten years experience. Neurochirurgia (Stuttg) 1987; 30(5): 135-8. [PMID: 3683699]

[23] Buchfelder M, Schlaffer SM, Lin F, Kleindienst A. Surgery for craniopharyngioma. Pituitary 2013; 16(1): 18-25. [http://dx.doi.org/10.1007/s11102-012-0414-8] [PMID: 22836237]

[24] Caldarelli M, di Rocco C, Papacci F, Colosimo C Jr. Management of recurrent craniopharyngioma. Acta Neurochir (Wien) 1998; 140(5): 447-54. [http://dx.doi.org/10.1007/s007010050123] [PMID: 9728244]

[25] Cavallo LM, Prevedello D, Esposito F, Laws EJ, Dusick JR, Messina A, *et al.* The role of the endoscope in the transsphenoidal management of cystic lesions of the sellar region Neurosurg Rev 2008; 31: 55-64.

[26] Cavazzuti V, Fischer EG, Welch K, Belli JA, Winston KR. Neurological and psychophysiological sequelae following different treatments of craniopharyngioma in children. J Neurosurg 1983; 59(3): 409-17. [http://dx.doi.org/10.3171/jns.1983.59.3.0409] [PMID: 6886754]

[27] Chakrabarti I, Amar AP, Couldwell W, Weiss MH. Long-term neurological, visual, and endocrine outcomes following transnasal resection of craniopharyngioma. J Neurosurg 2005; 102(4): 650-7. [http://dx.doi.org/10.3171/jns.2005.102.4.0650] [PMID: 15871507]

[28] Chan M, Herrera SR, Neckrysh S, Wallace A, Valyi-Nagy T, Charbel FT. Primitive neuroectodermal tumor after radiation therapy for craniopharyngioma. Neurosurg Focus 2011; 30(1): E3.

[http://dx.doi.org/10.3171/2010.11.FOCUS10224] [PMID: 21194276]

[29] Chapman SJ, Neville BG, Schurr PH. Craniopharyngioma in childhood: the nature and management of early postoperative fluid and electrolyte disturbance. Dev Med Child Neurol 1978; 20(5): 598-604. [http://dx.doi.org/10.1111/j.1469-8749.1978.tb15278.x] [PMID: 729907]

[30] Chatzisotiriou AS, Selviaridis PK, Kontopoulos VA, Kontopoulos AV, Patsalas IA. Delayed persistent hyperthermia after resection of a craniopharyngioma. Pediatr Neurosurg 2004; 40(4): 196-202. [http://dx.doi.org/10.1159/000081939] [PMID: 15608494]

[31] Chen C, Okera S, Davies PE, Selva D, Crompton JL. Craniopharyngioma: a review of long-term visual outcome. Clin Experiment Ophthalmol 2003; 31(3): 220-8. [http://dx.doi.org/10.1046/j.1442-9071.2003.00648.x] [PMID: 12786772]

[32] Chin HW, Maruyama Y, Young B. The role of radiation treatment in craniopharyngioma. Strahlentherapie 1983; 159(12): 741-4. [PMID: 6665811]

[33] Chiou SM, Lunsford LD, Niranjan A, Kondziolka D, Flickinger JC. Stereotactic radiosurgery of residual or recurrent craniopharyngioma, after surgery, with or without radiation therapy. Neuro-oncol 2001; 3(3): 159-66. [PMID: 11465396]

[34] Chung WY, Pan DH, Shiau CY, Guo WY, Wang LW. Gamma knife radiosurgery for craniopharyngiomas. J Neurosurg 2000; 93 (Suppl. 3): 47-56. [PMID: 11143262]

[35] Chung WY, Pan HC, Guo WY, *et al.* Protection of visual pathway in gamma knife radiosurgery for craniopharyngiomas. Stereotact Funct Neurosurg 1998; 70 (Suppl. 1): 139-51. [http://dx.doi.org/10.1159/000056416] [PMID: 9782245]

[36] Clark AJ, Cage TA, Aranda D, Parsa AT, Auguste KI, Gupta N. Treatment-related morbidity and the management of pediatric craniopharyngioma: a systematic review. J Neurosurg Pediatr 2012; 10(4): 293-301. [http://dx.doi.org/10.3171/2012.7.PEDS11436] [PMID: 22920295]

[37] Clark AJ, Cage TA, Aranda D, *et al.* A systematic review of the results of surgery and radiotherapy on tumor control for pediatric craniopharyngioma. Childs Nerv Syst 2013; 29(2): 231-8. [http://dx.doi.org/10.1007/s00381-012-1926-2] [PMID: 23089933]

[38] Clayton PE, Price DA, Shalet SM, Gattemaneni HR. Craniopharyngioma recurrence and growth hormone therapy. Lancet 1988; 1(8586): 642. [http://dx.doi.org/10.1016/S0140-6736(88)91434-1] [PMID: 2894566]

[39] Cohen M, Bartels U, Branson H, Kulkarni AV, Hamilton J. Trends in treatment and outcomes of pediatric craniopharyngioma, 1975-2011. Neuro-oncol 2013; 15(6): 767-74. [http://dx.doi.org/10.1093/neuonc/not026] [PMID: 23486689]

[40] Colleran K, Sanchez-Goettler L, Sloan A. Hypothalamic obesity complicated by adipsic central diabetes insipidus following surgical resection of a craniopharyngioma. J Clin Hypertens (Greenwich) 2009; 11(10): 608-10. [http://dx.doi.org/10.1111/j.1751-7176.2009.00057.x] [PMID: 19817945]

[41] de Vetten L, Bocca G. Systemic effects of hypothermia due to hypothalamic dysfunction after resection of a craniopharyngioma: case report and review of literature. Neuropediatrics 2013; 44(3): 159-62. [PMID: 23047234]

[42] De Vile CJ, Grant DB, Kendall BE, *et al.* Management of childhood craniopharyngioma: can the morbidity of radical surgery be predicted? J Neurosurg 1996; 85(1): 73-81. [http://dx.doi.org/10.3171/jns.1996.85.1.0073] [PMID: 8683285]

[43] Dehdashti AR, de Tribolet N. Frontobasal interhemispheric trans-lamina terminalis approach for

suprasellar lesions. Neurosurgery 2008; 62(6) (Suppl. 3): 1233-9.
[PMID: 18695544]

[44] Dejardin V, Jaumain P, Stragier A, Boschi A. [Craniopharyngioma: ophthalmological manifestations and prognosis after treatment]. Bull Soc Belge Ophtalmol 1999; 271: 85-90. [Craniopharyngioma: ophthalmological manifestations and prognosis after treatment].
[PMID: 10355164]

[45] Delgado L, Castillo C, Ramires F, Viñas FC. Treatment of giant cystic craniopharyngiomas. J Clin Neurosci 1999; 6(3): 239-41.
[http://dx.doi.org/10.1016/S0967-5868(99)90511-8] [PMID: 18639159]

[46] Di Pinto M, Conklin HM, Li C, Merchant TE. Learning and memory following conformal radiation therapy for pediatric craniopharyngioma and low-grade glioma. Int J Radiat Oncol Biol Phys 2012; 84(3): e363-9.
[http://dx.doi.org/10.1016/j.ijrobp.2012.03.066] [PMID: 22867897]

[47] Di Rocco C, Caldarelli M, Tamburrini G, Massimi L. Surgical management of craniopharyngiomas--experience with a pediatric series. J Pediatr Endocrinol Metab 2006; 19 (Suppl. 1): 355-66.
[PMID: 16700311]

[48] DiPatri AJ Jr, Prabhu V. A history of the treatment of craniopharyngiomas. Childs Nerv Syst 2005; 21(8-9): 606-21.
[http://dx.doi.org/10.1007/s00381-005-1224-3] [PMID: 16044342]

[49] Djordjević M, Djordjević Z, Janićijević M, Nestorović B, Stefanović B, Ivkov M. Surgical treatment of craniopharyngiomas in children. Acta Neurochir Suppl (Wien) 1979; 28(2): 344-7.
[PMID: 290201]

[50] Dobracki A, Woolf P. Multiple head and neck tumors following treatment for craniopharyngioma. Pituitary 2011; 14(4): 382-3.
[http://dx.doi.org/10.1007/s11102-009-0177-z] [PMID: 19357951]

[51] Dolson EP, Conklin HM, Li C, Xiong X, Merchant TE. Predicting behavioral problems in craniopharyngioma survivors after conformal radiation therapy. Pediatr Blood Cancer 2009; 52(7): 860-4.
[http://dx.doi.org/10.1002/pbc.21947] [PMID: 19191345]

[52] Duff J, Meyer FB, Ilstrup DM, Laws EJ, Schleck CD, Scheithauer BW. Long-term outcomes for surgically resected craniopharyngiomas. Neurosurgery 2000; 46: 291-305.

[53] Elfving M, Lundgren J, Englund E, Strömblad LG, Erfurth EM. Ectopic recurrence of a craniopharyngioma in a 15-year-old girl 9 years after surgery and conventional radiotherapy: case report. Childs Nerv Syst 2011; 27(5): 845-51.
[http://dx.doi.org/10.1007/s00381-010-1375-8] [PMID: 21221975]

[54] Elliott RE, Jane JJ, Wisoff JH. Surgical management of craniopharyngiomas in children: meta-analysis and comparison of transcranial and transsphenoidal approaches. Neurosurgery 2011; 69: 630-43.

[55] Elliott RE, Moshel YA, Wisoff JH. Minimal residual calcification and recurrence after gross-total resection of craniopharyngioma in children. J Neurosurg Pediatr 2009; 3(4): 276-83.
[http://dx.doi.org/10.3171/2009.1.PEDS08335] [PMID: 19338405]

[56] Elliott RE, Moshel YA, Wisoff JH. Surgical treatment of ectopic recurrence of craniopharyngioma. Report of 4 cases. J Neurosurg Pediatr 2009; 4(2): 105-12.
[http://dx.doi.org/10.3171/2009.3.PEDS0948] [PMID: 19645541]

[57] Elliott RE, Sands SA, Strom RG, Wisoff JH. Craniopharyngioma Clinical Status Scale: a standardized metric of preoperative function and posttreatment outcome. Neurosurg Focus 2010; 28(4): E2.
[http://dx.doi.org/10.3171/2010.2.FOCUS09304] [PMID: 20367359]

[58] Elwatidy SM. Adult craniopharyngioma. Clinical, radiological presentation and outcome of management. Neurosciences (Riyadh) 2004; 9(4): 271-5.

[PMID: 23377247]

[59] Elwatidy SM, Jamjoom ZA, Jamjoom AB, Yakoub AO. Craniopharyngioma. Analysis of factors that affect the outcome. Saudi Med J 2002; 23(1): 34-8.
[PMID: 11938361]

[60] Erfurth EM, Holmer H, Fjalldal SB. Mortality and morbidity in adult craniopharyngioma. Pituitary 2013; 16(1): 46-55.
[http://dx.doi.org/10.1007/s11102-012-0428-2] [PMID: 22961634]

[61] Erşahin Y, Yurtseven T, Ozgiray E, Mutluer S. Craniopharyngiomas in children: Turkey experience. Childs Nerv Syst 2005; 21(8-9): 766-72.
[http://dx.doi.org/10.1007/s00381-005-1187-4] [PMID: 16001286]

[62] Fahlbusch R, Honegger J, Paulus W, Huk W, Buchfelder M. Surgical treatment of craniopharyngiomas: experience with 168 patients. J Neurosurg 1999; 90(2): 237-50.
[http://dx.doi.org/10.3171/jns.1999.90.2.0237] [PMID: 9950494]

[63] Feldkamp J, Scherbaum WA. [Growth factor substitution after radical removal of craniopharyngioma]. Dtsch Med Wochenschr 1997; 122(42): 1298-9. [Growth factor substitution after radical removal of craniopharyngioma].
[PMID: 9378068]

[64] Fischer EG, Welch K, Shillito J Jr, Winston KR, Tarbell NJ. Craniopharyngiomas in children. Long-term effects of conservative surgical procedures combined with radiation therapy. J Neurosurg 1990; 73(4): 534-40.
[http://dx.doi.org/10.3171/jns.1990.73.4.0534] [PMID: 2398383]

[65] Flickinger JC, Lunsford LD, Singer J, Cano ER, Deutsch M. Megavoltage external beam irradiation of craniopharyngiomas: analysis of tumor control and morbidity. Int J Radiat Oncol Biol Phys 1990; 19(1): 117-22.
[http://dx.doi.org/10.1016/0360-3016(90)90143-8] [PMID: 2116387]

[66] Frank G, Pasquini E, Doglietto F, Mazzatenta D, Sciarretta V, Farneti G, *et al.* he endoscopic extended transsphenoidal approach for craniopharyngiomas. Neurosurgery 2006; 59: S75-83.

[67] Frank G, Pasquini E, Mazzatenta D. Extended transsphenoidal approach. J Neurosurg 2001; 95(5): 917-8.
[PMID: 11702890]

[68] Fujitsu K, Saijo M, Aoki F, Fujii S, Mochimatsu Y, Gondo G. Cranio-nasal median splitting for radical resection of craniopharyngioma. Neurol Res 1992; 14(4): 345-51.
[http://dx.doi.org/10.1080/01616412.1992.11740082] [PMID: 1360632]

[69] Geffner M, Lundberg M, Koltowska-Häggström M, *et al.* Changes in height, weight, and body mass index in children with craniopharyngioma after three years of growth hormone therapy: analysis of KIGS (Pfizer International Growth Database). J Clin Endocrinol Metab 2004; 89(11): 5435-40.
[http://dx.doi.org/10.1210/jc.2004-0667] [PMID: 15531494]

[70] Ghatak NR, White BE. Delayed radiation necrosis of the hypothalamus. Report of a case simulating recurrent craniopharyngioma. Arch Neurol 1969; 21(4): 425-30.
[http://dx.doi.org/10.1001/archneur.1969.00480160097011] [PMID: 5821004]

[71] Ghirardello S, Hopper N, Albanese A, Maghnie M. Diabetes insipidus in craniopharyngioma: postoperative management of water and electrolyte disorders. J Pediatr Endocrinol Metab 2006; 19 (Suppl. 1): 413-21.
[PMID: 16700319]

[72] Gleeson H, Amin R, Maghnie M. 'Do no harm': management of craniopharyngioma. Eur J Endocrinol 2008; 159 (Suppl. 1): S95-9.
[http://dx.doi.org/10.1530/EJE-08-0400] [PMID: 18775978]

[73] Gopalan R, Dassoulas K, Rainey J, Sherman JH, Sheehan JP. Evaluation of the role of Gamma Knife

surgery in the treatment of craniopharyngiomas. Neurosurg Focus 2008; 24(5): E5.
[http://dx.doi.org/10.3171/FOC/2008/24/5/E5] [PMID: 18447744]

[74] Gościński I. [Craniopharyngioma in childhood. Significance of the extent of surgical resection and adjuvant megavoltage irradiation for event-free survival]. Neurol Neurochir Pol 1997; 31(3): 635-6. [Craniopharyngioma in childhood. Significance of the extent of surgical resection and adjuvant megavoltage irradiation for event-free survival].
[PMID: 9446057]

[75] Gucev ZS, Danilovski D, Tasic V, *et al.* Childhood craniopharyngioma in Macedonia: incidence and outcome after subtotal resection and cranial irradiation. World J Pediatr 2011; 7(1): 74-8.
[http://dx.doi.org/10.1007/s12519-011-0250-3] [PMID: 21191780]

[76] Habrand JL, Saran F, Alapetite C, Noel G, El Boustany R, Grill J. Radiation therapy in the management of craniopharyngioma: current concepts and future developments. J Pediatr Endocrinol Metab 2006; 19 (Suppl. 1): 389-94.
[PMID: 16700315]

[77] Halac I, Zimmerman D. Endocrine manifestations of craniopharyngioma. Childs Nerv Syst 2005; 21(8-9): 640-8.
[http://dx.doi.org/10.1007/s00381-005-1246-x] [PMID: 16047216]

[78] Hamberger CA, Hammer G, Norlen G, Sjogren B. Surgical treatment of craniopharyngioma; radical removal by the transantrosphenoidal approach. Acta Otolaryngol 1960; 52: 285-92.
[http://dx.doi.org/10.3109/00016486009123151] [PMID: 13710959]

[79] Hamilton JK, Conwell LS, Syme C, Ahmet A, Jeffery A, Daneman D. Hypothalamic Obesity following Craniopharyngioma Surgery: Results of a Pilot Trial of Combined Diazoxide and Metformin Therapy. Int J Pediatr Endocrinol 2011; 2011: 417949.
[http://dx.doi.org/10.1155/2011/417949] [PMID: 21603206]

[80] Harris JR, Levene MB. Visual complications following irradiation for pituitary adenomas and craniopharyngiomas. Radiology 1976; 120(1): 167-71.
[http://dx.doi.org/10.1148/120.1.167] [PMID: 935443]

[81] Harwood-Nash DC. Neuroimaging of childhood craniopharyngioma. Pediatr Neurosurg 1994; 21 (Suppl. 1): 2-10.
[http://dx.doi.org/10.1159/000120853] [PMID: 7841074]

[82] Hasegawa T, Kondziolka D, Hadjipanayis CG, Lunsford LD. Management of cystic craniopharyngiomas with phosphorus-32 intracavitary irradiation. Neurosurgery 2004; 54: 813-22.

[83] Hashizume C, Mori Y, Kobayashi T, Shibamoto Y, Nagai A, Hayashi N. Stereotactic radiotherapy using Novalis for craniopharyngioma adjacent to optic pathways. J Neurooncol 2010; 98(2): 239-47.
[http://dx.doi.org/10.1007/s11060-010-0180-2] [PMID: 20422439]

[84] Hoffman HJ, De Silva M, Humphreys RP, Drake JM, Smith ML, Blaser SI. Aggressive surgical management of craniopharyngiomas in children. J Neurosurg 1992; 76(1): 47-52.
[http://dx.doi.org/10.3171/jns.1992.76.1.0047] [PMID: 1727168]

[85] Hofmann BM, Höllig A, Strauss C, Buslei R, Buchfelder M, Fahlbusch R. Results after treatment of craniopharyngiomas: further experiences with 73 patients since 1997. J Neurosurg 2012; 116(2): 373-84.
[http://dx.doi.org/10.3171/2011.6.JNS081451] [PMID: 21942724]

[86] Honegger J, Barocka A, Sadri B, Fahlbusch R. Neuropsychological results of craniopharyngioma surgery in adults: a prospective study. Surg Neurol 1998; 50: 19-29.

[87] Honegger J, Buchfelder M, Fahlbusch R. Surgical treatment of craniopharyngiomas: endocrinological results. J Neurosurg 1999; 90(2): 251-7.
[http://dx.doi.org/10.3171/jns.1999.90.2.0251] [PMID: 9950495]

[88] Hoorn EJ, Zietse R. Water balance disorders after neurosurgery: the triphasic response revisited. NDT

Plus 2010; 3(1): 42-4.
[PMID: 20090880]

[89] Huk WJ, Mahlstedt J. Intracystic radiotherapy (90Y) of craniopharyngiomas: CT-guided stereotaxic implantation of indwelling drainage system. AJNR Am J Neuroradiol 1983; 4(3): 803-6.
[PMID: 6410858]

[90] Illum P, Elbrond O, Nehen AM. Surgical treatment of nasophrayngeal craniopharyngioma. Radical removal by the transpalatal approach. J Laryngol Otol 1977; 91(3): 227-33.
[http://dx.doi.org/10.1017/S0022215100083602] [PMID: 850102]

[91] Isaac MA, Hahn SS, Kim JA, Bogart JA, Chung CT. Management of craniopharyngioma. Cancer J 2001; 7(6): 516-20.
[PMID: 11769865]

[92] Israel ZH, Pomeranz S. Intracranial craniopharyngioma seeding following radical resection. Pediatr Neurosurg 1995; 22(4): 210-3.
[http://dx.doi.org/10.1159/000120903] [PMID: 7619722]

[93] Jane JA Jr, Kiehna E, Payne SC, Early SV, Laws ER Jr. Early outcomes of endoscopic transsphenoidal surgery for adult craniopharyngiomas. Neurosurg Focus 2010; 28(4): E9.
[http://dx.doi.org/10.3171/2010.1.FOCUS09319] [PMID: 20367523]

[94] Jane JA Jr, Prevedello DM, Alden TD, Laws ER Jr. The transsphenoidal resection of pediatric craniopharyngiomas: a case series. J Neurosurg Pediatr 2010; 5(1): 49-60.
[http://dx.doi.org/10.3171/2009.7.PEDS09252] [PMID: 20043736]

[95] Jeon C, Kim S, Shin HJ, *et al.* The therapeutic efficacy of fractionated radiotherapy and gamma-knife radiosurgery for craniopharyngiomas. J Clin Neurosci 2011; 18(12): 1621-5.
[http://dx.doi.org/10.1016/j.jocn.2011.03.028] [PMID: 22015100]

[96] Julow J, Lányi F, Hajda M, *et al.* The radiotherapy of cystic craniopharyngioma with intracystic installation of 90Y silicate colloid. Acta Neurochir (Wien) 1985; 74(3-4): 94-9.
[http://dx.doi.org/10.1007/BF01418795] [PMID: 3984798]

[97] Julow J, Lányi F, Hajda M, *et al.* Stereotactic intracavitary irradiation of cystic craniopharyngiomas with yttrium-90 isotope. Prog Neurol Surg 2007; 20: 289-96.
[http://dx.doi.org/10.1159/000100172] [PMID: 17317997]

[98] Julow JV. Intracystic irradiation for craniopharyngiomas. Pituitary 2013; 16(1): 34-45.
[http://dx.doi.org/10.1007/s11102-012-0442-4] [PMID: 23196808]

[99] Jung TY, Jung S, Jang WY, Moon KS, Kim IY, Kang SS. Operative outcomes and adjuvant treatment of purely third ventricle craniopharyngioma after a transcallosal approach. Br J Neurosurg 2012; 26(3): 355-60.
[http://dx.doi.org/10.3109/02688697.2011.631615] [PMID: 22103565]

[100] Kadri H, Mawla AA. Endoscopy-assisted microsurgical total resection of craniopharyngioma in childhood. Minim Invasive Neurosurg 2006; 49(6): 369-72.
[http://dx.doi.org/10.1055/s-2006-961820] [PMID: 17323266]

[101] Kanesaka N, Mikami R, Nakayama H, *et al.* Preliminary results of fractionated stereotactic radiotherapy after cyst drainage for craniopharyngioma in adults. Int J Radiat Oncol Biol Phys 2012; 82(4): 1356-60.
[http://dx.doi.org/10.1016/j.ijrobp.2011.05.014] [PMID: 21719210]

[102] Karaiskos I, Galani L, Baziaka F, Giamarellou H. Intraventricular and intrathecal colistin as the last therapeutic resort for the treatment of multidrug-resistant and extensively drug-resistant Acinetobacter baumannii ventriculitis and meningitis: a literature review. Int J Antimicrob Agents 2013; 41(6): 499-508.
[http://dx.doi.org/10.1016/j.ijantimicag.2013.02.006] [PMID: 23507414]

[103] Karavitaki N. Hypopituitarism oddities: craniopharyngiomas. Horm Res 2007; 68 (Suppl. 5): 151-3.

[PMID: 18174734]

[104] Karavitaki N, Brufani C, Warner JT, *et al.* Craniopharyngiomas in children and adults: systematic analysis of 121 cases with long-term follow-up. Clin Endocrinol (Oxf) 2005; 62(4): 397-409. [http://dx.doi.org/10.1111/j.1365-2265.2005.02231.x] [PMID: 15807869]

[105] Karavitaki N, Wass JA. Craniopharyngiomas. Endocrinol Metab Clin North Am 2008; 37(1): 173-193, ix-x. [http://dx.doi.org/10.1016/j.ecl.2007.10.012] [PMID: 18226736]

[106] Katz EL. Late results of radical excision of craniopharyngiomas in children. J Neurosurg 1975; 42(1): 86-93. [http://dx.doi.org/10.3171/jns.1975.42.1.0086] [PMID: 1110394]

[107] Kawano N, Ohwada T, Yada K. Radical removal of craniopharyngioma: a long-term follow-up. Neurol Med Chir (Tokyo) 1993; 33(8): 543-6. [http://dx.doi.org/10.2176/nmc.33.543] [PMID: 7692326]

[108] Khamlichi AE, Melhaoui A, Arkha Y, Jiddane M, Gueddari BK. Role of gamma knife radiosurgery in the management of pituitary adenomas and craniopharyngiomas. Acta Neurochir Suppl (Wien) 2013; 116: 49-54. [PMID: 23417458]

[109] Kickingereder P, Maarouf M, El Majdoub F, *et al.* Intracavitary brachytherapy using stereotactically applied phosphorus-32 colloid for treatment of cystic craniopharyngiomas in 53 patients. J Neurooncol 2012; 109(2): 365-74. [http://dx.doi.org/10.1007/s11060-012-0902-8] [PMID: 22717668]

[110] Kiehna EN, Merchant TE. Radiation therapy for pediatric craniopharyngioma. Neurosurg Focus 2010; 28(4): E10. [http://dx.doi.org/10.3171/2010.1.FOCUS09297] [PMID: 20367354]

[111] Kim SK, Wang KC, Shin SH, Choe G, Chi JG, Cho BK. Radical excision of pediatric craniopharyngioma: recurrence pattern and prognostic factors. Childs Nerv Syst 2001; 17: 531-7.

[112] Kobayashi T. Long-term results of gamma knife radiosurgery for 100 consecutive cases of craniopharyngioma and a treatment strategy. Prog Neurol Surg 2009; 22: 63-76. [http://dx.doi.org/10.1159/000163383] [PMID: 18948720]

[113] Kobayashi T, Kida Y, Mori Y, Hasegawa T. Long-term results of gamma knife surgery for the treatment of craniopharyngioma in 98 consecutive cases. J Neurosurg 2005; 103(6) (Suppl.): 482-8. [PMID: 16383245]

[114] Kobayashi T, Mori Y, Tsugawa T, Hashizume C, Takahashi H. Prognostic factors for tumor recurrence after gamma knife radiosurgery of partially resected and recurrent craniopharyngiomas. Nagoya J Med Sci 2012; 74(1-2): 141-7. [PMID: 22515120]

[115] Kobayashi T, Tanaka T, Kida Y. Stereotactic gamma radiosurgery of craniopharyngiomas. Pediatr Neurosurg 1994; 21 (Suppl. 1): 69-74. [http://dx.doi.org/10.1159/000120865] [PMID: 7841081]

[116] Konovalov AN, Vikhert TM, Korshunov AG, Gorelyshev SK. Vopr Neirokhir 1988; •••: 7-12. [Evaluation of the radicalness of the removal of craniopharyngioma of the 3d ventricle in children and the possible sources of their continued growth and recurrence].

[117] Kortmann RD. Different approaches in radiation therapy of craniopharyngioma. Front Endocrinol (Lausanne) 2011; 2: 100. [http://dx.doi.org/10.3389/fendo.2011.00100] [PMID: 22654836]

[118] Laffond C, Dellatolas G, Alapetite C, *et al.* Quality-of-life, mood and executive functioning after childhood craniopharyngioma treated with surgery and proton beam therapy. Brain Inj 2012; 26(3): 270-81.

[http://dx.doi.org/10.3109/02699052.2011.648709] [PMID: 22372414]

[119] Lannering B, Westgren U. [Radical or conservative surgery in craniopharyngioma? Importance of individualized treatment!]. Lakartidningen 1995; 92(22): 2301-5. [Radical or conservative surgery in craniopharyngioma? Importance of individualized treatment!]. [PMID: 7783489]

[120] Larijani B, Bastanhagh MH, Pajouhi M, Kargar Shadab F, Vasigh A, Aghakhani S. Presentation and outcome of 93 cases of craniopharyngioma. Eur J Cancer Care (Engl) 2004; 13(1): 11-5. [http://dx.doi.org/10.1111/j.1365-2354.2003.00433.x] [PMID: 14961770]

[121] Laser BS, Merchant TE, Indelicato DJ, Hua CH, Shulkin BL, Snyder SE. Evaluation of children with craniopharyngioma using carbon-11 methionine PET prior to proton therapy. Neuro-oncol 2013; 15(4): 506-10. [http://dx.doi.org/10.1093/neuonc/nos321] [PMID: 23408862]

[122] Laws ER Jr. Surgical outcome in 90 patients with craniopharyngiomas: an evaluation of the transsphenoidal approach. World Neurosurg 2010; 74(2-3): 254-5. [http://dx.doi.org/10.1016/j.wneu.2010.07.033] [PMID: 21492549]

[123] Leber KA, Berglöff J, Pendl G. Dose-response tolerance of the visual pathways and cranial nerves of the cavernous sinus to stereotactic radiosurgery. J Neurosurg 1998; 88(1): 43-50. [http://dx.doi.org/10.3171/jns.1998.88.1.0043] [PMID: 9420071]

[124] Lee MJ, Hwang JM. Initial visual field as a predictor of recurrence and postoperative visual outcome in children with craniopharyngioma. J Pediatr Ophthalmol Strabismus 2012; 49(1): 38-42. [http://dx.doi.org/10.3928/01913913-20110208-03] [PMID: 21323242]

[125] Lehrnbecher T, Müller-Scholden J, Danhauser-Leistner I, Sörensen N, von Stockhausen HB. Perioperative fluid and electrolyte management in children undergoing surgery for craniopharyngioma. A 10-year experience in a single institution. Childs Nerv Syst 1998; 14(6): 276-9. [http://dx.doi.org/10.1007/s003810050224] [PMID: 9694340]

[126] Li GM, Sun XJ, Shao P. Postoperative pituitary hormonal disturbances and hormone replacement therapy time and dosage in children with craniopharyngiomas. Chin Med J (Engl) 2008; 121(20): 2077-82. [PMID: 19080279]

[127] Lin LL, El Naqa I, Leonard JR, *et al.* Long-term outcome in children treated for craniopharyngioma with and without radiotherapy. J Neurosurg Pediatr 2008; 1(2): 126-30. [http://dx.doi.org/10.3171/PED/2008/1/2/126] [PMID: 18352781]

[128] Liu AK, Bagrosky B, Fenton LZ, *et al.* Vascular abnormalities in pediatric craniopharyngioma patients treated with radiation therapy. Pediatr Blood Cancer 2009; 52(2): 227-30. [http://dx.doi.org/10.1002/pbc.21787] [PMID: 18937328]

[129] Liu JK. Modified one-piece extended transbasal approach for translamina terminalis resection of retrochiasmatic third ventricular craniopharyngioma. Neurosurg Focus 2013; 34(1) (Suppl.): 1. [PMID: 23282153]

[130] Liu JK, Christiano LD, Patel SK, Eloy JA. Surgical nuances for removal of retrochiasmatic craniopharyngioma via the endoscopic endonasal extended transsphenoidal transplanum transtuberculum approach. Neurosurg Focus 2011; 30(4): E14. [http://dx.doi.org/10.3171/2011.1.FOCUS10297] [PMID: 21456925]

[131] Liu Z, Tian Z, Yu X, *et al.* Stereotactic intratumour irradiation with nuclide for craniopharyngiomas. Chin Med J (Engl) 1996; 109(3): 219-22. [PMID: 8758313]

[132] Liubinas SV, Munshey AS, Kaye AH. Management of recurrent craniopharyngioma. J Clin Neurosci 2011; 18(4): 451-7. [http://dx.doi.org/10.1016/j.jocn.2010.10.004] [PMID: 21316970]

[133] Lonjon M, Dran G, Casagrande F, Vandenbos F, Mas JC, Richelme C. Prenatal diagnosis of a craniopharyngioma: a new case with radical surgery and review. Childs Nerv Syst 2005; 21(3): 177-80.
[http://dx.doi.org/10.1007/s00381-004-1019-y] [PMID: 15290187]

[134] Lopez SJ, Garcia GE, Martinez-Aedo MJ, Martinez VA. An Esp Pediatr 2000; 53: 64-6. [Excessive growth and growth hormone deficiency after treatment for craniopharyngioma].
[http://dx.doi.org/10.1016/S1695-4033(00)77418-2] [PMID: 10998409]

[135] Lunsford LD, Pollock BE, Kondziolka DS, Levine G, Flickinger JC. Stereotactic options in the management of craniopharyngioma. Pediatr Neurosurg 1994; 21 (Suppl. 1): 90-7.
[http://dx.doi.org/10.1159/000120868] [PMID: 7841084]

[136] Lustig RH. Hypothalamic obesity after craniopharyngioma: mechanisms, diagnosis, and treatment. Front Endocrinol (Lausanne) 2011; 2: 60.
[http://dx.doi.org/10.3389/fendo.2011.00060] [PMID: 22654817]

[137] Luu QT, Loredo LN, Archambeau JO, Yonemoto LT, Slater JM, Slater JD. Fractionated proton radiation treatment for pediatric craniopharyngioma: preliminary report. Cancer J 2006; 12(2): 155-9.
[PMID: 16630407]

[138] Masson-Cote L, Masucci GL, Atenafu EG, *et al.* Long-term outcomes for adult craniopharyngioma following radiation therapy. Acta Oncol 2013; 52(1): 153-8.
[http://dx.doi.org/10.3109/0284186X.2012.685525] [PMID: 22568405]

[139] Matson DD, Crigler JF Jr. Radical treatment of craniopharyngioma. Ann Surg 1960; 152: 699-704.
[http://dx.doi.org/10.1097/00000658-196010000-00013] [PMID: 13768199]

[140] Merchant TE. Craniopharyngioma radiotherapy: endocrine and cognitive effects. J Pediatr Endocrinol Metab 2006; 19 (Suppl. 1): 439-46.
[PMID: 16700322]

[141] Mokry M. Craniopharyngiomas: A six year experience with Gamma Knife radiosurgery. Stereotact Funct Neurosurg 1999; 72 (Suppl. 1): 140-9.
[http://dx.doi.org/10.1159/000056450] [PMID: 10681702]

[142] Mortini P, Losa M, Pozzobon G, *et al.* Neurosurgical treatment of craniopharyngioma in adults and children: early and long-term results in a large case series. J Neurosurg 2011; 114(5): 1350-9.
[http://dx.doi.org/10.3171/2010.11.JNS10670] [PMID: 21214336]

[143] Müller HL. Childhood craniopharyngioma. Pituitary 2013; 16(1): 56-67.
[http://dx.doi.org/10.1007/s11102-012-0401-0] [PMID: 22678820]

[144] Müller HL, Faldum A, Etavard-Gorris N, *et al.* Functional capacity, obesity and hypothalamic involvement: cross-sectional study on 212 patients with childhood craniopharyngioma. Klin Padiatr 2003; 215(6): 310-4.
[http://dx.doi.org/10.1055/s-2003-45499] [PMID: 14677094]

[145] Müller HL, Gebhardt U, Etavard-Gorris N, Kolb R, Warmuth-Metz M, Sörensen N. Current strategies in diagnostics and endocrine treatment of patients with childhood craniopharyngioma during follow-up--recommendations in KRANIOPHARYNGEOM 2000. Onkologie 2005; 28(3): 150-6.
[PMID: 15772466]

[146] Müller HL, Heinrich M, Bueb K, *et al.* Perioperative dexamethasone treatment in childhood craniopharyngioma--influence on short-term and long-term weight gain. Exp Clin Endocrinol Diabetes 2003; 111(6): 330-4.
[http://dx.doi.org/10.1055/s-2003-42722] [PMID: 14520598]

[147] Müller-Scholden J, Lehrnbecher T, Müller HL, *et al.* Radical surgery in a neonate with craniopharyngioma. report of a case. Pediatr Neurosurg 2000; 33(5): 265-9.
[http://dx.doi.org/10.1159/000055967] [PMID: 11155065]

[148] Mutlukan E, Cullen JF. Visual outcome after craniopharyngioma. Ophthalmology 1990; 97(5): 539-40.
[http://dx.doi.org/10.1016/S0161-6420(13)31846-6] [PMID: 2386576]

[149] Nagata T, Goto T, Ichinose T, Mitsuhashi Y, Tsuyuguchi N, Ohata K. Pathological findings of fusiform dilation of the internal carotid artery following radical dissection of a craniopharyngioma. J Neurosurg Pediatr 2010; 6(6): 567-71.
[http://dx.doi.org/10.3171/2010.9.PEDS10280] [PMID: 21121732]

[150] Nicolato A, Foroni R, Rosta L, Gerosa M, Bricolo A. Multimodality stereotactic approach to the treatment of cystic craniopharyngiomas. Minim Invasive Neurosurg 2004; 47(1): 32-40.
[http://dx.doi.org/10.1055/s-2003-812467] [PMID: 15100930]

[151] Nishizawa S, Ohta S, Oki Y. Spontaneous resolution of diabetes insipidus after pituitary stalk sectioning during surgery for large craniopharyngioma. Endocrinological evaluation and clinical implications for surgical strategy. Neurol Med Chir (Tokyo) 2006; 46: 126-35.

[152] Olsson DS, Buchfelder M, Wiendieck K, *et al.* Tumour recurrence and enlargement in patients with craniopharyngioma with and without GH replacement therapy during more than 10 years of follow-up. Eur J Endocrinol 2012; 166(6): 1061-8.
[http://dx.doi.org/10.1530/EJE-12-0077] [PMID: 22457235]

[153] Page-Wilson G, Wardlaw SL, Khandji AG, Korner J. Hypothalamic obesity in patients with craniopharyngioma: treatment approaches and the emerging role of gastric bypass surgery. Pituitary 2012; 15(1): 84-92.
[http://dx.doi.org/10.1007/s11102-011-0349-5] [PMID: 21935755]

[154] Pan DH, Lee LS, Huang CI, Wong TT. Stereotactic internal irradiation for cystic craniopharyngiomas: a 6-year experience. Stereotact Funct Neurosurg 1990; 54-55: 525-30.
[http://dx.doi.org/10.1159/000100267] [PMID: 2080379]

[155] Parízek J, Malec R, Německová J. A contribution to the problem of radical surgery in craniopharyngioma. Sb Ved Pr Lek Fak Karlovy Univerzity Hradci Kralove 1973; 16(4-5): 301-4.
[PMID: 4531726]

[156] Park YS, Chang JH, Park YG, Kim DS. Recurrence rates after neuroendoscopic fenestration and Gamma Knife surgery in comparison with subtotal resection and Gamma Knife surgery for the treatment of cystic craniopharyngiomas. J Neurosurg 2011; 114(5): 1360-8.
[http://dx.doi.org/10.3171/2009.9.JNS09301] [PMID: 19877807]

[157] Pedreira CC, Stargatt R, Maroulis H, *et al.* Health related quality of life and psychological outcome in patients treated for craniopharyngioma in childhood. J Pediatr Endocrinol Metab 2006; 19(1): 15-24.
[http://dx.doi.org/10.1515/JPEM.2006.19.1.15] [PMID: 16509524]

[158] Pekmezci M, Louie J, Gupta N, Bloomer MM, Tihan T. Clinicopathological characteristics of adamantinomatous and papillary craniopharyngiomas: University of California, San Francisco experience 1985-2005. Neurosurgery 2010; 67: 1341-9.

[159] Pemberton LS, Dougal M, Magee B, Gattamaneni HR. Experience of external beam radiotherapy given adjuvantly or at relapse following surgery for craniopharyngioma. Radiother Oncol 2005; 77(1): 99-104.
[http://dx.doi.org/10.1016/j.radonc.2005.04.015] [PMID: 16216361]

[160] Pereira AM, Schmid EM, Schutte PJ, *et al.* High prevalence of long-term cardiovascular, neurological and psychosocial morbidity after treatment for craniopharyngioma. Clin Endocrinol (Oxf) 2005; 62(2): 197-204.
[http://dx.doi.org/10.1111/j.1365-2265.2004.02196.x] [PMID: 15670196]

[161] Pollock BE, Lunsford LD, Kondziolka D, Levine G, Flickinger JC. Phosphorus-32 intracavitary irradiation of cystic craniopharyngiomas: current technique and long-term results. Int J Radiat Oncol Biol Phys 1995; 33(2): 437-46.

[http://dx.doi.org/10.1016/0360-3016(95)00175-X] [PMID: 7673031]

[162] Poretti A, Grotzer MA, Ribi K, Schönle E, Boltshauser E. Outcome of craniopharyngioma in children: long-term complications and quality of life. Dev Med Child Neurol 2004; 46(4): 220-9. [http://dx.doi.org/10.1111/j.1469-8749.2004.tb00476.x] [PMID: 15077699]

[163] Price DA, Jönsson P. Effect of growth hormone treatment in children with craniopharyngioma with reference to the KIGS (Kabi International Growth Study) database. Acta Paediatr Suppl 1996; 417: 83-5.
[http://dx.doi.org/10.1111/j.1651-2227.1996.tb14307.x] [PMID: 9055921]

[164] Puget S. Treatment strategies in childhood craniopharyngioma. Front Endocrinol (Lausanne) 2012; 3: 64.
[http://dx.doi.org/10.3389/fendo.2012.00064] [PMID: 22679439]

[165] Qi S, Huang G, Pan J, *et al.* Involvement of osteopontin as a core protein in craniopharyngioma calcification formation. J Neurooncol 2010; 98(1): 21-30.
[http://dx.doi.org/10.1007/s11060-009-0053-8] [PMID: 19902145]

[166] Qi S, Pan J, Lu Y, *et al.* The impact of the site of origin and rate of tumour growth on clinical outcome in children with craniopharyngiomas. Clin Endocrinol (Oxf) 2012; 76(1): 103-10.
[http://dx.doi.org/10.1111/j.1365-2265.2011.04172.x] [PMID: 21752042]

[167] Raimondi AJ, Rougerie J. A critical review of personal experiences with craniopharyngioma: clinical history, surgical technique and operative results. 1983. Pediatr Neurosurg 1994; 21: 134-54.

[168] Rajan B, Ashley S, Thomas DG, Marsh H, Britton J, Brada M. Craniopharyngioma: improving outcome by early recognition and treatment of acute complications. Int J Radiat Oncol Biol Phys 1997; 37(3): 517-21.
[http://dx.doi.org/10.1016/S0360-3016(96)00537-8] [PMID: 9112447]

[169] Riva D, Pantaleoni C, Devoti M, Saletti V, Nichelli F, Giorgi C. Late neuropsychological and behavioural outcome of children surgically treated for craniopharyngioma. Childs Nerv Syst 1998; 14(4-5): 179-84.
[http://dx.doi.org/10.1007/s003810050207] [PMID: 9660119]

[170] Roderick E, Karavitaki N, Wass JA. Craniopharyngiomas. Historical aspects of their management. Hormones (Athens) 2008; 7(3): 271-4.
[http://dx.doi.org/10.14310/horm.2002.1208] [PMID: 18694868]

[171] Romodanov AP, Zozulia I, Patsko I. Vopr Neirokhir 1980; •••: 3-9. [Experience with radical surgery for craniopharyngiomas].

[172] Rosenthal R, Gamroth A, Sturm V, Wowra B, van Kaick G. [Cystic craniopharyngiomas: computed tomography in the pretherapeutic evaluation and control of treatment results following intracystic contact irradiation]. Strahlenther Onkol 1987; 163(9): 621-5. [Cystic craniopharyngiomas: computed tomography in the pretherapeutic evaluation and control of treatment results following intracystic contact irradiation].
[PMID: 3660228]

[173] Sääf M, Thorén M, Bergstrand CG, *et al.* Treatment of craniopharyngiomas--the stereotactic approach in a ten to twenty-three years' perspective. II. Psychosocial situation and pituitary function. Acta Neurochir (Wien) 1989; 99(3-4): 97-103.
[http://dx.doi.org/10.1007/BF01402315] [PMID: 2672706]

[174] Sagoh M, Murakami H, Hirose Y, Mayanagi K. Occlusive cerebrovasculopathy after internal radiation and bleomycin therapy for craniopharyngioma--case report. Neurol Med Chir (Tokyo) 1997; 37(12): 920-3.
[http://dx.doi.org/10.2176/nmc.37.920] [PMID: 9465592]

[175] Saleem MA, Hashim AS, Rashid A, Ali M. Role of gamma knife radiosurgery in multimodality management of craniopharyngioma. Acta Neurochir Suppl (Wien) 2013; 116: 55-60.

[PMID: 23417459]

[176] Schefter JK, Allen G, Cmelak AJ, *et al.* The utility of external beam radiation and intracystic 32P radiation in the treatment of craniopharyngiomas. J Neurooncol 2002; 56(1): 69-78. [http://dx.doi.org/10.1023/A:1014467721132] [PMID: 11949829]

[177] Scott RM, Hetelekidis S, Barnes PD, Goumnerova L, Tarbell NJ. Surgery, radiation, and combination therapy in the treatment of childhood craniopharyngioma--a 20-year experience. Pediatr Neurosurg 1994; 21 (Suppl. 1): 75-81. [http://dx.doi.org/10.1159/000120866] [PMID: 7841082]

[178] Shi X, Huang W, Wang Z. Preservation of the hypothalamic structures in the total resection of craniopharyngioma. Chin Med Sci J 2001; 16(4): 218-22. [PMID: 12903760]

[179] Shi Z, Esiashvili N, Janss AJ, *et al.* Transient enlargement of craniopharyngioma after radiation therapy: pattern of magnetic resonance imaging response following radiation. J Neurooncol 2012; 109(2): 349-55. [http://dx.doi.org/10.1007/s11060-012-0900-x] [PMID: 22692563]

[180] Shillito J Jr. Treatment of craniopharyngioma. Clin Neurosurg 1986; 33: 533-46. [PMID: 3791815]

[181] Steinbok P, Hukin J. Intracystic treatments for craniopharyngioma. Neurosurg Focus 2010; 28(4): E13. [http://dx.doi.org/10.3171/2010.1.FOCUS09315] [PMID: 20367357]

[182] Sweet WH. Radical surgical treatment of craniopharyngioma. Clin Neurosurg 1976; 23: 52-79. [PMID: 975700]

[183] Symon L. An approach to radical excision of craniopharyngioma by the temporal route. Pediatr Neurosurg 1994; 21 (Suppl. 1): 64-8. [http://dx.doi.org/10.1159/000120864] [PMID: 7841080]

[184] Symon L, Pell MF, Habib AH. Radical excision of craniopharyngioma by the temporal route: a review of 50 patients. Br J Neurosurg 1991; 5(6): 539-49. [http://dx.doi.org/10.3109/02688699109002877] [PMID: 1772600]

[185] Symon L, Sprich W. Radical excision of craniopharyngioma. Results in 20 patients. J Neurosurg 1985; 62(2): 174-81. [http://dx.doi.org/10.3171/jns.1985.62.2.0174] [PMID: 3968556]

[186] Thomsett MJ, Conte FA, Kaplan SL, Grumbach MM. Endocrine and neurologic outcome in childhood craniopharyngioma: Review of effect of treatment in 42 patients. J Pediatr 1980; 97(5): 728-35. [http://dx.doi.org/10.1016/S0022-3476(80)80254-X] [PMID: 7431164]

[187] Tian ZM. Stereotactic intracavitary irradiation of huge cystic craniopharyngiomas Zhonghua Wai Ke Za Zhi 1992; 30: 102-25.

[188] Toumba M, Stanhope R. Quality of life and psychological outcome in patients treated for craniopharyngioma. J Pediatr Endocrinol Metab 2006; 19(1): 11-3. [http://dx.doi.org/10.1515/JPEM.2006.19.1.11] [PMID: 16509523]

[189] Trivin C, Busiah K, Mahlaoui N, *et al.* Childhood craniopharyngioma: greater hypothalamic involvement before surgery is associated with higher homeostasis model insulin resistance index. BMC Pediatr 2009; 9: 24. [http://dx.doi.org/10.1186/1471-2431-9-24] [PMID: 19341477]

[190] Ulfarsson E, Lindquist C, Roberts M, *et al.* Gamma knife radiosurgery for craniopharyngiomas: long-term results in the first Swedish patients. J Neurosurg 2002; 97(5) (Suppl.): 613-22. [PMID: 12507107]

[191] Van Effenterre R, Boch AL. Craniopharyngioma in adults and children: a study of 122 surgical cases. J Neurosurg 2002; 97(1): 3-11.

[http://dx.doi.org/10.3171/jns.2002.97.1.0003] [PMID: 12134929]

[192] Varlotto JM, Flickinger JC, Kondziolka D, Lunsford LD, Deutsch M. External beam irradiation of craniopharyngiomas: long-term analysis of tumor control and morbidity. Int J Radiat Oncol Biol Phys 2002; 54(2): 492-9.
[http://dx.doi.org/10.1016/S0360-3016(02)02965-6] [PMID: 12243827]

[193] Walczak M, Pawlaczyk J. [Hypothalamic dysfunction and Glinski-Simmonds syndrome caused by craniopharyngioma of the 3d ventricle fundus in a 14-year-old girl]. Endokrynol Pol 1969; 20(2): 103-8. [Hypothalamic dysfunction and Glinski-Simmonds syndrome caused by craniopharyngioma of the 3d ventricle fundus in a 14-year-old girl].
[PMID: 5782271]

[194] Wang L, Zhao SF, Zhang W, Zhang MZ. Treatment of alternated water-electrolyte balance and endocrine status after removal of craniopharyngioma in adults. Chin Med J (Engl) 2006; 119(16): 1348-52.
[PMID: 16934180]

[195] Wara WM, Sneed PK, Larson DA. The role of radiation therapy in the treatment of craniopharyngioma. Pediatr Neurosurg 1994; 21 (Suppl. 1): 98-100.
[http://dx.doi.org/10.1159/000120869] [PMID: 7841085]

[196] Watanabe T, Sato T, Ichikawa M, Sakuma J, Saito K, Nagatani T. [Surgical approach for craniopharyngioma bifrontal basal interhemispheric approach/extended endonasal endoscopic approach]. No Shinkei Geka 2011; 39(9): 849-57. [Surgical approach for craniopharyngioma bifrontal basal interhemispheric approach/extended endonasal endoscopic approach].
[PMID: 21873739]

[197] Winkfield KM, Linsenmeier C, Yock TI, *et al.* Surveillance of craniopharyngioma cyst growth in children treated with proton radiotherapy. Int J Radiat Oncol Biol Phys 2009; 73(3): 716-21.
[http://dx.doi.org/10.1016/j.ijrobp.2008.05.010] [PMID: 18676089]

[198] Winkfield KM, Tsai HK, Yao X, *et al.* Long-term clinical outcomes following treatment of childhood craniopharyngioma. Pediatr Blood Cancer 2011; 56(7): 1120-6.
[http://dx.doi.org/10.1002/pbc.22884] [PMID: 21488157]

[199] Xu Z, Yen CP, Schlesinger D, Sheehan J. Outcomes of Gamma Knife surgery for craniopharyngiomas. J Neurooncol 2011; 104(1): 305-13.
[http://dx.doi.org/10.1007/s11060-010-0494-0] [PMID: 21153860]

[200] Yamada S, Fukuhara N, Oyama K, *et al.* Surgical outcome in 90 patients with craniopharyngioma: an evaluation of transsphenoidal surgery. World Neurosurg 2010; 74(2-3): 320-30.
[http://dx.doi.org/10.1016/j.wneu.2010.06.014] [PMID: 21492566]

[201] Yamada S, Fukuhara N, Oyama K, *et al.* Surgical outcome in 90 patients with craniopharyngioma: an evaluation of transsphenoidal surgery. World Neurosurg 2010; 74(2-3): 320-30.
[http://dx.doi.org/10.1016/j.wneu.2010.06.014] [PMID: 21492566]

[202] Yang I, Sughrue ME, Rutkowski MJ, *et al.* Craniopharyngioma: a comparison of tumor control with various treatment strategies. Neurosurg Focus 2010; 28(4): E5.
[http://dx.doi.org/10.3171/2010.1.FOCUS09307] [PMID: 20367362]

[203] Yomo S, Hayashi M, Chernov M, *et al.* Stereotactic radiosurgery of residual or recurrent craniopharyngioma: new treatment concept using Leksell gamma knife model C with automatic positioning system. Stereotact Funct Neurosurg 2009; 87(6): 360-7.
[http://dx.doi.org/10.1159/000236370] [PMID: 19752595]

[204] Yu X, Liu Z, Li S. Combined treatment with stereotactic intracavitary irradiation and gamma knife surgery for craniopharyngiomas. Stereotact Funct Neurosurg 2000; 75(2-3): 117-22.
[http://dx.doi.org/10.1159/000048392] [PMID: 11740179]

[205] Zada G, Cappabianca P. Transsphenoidal surgery for craniopharyngiomas: the lessons of experience,

timing, and restraint. World Neurosurg 2010; 74(2-3): 256-8. [http://dx.doi.org/10.1016/j.wneu.2010.06.027] [PMID: 21492550]

[206] Zhao R, Deng J, Liang X, Zeng J, Chen X, Wang J. Treatment of cystic craniopharyngioma with phosphorus-32 intracavitary irradiation. Childs Nerv Syst 2010; 26(5): 669-74. [http://dx.doi.org/10.1007/s00381-009-1025-1] [PMID: 19904543]

[207] Zuccaro G. Radical resection of craniopharyngioma. Childs Nerv Syst 2005; 21(8-9): 679-90. [http://dx.doi.org/10.1007/s00381-005-1201-x] [PMID: 16133275]

[208] Zuccaro G, Jaimovich R, Mantese B, Monges J. Complications in paediatric craniopharyngioma treatment. Childs Nerv Syst 1996; 12: 385-91.

CHAPTER 5

Experimental Craniopharyngioma Research

Guang-long Huang[1,*] and **Jie Zhou**[2]

[1] *Department of Neurosurgery, Nanfang Neurosurgery Research Institution, Nanfang Hospital, Southern Medical University, 1838 North Guangzhou Avenue, Guangzhou, China*

[2] *Department of Neurosurgery, The First Affiliated Hospital of Sichuan Medical University, 25 Taiping Road, Luzhou, China*

Abstract: Craniopharyngioma, an intracranial, extra-axial, epithelial tumor of the sellar or parasellar region that grows along the craniopharyngeal duct, was established in 1904 as a distinct tumor type by the Austrian neuropathologist Jakob Erdheim. Though classified as a Grade I tumor by the World Health Organization, craniopharyngioma can cause significant morbidity through its intimate involvement with and mass effects on surrounding critical structures, including the hypothalamus, pituitary gland, and optic chiasm, and its tendency to recur even after successful therapy. Many extensive and in-depth studies of craniopharyngioma have been conducted; however, during the past century, studies of the genetic and molecular basis of the two major craniopharyngioma subtypes (adamantinomatous and squamous papillary) have been limited because of the benign histology, epidemiological rarity (relative to malignant tumors), and lack of a tumor research platform and technical conditions associated with these lesions. Therefore, consensus remains lacking with respect to the etiology, pathological features, pathogenesis, and biological characteristics of these formidable neoplasms. In this chapter, we reviewed experimental craniopharyngioma research.

Keywords: Craniopharyngioma, EMT, Experimental research, Inflammation, mice model.

INTRODUCTION

Craniopharyngioma, an intracranial, extra-axial, epithelial tumor of the sellar or parasellar region that grows along the craniopharyngeal duct [1], was established in 1904 as a distinct tumor type by the Austrian neuropathologist Jakob Erdheim [2]. Though classified as a Grade I tumor by the World Health Organization, craniopharyngioma can cause significant morbidity through its intimate involvement with and mass effects on surrounding critical structures, including

* **Corresponding author Guang-long Huang**: Department of Neurosurgery, Nanfang Neurosurgery Research Institution, Nanfang Hospital, Southern Medical University, 1838 North Guangzhou Avenue, Guangzhou, China; Tel/Fax: +8620-61641806; E-mail: 223905569@qq.com

the hypothalamus, pituitary gland, and optic chiasm, and its tendency to recur even after successful therapy. Many extensive and in-depth studies of craniopharyngioma have been conducted [3 - 6]; however, during the past century, studies of the genetic and molecular basis of the two major craniopharyngioma subtypes (adamantinomatous [ACP] and squamous papillary [SPCP]) have been limited because of the benign histology, epidemiological rarity (relative to malignant tumors), and lack of a tumor research platform and technical conditions associated with these lesions. Therefore, consensus remains lacking with respect to the etiology, pathological features, pathogenesis, and biological characteristics of these formidable neoplasms.

CELL CULTURE AND TUMORIGENICITY *IN VIVO*

Cell Culture *in Vitro*

Craniopharyngiomas remain one of most challenging and often enigmatic tumors; they are often associated with unfavorable and occasionally disastrous sequelae despite of benign histological appearance. Development of a cellular model of this tumor might provide a platform for evaluating potential therapies prior to clinical trials in humans. Despite more than 50 years of experience with epithelial tumors in culture, no ideal craniopharyngioma cell line currently exists because of this tumor's benign histology. During the most recent 20 years, some scholars have investigated the behavior of craniopharyngioma in culture and performed some functional experiments in vitro based on cell models, particularly of the adamantinomatous subtype. Honegger and colleagues were the first to demonstrate the systemic culture of craniopharyngioma cells to produce cell lines. These researchers successfully cultured craniopharyngioma cells and identified the expression of progesterone receptor (PR) mRNA in at least some human craniopharyngiomas; furthermore, they demonstrated that treating craniopharyngioma cell cultures with progesterone led to increased tumor cell proliferation [7]. In 2005 Ulfarsson also reported culturing craniopharyngioma cells using a similar method as that described for keratinocytes by Green [8]. In that study, all nine cultured cell lines expressed cytokeratin (CK) 7, a well-documented marker of craniopharyngioma cells, irrespective of histological subtype. Ulfarsson subsequently disclosed that tumor cells expressing high levels of the insulin-like growth factor-1 receptor (IGF-IR), but not those expressing low levels, responded promptly with the decreased level of Akt phosphorylation, followed by growth arrest Fig. (**1**) [9]. In 2010, Hölsken cultured ACP cell lines according to the method described by Ulfarsson and reported that all lines expressed KL-1, a well-documented epithelial cell marker. Subsequent migration experiments demonstrated significantly reduced in vitro tumor cell motility following transfection with fascin-specific small interfering RNA (siRNA);

additionally, an epidermal growth factor receptor (EGFR) inhibitor (gefatinib) reduced fascin expression and inhibited tumor cell migration in vitro Fig. (**2**) [10, 11]. The present authors have also investigated ACP cell culture. For example, we identified all ACP cells according to their immunoreactivity for pan-CK, a well-documented epithelial cell marker. The epithelial origin of ACP cells was demonstrated on the basis of an epithelial-like morphology and pan-CK phenotype (Fig. **1**). Simultaneously, researchers mainly focused on the culture method and molecular oncogenesis of ACP cells, the latter of which is primarily involved in development of the adamantinomatous subtype; otherwise, the characteristics and molecular pathogenesis of SPCP remains unknown.

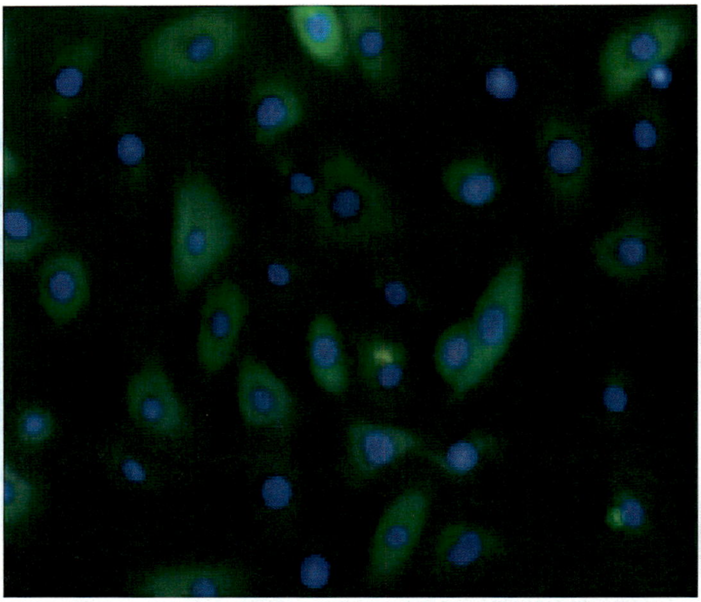

Fig. (1). Pan-CK immunostaining of craniopharyngioma cell lines (200× magnification).

Recently, Brastianos *et al.* identified BRAF mutations in SPCPs *via* exome sequencing [12]. The researchers identified mutations in CTNNB1 (Fig. **2**), the gene encoding β-catenin, in nearly all examined ACPs (11/12, 92%) and recurrent BRAF (p.Val600Glu) mutations in all SPCPs (3/3, 100%).They also found BRAF p.Val600Glu mutation in 95% of SPCPs (36/39 tumors) and CTNNB1 mutations in 96% of ACPs (51/53 tumors) by targeted genotyping. The CTNNB1 and BRAF mutations were exclusive in each tumor subtype, and no other recurrent mutations or genomic aberrations were detected. However, Sarah *et al.* demonstrated that although the majority of ACPs do not contain BRAF mutations, while this mutation is not exclusive to SPCP and can coexist with CTNNB1 mutations after they examined 37 CPs. The other research [13] indicated that BRAF V600E mutations might be characteristic for papillary craniopharyngioma and may coexist with CTNNB1-mutated adamantinomatous craniopharyngioma.

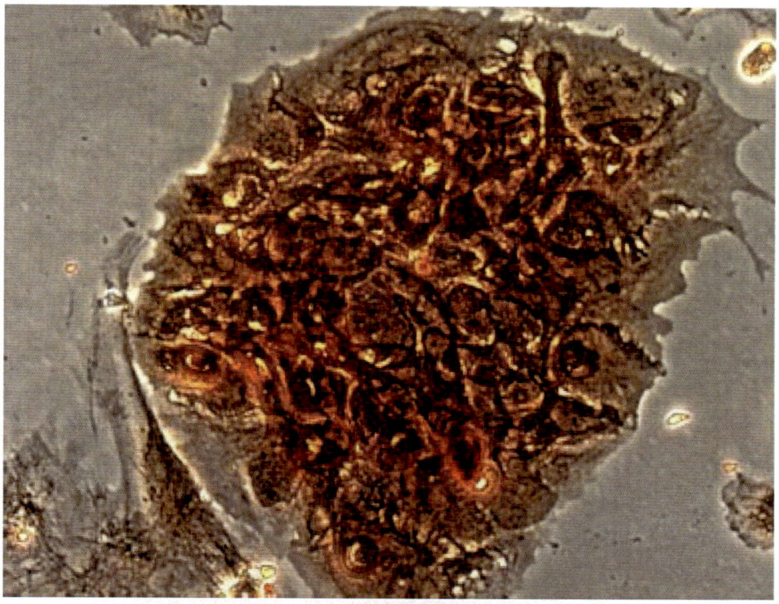

Fig. (2). β-catenin in primary ACP cell cultures.

In craniopharyngioma, the role played by BRAF mutation remains unknown. However, BRAF mutation is a predictor of worse prognosis in many other cancers, including melanoma and papillary thyroid carcinoma. The US Food and Drug Administration (FDA) has approved the use of drugs targeting the BRAF pVal600Glu mutation for melanoma treatment; the use of these drugs for the treatment of craniopharyngioma, especially the SPCP subtype, should be considered.

Tumorigenicity *In Vivo*

In 1979 Bullard subcutaneously transplanted two human craniopharyngiomas into six athymic "nude" mice. Morphologically characteristic craniopharyngiomas grew in five of these animals. The tumors that grew in mice maintained the same adamantinomatous architecture, epithelial nests, and keratinized nodules, characteristic of human craniopharyngiomas, that were present in the original surgical samples and were sufficient to allow transplantation into a second generation of animals [14]. In 2005 Xu collected 12 craniopharyngioma tissues and transplanted them subcutaneously under the front limbs of 24 nude mice. The overall successful transplantation rate was 39.58%; the individual rates of ACP and SPCP were 58.33% and 20.83%, respectively. However, the authors also noted that their animal model was not suited for further experimentation, given the low success rates [15]. In 2011 the English scholars Gaston-Massuet and Andoniadou produced a mouse model by using a degradation-resistant form of b-catenin in Rathke's pouch progenitor cells,which indicate that wnt pathway may play a significant role in ACP formation (Fig. **3**) [16, 17]. The development of a genetically engineered animal model of this tumor might provide a platform for exploring the pathogenesis and biological characteristics of craniopharyngioma. Advances in our understanding of the molecular pathogenesis of tumor recurrence have also been made and have provided clues regarding the development of target therapies that could improve optimal response rates. Moreover, these studies will guide the development of genetically engineered animal models that will more accurately recapitulate human craniopharyngiomas, thus providing an unprecedented ability to develop and validate optimal treatment regimens for patients with craniopharyngiomas.

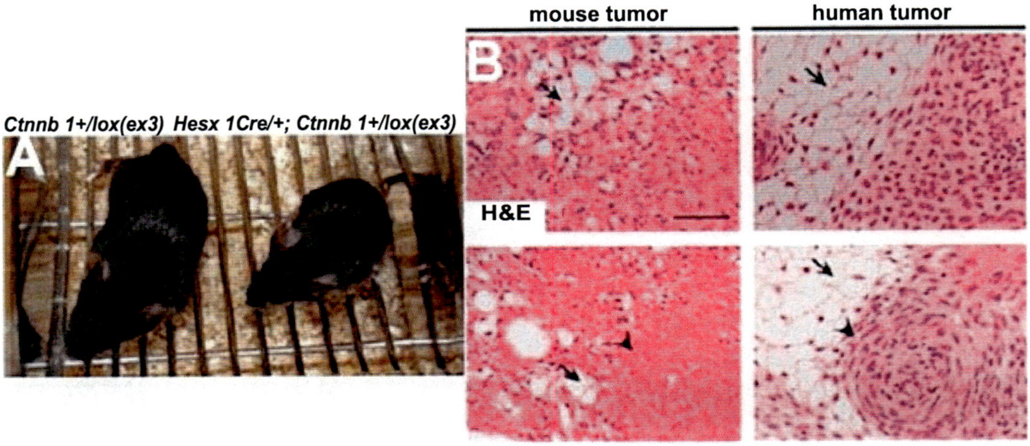

Fig. (3). Hesx1Cre/+; Ctnnb1+/lox(ex3) mice develop hypopituitarism and pituitary tumors that resemble human ACP. (A) A 5-week-old heterozygous mutant exhibits marked dwarfism relative to a sex-matched control littermate. Hematoxylin/eosin (H.E.) staining of histological sections from a human ACP (Right) and murine tumor (Left) showing the presence of microcystic changes (stellate reticulum; arrows) and nodular structures (cell clusters; arrowheads) in both (From Gaston-Massuet, C., *et al.* Increased Wingless (WNT) signaling in pituitary progenitor/stem cells gives rise to pituitary tumors in mice and humans. Reference from PNAS U S A, 2011. 108(28): p. 11482-11487).

CRANIOPHARYNGIOMA AND INFLAMMATION

Craniopharyngiomas are formidable and complex benign epithelial tumors of the sellar region. Given their benign nature, total surgical resection is the treatment of choice to achieve a cure and prevent recurrence [18, 19]. However, the aggressive behavior of these tumors and the associated potential for adhesion to adjacent brain structures favor significant regrowth or recurrence even after complete resection, particularly of the adamantinomatous subtype [5]. Some studies involving series of craniopharyngiomas have also reported a better outcome for the papillary subtype [20, 21]. Unfortunately, the underlying mechanisms are not clear.

The adamantinomatous subtype comprises cystic and/or solid components, necrotic debris, fibrous tissue, and calcification, whereas the papillary subtype usually comprises solid components [22]. Kulkarni reported that the spontaneous rupture of ACP cysts and cyst fluid spillage during surgery could cause aseptic meningitis [23]. Moreover, intense fibrillary gliosis, which is histologically rich in Rosenthal fibers and infiltrating inflammatory cells (mainly lymphocytes, neutrophils, and eosinophilic granulocytes), is frequently present in the parenchyma surrounding ACP but not SPCP [24, 25]. It is now becoming clear that the tumor microenvironment is largely directed by inflammatory cells. Chronic inflammation, which has been implicated in all stages of carcinogenesis, from initiation and promotion to progression, represents a major pathological basis for the majority of human malignancies. In our previous study, inflammation in craniopharyngiomas was associated with the pathological classification, rate of total resection, calcification, and postoperative hypothalamic function [26]. Either the tumor or stromal cells may produce certain inflammatory cytokine(s); these cytokines participate in complex inflammatory signaling that facilitates the extravasation of tumor cells through the stroma, thereby fostering tumor progression. Our earlier study, as well as a study by Mori, strongly implicated that in the context of ACP, interleukin (IL) 6 might be a key among the various cytokines with respect to inflammation [26, 27]. Moreover, another author reported that serum IL-6, IL-8, and macrophage inflammatory protein 1-alpha worked synergistically to regulate tumor progression [28].

Studies of the molecular mechanics of inflammation in the context of craniopharyngioma are uncommon. In our study, we demonstrated that autocrine and/or paracrine sources of IL-6 might play important roles in the regulation of the biological characteristics associated with ACP. We found that IL-6 promoted the migration of ACP cells in an assay of primary cultured ACP cells but did not stimulate tumor cell proliferation.

CRANIOPHARYNGIOMA AND THE EPITHELIAL-MESENCHYMAL TRANSITION (EMT)

Together with our previous results, we found that the epithelial-mesenchymal transition (EMT) played a potential role in the pathogenesis and development of craniopharyngiomas, especially ACPs. Overexpression of vimentin and decreased expression of E-cadherin were observed in ACPs and was related to tumor recurrence and poor postoperative hypothalamic function. A rapid, dose-dependent increase in vimentin and decrease in E-cadherin were observed after stimulating ACP cells with IL-6, and this expression pattern was inverted when the cells were treated with an IL-6 neutralizing antibody. Therefore, the EMT might play a role in IL-6-mediated migration, and an IL-6-mediated EMT phenotype in some cancer cells has been clinically associated with poor outcomes in numerous types of human carcinomas, including breast and biliary tract cancers [29]. As mentioned above, the Wnt pathway may play a role in ACP tumorigenicity. However, abnormal Wnt pathway signaling may also contribute to EMT. Rolf *et al.* found that in ACP, nuclear β-catenin expression was restricted to cohesive cell clusters within whorl-like areas and to transitional cells adjacent to the extracellular matrix. Nuclear β-catenin accumulation can upregulate the expression of EMT-associated transcription factors such as Snail and Twist and can also induce EMT. Further studies are needed to fully determine the cause of nuclear β-catenin expression restriction in ACP and the role of the extracellular matrix in ACP progression (Fig. **4**).

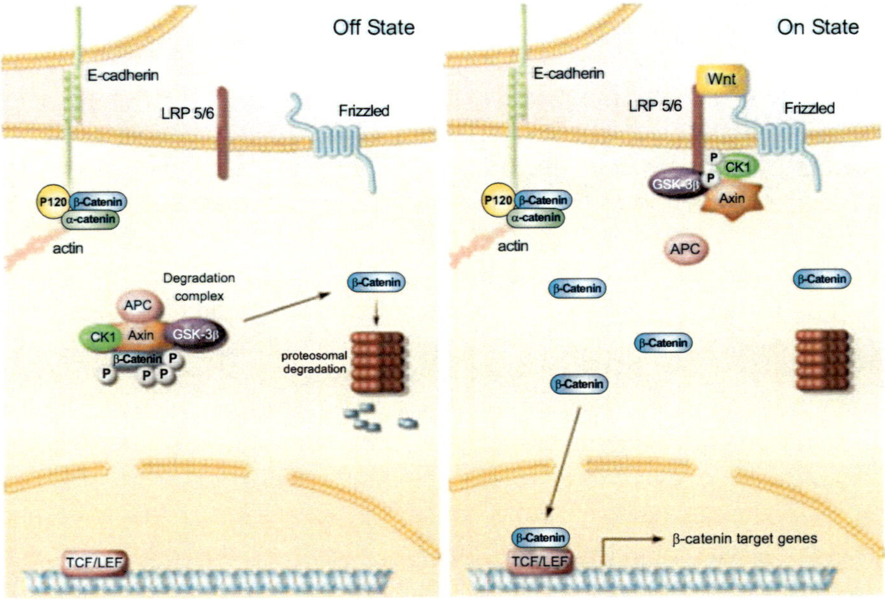

Fig. (4). WNT signaling pathway [29]. This pathway is maintained in the off state by the β-catenin degradation complex and proteasome. When a Wnt ligand is present, the complex cannot assemble and β-catenin translocates to the nucleus to initiate transcription of its target genes. Mutations in exon 3 of the β-catenin gene CTNNB1 prevent complex formation, leading to constitutively active Wnt signaling.

In contrast, Mori considered it impractical to attempt to reduce adhesions between craniopharyngiomas and the surrounding parenchyma by administering anti-inflammatory drugs because strong adhesions have already been established by the time a clinical diagnosis is made. In clinical practice, we identified some adhesions between the tumor and parenchyma (third ventricle floor) that were easily dissected, whereas others could hardly be separated without damaging the parenchyma. The reason for this difference remains unknown.

CONFLICT OF INTEREST

The authors (editor) declares no conflict of interest, financial or otherwise.

ACKNOWLEDGEMENTS

Declared none.

REFERENCES

[1] Karavitaki N, Cudlip S, Adams CB, Wass JA. Craniopharyngiomas. Endocr Rev 2006; 27(4): 371-97. [http://dx.doi.org/10.1210/er.2006-0002] [PMID: 16543382]

[2] Lindholm J, Nielsen EH. Craniopharyngioma: historical notes. Pituitary 2009; 12(4): 352-9. [http://dx.doi.org/10.1007/s11102-008-0165-8] [PMID: 19130248]

[3] Adamson TE, Wiestler OD, Kleihues P, Yaşargil MG. Correlation of clinical and pathological features in surgically treated craniopharyngiomas. J Neurosurg 1990; 73(1): 12-7. [http://dx.doi.org/10.3171/jns.1990.73.1.0012] [PMID: 2352012]

[4] Weiner HL, Wisoff JH, Rosenberg ME, *et al.* Craniopharyngiomas: a clinicopathological analysis of factors predictive of recurrence and functional outcome. Neurosurgery 1994; 35(6): 1001-10. [http://dx.doi.org/10.1227/00006123-199412000-00001] [PMID: 7885544]

[5] Van Effenterre R, Boch AL. Craniopharyngioma in adults and children: a study of 122 surgical cases. J Neurosurg 2002; 97(1): 3-11. [http://dx.doi.org/10.3171/jns.2002.97.1.0003] [PMID: 12134929]

[6] Müller HL. Childhood craniopharyngioma--current concepts in diagnosis, therapy and follow-up. Nat Rev Endocrinol 2010; 6(11): 609-18. [http://dx.doi.org/10.1038/nrendo.2010.168] [PMID: 20877295]

[7] Honegger J, Renner C, Fahlbusch R, Adams EF. Progesterone receptor gene expression in craniopharyngiomas and evidence for biological activity. Neurosurgery 1997; 41(6): 1359-63. [http://dx.doi.org/10.1097/00006123-199712000-00022] [PMID: 9402587]

[8] Green H, Kehinde O, Thomas J. Growth of cultured human epidermal cells into multiple epithelia suitable for grafting. Proc Natl Acad Sci USA 1979; 76(11): 5665-8. [http://dx.doi.org/10.1073/pnas.76.11.5665] [PMID: 293669]

[9] Ulfarsson E, Karström A, Yin S. Cancer Res 2005; 11(13): 4674-80.

[10] Hölsken A, Buchfelder M, Fahlbusch R, Blümcke I, Buslei R. Tumour cell migration in adamantinomatous craniopharyngiomas is promoted by activated Wnt-signalling. Acta Neuropathol 2010; 119(5): 631-9. [http://dx.doi.org/10.1007/s00401-010-0642-9] [PMID: 20131060]

[11] Hölsken A, Gebhardt M, Buchfelder M, Fahlbusch R, Blümcke I, Buslei R. EGFR signaling regulates tumor cell migration in craniopharyngiomas. Clin Cancer Res 2011; 17(13): 4367-77. [http://dx.doi.org/10.1158/1078-0432.CCR-10-2811] [PMID: 21562037]

[12] Brastianos PK, Taylor-Weiner A, Manley PE, *et al.* Exome sequencing identifies BRAF mutations in papillary craniopharyngiomas. Nat Genet 2014; 46(2): 161-5. [http://dx.doi.org/10.1038/ng.2868] [PMID: 24413733]

[13] Larkin SJ, Preda V, Karavitaki N, Grossman A, Ansorge O. BRAF V600E mutations are characteristic for papillary craniopharyngioma and may coexist with CTNNB1-mutated adamantinomatous craniopharyngioma. Acta Neuropathol 2014; 127(6): 927-9. [http://dx.doi.org/10.1007/s00401-014-1270-6] [PMID: 24715106]

[14] Bullard DE, Bigner DD. Heterotransplantation of human craniopharyngiomas in athymic "nude" mice. Neurosurgery 1979; 4(4): 308-14. [http://dx.doi.org/10.1227/00006123-197904000-00006] [PMID: 450229]

[15] Xu J, You C, Zhang S, *et al.* Angiogenesis and cell proliferation in human craniopharyngioma xenografts in nude mice. J Neurosurg 2006; 105(4) (Suppl.): 306-10. [PMID: 17328281]

[16] Gaston-Massuet C, Andoniadou CL, Signore M, *et al.* Increased Wingless (Wnt) signaling in pituitary progenitor/stem cells gives rise to pituitary tumors in mice and humans. Proc Natl Acad Sci USA 2011; 108(28): 11482-7. [http://dx.doi.org/10.1073/pnas.1101553108] [PMID: 21636786]

[17] Andoniadou CL, Gaston-Massuet C, Reddy R, *et al.* Identification of novel pathways involved in the pathogenesis of human adamantinomatous craniopharyngioma. Acta Neuropathol 2012; 124(2): 259-71. [http://dx.doi.org/10.1007/s00401-012-0957-9] [PMID: 22349813]

[18] Yaşargil MG, Curcic M, Kis M, Siegenthaler G, Teddy PJ, Roth P. Total removal of craniopharyngiomas. Approaches and long-term results in 144 patients. J Neurosurg 1990; 73(1): 3-11. [http://dx.doi.org/10.3171/jns.1990.73.1.0003] [PMID: 2352020]

[19] Karavitaki N, Wass JA. Craniopharyngiomas. Endocrinol Metab Clin North Am 2008; 37(1): 173-193, ix-x. [http://dx.doi.org/10.1016/j.ecl.2007.10.012] [PMID: 18226736]

[20] Szeifert GT, Sipos L, Horváth M, *et al.* Pathological characteristics of surgically removed craniopharyngiomas: analysis of 131 cases. Acta Neurochir (Wien) 1993; 124(2-4): 139-43. [http://dx.doi.org/10.1007/BF01401137] [PMID: 7508161]

[21] Garnett MR, Puget S, Grill J, Sainte-Rose C. Craniopharyngioma. Orphanet J Rare Dis 2007; 10(2): 18.

[22] Kulkarni V, Daniel RT, Pranatartiharan R. Spontaneous intraventricular rupture of craniopharyngioma cyst Urg Neurol 2000; 54(3): 249-53. discussion 253.

[23] Kasai H, Hirano A, Llena JF, Kawamoto K. A histopathological study of craniopharyngioma with special reference to its stroma and surrounding tissue. Brain Tumor Pathol 1997; 14(1): 41-5. [http://dx.doi.org/10.1007/BF02478867] [PMID: 9384801]

[24] Nishio Y, Takashima S, Taguchi Y, *et al.* [A case of craniopharyngioma with chemical meningitis as an initial symptom]. No To Shinkei 2001; 53(10): 957-60. [PMID: 11725506]

[25] Zhou J, Qi ST, Chen LG, *et al.* The expression of inflammatory cytokines in different inflammatory levels of adamantinomatous Craniopharyngioma Natl Med J China 2013; 93(31): 2499-502.

[26] Mori M, Takeshima H, Kuratsu J. Expression of interleukin-6 in human craniopharyngiomas: a possible inducer of tumor-associated inflammation. Int J Mol Med 2004; 14(4): 505-9. [PMID: 15375575]

[27] Liu ZZ, Ding XR. BJ YUAN, J Shi, XX KANG. Survey of the serum IL-6, IL-8,MIP-1α concentration in children with craniopharyngioma. ZhongGuo MianYiXue ZaZhi 2012; 28: 78-80.

[28] Sullivan NJ, Sasser AK, Axel AE, *et al.* Interleukin-6 induces an epithelial-mesenchymal transition phenotype in human breast cancer cells. Oncogene 2009; 28(33): 2940-7. [http://dx.doi.org/10.1038/onc.2009.180] [PMID: 19581928]

[29] Yamada D, Kobayashi S, Wada H, *et al.* Role of crosstalk between interleukin-6 and transforming growth factor-beta 1 in epithelial-mesenchymal transition and chemoresistance in biliary tract cancer. Eur J Cancer 2013; 49(7): 1725-40.
[http://dx.doi.org/10.1016/j.ejca.2012.12.002] [PMID: 23298711]

CHAPTER 6

Anatomy Based on Pterional Approach and its Extension Approach for Surgery of Craniopharyngioma

Yuntao Lu

Department of Neurosurgery, Nanfang Neurosurgery Research Institution, Nanfang Hospital, Southern Medical University, 1838 North Guangzhou Avenue, Guangzhou, China

Abstract: As the surrounding vital constructures, such as pituitary stalk, hypothalamus, third verntricule, et al, the surgery of craniopharyngioma (CP) is one of the most difficult in the field of neurosurgery. Better understanding the anatomy of sellar region, especially the related constructures to the possible origin site of CP are particularly important. In this chapter, we focus depicted the anatomy of sellar region based on the pterional approach, which is the most common surgical approach used in resection of CP. Within the description, we added the understandings about the surgical skills when removal the CP. Moreover, the morphology of tumor was analyzed and the reason of choosing pterional and its extension approach were also discussed.

Keywords: Anatomy, Craniopharyngioma, Craniotomy, Pterional approach.

PTERIONAL APPROACH AND ITS EXTENSION

Historical Overview

Pterional craniotomy was first devised and proposed by Yaşargil in 1970 [1, 2] and was based on the pioneering work conducted by previous scholars such as Parkinson *et al.* [3 - 7]. The emergence of this approach is considered a landmark micro-neurosurgical development. This craniotomy can specifically expose the entire anterior part of the frontotemporal lobe [8, 9], entire sylvian fissure opening [10], circle of Willis, anterior cisterns under the encephalon [4], and cavernous sinus (CS) while requiring less brain retraction. Even today, pterional craniotomy and the trans-sylvian approach are considered very important and are widely used in neurosurgical practice. Especially for surgical removal of craniopharyngioma,

* **Corresponding author Yuntao Lu**: Department of Neurosurgery, Nanfang Neurosurgery Research Institution, Nanfang Hospital, Southern Medical University, 1838 North Guangzhou Avenue, Guangzhou, China; Tel/Fax: +8620-61641806; E-mail: panjundu@hotmail.com

Songtao Qi (Ed.)

as the tumor have close relationship to the neurovascular structures in sellar region. The pterional approach is the most important and convenience corridor to expose this region. During the several decades following its introduction, the standard pterional approach has undergone much systematic modification by several scholars [11, 12]. As a result, some extended approaches based on the standard pterional approach have been proposed. For example, craniotomy was extended to the lateral part of the frontal bone to enlarge the exposure of the frontal lobe base, and a temporal extension was used to increase the base of the temporal lobe and lateral midbrain [13]. Moreover, after combining the technique with a cranial base approach, supraorbital craniotomy [14, 15] and orbitofrontozygomatic craniotomy [16], which are also based on exposure *via* the pterional approach, emerged for use in the treatment of lesions involving both intracranial and orbital spaces. All the above reasons indicated that the pterional and it's extended approach is the most important for surgical management of craniopharyngioma.

Position and Surgical Technique

Recently, Chaddad-Neto [17] summarized the tips and tricks of pterional craniotomy and provided details about the procedures. In general, the patient should be placed in a supine position with bilateral limbs in a neutral position. After removal of head supports, the head and neck should be held in suspension and fixed securely with three Mayfield head pins or a Sugita headrest. The cranial level should be above the height of the right atrium to facilitate venous blood return. Notably, close attention should be paid to the pin positions to prevent the operative holder from obstructing the surgeon's view of the procedures. The ipsilateral pin should be placed on the mastoid region while avoiding the air cells. The two contralateral pins should be set on the contralateral superior temporal line above the temporal muscle. Pin placement should be avoided on the paranasal sinus, mastoid gasification cells, and squamous part of temporal bone because of the weak external bone lamella. Moreover, the pin should not be placed on the temporal muscle; as this cannot be penetrated, the pin will not contact a bony surface. Strive to maintain a line from the ipsilateral pin on the mastoid and the contralateral anterior pins in parallel positions on the superior temporal line in order to avoid any head movement, especially when using fish hooks for tight retraction of the cranial skin and muscle flaps.

The proper surgical head position should be regulated following the five steps of traction, lifting, deflection, rotation, and torsion. Firstly, the patient's head, along with the Mayfield holder, should be retracted towards the surgeons. Next, the head level should be lifted above the right atrial position. According to operation requirements, the head and neck should be deflected and rotated. In general, the classical pterional approach required a contralateral head rotation of 45° with hypsokinesis of 10-15°. However, if a subfrontal approach is added, the rotation should be decreased to 35-40° degrees and if the subtemporal corridor is used, the rotation should be increased to 60°. Torsion should be emphasized, as many surgeons have ignored this procedure. This step can increase the angles between the head, neck, and ipsilateral shoulder, thus facilitating improved proximity of the neurosurgeon to the surgical region and aiding surgical manipulation.

Anatomical Figures (Figs. 1-8)

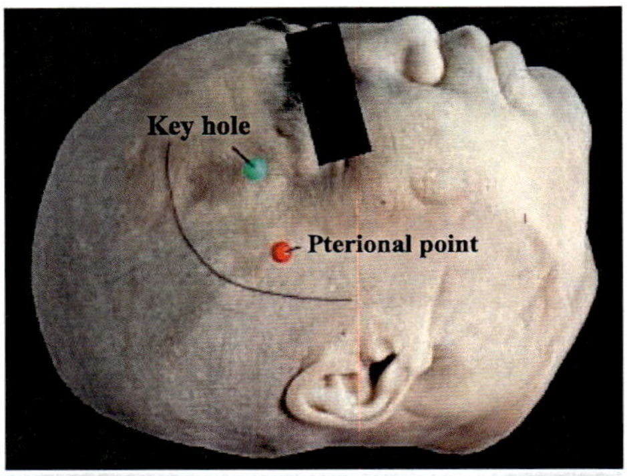

Fig. (1). Surgical incision of the standard pterional approach. The incision originates 1–1.5 cm in front of the tragus while avoiding the main trunk of the superficial temporal artery. Within the hairline, the incision course remains vertical to the zygomatic arch until the superior temporal line and then turns forward, ending 2.5 cm beside the midline. The incision should include the location of the pterional point. The locations of the keyhole (frontal angle) and pterional point are indicated in the (Fig. **2**).

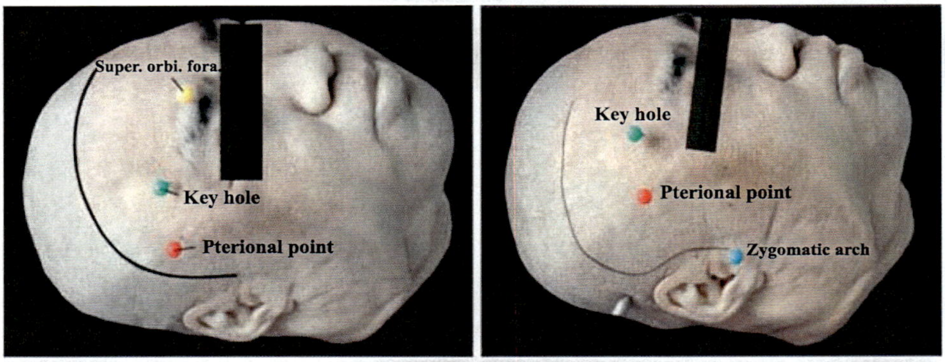

Fig. (2). Pterional extended approach. Depending on the lesion involvement, the classic pterional incision can be modified forward (frontal side) and backward (temporal side). For frontal extension, the incision can be elongated to the skin above the superior orbital foramen (Super. orbi. fora.) and inside the hairline. In this scenario, the skin flap can be retracted forward to expose the frontal bone lateral to the superior orbital foramen. In sequence, both the pterional bone flap and ipsilateral subfrontal approach can be exposed. The incision can be adapted to a question-mark shape that extends temporally and traverses above the auricular, thus providing exposure *via* a combined pterional and subtemporal approach.

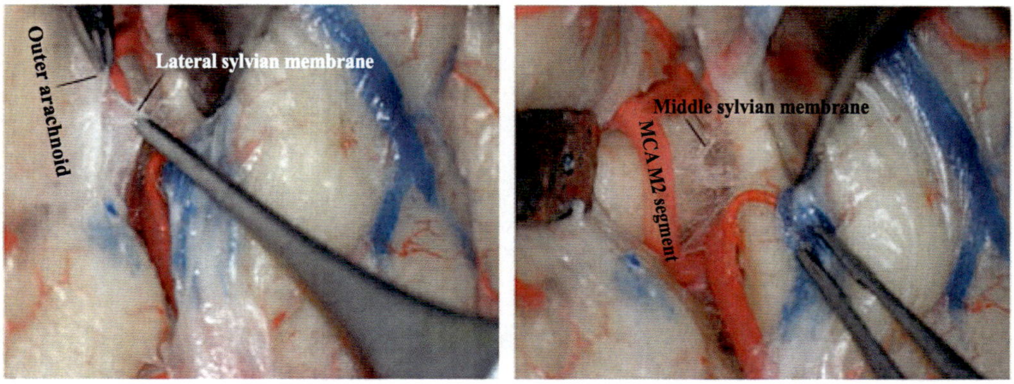

Fig. (3). Separation of the sylvian fissure. Further opening of the lateral sylvian membrane exposes the M2 and M3 segments of the middle cranial artery (MCA). Meanwhile, beneath the M2 segment, the middle sylvian membrane is found to connect the median aspect of the frontal lobe to the temporal lobe.

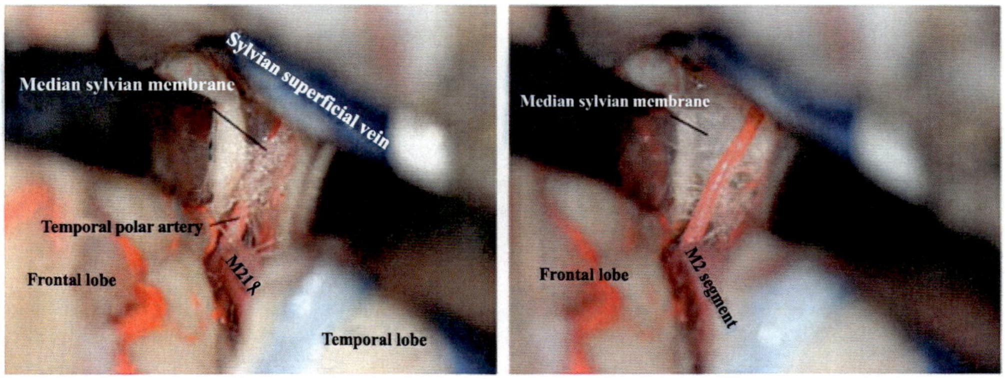

Fig. (4). Separation of the sylvian fissure. After opening the median sylvian membrane and further dissection, the temporal polar artery that originates from M2 segment of middle cerebral artery is covered by the median sylvian membrane. This median membrane tightly connects the temporal pole and basement of the frontal lobe. Following further opening of superficial temporal polar artery membrane, the median sylvian is shown to close the internal carotid cistern.

Separation of the sylvian fissure. Normally, the frontal side of the sylvian superficial vein is selected for separation because it provides the main drainage of venous blood to the sphenoparietal sinus. The branches toward the frontal side need to be cut. When opening the outer arachnoid, the far lateral sylvian membrane (inner arachnoid) covers the surface of the superficial vein. The far lateral sylvian membrane, or the lateral sylvian membrane adhered from frontal lobe to the temporal lobe, is dissected further. The M2 and M3 segments of the middle cerebral artery course beneath the lateral sylvian membrane.

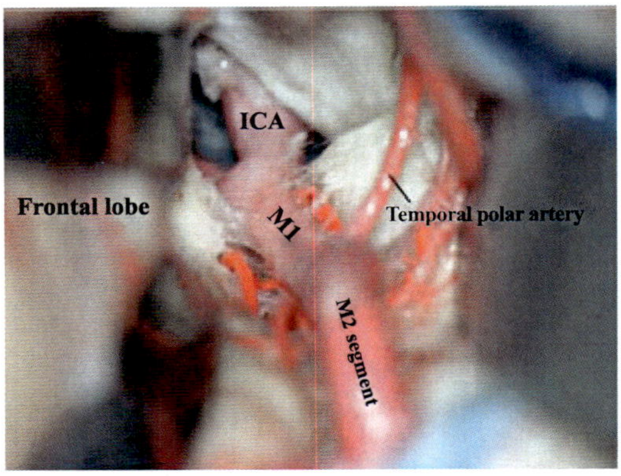

Fig. (5). Separation of the sylvian fissure. When opening the median sylvian membrane and lateral wall of the internal carotid cistern, the internal carotid artery (ICA) and M1 segment of the middle cerebral artery are exposed. Meanwhile, many arachnoid trabeculae from the frontal basement and temporal pole connect the ICA and M1 segment to secure arteries within the internal carotid cistern.

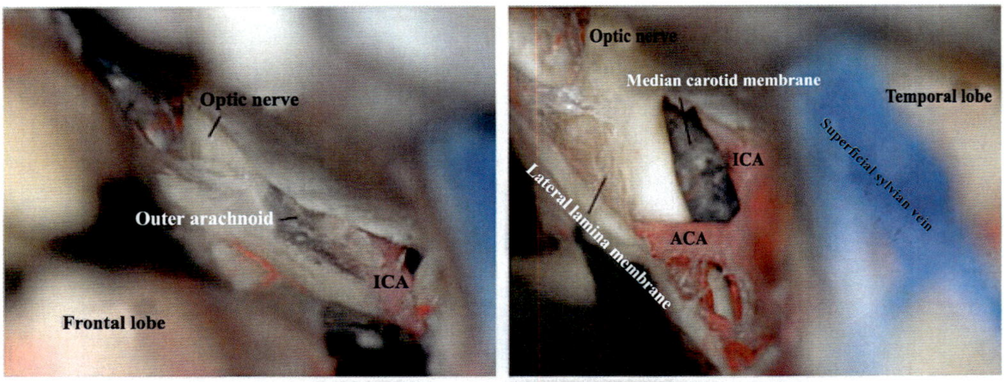

Fig. (6). After lifting the frontal lobe, the basal membrane arachnoid (outer arachnoid) covering the surface of the optic nerve can be observed. Further opening of this membrane exposes structures located within the optic chiasm and ICA cisterns, including the ipsilateral ICA and A1 segment of the anterior cerebral artery (ACA) with its perforating arteries. In the meantime, the median wall of the ICA cistern can be identified as the lateral lamina membrane. The A1 segment perforates the lateral lamina membrane and enters the lamina terminalis cistern. Through the second space (optic-ICA space), the median carotid membrane is shown to compose the ICA cistern floor.

PTERIONAL APPROACH WITH SUB-TEMPORAL EXTENSION

The subtemporal approach was first used at the end of the 19th century; however, the first attempt to treat a trigeminal nerve lesion *via* this approach was made by Frazier in 1901 [18, 19]. In 1905, Cushing reported a 5% mortality rate for this approach, indicating a significant improvement in the quality of treatment for middle cranial fossa lesions. The subtemporal approach has been accepted widely since the fifth decade of the 20th century. In 1962, Kurze attempted the subtemporal extradural approach, or middle cranial fossa approach, to investigate the internal acoustic meatus as well as the cerebellopontine angle region. In 1968, Drake [20] reported clasping a basilar artery (BA) aneurysm *via* this approach. Both Glasscock and Kawase modified this approach in accordance with anatomical development and an understanding of the temporal region and drilled the Glasscock and Kawase triangle of petrous bone to ligate the petrous segment of the internal carotid artery, clasp a BA aneurysm, and remove petroclival region tumors.

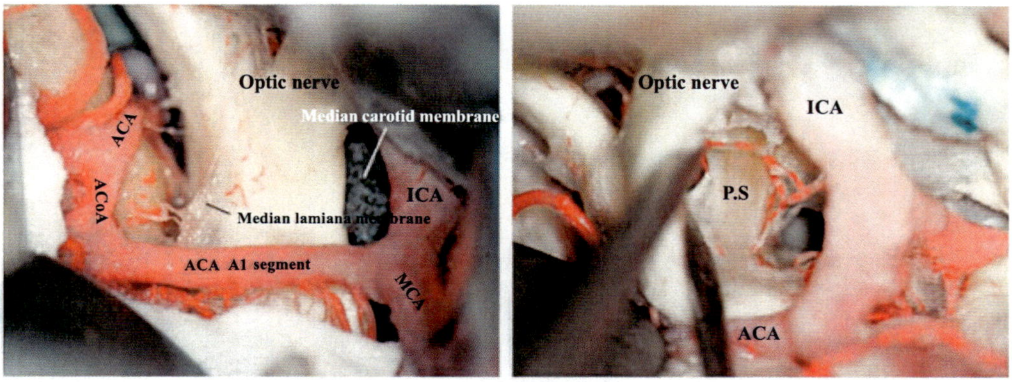

Fig. (7). After further dissection of the lateral lamina membrane, the entire ipsilateral ACA A1 segment, anterior communicating artery (ACoA), and contralateral ACA are exposed. The lamina terminalis, median lamina membrane, and Heubner recurrent artery can also be observed. Lifting of the ipsilateral optical nerve and dissection of the median carotid membrane exposes the pituitary stalk (P.S.) and superior hypophyseal artery, which originates from the ICA.

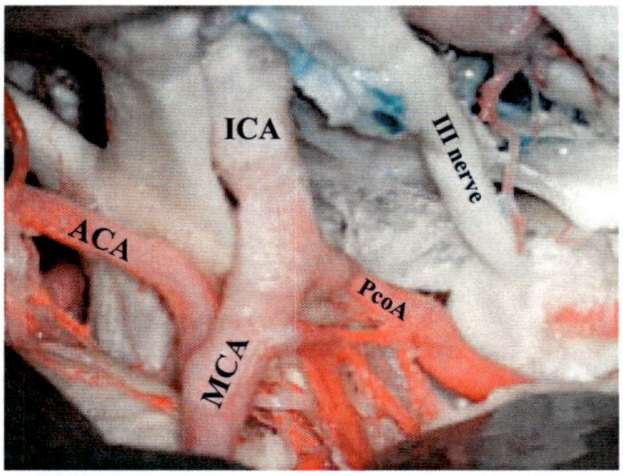

Fig. (8). Entire view of the sellar region after total separation. The posterior communicating artery (PcoA), anterior choroidal artery, and perforating arteries are exposed. In addition to vascular structures, the ipsilateral cranial nerve III and Liliequist membrane can be identified. Opening the CS roof also exposes the CS-ICA and meningohypophyseal trunk.

To extend exposure with this approach, Goel [21] enlarged dissection of the zygomatic arch, upper wall of the external acoustic meatus to complete the removal of a petroclival region tumor. In 1985, Fujitsu [22] removed the zygomatic arch and part of the lateral orbital wall together with the subtemporal approach to treat lesions located inside the interpeduncular cistern. In the following several decades, these extended approaches [23, 24] have been widely used and modified still further to provide greater exposure. The pterional approach with subtemporal extension is usually used to expose the sellar and parasellar region, edge of the tentorium, anterior part of the petrous bone when incising the tentorium, and interpeduncular region [25 - 29].

Anatomical Figures (Figs. 9-16)

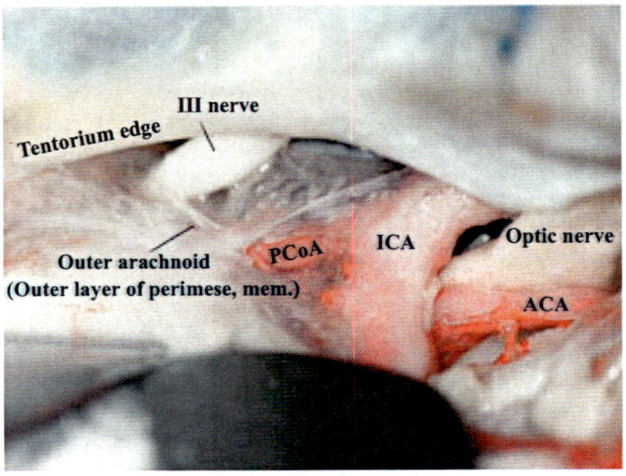

Fig. (9). When lifting the temporal lobe, the outer layer of the perimesencephalic membrane (Peimese. Mem.) can be observed. The III cranial nerve penetrates the outer arachnoid and then courses into the CS. The PCoA from the ICA courses under the outer arachnoid.

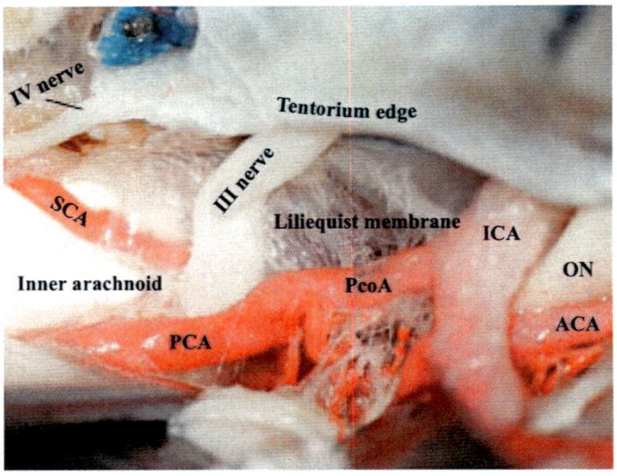

Fig. (10). After dissecting the tentorium behind the trochlear nerve entrance and opening the outer arachnoid, the PcoA and its perforating arteries are observed within the oculomotor cistern. The Liliequist membrane (diencephal lobe and mesencephal lobe) comprises the anteromedial wall of the oculomotor cistern. Meanwhile, the inner layer of the perimesencephalic membrane covers the supercerebellar artery (SCA) and posterior carotid artery (PCA).

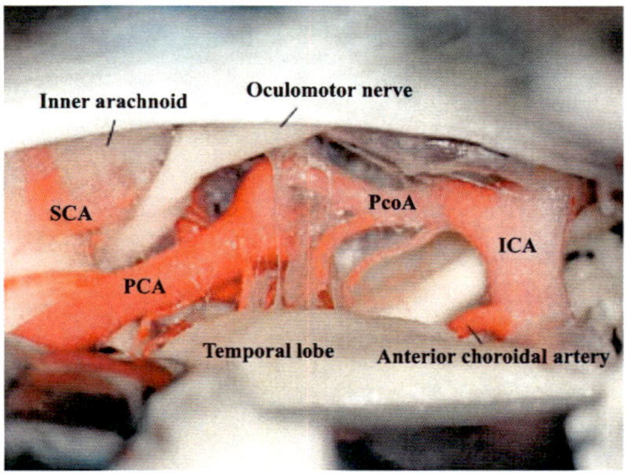

Fig. (11). Forward separation exposes the ICA, PcoA, PCA, and anterior choroidal artery. The optic nerve ventral structures are also visible.

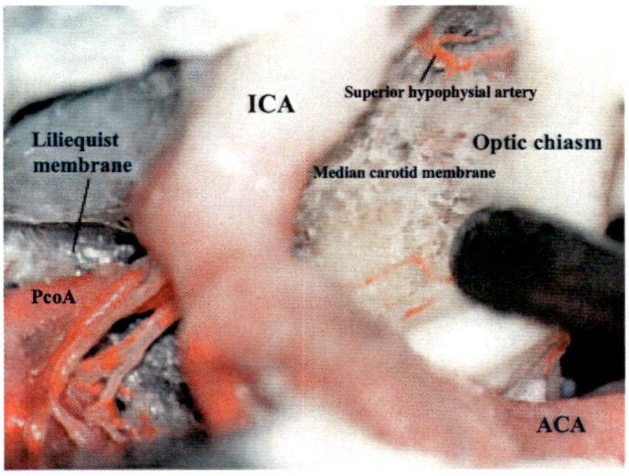

Fig. (12). Separation through the second space (optic-carotid space) exposes the median carotid membrane located at the ventral optic chiasm; this separates the ICA cistern and optic chiasm cistern. The Liliequist membrane is located behind the dorsum sellae.

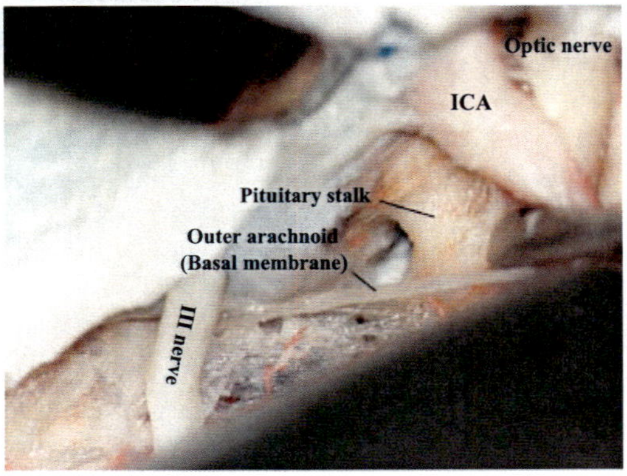

Fig. (13). Retraction of the ICA to expose the arachnoidal sleeve of the pituitary stalk, which originates from the outer arachnoid (basal arachnoid membrane). The Liliequist membrane is shown to form the anteromedial wall of the oculomotor cistern.

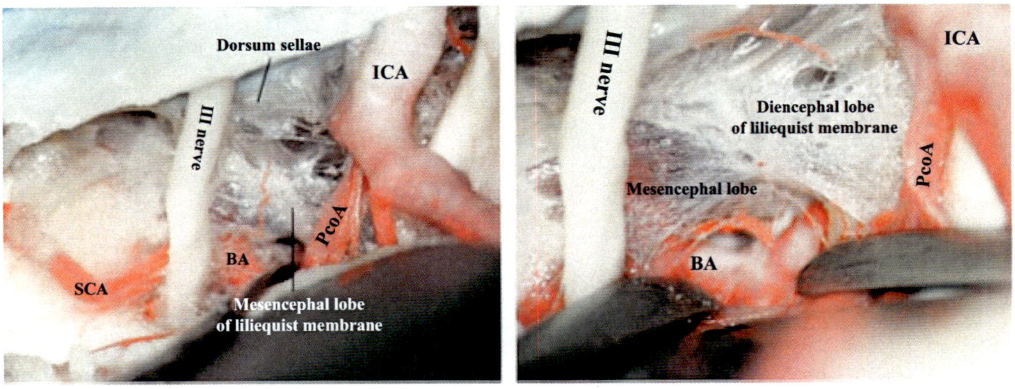

Fig. (14). The diencephal lobe and mesencephal lobes of the Liliequist membrane comprise the anteromedial wall of the oculomotor cistern. The diencephal lobe connects the dorsum sellae and mammillary body, whereas the mesencephal lobe connects the dorsum sellae and BA tip.

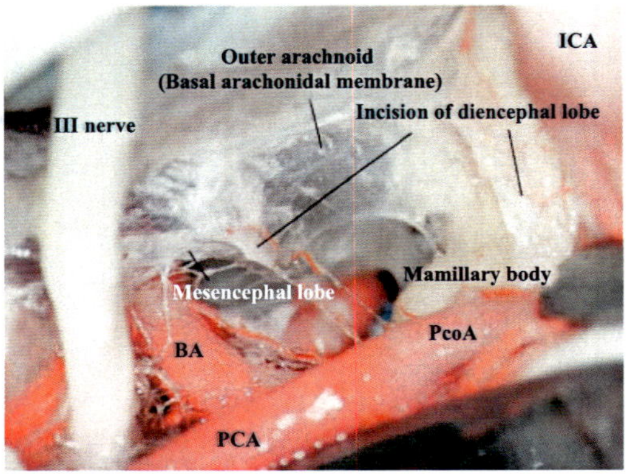

Fig. (15). After dissecting the diencephal lobe of the Liliequist membrane, the mammillary bodies, BA, and PCA are clearly exposed. The mesencephal lobe originates from the dorsum sellae and connects the BA tip.

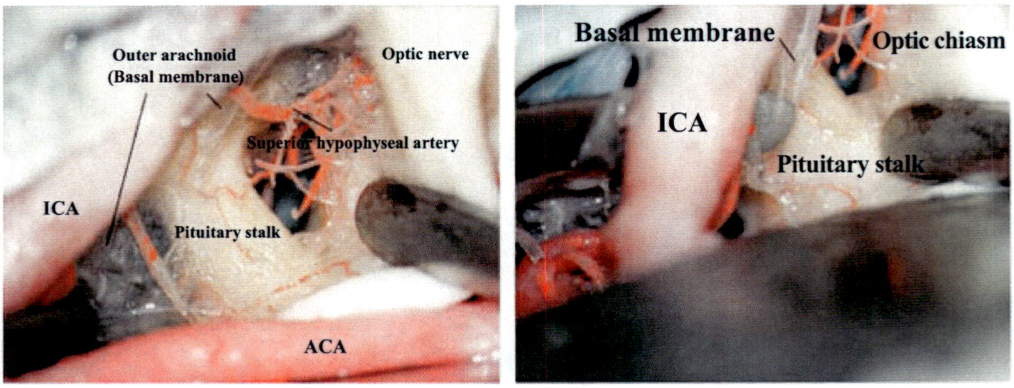

Fig. (16). Opening the median carotid membrane exposes the pituitary stalk, superior hypophyseal artery, and ventral optic chiasm. Moreover, the basal arachnoid membrane forms the membranous sleeve of the pituitary stalk.

SURGERY OF CRANIOPHARYNGIOMA

Pterional approach might be the most classic and frequently used approach in Neurosurgery. The approach can provide enough exposure for the surgical space of sellar region through dissection of the nature corridor. As tumor located at sellar region, pterional and it's extension approaches certainly play indispensable role to treat craniopharyngioma. As our opinion, for purely extra-axial CP Figs. (**17** and **18**), the pterional approach was first choice as it can avoid the dissection of the nervous tissue.

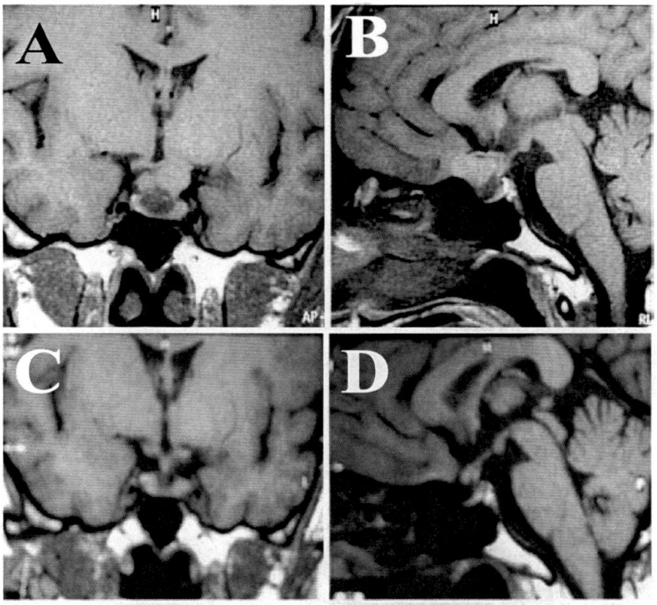

Fig. (17). A 37-year-old female patient presented with decreased visual accuracy in the left eye for 6 months. Physical examination revealed no significant positive results except for temporal hemianopia and decreased vision in the left eye. Presurgical and postsurgical magnetic resonance imaging (MRI) of the present case. **A-B.** Sagittal and coronal MRI scans indicated that the tumor mainly occupied the prechiasmatic subarachnoid cistern space. The site of tumor origin was located in the middle segment of the pituitary stalk. **C-D.** Postsurgical MRI revealed total tumor removal with good pituitary stalk preservation.

For such kind of purely extra-axial CP, patients always suffered with only minor and partial hypopituitarism, and without significant hypothalamic dysfunction. The visual defect was limited and reversible. So the surgical aims should be 1) Total tumor removal; 2) Attempted preservation of hypothalamus–infundibulum–pituitary axis continuity to the extent possible.

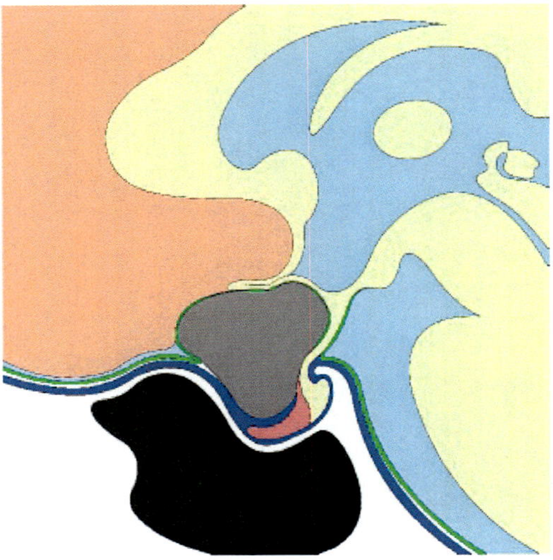

Fig. (18). Schematic Fig. (revealing the tumor morphology and its relationship with the surrounding structures. Blue line: Dura mater (Diaphragm and sellar floor dura); Green line: Arachnoid mater. Notably, as the extra-arachonidal origination, the tumor surface was covered by a layer of arachnoid membrane.

As concerned with the tumoral growth pattern, a typical extra-axial CP with purely subarachnoid intracisternal location might originate from the subarachnoid segment of the pituitary stalk (PS). The lesion predominantly occupied the chiasmatic arachnoidal cistern with external growth from the third ventricle floor (3rd VF). The majority of the PS was intact except at the site of tumor origin. The basilar membranous arachnoid covered the tumor surface and provided an interface between the tumor and adjacent neurovascular structures. Given the tumor's cisternal occupation, an extra-axial route was selected. During surgery after dissecting the lateral fissure, the suprasellar tumor was exposed. Significant arachnoidal septation existed between the tumor and optic nerves. The site of tumor origin was located at the lower segment of the PS (Fig. **19**).

As most of CP will have close relation to the optic nerves and also pre-chiasmatic space. Lateral frontal extension of pterional approach can use the sub-frontal corridor and also classical sylvian fissure spaces to provide extra-exposure to the lamina terminalis, the contra-lateral optic nerve, and even ICA. So pterional with it lateral frontal extension was most frequently and commonly used. In some cases, the pterional combined with bilateral frontal expanding need to be selected to provide extra-exposure by usage of interhemispheric corridor (Fig. **20**). Meanwhile, the infundibulo-tuberal CP will sometimes combine with extended sub-arachnoidal expanding, Under this situation, pterional approach can provided both intra-axial exposure by opening lamina terminalis and also extra-axial exposure.

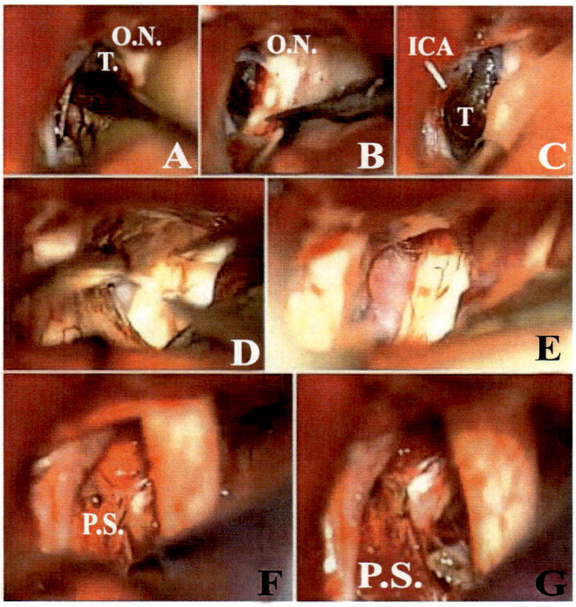

Fig. (19). Intraoperative findings. **A-E.** A significant arachnoidal interface existed between the tumor, internal carotid artery, and bilateral optic nerves. The tumor was safely separated along this interface. **F-G.** The site of tumor origin was located at the lower segment of the pituitary stalk.

As the sample of Fig. (**20**), this cystic tumor involved several subarachnoid spaces, including the chiasmatic cistern, exterior and interior carotid artery cisterns (left side), and olfactory cistern (Fig. **21**). Part of the cystic wall intruded into the ventral aspect of the frontal lobe. The left-side internal carotid artery (ICA) and its branches as well as cranial nerve III were surrounded by the tumor, which required sharp surgical dissection. Coarse calcification had tightly adhered to the PS and possible to the left carotid artery. However, even with extremely frontal expanding, this main body of this kind of CP was still intra-cisternal location with similar with purely extra-aixal CP. The origination site was still the subarachonidal segment of pituitary stalk. So the surgical aim was still total tumor removal while attempting to anatomically preserve hypothalamus–infundibulum–pituitary axis continuity.

During the surgery by the right-side pterional with lateral frontal expanding approach (Fig. **22**), we found a identifiable membranous interface between tumor and optic nerves, ICA, and its branches. The only place where closely relationship between tumor to the nervous tissue happened was the origination site at the middle and upper segment of pituitary stalk.

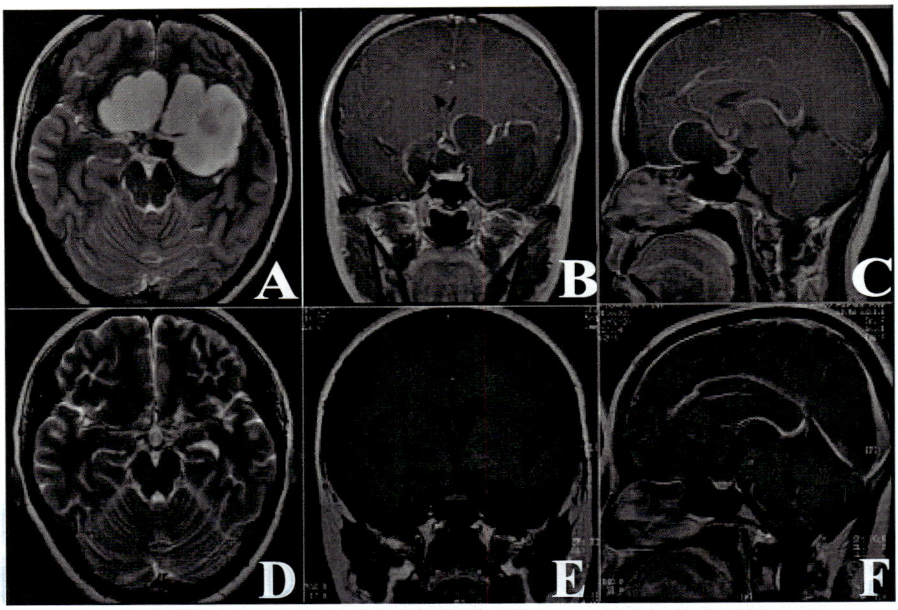

Fig. (20). A 24-year-old female patient with a 2-year history of menstrual disorders and a 2-month history of amenorrhea. She experienced repeated headaches, decreased visual accuracy, and olfactory dysfunction for 1 month without nausea or vomiting. **A-C.** Presurgical MRI indicated a cystic tumor mainly located at the optic chiasmatic cistern with extensive expansion to the anterior cranial fossa and right-side middle fossa through the enlarged first space. The pituitary stalk is located at the right posterior side of the tumor. **D-F.** Postsurgical MRI indicated total tumor removal with preservation of the pituitary stalk and third ventricle floor.

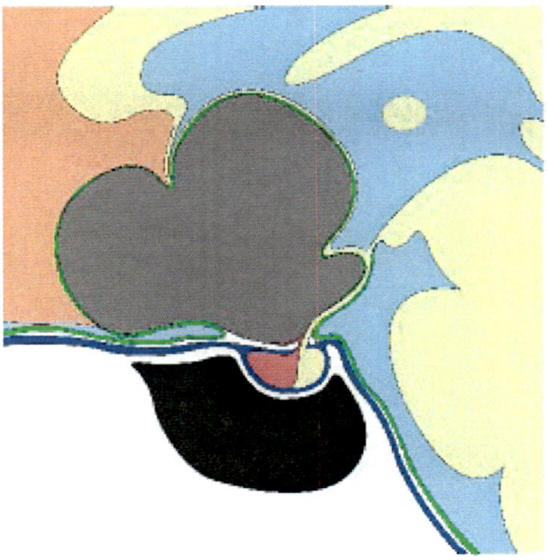

Fig. (21). Schematic Fig. (demonstrating the tumor morphology and relationships with the surrounding structures. Blue line: Dura mater (Diaphragm and sellar floor dura); Green line: Arachnoid mater. Notably, as the extra-arachonidal origination, the tumor surface was covered by a layer of arachnoid membrane. It might provide a separating interface from the surrounding structures except the origination site.

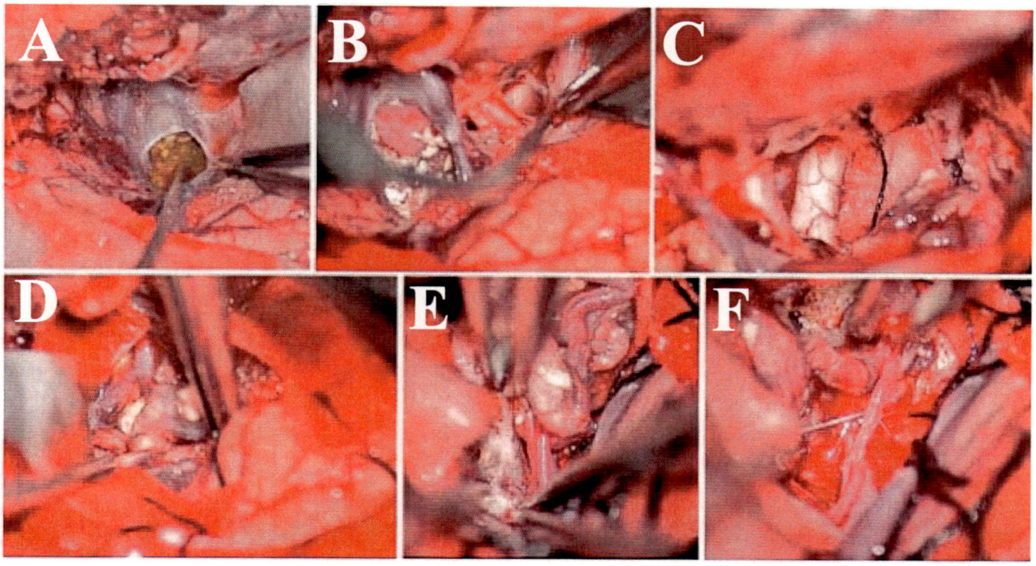

Fig. (22). Intraoperative findings. **A:** After craniotomy, the lateral fissure was dissected to expose the tumor. The huge cystic tumor was located beneath the arachnoid membrane. Therefore, the tumor had expanded along the potential space between the frontal lobe and arachnoid, causing tight adhesion between the tumor cystic wall and nervous tissue that required sharp dissection. Punctate calcification was observed on the tumor wall. **B-C** After sharp dissection, the bilateral optical nerves were exposed. **D.** The calcified tumor had adhered tightly to the left side of the internal carotid artery (ICA) and its branches, thus presenting significant challenges to surgical removal. **E-F.** The ICA branches were separated from the tumor and preserved well.

For CP with posterior expanding to occupy the inter-peduncular cistern, prepontile cistern or even reaching upper cervical cistern Figs. (**23** and **24**), classic pterional approach should be modified by extending to the sub-temporal exposure. Under this condition, the sub-temporal corridor must be used, and the tentorium sometimes should be dissected to provide extra infra-tentorial exposure.

Although posterior expanding, the tumor had still mainly developed within subarachnoid space without involving the hypothalamic structure (Fig. **25**). The Liliequist membrane still separated tumor to the basilar artery and its' branches. Normally, tumor protruded to the posterior fossa through later side of pituitary stalk with originate site of CP always located at the side-place of PS. So the surgical aim was still radical tumor removal. A right-side pterional approach with sub-temporal expanding was used to remove the tumor.

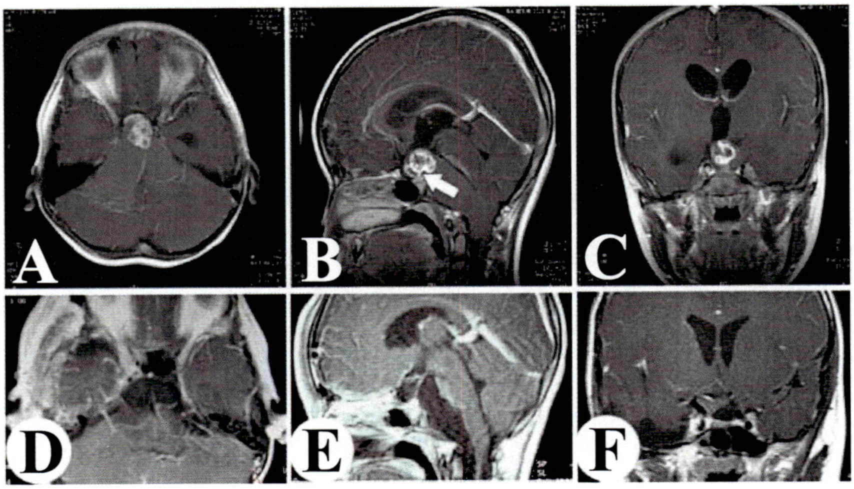

Fig. (23). A 6-year-old male patient with a 2-month history of progressively aggravated headache and a 10-day history of nausea and vomiting. The patient exhibited normal consciousness. Endocrinological detection indicated slightly increased FSH and PRL levels. **A-C.** Presurgical MRI indicated a huge mixed cystic-solid tumor in the suprasellar region with extensive expansion toward the posterior cranial fossa. The lower part of the tumor reached the C2 segment. The brain stem and upper cervical spinal cord were significantly compressed backward. The lower part of the pituitary stalk was observed on enhanced T1-weighted images (white arrow). The optic chiasm and anterior communicating artery complex were displaced upward and anteriorly. **D-F.** Postsurgical MRI scan confirmed total tumor removal. The third ventricle floor was preserved.

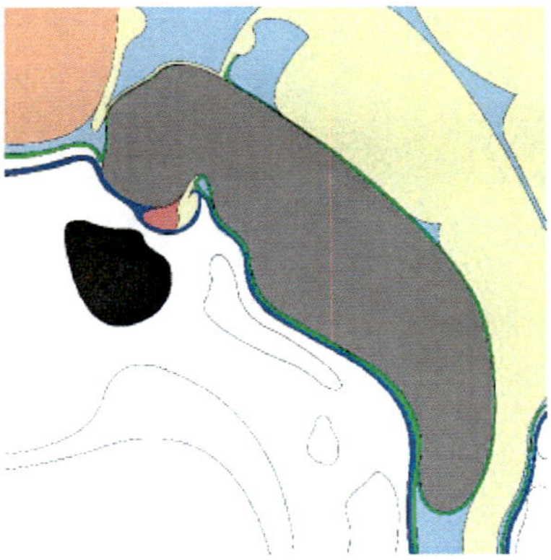

Fig. (24). Schematic Fig. (demonstrating the tumor morphology and relationship with the surrounding structures. Blue line: Dura mater (Diaphragm and sellar floor dura); Green line: Arachnoid mater. Notably, the related compact Liliequist membrane provided a clear interface and block the adherence of tumor to the surrounding structures in the posterior cranial fossa.

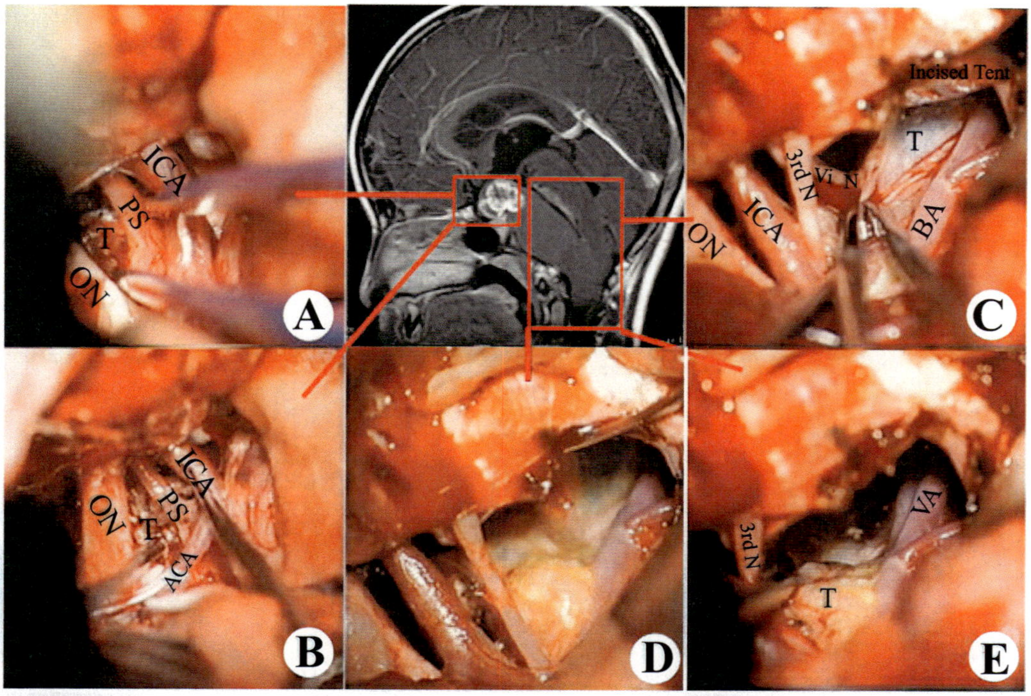

Fig. (25). Intraoperative findings. **A-B.** The suprasellar part of the tumor was exposed through the internal carotid artery-optic nerve space. The tumor adhered closely to the surrounding neurovascular structures and originated from the infundibular part of the hypothalamus and pituitary stalk. **C.** Tumor expansion resulted in a large surgical manipulation space. Through the enlarged space behind cranial nerve III, expansion of the cystic tumor to the posterior cranial fossa was observed. **D-E.** To increase exposure of the posterior cranial fossa, an incision was made to open the tentorium. The tumor was separated along the cystic wall. Sharp dissection was used to remove the section of tumor that adhered tightly to the brain stem and vascular structures.

CONFLICT OF INTEREST

The author (editor) declares no conflict of interest, financial or otherwise.

ACKNOWLEDGEMENTS

We should acknowledge Dr. Shi Jin for preparing the cadaver specimens and assistant about the anatomical studies.

REFERENCES

[1] Krayenbühl HA, Yaşargil MG, Flamm ES, Tew JM Jr. Microsurgical treatment of intracranial saccular aneurysms. J Neurosurg 1972; 37(6): 678-86. [http://dx.doi.org/10.3171/jns.1972.37.6.0678] [PMID: 4654697]

[2] Yasargil MG, Antic J, Laciga R, Jain KK, Hodosh RM, Smith RD. Microsurgical pterional approach to aneurysms of the basilar bifurcation. Surg Neurol 1976; 6(2): 83-91. [PMID: 951657]

[3] Yasargil MG, Fox JL. The microsurgical approach to intracranial aneurysms. Surg Neurol 1975; 3(1): 7-14.
[PMID: 1111150]

[4] Yasargil MG, Kasdaglis K, Jain KK, Weber HP. Anatomical observations of the subarachnoid cisterns of the brain during surgery. J Neurosurg 1976; 44(3): 298-302.
[http://dx.doi.org/10.3171/jns.1976.44.3.0298] [PMID: 1082498]

[5] Yaşargil MG. A legacy of microneurosurgery: memoirs, lessons, and axioms. Neurosurgery 1999; 45(5): 1025-92.
[http://dx.doi.org/10.1097/00006123-199911000-00014] [PMID: 10549924]

[6] Parkinson D. A surgical approach to the cavernous portion of the carotid artery. Anatomical studies and case report. J Neurosurg 1965; 23(5): 474-83.
[http://dx.doi.org/10.3171/jns.1965.23.5.0474] [PMID: 5858438]

[7] Parkinson D. Transcavernous repair of carotid cavernous fistula. Case report. J Neurosurg 1967; 26(4): 420-4.
[http://dx.doi.org/10.3171/jns.1967.26.4.0420] [PMID: 6021346]

[8] Chaddad K, Carvalhal R, de Oliveira E. A craniotomia pterional, description passo a passo. Arq Neuropsiquiatr 2007; (65): 101-6.
[http://dx.doi.org/10.1590/S0004-282X2007000100021]

[9] Yaşargil MG. Personal considerations on the history of microneurosurgery. J Neurosurg 2010; 112(6): 1163-75.
[http://dx.doi.org/10.3171/2009.7.JNS091124] [PMID: 19747053]

[10] Türe U, Yaşargil DC, Al-Mefty O, Yaşargil MG. Topographic anatomy of the insular region. J Neurosurg 1999; 90(4): 720-33.
[http://dx.doi.org/10.3171/jns.1999.90.4.0720] [PMID: 10193618]

[11] Figueiredo EG, Oliveira AM, Plese JP, Teixeira MJ. Perspective of the frontolateral craniotomies. Arq Neuropsiquiatr 2010; 68(3): 430-2.
[http://dx.doi.org/10.1590/S0004-282X2010000300020] [PMID: 20602050]

[12] Kim E, Delashaw JJ. Osteoplastic pterional craniotomy revisited. Neurosurgery 2011; 68(1 Suppl Operative): 125-9. discussion 129
[http://dx.doi.org/10.1227/NEU.0b013e318207b3e3]

[13] Mariniello G, de Divitiis O, Seneca V, Maiuri F. Classical pterional compared to the extended skull base approach for the removal of clinoidal meningiomas. J Clin Neurosci 2012; 19(12): 1646-50.
[http://dx.doi.org/10.1016/j.jocn.2011.12.033] [PMID: 23063496]

[14] Shimano H, Nagasawa S, Kawabata S, Ogawa R, Ohta T. Surgical strategy for meningioma extension into the optic canal. Neurol Med Chir (Tokyo) 2000; 40(9): 447-51.
[http://dx.doi.org/10.2176/nmc.40.447] [PMID: 11021075]

[15] Rohde V, Schaller K, Hassler W. The combined pterional and orbitocygomatic approach to extensive tumours of the lateral and latero-basal orbit and orbital apex. Acta Neurochir (Wien) 1995; 132(1-3): 127-30.
[http://dx.doi.org/10.1007/BF01404859] [PMID: 7754846]

[16] McDermott MW, Durity FA, Rootman J, Woodhurst WB. Combined frontotemporal-orbitozygomatic approach for tumors of the sphenoid wing and orbit. Neurosurgery 1990; 26(1): 107-16.
[http://dx.doi.org/10.1227/00006123-199001000-00015] [PMID: 2152976]

[17] Chaddad-Neto F, Campos Filho JM, Dória-Netto HL, Faria MH, Ribas GC, Oliveira E. The pterional craniotomy: tips and tricks. Arq Neuropsiquiatr 2012; 70(9): 727-32.
[http://dx.doi.org/10.1590/S0004-282X2012000900015] [PMID: 22990732]

[18] Spiller WG. Pathological report on a case of dermatitis vesiculo-bullosa et gangraenosa mutilans

manuum (duhring), with a consideration of the relations of vascular and nervous changes to spontaneous gangrene and ray naud's disease. J Exp Med 1900; 5(1): 91-100. [http://dx.doi.org/10.1084/jem.5.1.91] [PMID: 19866938]

[19] Spiller WG. The pathological changes in the nerye System in a Case of Lead Poisoning. J Med Res 1903; 10(1): 142-152.1, 1. [PMID: 19971557]

[20] Drake CG. The surgical treatment of aneurysms of the basilar artery. J Neurosurg 1968; 29(4): 436-46. [http://dx.doi.org/10.3171/jns.1968.29.4.0436] [PMID: 4880820]

[21] Goel A. Extended lateral subtemporal approach for petroclival meningiomas: report of experience with 24 cases. Br J Neurosurg 1999; 13(3): 270-5. [http://dx.doi.org/10.1080/02688699943673] [PMID: 10562837]

[22] Fujitsu K, Kuwabara T. Zygomatic approach for lesions in the interpeduncular cistern. J Neurosurg 1985; 62(3): 340-3. [http://dx.doi.org/10.3171/jns.1985.62.3.0340] [PMID: 3973701]

[23] Hakuba A, Liu S, Nishimura S. The orbitozygomatic infratemporal approach: a new surgical technique. Surg Neurol 1986; 26(3): 271-6. [http://dx.doi.org/10.1016/0090-3019(86)90161-8] [PMID: 3738722]

[24] Hakuba A, Tanaka K, Suzuki T, Nishimura S. A combined orbitozygomatic infratemporal epidural and subdural approach for lesions involving the entire cavernous sinus. J Neurosurg 1989; 71(5 Pt 1): 699-704. [http://dx.doi.org/10.3171/jns.1989.71.5.0699] [PMID: 2809723]

[25] Day JD, Fukushima T, Giannotta SL. Innovations in surgical approach: lateral cranial base approaches. Clin Neurosurg 1996; 43: 72-90. [PMID: 9247796]

[26] Froelich S, *et al.* Extension of the one-piece orbitozygomatic frontotemporal approach to the glenoid fossa: cadaveric study. Cadaveric study Neurosurgery 2008; 62(5 Suppl 2): 312-7. [http://dx.doi.org/10.1227/01.neu.0000326012.91939.fb]

[27] Goel A. Extended middle fossa approach for petroclival lesions. Acta Neurochir (Wien) 1995; 135(1-2): 78-83. [http://dx.doi.org/10.1007/BF02307418] [PMID: 8748796]

[28] Zhao JC, Liu JK. Transzygomatic extended middle fossa approach for upper petroclival skull base lesions. Neurosurg Focus 2008; 25(6): E5. Discussion E5 [http://dx.doi.org/10.3171/FOC.2008.25.12.E5]

[29] Sakata S, Fujii K, Matsushima T, *et al.* Aneurysm of the posterior cerebral artery: report of eleven cases--surgical approaches and procedures. Neurosurgery 1993; 32(2): 163-7. [http://dx.doi.org/10.1227/00006123-199302000-00002] [PMID: 8437652]

CHAPTER 7

Anatomy Based on Interhemispheric Approach for Surgery of Craniopharyngioma

Yuntao Lu*

Department of Neurosurgery, Nanfang Neurosurgery Research Institution, Nanfang Hospital, Southern Medical University, 1838 North Guangzhou Avenue, Guangzhou, China

Abstract: In this chapter, based on interhemispheric approaches including the corridor through fronto-basal, anterior part of interhemispheric space and also through inter-fonix corridor, we illustrated the advantage of different approaches. And the related structures such as, pituitary gland, pituitary stalk, and hypothalamus were depicted under such surgical view. The other accessory structures, for example, optic pathway, sphenoid sinus and also the cavernous sinus were described as well. Moreover, the morphological features of craniopharyngioma were analyzed and then how to choose the most appropriate approaches was discussed.

Keywords: Anatomy, Craniopharyngioma, Craniotomy, Interhemispheric approach.

FRONTOBASAL INTERHEMISPHERIC APPROACH

Historical Overview

As summarized by Zeleny in 1984 [1], frontal craniotomy initially opened only the anterior wall of the frontal sinus to treat lesions inside the sinus. In 1926, Dandy [2] further removed the posterior wall of the frontal sinus to expose and repair CSF leakage. In subsequent decades, several scholars developed and modified this craniotomy to propose a trans-frontal base approach. In 1981, Suzuki [3] first used a subfrontal approach to complete the treatment of an AcoA aneurysm. As it provides a direct route to the anterior cranial fossa and sellar region floor, the subfrontal approach was widely accepted for the treatment of lesions in the anterior cranial fossa and intra- or supra-sellar region. However, the subfrontal or single trans-callosal approach was quite difficult for some lesions

* **Corresponding author Yuntao Lu**: Department of Neurosurgery, Nanfang Neurosurgery Research Institution, Nanfang Hospital, Southern Medical University, 1838 North Guangzhou Avenue, Guangzhou, China; Tel/Fax: +8620-61641806; E-mail: lllu2000yun@gmail.com

Songtao Qi (Ed.)

such as craniopharyngioma originating from the sellar region with suprasellar cistern involvement and protrusion into the third or even lateral ventricle [4, 5].

Fahlbusch *et al.* [4], Oi *et al.* [5], and Suzuki *et al.* [6] described using an interhemispheric approach to treat such lesions. Subsequently, other scholars [7 - 9] proposed a frontobasal combined interhemispheric approach and suggested that this combined approach could provide a good view of infundibulohypophyseal axial structures, would tend not to require strong retraction of the frontal lobes, and could preserve the olfactory tracts [10 - 12]. In cases of suprasellar region lesions that inferoposteriorly displace the third ventricle, this approach provides a wide operative field in which to expose the lamina terminalis without causing significant damage to brain tissues. Using a trans-lamina terminalis approach, lesions with partial third ventricular cavity involvement can also be removed.

Position and Surgical Technique

Patients should be placed in the supine position after general anesthesia and intubation. The neck should be deflexed approximately 10–15° degrees to rotate the vertex towards the floor. The head should be placed in a slight extension. Use three or four head pins and a Mayfield holder to fix the head safely.

Anatomical Figures (Figs. 1-9)

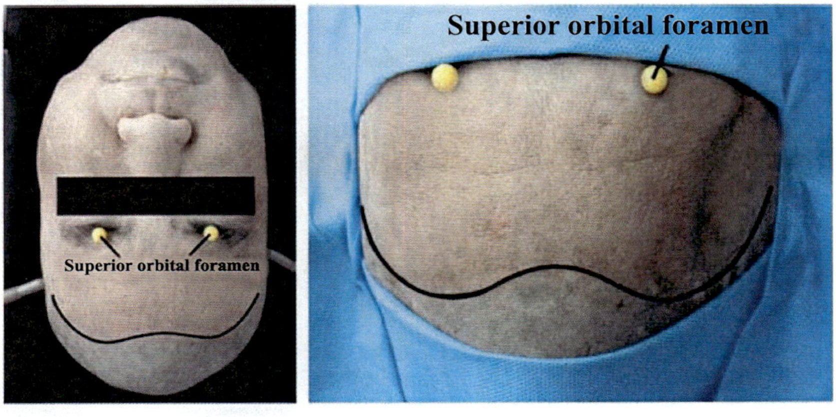

Fig. (1). Skin incision of the frontobasal interhemispheric approach. The incision is located 1 cm inside the frontal hairline, originating from the posterior part of the frontal angle, and courses inside the hairline to the contralateral side.

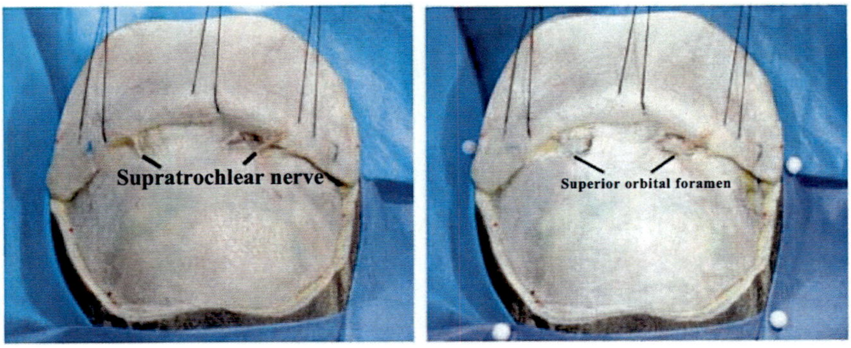

Fig. (2). Separation of the skin flap beneath the galea aponeurotica and forward retraction. The supratrochlear nerves and supraorbital artery are exposed. A round periosteal incision is made around the superior orbital foramen. The periosteal flap is separated together with the nerve and artery and turned open.

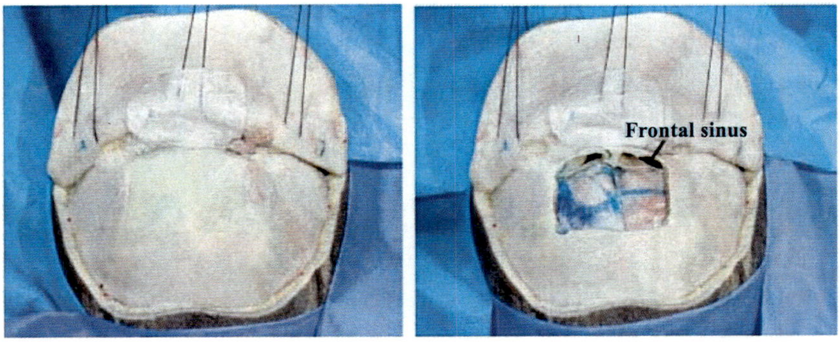

Fig. (3). A periosteal incision is made at the median edge of the superior orbital foramen. The upper border of the periosteal flap extended 3–4 cm from the orbital margin. After separation under the periosteum and forward retraction, the flap can be used to seal the frontal sinus. Two burr holes are made at the two frontal angles, after which a mill is used to establish the free bone flap. In general, the frontal sinus is opened during craniotomy, as shown in the Fig. (**4**).

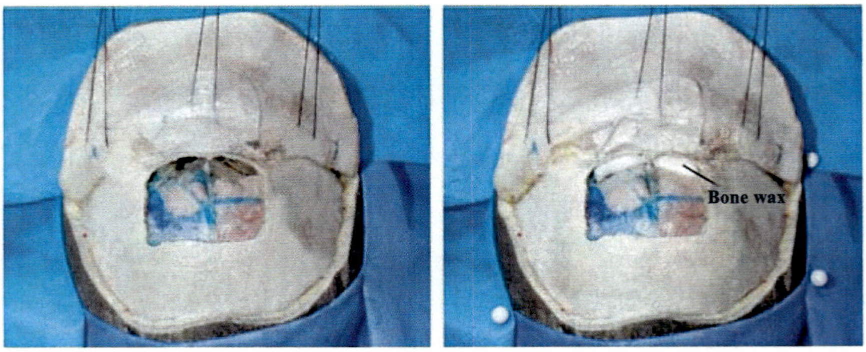

Fig. (4). A bone rongeur is used to remove the inner wall or frontal sinus, and the frontal sinus mucosa is separated to the extent possible. Iodine tincture and alcohol are used to sterilize the sinus. Subsequently, bone wax containing antibiotic powder is used to fill the sinus to avoid infection.

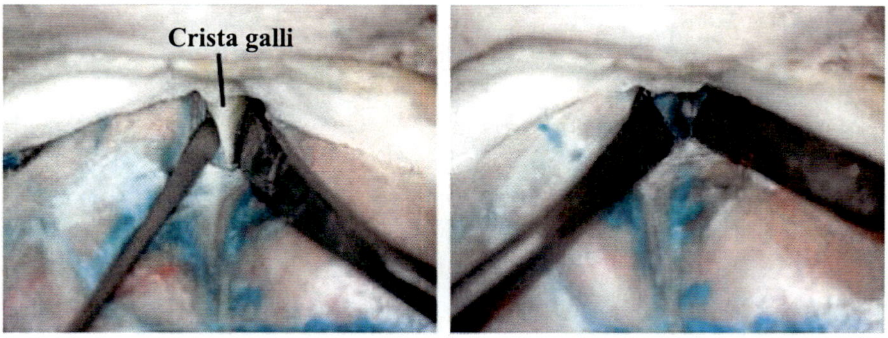

Fig. (5). The crista galli is separated extradurally at the frontal base midline. In some patients, the crista galli is extremely large and penetrates inside the dura mater. In this scenario, scissors and a sharp-point knife are needed to perform a sharp separation. A drill is used for total crista galli removal to reduce the obstruction of the exposure to the frontal basement.

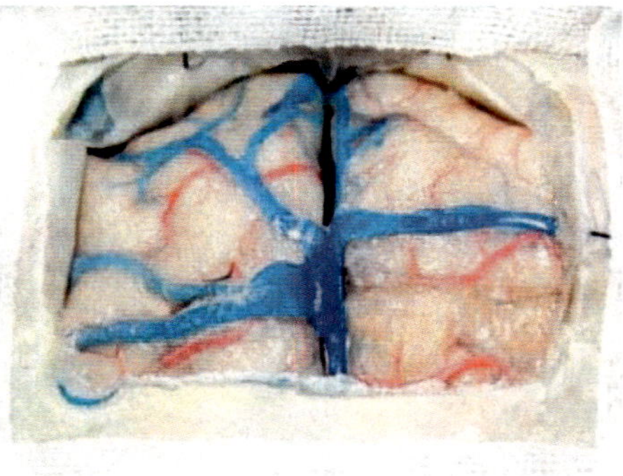

Fig. (6). The dural incision is made approximately 1.5–2 cm from the anterior border of the bone windows. Subsequently, the anterior part of the superior sagittal sinus was ruptured. Bilateral round incisions were made, after which the cerebral falx was dissected deeply to retract the dural flap forward. The surrounding dura was cut radically to expose the frontal lobes.

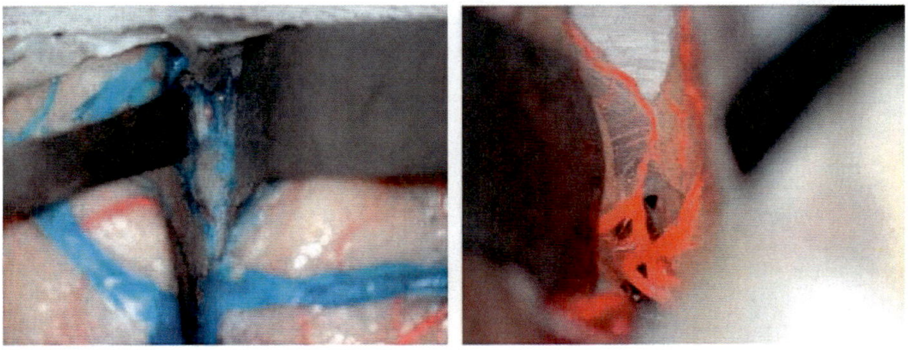

Fig. (7). Retraction of the bilateral frontal lobes with a brain spatula exposes the arachnoidal trabecula and membrane between the two lobes. Occasionally, the median aspects of the two frontal lobes can penetrate each other, thus it is important to pay attention to the trabecular distribution as the separation interface. Further dissection exposes the basal arachnoid membrane located at the frontal basement (outer arachnoid).

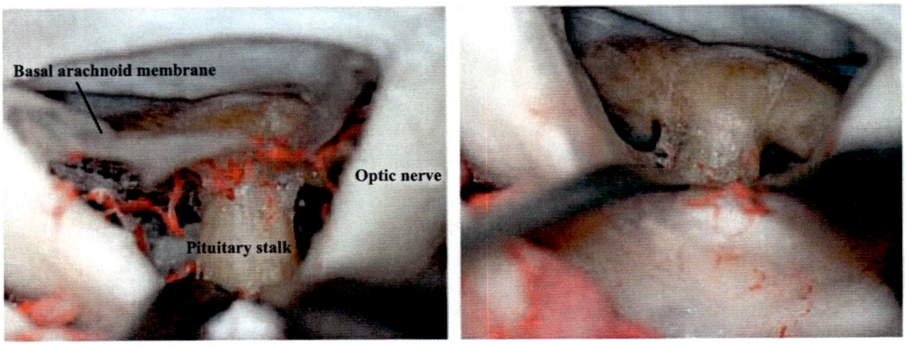

Fig. (8). After total separation of the bilateral frontobasal arachnoid, the basal arachnoidal membrane is shown to course towards the ventral optic chiasm and form the arachnoidal sleeve of the pituitary stalk. Upward retraction of the basal arachnoid membrane divides the pituitary stalk into two segments, extra- and intra-arachnoidal, by the sleeve.

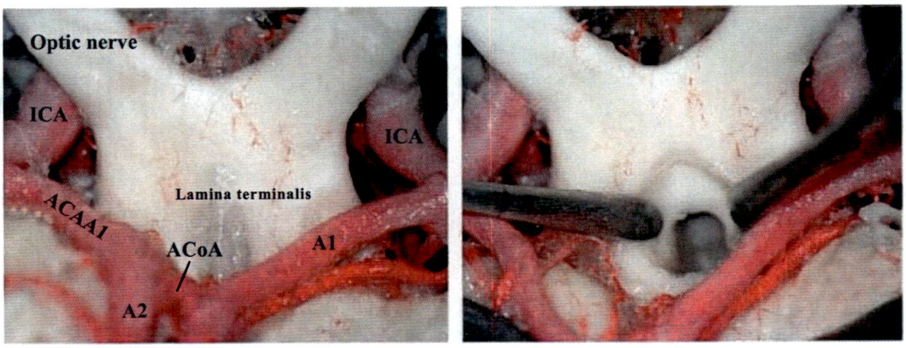

Fig. (9). Continuous backward separation to expose anatomical structures of the total sellar region, including bilateral optic nerves, chiasm, ICA, A1 segment of ACA, ACoA, and lamina terminalis. In this case, the AcoA is relatively retro-located, and thus the terminalis was easily exposed and opened. The third ventricular cavity was entered upon opening the terminalis.

TRANSCALLOSAL AND INTERFONIX APPROACH

Historical Overview

In 1922, Dandy [13] first used the trans-callosal approach to reach the third ventricle. In 1979, Hirsch and Delandcheer [14] reported making a trans-choroid fissure by rupturing the vena thalamostriata, retracting the foramen of Monro, and then lifting the choroid flex, fornix body, and internal cerebral vein to remove tumors inside the third ventricle. In 1980, Viale *et al.* [15] proposed that the vena thalamostriata should be protected from injury by retracting only the choroid flex and fornix body contralaterally and then entering the top of the third ventricle. For a trans-callosal approach landmark, in 1982, Apuzzo [16] first proposed an approach involving the trans-callosal inter-space of the septum pellucidum-inner fornix to remove lesions in the third ventricle. Following continuous attempts and development, this approach was widely accepted because of the lower injury rates and provision of a direct route and wide surgical view [17, 18]. This approach uses the natural anatomical corridor in the midline with great advantage to expose the anterior and middle parts of the third ventricle. Therefore, this approach has been widely used to remove primary or secondary tumors protruding into and occupying the anterior or middle part of the third ventricle.

Position and Surgical Technique

The patient is placed in the supine position with the head deflexed upward approximately 10–15°. The head can be rotated from 0° to 60° depending on the lesion location. Normally, a frontal and parietal horseshoe-shaped skin incision is made with anterior branches 4 cm ahead of the coronal suture and posterior branches 2 cm behind the coronal suture. The incision is contralateral to 1 cm before the median. Several elements (see the following) restrict exposure with this approach. After opening the bone flap, the median cerebral tissue aspect must be retracted. In general, the retraction should not exceed 5 cm in length and 2.5 cm in width to avoid brain tissue injury. However, bridge veins always restrict exposure. Several publications have reported a relatively safe area; this is normally 4–5-cm ahead of the coronal suture, where few bridge veins are thought to enter. However, several veins have been observed 2 cm behind the coronal suture. In a Chinese population, some scholars found a safe area at 32.6 mm anterior and 7.5 mm posterior of the coronal suture was safety area. Our experiences indicate that bridge veins always course within the arachnoid mater; if the membrane is carefully dissected, an additional exposure of 1-1.5 cm can be provided.

The second restriction element is dissection of the callosum. Normally, the pars geniculate and splenium of callosum are thought to have important functions as communication fibers. Therefore, injury to those parts will cause severe memory dysfunction. Woiciechowsky *et al.* [19] reported that the callosum incision should not exceed 2 cm when using the trans-callosal approach. However, a 2-cm incision does not always provide sufficient exposure during the operation. Later, some scholars proposed that an incision shorter than 3 cm would not cause significant dysfunction. In general, a callosum incision of approximately 2.5 cm can provide the required surgical view.

The size of the foramen of Monro is the other element if third ventricle manipulation is performed through this foramen. Usually, in patients with hydrocephalus the foramen of Monro is enlarged and thus provides a wide route for surgical manipulation. However, the normal-sized foramen does not always provide a sufficiently large exposure. The anterior fornix column cannot be cut to enlarge the foramen. However, the posterior fornix tenia can be opened slightly.

However, the septal and thalamostriata veins always obstruct posterior enlargement, and these should not be injured, given the high risk of severe thalamic edema and memory dysfunction. In general, the inter-fornix approach is thought to provide a larger surgical field. Notably, however, an extensively posterior psalterium incision should be avoided to prevent memory dysfunction.

Approach Figures (Figs. 10-15)

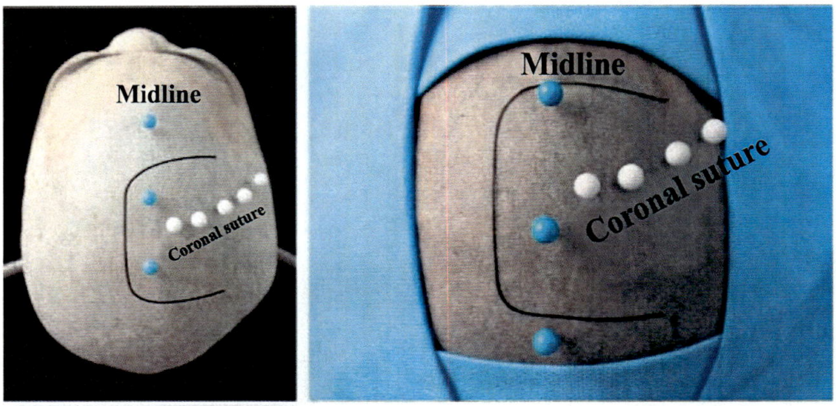

Fig. (10). The skin incision is horseshoe shaped. First, the coronal suture should be located and, in general, the distance from the coronal suture to the nasal root is 12–13 cm. The incision is made across the midline and is approximately 1 cm, with the coronal suture located at the anterior third to half of the incision.

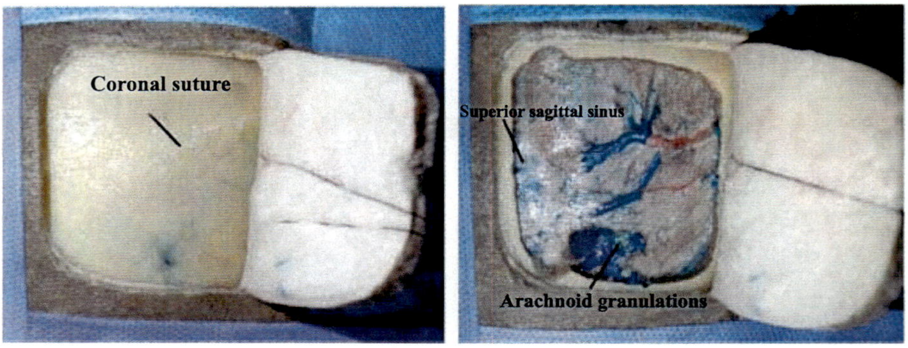

Fig. (11). After opening the skin, galea aponeurotica, and periosteum, the skin flap is separated under the periosteum. The coronal suture is located at the anterior third of the bone windows. After drilling two burr holes beside the superior sagittal sinus, mills were used to form the bone flap and expose the sinus. Two bridge veins and abundant arachnoid granulations were observed with drainage to the superior sagittal sinus.

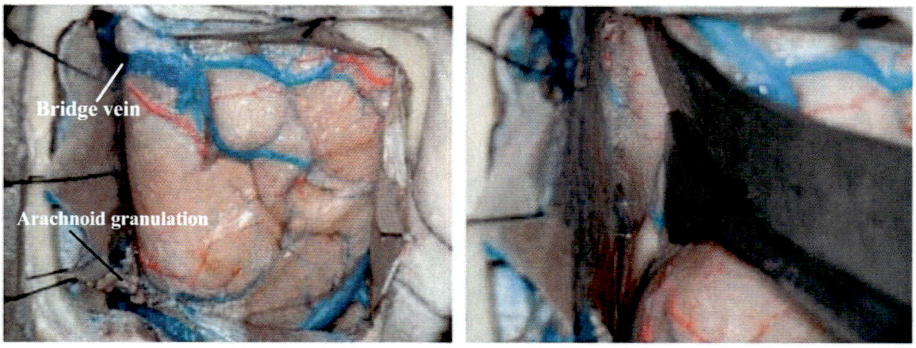

Fig. (12). Display of the entire view after opening the dura mater. The outer arachnoid is observed to connect the bilateral frontal lobes under the cerebral falx when the frontal lobe is retracted.

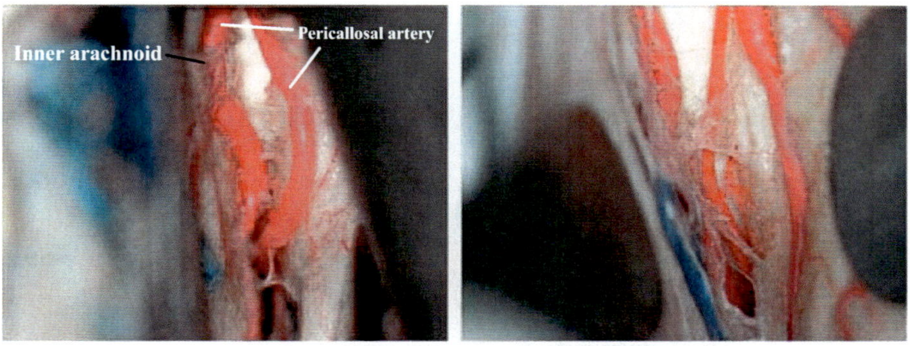

Fig. (13). Further division of the arachnoidal septation exposes the bilateral pericallosal arteries. An inner arachnoid membrane separates the two arteries. During separation, attempt to the enter corpus callosum between the two arteries to avoid injuring the branches.

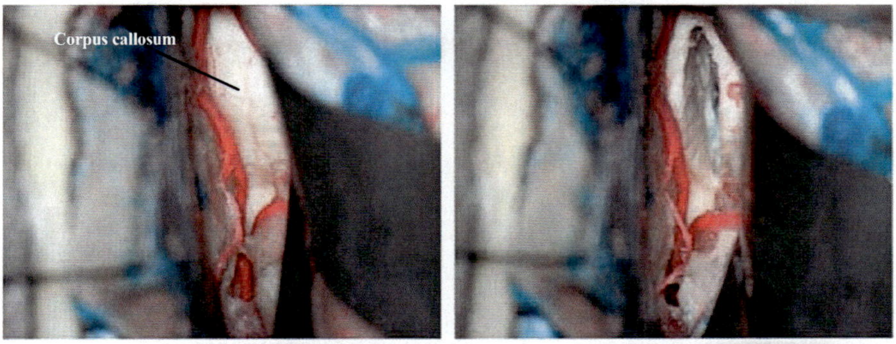

Fig. (14). The ipsilateral pericallosal artery is protected by the retractor to enlarge the callosum exposure. A 2-cm-long incision is made in the callosum. Notably, the incision should not exceed 3 cm to avoid severe injury to the communication fibers.

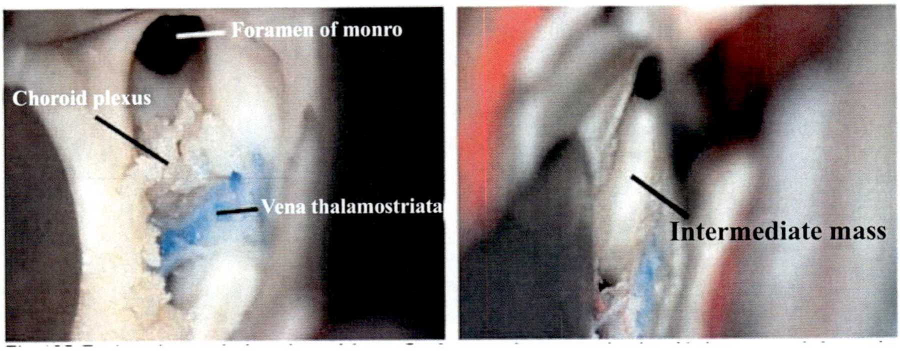

Fig. (15). For lateral entry, the lateral ventricle can first be opened to expose the choroid plexus, vena thalamostriata, and foramen of Monro. For midline entry through the interfornix space, the third ventricle can be entered directly. Intermediate masses can be exposed inside the ventricular cavity.

SURGERY FOR CRANIOPHARYNGIOMA

Frontobasal interhemispheric approach (FIH) might be the most frequent used corridor to dissect CP with variant growth pattern. For infradiaphragmatic tumor, the pre-chiasmatic space always enlarged, which can be directly exposed through this approach Fig. (**16**). Sometimes, tumor might protrude upwards to the superior of chiasm and AcoA Fig. (**17**). The FIH have its advantage to expose the AcoA complex and also the terminalis space as well.

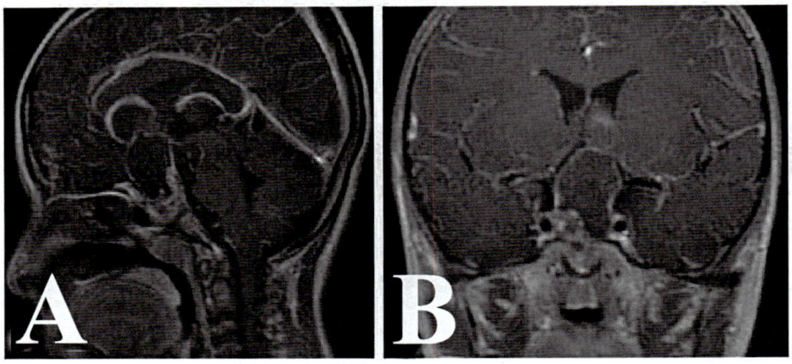

Fig. (16). A predominantly cystic intra- and suprasellar mass. Presurgical magnetic resonance imaging indicated a predominantly cystic tumor in the suprasellar region with upward expansion of a daughter cyst behind the anterior communicating artery. The anterior communicating (AcoA) and anterior carotid arteries (ACA) formed a snowman shape at the top of the cystic tumor. On enhanced MRI, the cystic tumor wall was significantly enhanced roundly. On a coronal scan, a solid tumor was observed on the right side of the pituitary fossa near the medial wall of the CS. No obstructive hydrocephalus consequent to the tumor growth pattern and expansion was observed.

During the surgery, the identification of the origin site of tumor was still the most important. The pituitary stalk was always behind or bias to lateral side of tumor. As infra-diaphragmatic CP for example, the originate site of tumor always located at the middle and lower segment of pituitary stalk. The distal pituitary stalk was always found to fuse with the tumor capsule at the border of the diaphragmatic foramen Fig. (**18**). Under this situation, the infundibulo-tuberalis was inflattened or displaced. In operation, the identification of the membranous structure, which separated the tumor to the posterior lobe of pituitary gland, was quite important. The interface will ensure the total removal of tumor and protection of stalk and neuro-hypophysis. Sometimes it was difficult to preserve the PS continuity as the distal segment of the PS was ruptured where the stalk and tumor capsule had fused.

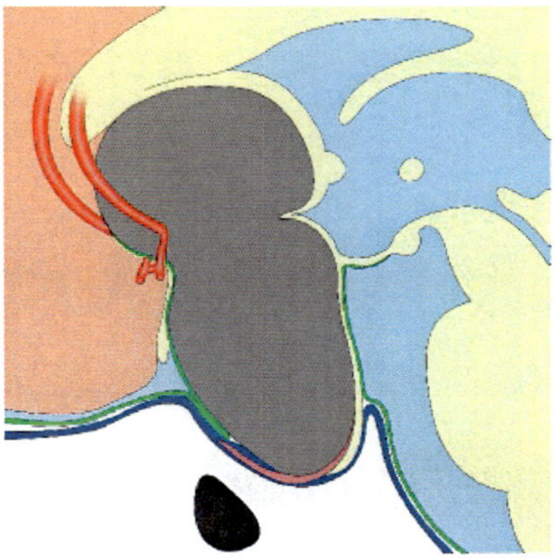

Fig. (17). Schematic Fig. (demonstrating the tumor morphology and relationships with the surrounding structures. Blue line: Dura mater (Diaphragm and sellar floor dura); Green line: Arachnoid mater.

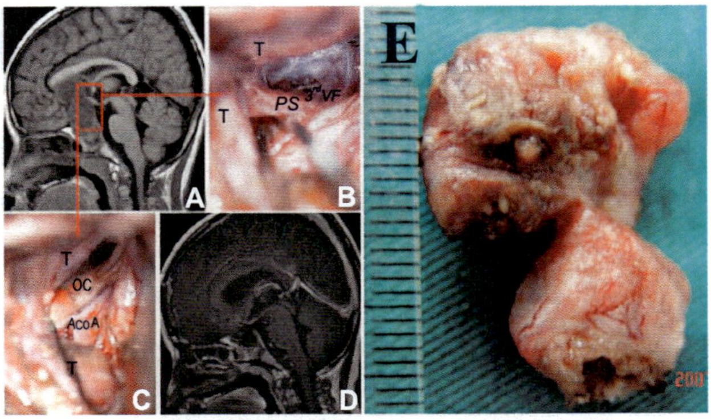

Fig. (18). Tumor exposure *via* the frontobasal interhemispheric approach. **A.** The bilateral frontal lobes and hemispheric fissure were visible after completing the craniotomy. **B.** The suprasellar tumor capsule along with the evaluated DS were identified through the prechiasmatic space. **C.** Intrasurgical photographs showing the tumor–stalk relationship: the lower part of the stalk had fused with the superoposterior part of the tumor capsule (**B**). Note that the third ventricle floor (3rd VF) remained intact. The protruding suprasellar tumor encased the anterior communicating artery (AcoA) complex (**C**), necessitating sharp dissection to release the tumor. **D.** Postoperative sagittal T1-weighted magnetic resonance image confirming total tumor removal. The 3rd VF remained intact. **E.** The tumor was removed completely en bloc. OC: optic chiasm; PS: pituitary stalk; T: tumor.

On the other hand, for the infundibulo-tuberal CP, FIH can also provide enough exposure by usage both extra-axial space (pre-chiasmatic space, ICA-optic nerve space, and also the ICA-Oculomotor nerve space) and intra-axial space (Lamina terminalis). The originate site of this type of tumor always located at the upper segment of pituitary stalk or infundibulo-tuberalis Figs. (**19**, **20**). After dissection of the lamina terminalis, the identification of the third ventricular floor nervous tissue was extremely important Fig. (**21**). Sometimes, the presurgical MRI coronal images could provide some vital information or clue. Carefully reading the series images and correspondingly intraoperative dissection might helpful to protect those nervous tissue with avoiding the hypothalamic reaction after surgery.

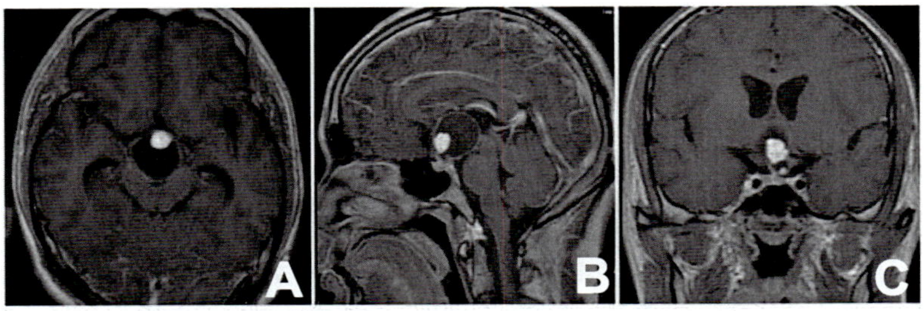

Fig. (19). Preoperative sagittal and coronal contrast-enhanced T1-weighted magnetic resonance imaging of a 27-year-old man demonstrates the typical pattern of a mixed cystic-solid formation in a squamous papillary craniopharyngioma with an infundibulotuberal growth pattern. The main tumor body occupied the third ventricular cavity, and most residual hypothalamic pituitary fibers were located at the anterior of the tumor. The solid tumor was located at the infundibulum, a possible site of origin. The lower segment of the PS was normal. The solid tumor is located inside the cyst, in contrast to the lobulated cysts observed in the adamantinomatous variant.

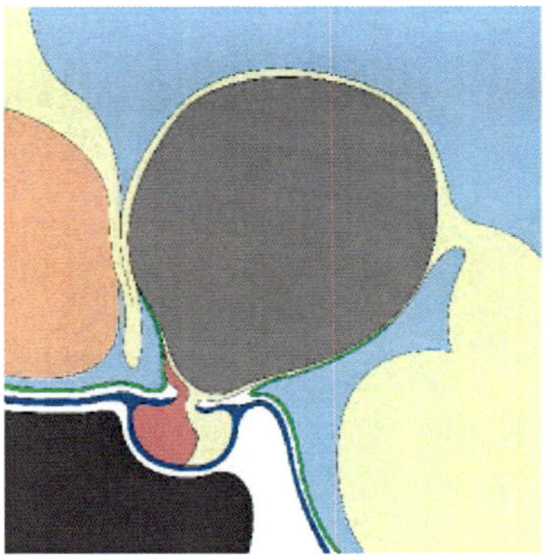

Fig. (20). Schematic Fig. (demonstrating the tumor morphology and relationships with the surrounding structures. Regarding morphological features, the tumor was a typical adult infundibulotuberal CP. However, the main growth direction was posterior with an upward extension. As a result, the main infundibular structure and pituitary fibers were located anteriorly to the tumor. The site of origin was at the posterior of the infundibulum and under the pia mater with big possible.

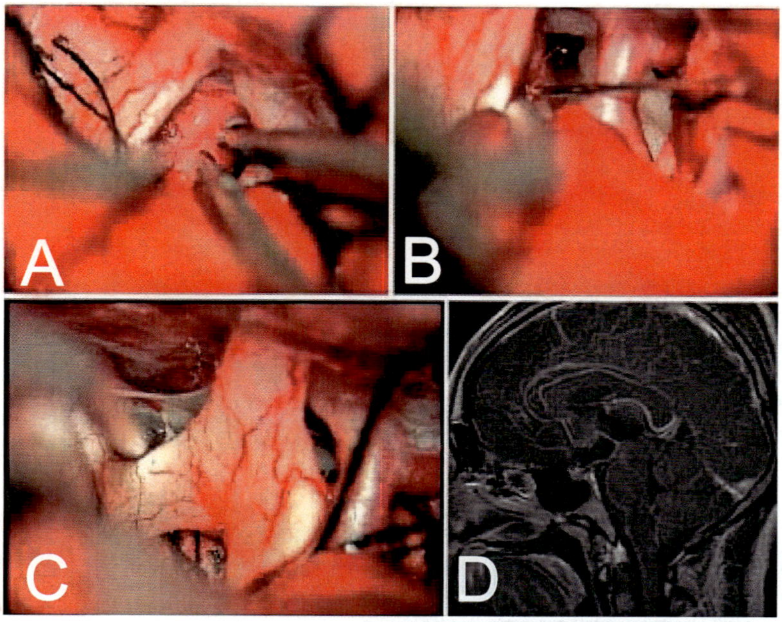

Fig. (21). Intraoperative findings and postsurgical magnetic resonance imaging (MRI). **A.** Through the optic-internal carotid artery (ICA) space, the infundibular part of the pituitary stalk was flattened and served as the site of tumor origin. The lower segment of the pituitary stalk remained intact. **B.** Cystic fluid was suctioned to reduce the tumor volume. **C.** The lamina terminalis was opened to remove the tumor. **D.** Postsurgical MRI confirmed total tumor removal. The hypothalamic–pituitary stalk continuity was preserved.

As concerned with the application of the FIH approach, if the tumor was "extra- and intra-ventricular type" as described by Pascual, the extra-axial space must be used to dissect the intra-arachnoidal cistern part of tumor. Under this situation, in order to gross total removal of tumor, the defection of the 3rd VF might happen. Regarding morphological features, although variant extension directions were observed in this type of CP, the site of origin remained at the infundibulum and under the pia mater Figs. (**22-24**). The tumor had remained external to the ventricular system. The 3rd VF structure was invaginated and inflated by the tumor, but the ependymal layer remained intact. In this situation, although opening of the lamina terminalis was required to remove the upward tumor growth, the residual 3rd VF nervous tissue should be preserved as much as possible. For the backward tumor growth, which might occupy the interpeduncular cistern, septation of Liliequist's membrane between the tumor and brain stem and the basilar artery and its branches allowed relatively safe tumor removal. Notably, several arachnoidal trabeculae connected the artery branches to the arachnoid mater. During surgery, these branches might have been dissected while pulling the tumor. Therefore, dissection of these transverse trabeculae was needed to avoid arterial injury.

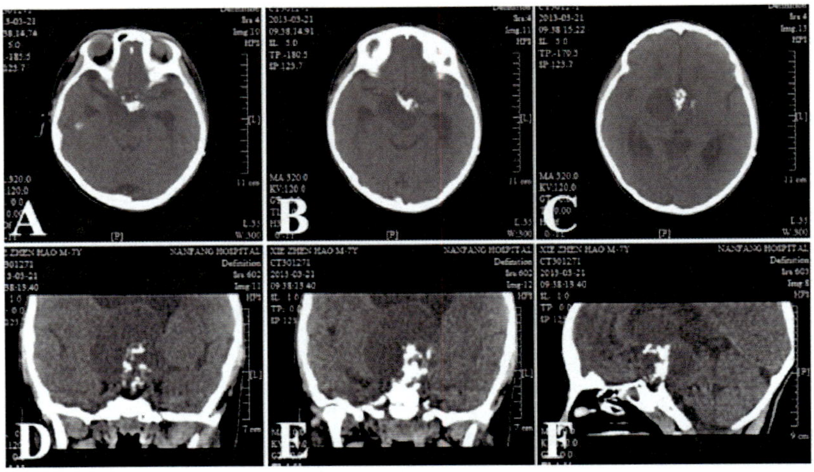

Fig. (22). A 7-year-old male patient presented with a 6-month history of progressively aggravated headache, dizziness, and decreased visual acuity. Presurgical computed tomography scans indicated a mixed cystic solid lesion occupying the intrasellar and suprasellar region along with a large calcification mass in the suprasellar region. The cystic tumor occupied the third ventricular cavity and had caused hydrocephalus. MRI showed a lesion that had originated from the infundibulotuberum with a cyst that had extended excessively upward to the third ventricular cavity and backward to the interpeduncular cistern.

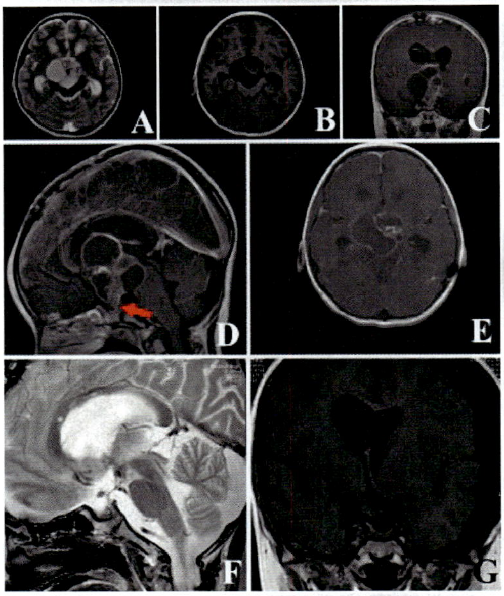

Fig. (23). Presurgical magnetic resonance imaging of case in Fig. (**22**).

Sometimes after dissecting the interhemispheric fissure, the AcoA was divided to increase exposure of the lamina terminalis space Fig. (**25**). The tumor had grown inside the nervous tissue layer of the 3rd VF, so the lamina terminalis and 3rd VF were spliced to dissect the tumor. The tumor was removed in a piecemeal manner, and the infundibulum and proximal segment of the PS, which were inflated by the tumor, were vertically incised to remove the tumor.

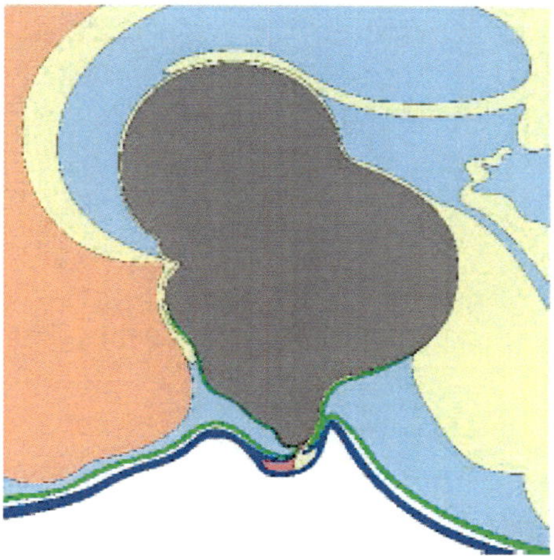

Fig. (24). Schematic Fig. (demonstrating the tumor morphology and relationships with the surrounding structures. Although the tumor had variant extension upwards and backwards with occupying the 3rd ventricular space, the tumor was not truly inside the third ventricular cavity. The 3rd VF structure was invaginated and inflated by the tumor, but the ependymal layer remained intact.

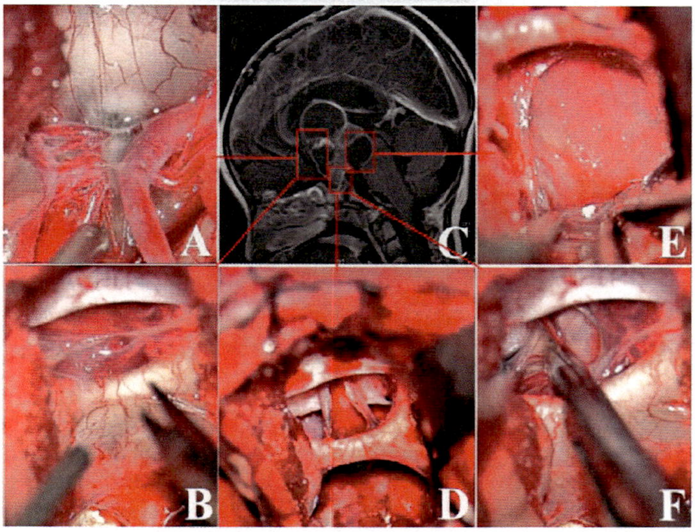

Fig. (25). Preoperative magnetic resonance imaging (MRI) and intraoperative images of a 7-year-old boy with a typical infundibulotuberal CP. Presurgical sagittal contrast-enhanced T1-weighted MRI after a flawed surgery *via* a trans-corpus callosum trans-fornix approach at a local hospital (**C**). Intraoperative images showing tumor removal. The anterior communicating artery was divided to enhance tumor exposure (**A**). After dissecting the arachnoid enveloping the pituitary stalk (**B**), the bulged pituitary stalk was exposed (**F**). The tumor was totally removed using a combined trans-lamina terminalis and extra-axial route. The pituitary stalk was split vertically to expose the tumor (**D**). Note the attenuated but uninterrupted third ventricle floor after tumor removal (**E**).

As concerned with transcallosal and inter-fonix approach (TSI), as a classic corridor to treat the occupation inside the third ventricle, the approach was commonly used to deal with the "intraventricular" CP in some clinical centers. However, as our opinion, we prefer FIH as described above, instead of this approach. As concerned of the terminology of "intraventricular" CP, we thought there was no strictly intra-ventricular tumor. The CP origin from the infundibulo-tuberalis with protruding inside the 3rd VF, so as result, there still are a layer of nervous tissue covering the surface of the tumor. The morphological construction can see also our article or the Chapter 12 of this book. The only situation for usage of TSI was the tumor companying with extremely posterior extension through the Monro's foramen and occupying the lateral ventricle. However, even in this kind of tumor, we preferred the trans-cortex ventricle approach to avoid the injury of callosal and fonix (Figs. **26-28**).

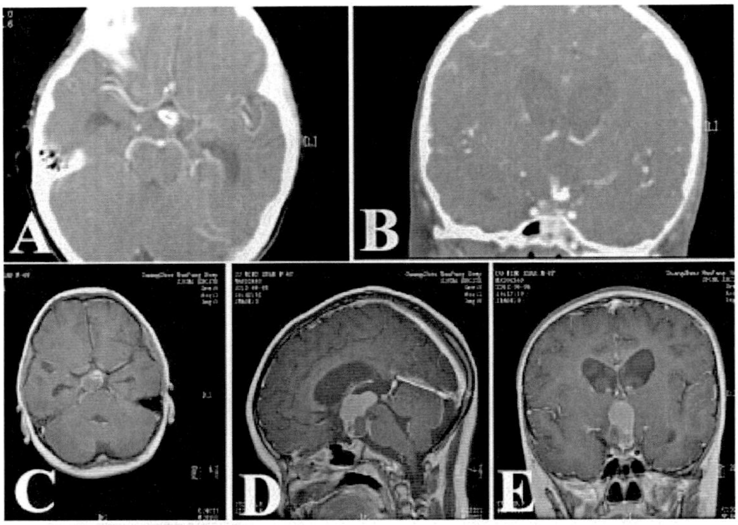

Fig. (26). A 7-year-old male patient presented with a 6-month history of headache, decreased visual acuity, polyuria, and polydipsia. Presurgical computed tomography (CT) and magnetic resonance imaging (MRI) of Case 5. **A-B.** Presurgical CT indicated a predominantly cystic tumor in the suprasellar region without significant calcification. The cystic tumor occupied the third ventricular cavity and had caused hydrocephalus. **C-E.** MRI indicated a suprasellar tumor that had originated from the infundibular part with invagination into the third ventricular floor and occupation of the third ventricular cavity. The cystic tumor extended backwards to occupy most of the third ventricular cavity and obstruct the foramen of Monro. The lower segment of the PS was normal.

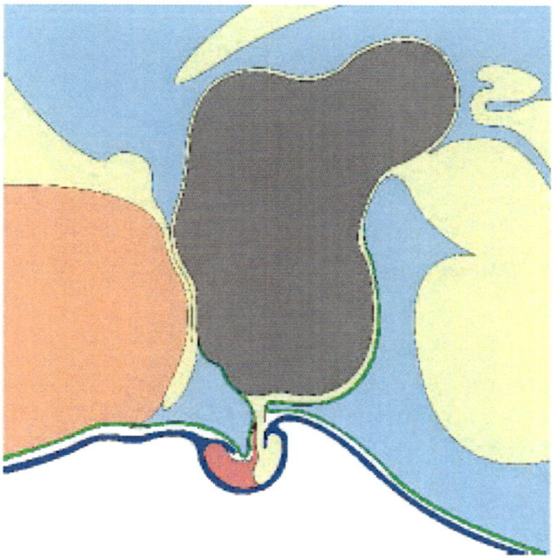

Fig. (27). Schematic Fig. (demonstrating the tumor morphology and relationships with the surrounding structures. Although in MRI, the tumor's location might be thought as inside the 3rd ventricular cavity, the truly morphological features of tumor were in the nervous tissue layer of the 3rd VF. The clearly identifiable interface between the tumor and hypothalamus can be found intra-operation. The intact 3rd VF and pituitary stalk were preserved.

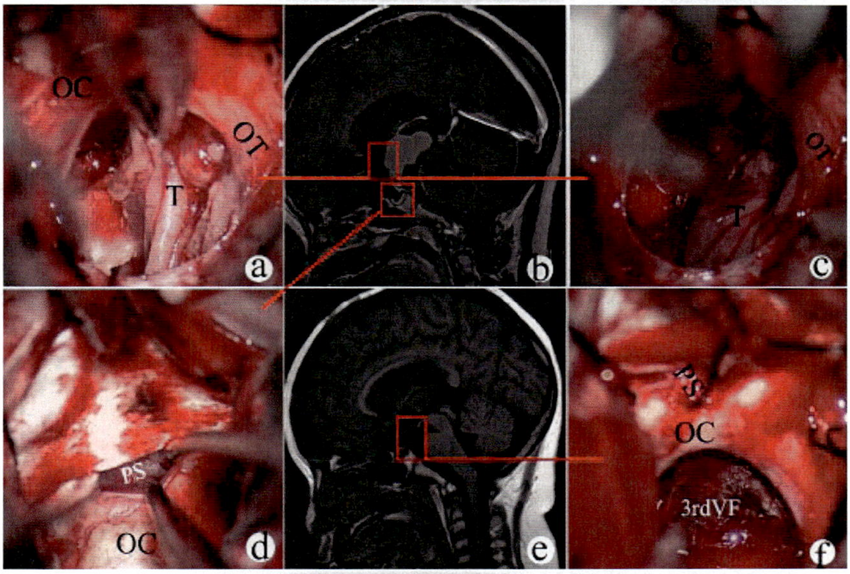

Fig. (28). Intraoperative findings. **A.** The lamina terminalis was opened to expose the tumor. The tumor was dissected along the interface between the tumor and nervous tissue layer of the third ventricular floor (3rd VF). **B.** Presurgical sagittal magnetic resonance imaging (MRI). **C.** The site of tumor origin remained at the infundibular part of the pituitary stalk, where the tumor was sharply dissected while attempting to preserve the hypothalamus–pituitary stalk axial continuity. **D.** A small prechiasmatic space was observed. **E.** Postsurgical sagittal MRI. **F.** The 3rd VF was well preserved after total tumor removal.

CONFLICT OF INTEREST

The author (editor) declares no conflict of interest, financial or otherwise.

ACKNOWLEDGEMENTS

We should acknowledge Dr. Shi Jin for preparing the cadaver specimens and assistant about the anatomical studies.

REFERENCES

[1] Zelený M, Voldrich Z, Navrátilová A, Soldán J. [Late development of osteoplastic flaps in operations on the frontal sinuses]. Cesk Otolaryngol 1984; 33(6): 333-5. [Late development of osteoplastic flaps in operations on the frontal sinuses].
[PMID: 6509592]

[2] Dandy W. Pneumocephalus (Intracranial pneumatocele or aerocel). Arch Surg 1926; (12): 949-82.
[http://dx.doi.org/10.1001/archsurg.1926.01130050003001]

[3] Suzuki J, Yoshimoto T, Mizoi K, Sato M. [Preservation of the olfactory tract following surgery on anterior communicating artery aneurysm using bifrontal craniotomy, and its functional prognosis (author's transl)]. No Shinkei Geka 1981; 9(8): 921-4. [Preservation of the olfactory tract following surgery on anterior communicating artery aneurysm using bifrontal craniotomy, and its functional prognosis (author's transl)].
[PMID: 7279130]

[4] Fahlbusch R, Honegger J, Paulus W, Huk W, Buchfelder M. Surgical treatment of craniopharyngiomas: experience with 168 patients. J Neurosurg 1999; 90(2): 237-50.
[http://dx.doi.org/10.3171/jns.1999.90.2.0237] [PMID: 9950494]

[5] Oi S, Samii M. [Operative techniques for tumors in the third ventricle]. Op. Tech Neurosurg 2003; (6): 205-14.
[http://dx.doi.org/10.1016/j.otns.2003.09.002]

[6] Suzuki J, Katakura R, Mori T. Interhemispheric approach through the lamina terminalis to tumors of the anterior part of the third ventricle. Surg Neurol 1984; 22(2): 157-63.
[http://dx.doi.org/10.1016/0090-3019(84)90044-2] [PMID: 6740479]

[7] Fuzitsu K. [Anterior interhemispheric approach to the diseases involving the third ventricle and/or the suprasellar region]. No Shinkei Geka 1998; 26(8): 667-77. [Anterior interhemispheric approach to the diseases involving the third ventricle and/or the suprasellar region].
[PMID: 9743995]

[8] Maira G, Anile C, Colosimo C, Cabezas D. Craniopharyngiomas of the third ventricle: trans-lamina terminalis approach. Neurosurgery 2000; 47(4): 857-63.
[http://dx.doi.org/10.1097/00006123-200010000-00014] [PMID: 11014425]

[9] Ohata K, Hakuba A, Nagai K, Morino M, Iwa Y. A biorbitofrontobasal interhemispheric approach for suprasellar lesions. Mt Sinai J Med 1997; 64(3): 217-21.
[PMID: 9145673]

[10] Shibuya M, Takayasu M, Suzuki Y, Saito K, Sugita K. Bifrontal basal interhemispheric approach to craniopharyngioma resection with or without division of the anterior communicating artery. J Neurosurg 1996; 84(6): 951-6.
[http://dx.doi.org/10.3171/jns.1996.84.6.0951] [PMID: 8847589]

[11] Shirane R, Ching-Chan S, Kusaka Y, Jokura H, Yoshimoto T. Surgical outcomes in 31 patients with craniopharyngiomas extending outside the suprasellar cistern: an evaluation of the frontobasal interhemispheric approach. J Neurosurg 2002; 96(4): 704-12.

[http://dx.doi.org/10.3171/jns.2002.96.4.0704] [PMID: 11990811]

[12] Dehdashti AR, de Tribolet N. Frontobasal interhemispheric trans-lamina terminalis approach for suprasellar lesions. Neurosurgery 2005; 56(2) (Suppl.): 418-24. [PMID: 15794839]

[13] Dandy WE. Diagnosis, localization and removal of tumors of the third ventricle. Bull Johns Hopkins Hosp 1922; 33: 188-9.

[14] Hirsch JF, Zouaoui A, Renier D, Pierre-Kahn A. A new surgical approach to the third ventricle with interruption of the striothalamic vein. Acta Neurochir (Wien) 1979; 47(3-4): 135-47. [http://dx.doi.org/10.1007/BF01406399] [PMID: 474208]

[15] Viale GL, Turtas S. The subchoroid approach to the third ventricle. Surg Neurol 1980; 14(1): 71-4. [PMID: 7414489]

[16] Apuzzo ML, Chikovani OK, Gott PS, *et al.* Transcallosal interforniceal approaches for lesions affecting the third ventricle: Surgical considerations and consequences. Neurosurgery 1982; 10: 547-54. [http://dx.doi.org/10.1227/00006123-198205000-00001] [PMID: 7099406]

[17] Erturk M, Kayalioglu G, Ozer MA, Ozgur T. Morphometry of the anterior third ventricle region as a guide for the transcallosal-interforniceal approach. Neurol Med Chir (Tokyo) 2004; 44(6): 288-92. [http://dx.doi.org/10.2176/nmc.44.288] [PMID: 15253543]

[18] Siwanuwatn R, Deshmukh P, Feiz-Erfan I, *et al.* Microsurgical anatomy of the transcallosal anterior interforniceal approach to the third ventricle. Neurosurgery 2005; 56(2) (Suppl.): 390-6. [PMID: 15794835]

[19] Woiciechowsky C, Vogel S, Lehmann R, Staudt J. Transcallosal removal of lesions affecting the third ventricle: an anatomic and clinical study. Neurosurgery 1995; 36(1): 117-22. [http://dx.doi.org/10.1227/00006123-199501000-00015] [PMID: 7708147]

CHAPTER 8

Anatomy Based on Transspenoidal Approaches for Surgery of Craniopharyngioma

Yuntao Lu*

Department of Neurosurgery, Nanfang Neurosurgery Research Institution, Nanfang Hospital, Southern Medical University, 1838 North Guangzhou Avenue, Guangzhou, China

Abstract: As the sellar region location, the trans-nasal transsphenoidal corridor was thought to be the most effective approach to reach the surgical area. In recent decade, the endoscopic surgery developed extremely rapidly. As the result, more and more scholars tried to use transsphenoidal and it extended approach to dissect the craniopharyngioma (CP). In this chapter, we provided the basic anatomical details concerning the endonasal transsphenoid approach and its expanded application for surgical removal of CP. Moreover, several clinical cases and the morphological features of CP were analyzed. Base on the different classification of CP, the appropriate application of this approach was discussed.

Keywords: Anatomy, Craniopharyngioma, Transsphenoidal approach.

TRANSNASAL TRANSSHPENOIDAL APPROACH AND EXTENSIONS

Historical Overview

In 1906, Schloffer [1] first conceived a trans-sphenoidal sinus approach and, in the following reported the complete removal of pituitary adenomas *via* a trans-nasal ethmoid sinus and trans-sphenoidal sinus approach. Two years later, Hirsch [2] used the trans-nasal trans-sphenoidal approach to remove pituitary adenomas. In 1913, Cushing [3] proposed the trans-sublip-septum-sphenoid (TSSS) approach. However, because of restrictions in the surgical instruments and illuminating equipment, tumor resection was incomplete and associated with high morbidity, which restricted the utilization of this approach. The TSSS approach was not improved until 1969, when Hardy [4] used a surgical microscope and intra-surgical X-ray monitor to support the trans-sphenoidal approach, which was then accepted widely. In recent years with development of the endoscope, many

* **Corresponding author Yuntao Lu**: Department of Neurosurgery, Nanfang Neurosurgery Research Institution, Nanfang Hospital, Southern Medical University, 1838 North Guangzhou Avenue, Guangzhou, China; Tel/Fax: +8620-61641806; E-mail: lllu2000yun@gmail.com

Songtao Qi (Ed.)

scholars have proposed an endoscopic trans-sphenoidal approach. In 1922, Jankowski [5] first incorporated endoscopy into this approach, and this modality was subsequently used widely to treat sellar region lesions.

In recent decades, the instruments and techniques associated with the trans-sphenoidal approach have improved continuously and tremendously, as described by Dandie *et al.* in 1996 [6], Kitano and Taneda in 1997 [7], Alfieri in 1999 [8], and Arita *et al.* in 2000 [9]. Moreover, in 2009, Yano *et al.* [10] used an endoscope through the bilateral nostrils corridors to obtain sufficient surgical space for third instrument manipulation. An extended trans-sphenoidal (ETS) approach has been used increasingly widely in recent years as a result of a deeper understanding of the sellar anatomy as reported by Frank *et al.* in 2001 [11], Catapano *et al.* in 2006 [12], and Wang *et al.* in 2010 [13]. Several publications in which the ETS approach was used to treat supra- and parasellar lesions (Abuzayed *et al.* 2010 [14]; Kim *et al.* 2011 [15]) and even lesions in the petrous apex (Zanation *et al.* 2009 [16]) and floor of the middle cranial fossa (Ceylan *et al.* 2009 [17]) have described surgical manipulation details. The follow-up outcomes of these patients indicate that the ETS approach might be an efficient and feasible way to expand the traditional trans-sphenoidal exposure.

Position and Surgical Technique

Patients are always placed in a supine position with the head deflexed and hypsokinesis of 15-20°. Generally, the neck is rotated contralaterally 10-15° to facilitate surgical manipulation. To date, several trans-sphenoidal approach methods have been reported, including the 1) TSSS, 2) trans-nasal columella-septum-sphenoid approach (TCSS), 3) endonasal-septum-sphenoid approach (ESS) and, more recently, 4) endonasal-sphenoid approach (ES). Among these techniques, ESS and ES have been used most widely because these are associated with only minor nasal cavity injury. In 1987 Griffith and Veerapen [18] first described the ESS approach; Cooke *et al.* later used this approach to remove pituitary adenomas. In 1996 and 1997, Rodziewicz *et al.* [19] and Yaniv and Rappaport [20] respectively, proposed the endoscopic ESS approach. ESS manipulation occurs as follows. A semi-lunar incision is made in the septum at the interface of the cartilaginous and osseous tissues. Next, the mucosa flap is lifted to expose the vomer bone, which is removed and saved for sellar floor reconstruction. Notably, the vomer bone can act as a landmark for the middle entrance; the anterior wall of sphenoid sinus is subsequently opened to expose the sellar floor. The ESS approach reduces nasal cavity injuries relative to TSSS and TCSS while providing sufficient exposure.

ES was first reported in 1996 by Carrau [21] and Jho [22], who used endoscopy to surgically remove pituitary adenomas. The single-nostril technique was always selected, and the left or right nostril was selected according to the nasal cavity width and tumor location. The bilateral-nostril technique can be used in patients with small nasal cavities. The details of approach are depicted as follows. The middle nasal concha is moved laterally or removed, and the endoscope is entered and placed at the sphenoethmoidal recess to identify the sphenoid sinus opening. After mucosal coagulation, the anterior wall and sinus septation are removed. The nasal septum is fractured and pushed towards the contralateral side to expose the sellar floor. Badie *et al.* [23] compared the ES, TSSS, and TCSS approaches and concluded that ES can provide a full view of the entire sinus and thus sufficient exposure when compared with TCSS and TSSS. These approaches do not differ significantly with respect to prognosis; however, the ES approach significantly reduces both the surgical duration and hospitalization period.

Approach Figures (Figs. 1-14)

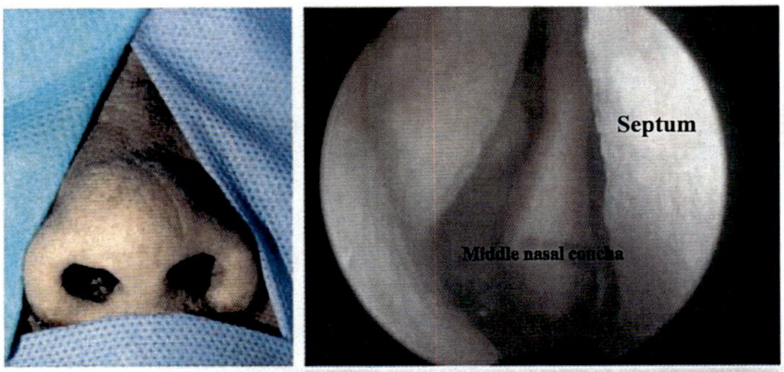

Fig. (1). Trans-nasal trans-sphenoidal approach normally uses the right nostril because the septum is usually flank-curved towards the left side, yielding a relatively larger right nasal cavity. The tumors location, sphenoidal septation, and pneumatic sinus condition can also affect the selection. Endoscopy is used to identify the middle nasal concha and septum.

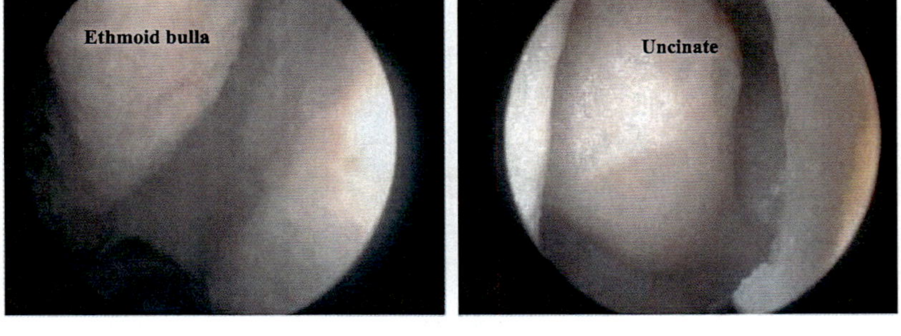

Fig. (2). The middle nasal meatus is entered under the concha to expose the ethmoid bulla and uncinate. After locating the uncinate median, the semi-lunar fissure forms an opening in the frontal sinus, maxillary sinus, and anterior ethmoid sinus group.

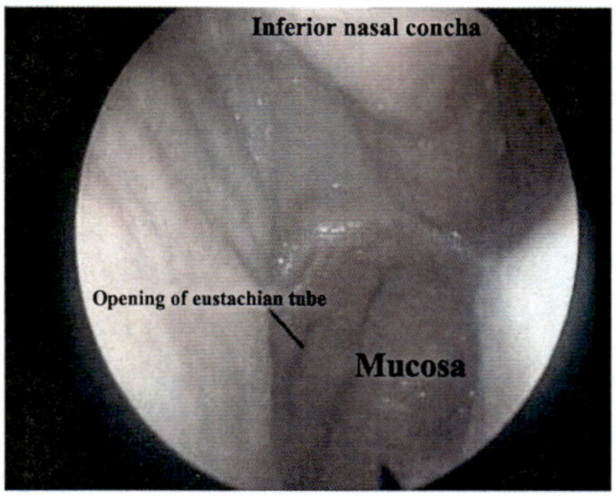

Fig. (3). Beneath the inferior nasal concha, the posterior nasal apertures, palatopharyngeal arch, and pharyngeal mucosa are exposed. The eustachian tube open can also be exposed laterally.

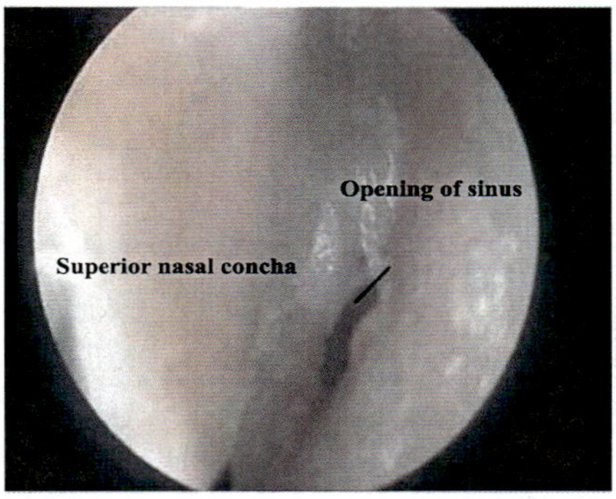

Fig. (4). The sphenoid sinus opening can be observed in the sphenoethmoidal recess at the conjunction of the superior nasal concha and septum. Normally, this opening is located 1–1.5 cm above the palatopharyngeal arch.

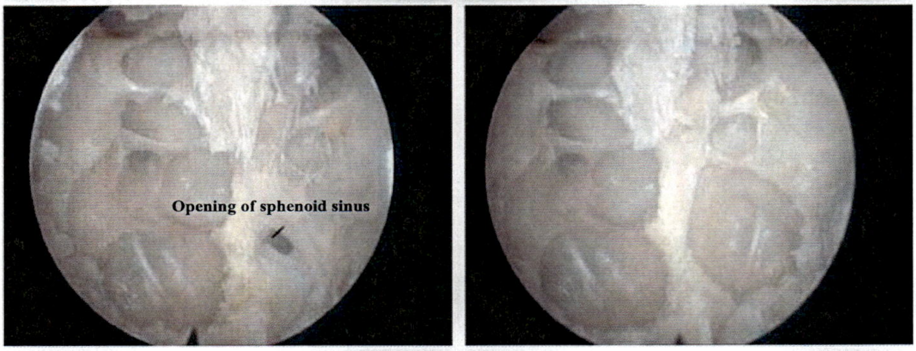

Fig. (5). Observation of poor sphenoidal sinus gasification (conchal type) *via* endoscopy; only the left-side sphenoid sinus opening can be identified. After removing the anterior sphenoid wall, no anatomical markers can be identified. The sellar floor is much thicker.

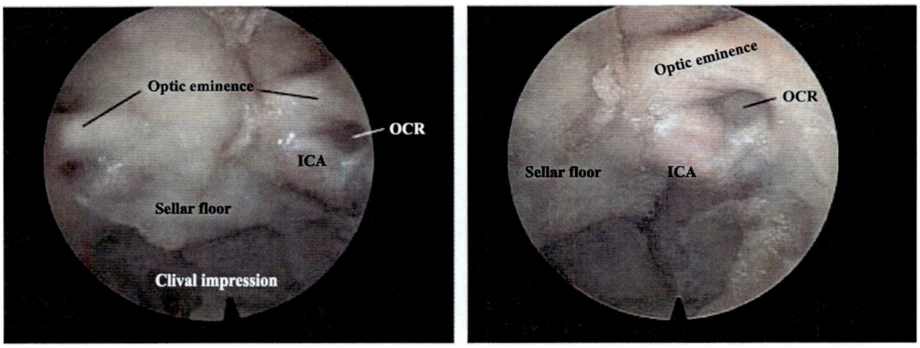

Fig. (6). Sphenoidal sinus with good gasification; after opening the anterior sinus wall, several bone markers are exposed on the sellar floor, including the bilateral ICA prominence, optic eminence, optic-carotid recess (OCR), and clival impression.

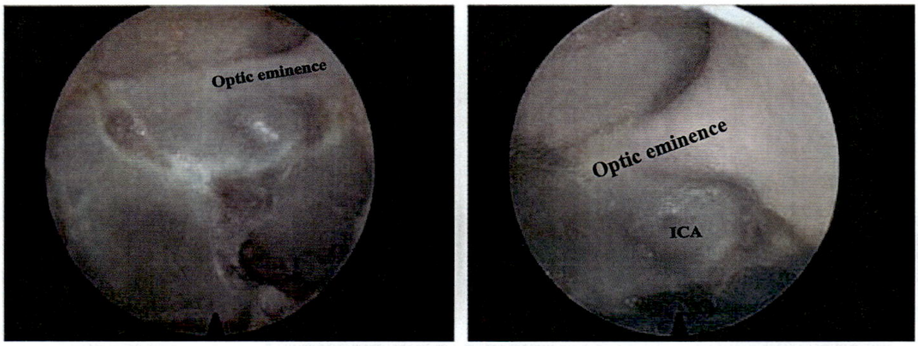

Fig. (7). In some cases with a partly pneumatic sinus, only a few markers can be identified after anterior wall removal. In this case, only the ipsilateral optic eminence and ICA prominence are exposed.

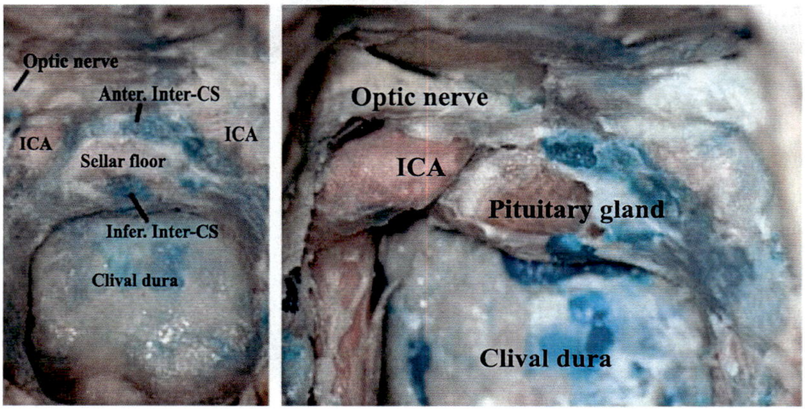

Fig. (8). After drilling the sellar floor bone, anatomical structures can be identified through the dura mater. The bilateral optic nerves, ICA, and anterior/inferior intercavernous sinuses can be observed. When one side of the sellar floor dura and CS is opened, the pituitary capsule is observed to envelop the gland. In the CS, the ICA can be identified with the sympathetic trunk on the surface.

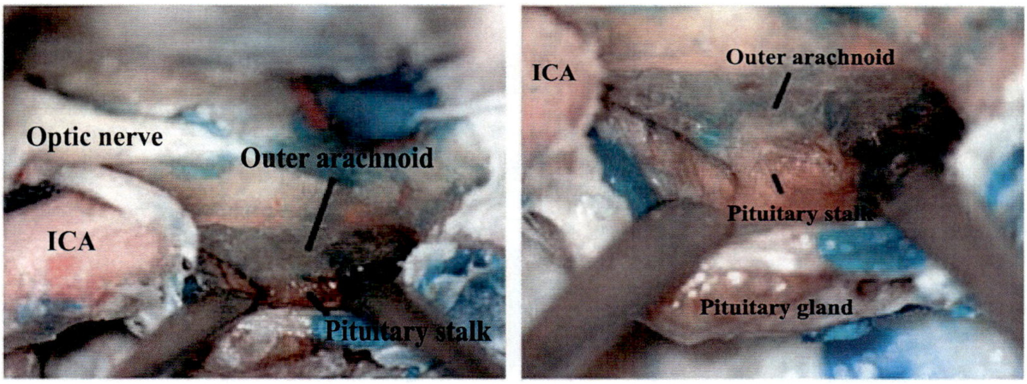

Fig. (9). The basal arachnoidal membrane (outer arachnoid) is exposed after opening the dura located at the tuberculum sellae and sphenoid platform. The basal membrane also forms an arachnoidal sleeve around the pituitary stalk.

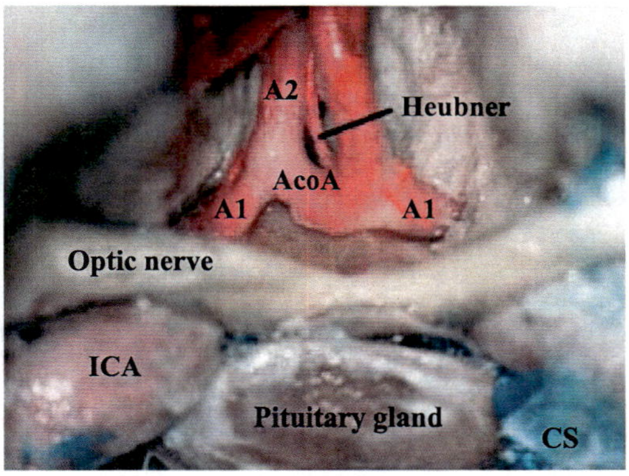

Fig. (10). Opening the basal arachnoid membrane and dissecting above the optic chiasm exposes the bilateral ACA, AcoA, and Heubner recurrent artery.

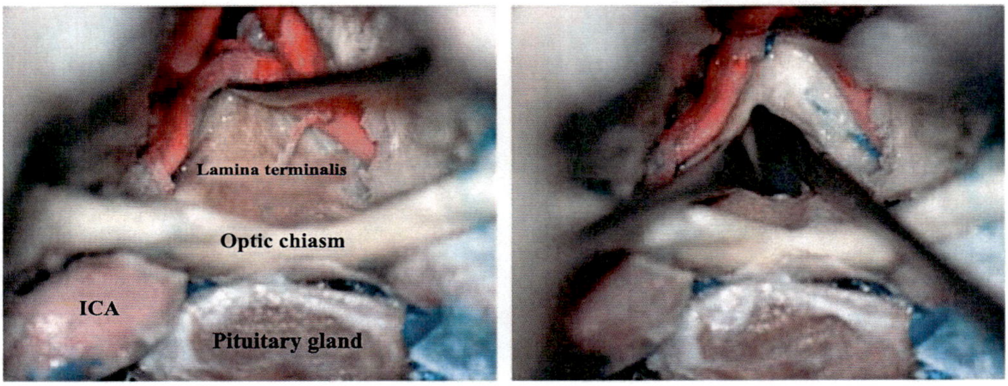

Fig. (11). The lamina terminalis can be exposed by lifting the AcoA. The third ventricle cavity can be entered by opening the terminalis.

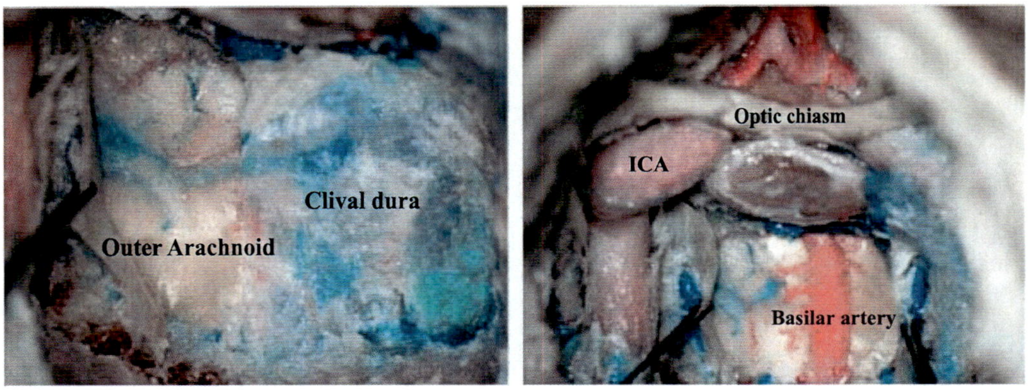

Fig. (12). Opening the clival dura exposes the arachnoid membrane covering the pons and BA.

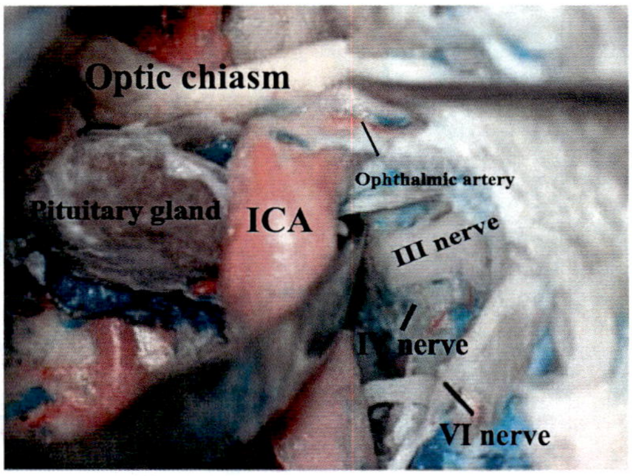

Fig. (13). One side of the CS was opened and the ICA retracted to expose the anatomical structures inside the CS. Abundant nerves are observed at the lateral ICA within the CS cavity; however, the oculomotor and trochlear nerves are located in the lateral walls of the CS. The ophthalmic artery is also exposed by retracting the dural ring of the ICA.

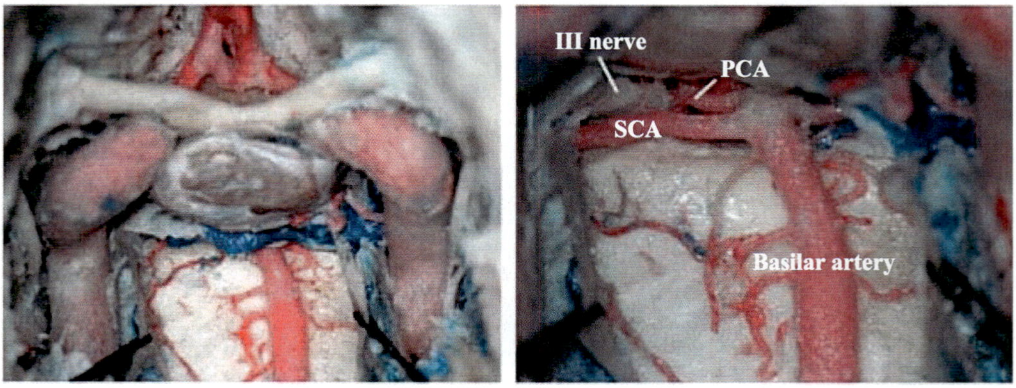

Fig. (14). Lifting the pituitary gland exposes the structures at the BA tip, including the bilateral SCA, PCA, and oculomotor nerves.

SURGERY OF CRANIOPHAYRNGIOMA

Transsphenoidal corridor is the closest and fastest approach to reach the sellar region, which is also the most minimal invasive approach to avoid the injury to the soft tissue and also brain tissue during the craniotomy. As result, this popular approach had been widely used to treat pituitary adenomas, Rathke's cyst, and meningiomas *et al.* Recent decades years, as reported by several publications, it was also used to surgical remove CP as well. However, craniopharyngioma was the special occupation of sellar region as multiple morphological variation. As our opinion, CP has totally different approach selection with compared to the pituitary adenomas. Moreover, extended transsphenoidal approach (ETS) certainly can't be used to treat all kinds of CP.

Since beginning, as being similar with pituitary adenomas, the sub-diaphragmatic location caused that the ETS approach was firstly used in the Infra-diaphragmatic CP. As theoretically, infra-diaphragmatic CP located below of the diaphragm (Fig. **15**). As results, during ETS surgery when opening the sellar floor dura, tumor will be directly exposed (Fig. **16**). However, sometimes the Id-CP will protrude through enlarged diaphragmatic foramen, which might cause close relationship to AcoA and its branches. Under this situation, ETS might cause some blinding surgical view to identify the accurate interface between tumor and AcoA complex. So we preferred trans-cranial surgery for this kind of tumor.

Intra-cisternal CP without extremely expanding was the best complication for usage of ETS. The ventral anterior exposure provided easy exposure to the ventral aspect of the optic chiasm and pituitary stalk. As the tumor located at the ventral of optical chiasm, ETS can avoid the retraction of nerves. Moreover, the originate site of this type of CP always at the middle or middle upper segment of pituitary stalk, which was easy to be dissected. Based on our experience, for intra-cisterna CP without extremely expanding to the frontal, temporal lobes or posterior cranial fossa, ETS was the best approach. However, when huge tumor with widely expanding, it should be more cautious to use ETS approach. As the trans-sphenoidal corridor can only provide a narrow exposure. For huge expanding tumor, there must be some surgical blind point, the branches of vessel might have close relationship to the tumor walls, if blindly dragging or pulling could cause vital bleeding. It was pretty difficult to stop the bleeding under ETS approach.

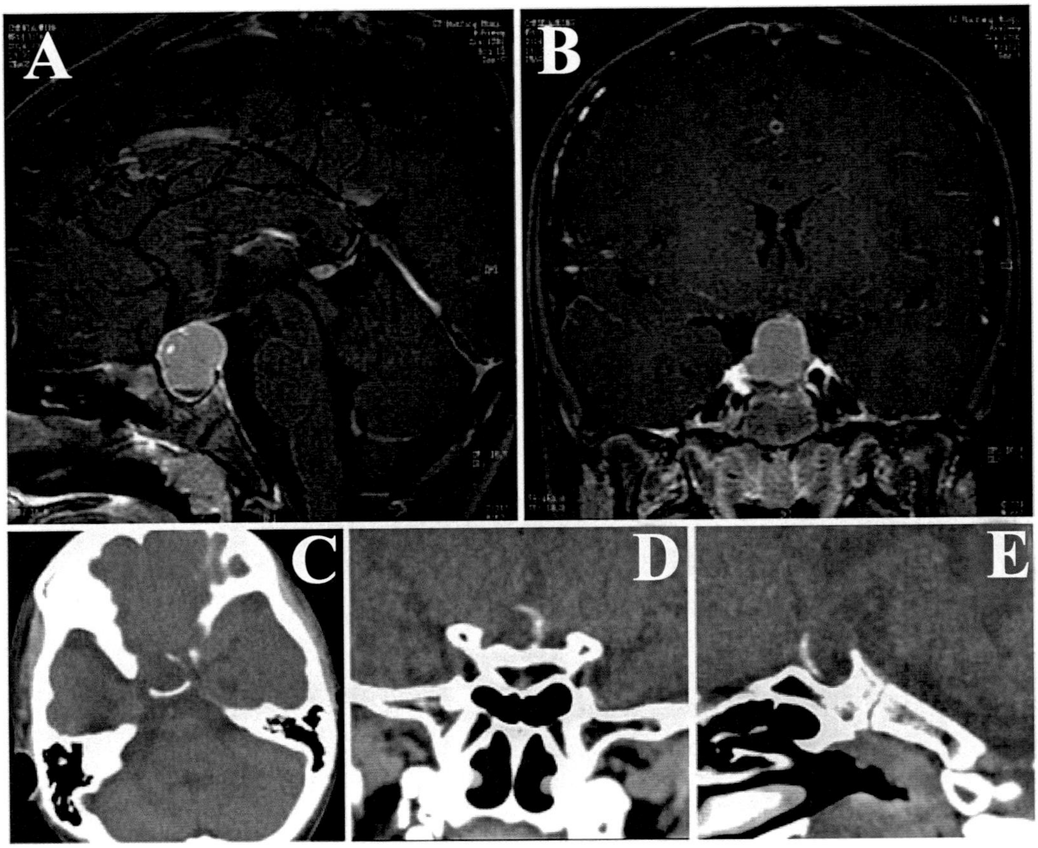

Fig. (15). This was a 6-year-old female with a 2 months history of headache. Presurgical radiological images. **A-B.** Magnetic resonance imaging revealed that the cystic predominant tumor had lifted the optic chiasm and anterior communicating artery upward. The cystic wall were enhanced significantly. The tumor was a typical Id-CP. **C, D and E.** Computed tomography indicated eggshell-shaped calcification was observed on the tumor cystic wall.

For infundibulo-tuberal CP, as tumor grew inside the nervous tissue layer of third ventricular floor, the main nerve nucleus might be displaced downwards. Under this situation, opening the ventral of 3rd VF will cause tremendous injury to the hypothalamic function. Opening the lamina terminalis and try to protect the residual nervous tissue of 3rd VF was the first choice. However, as the narrow surgical corridor and space, it was not easy to process the surgical manipulation at the superior of optical chiasm under ETS approach. Especially when CP expanded posterior extremely, the operator might have to pull and drag the cystic wall with the results of partial tumor residual. So as our opinion, for infundibulo-tuberal CP, especially posterior expanding tumor, we still preferred trans-cranial approach.

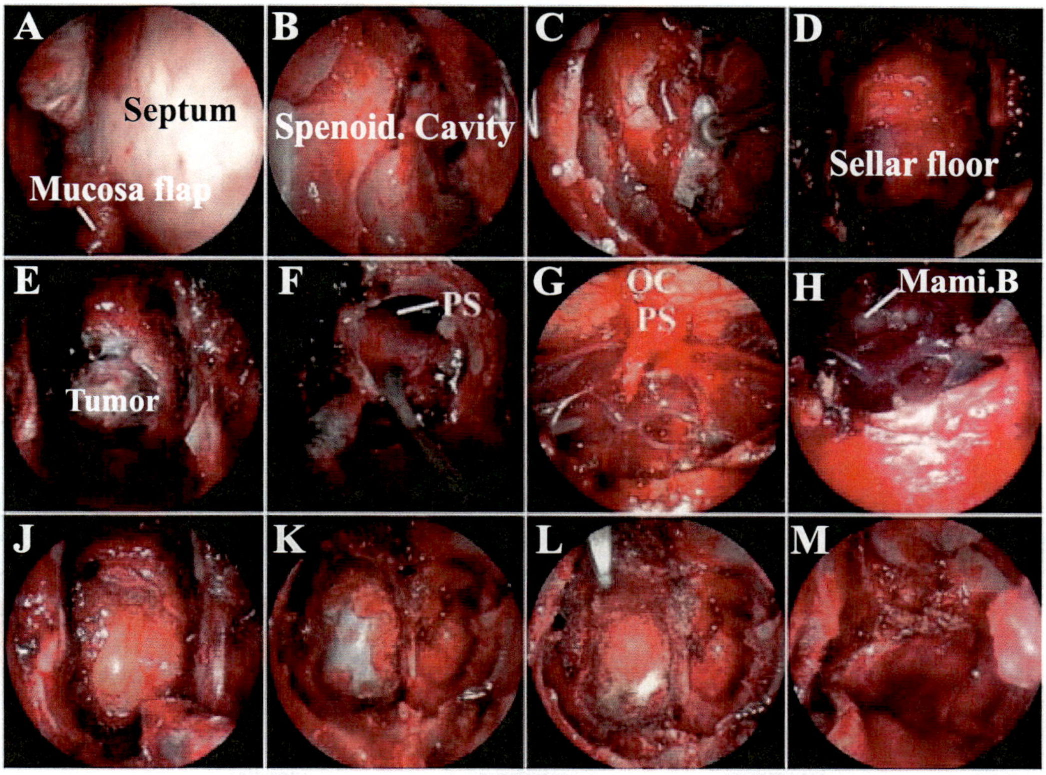

Fig. (16). Intraoperative findings. **A.** Mucosa flap was prepared for repatching the sellar floor. **B.** After removal of the anterior wall of sphenoidal sinus, the sinus cavity and sellar floor was exposed. **C.** High speed drill was used to open the sellar floor. **D.** After removing the bone of sellar floor and also the tuberculum sellae, the dura of sellar floor and anterior cranial floor was exposed. E. When opening the sellar floor dura, and thin layer of anterior lobe of pituitary gland was opened to expose the tumor. And a mass of calcification was observed on the anterior wall of tumor. F. At the top of tumor, the inflated pituitary stalk can be found. G. After totally tumor removal, the ventral aspect of optic chiasm and residual pituitary stalk was observed, and also the vascular structure. H. The bilateral mammillary bodies were also observed. J~M. After tumor removal, the fat, artificial dura, gelatin sponge and prepared mucosa flap were used for repairing the sellar floor.

CONFLICT OF INTEREST

The author (editor) declares no conflict of interest, financial or otherwise.

ACKNOWLEDGEMENTS

We should acknowledge Dr. Shi Jin for preparing the cadaver specimens and assistant about the anatomical studies.

REFERENCES

[1] Schloffer H. Erfolgreiche operation eines hypophysentumors auf nasalem wege. Wien Klin Wochenschr 1907; 20(6): 621-4.

[2] Hirsch O. Demonstration eines nach einer neuen methode operiten hypophysentumors. Verch Dtsch Ges Chir 1910; 39(1): 51-6.

[3] Cushing H. The pituitary body and its disorders of the hypophysis cerebi. Philadephia JB Lippincott 1913; pp. 292-315.

[4] Hardy J. Transphenoidal microsurgery of the normal and pathological pituitary. Clin Neurosurg 1969; 16(16): 185-217.
[PMID: 5811707]

[5] Jankowski R, Auque J, Simon C, Marchal JC, Hepner H, Wayoff M. Endoscopic pituitary tumor surgery. Laryngoscope 1992; 102(2): 198-202.
[http://dx.doi.org/10.1288/00005537-199202000-00016] [PMID: 1738293]

[6] Dandie GD, Pell MF, Atlas MD. Endoscopic transsphenoidal approach to the pituitary fossa technical note. J Clin Neurosci 1996; 3(1): 65-8.
[http://dx.doi.org/10.1016/S0967-5868(96)90085-5] [PMID: 18644266]

[7] Kitano M, Taneda M. [Endoscope assisted transsphenoidal approach for pituitary adenomas]. No Shinkei Geka 1997; 25(3): 197-203. [Endoscope assisted transsphenoidal approach for pituitary adenomas].
[PMID: 9058426]

[8] Alfieri A. Endoscopic endonasal transsphenoidal approach to the sellar region: technical evolution of the methodology and refinement of a dedicated instrumentation. J Neurosurg Sci 1999; 43(2): 85-92.
[PMID: 10735761]

[9] Arita K, Kurisu K, Tominaga A, *et al.* Transsphenoidal "cross court" approach using a slightly modified speculum to reach pituitary adenomas with lateral growth. Acta Neurochir (Wien) 2000; 142(9): 1055-8.
[http://dx.doi.org/10.1007/s007010070062] [PMID: 11086816]

[10] Yano S, Kawano T, Kudo M, *et al.* Endoscopic endonasal transsphenoidal approach through the bilateral nostrils for pituitary adenomas. Neurol Med Chir (Tokyo) 2009; 49(1): 1-7.
[http://dx.doi.org/10.2176/nmc.49.1] [PMID: 19168995]

[11] Frank G, Pasquini E, Mazzatenta D. Extended transsphenoidal approach. J Neurosurg 2001; 95(5): 917-8.
[PMID: 11702890]

[12] Catapano D, Sloffer CA, Frank G, Pasquini E, D'Angelo VA, Lanzino G. Comparison between the microscope and endoscope in the direct endonasal extended transsphenoidal approach: anatomical study. J Neurosurg 2006; 104(3): 419-25.
[http://dx.doi.org/10.3171/jns.2006.104.3.419] [PMID: 16572655]

[13] Wang Q, Lan Q, Lu XJ. Extended endoscopic endonasal transsphenoidal approach to the suprasellar region: anatomic study and clinical considerations. J Clin Neurosci 2010; 17(3): 342-6.
[http://dx.doi.org/10.1016/j.jocn.2009.05.032] [PMID: 20074954]

[14] Abuzayed B, Tanriover N, Gazioglu N, Ozlen F, Cetin G, Akar Z. Endoscopic anatomy and approaches of the cavernous sinus: cadaver study. Surg Radiol Anat 2010; 32(5): 499-508.
[http://dx.doi.org/10.1007/s00276-010-0651-3] [PMID: 20443000]

[15] Kim EH, Ahn JY, Kim SH. Technique and outcome of endoscopy-assisted microscopic extended transsphenoidal surgery for suprasellar craniopharyngiomas. J Neurosurg 2011; 114(5): 1338-49.
[http://dx.doi.org/10.3171/2010.11.JNS10612] [PMID: 21214338]

[16] Zanation AM, Snyderman CH, Carrau RL, Gardner PA, Prevedello DM, Kassam AB. Endoscopic endonasal surgery for petrous apex lesions. Laryngoscope 2009; 119(1): 19-25.
[http://dx.doi.org/10.1002/lary.20027] [PMID: 19117306]

[17] Ceylan S, Koc K, Anik I. Extended endoscopic approaches for midline skull-base lesions. Neurosurg

Rev 2009; 32(3): 309-19.
[http://dx.doi.org/10.1007/s10143-009-0201-9] [PMID: 19408020]

[18] Griffith HB, Veerapen R. A direct transnasal approach to the sphenoid sinus. Technical note. J Neurosurg 1987; 66(1): 140-2.
[http://dx.doi.org/10.3171/jns.1987.66.1.0140] [PMID: 3783248]

[19] Rodziewicz GS, Kelley RT, Kellman RM, Smith MV. Transnasal endoscopic surgery of the pituitary gland: technical note. Neurosurgery 1996; 39(1): 189-92.
[http://dx.doi.org/10.1097/00006123-199607000-00046] [PMID: 8805160]

[20] Yaniv E, Rappaport ZH. Endoscopic transseptal transsphenoidal surgery for pituitary tumors. Neurosurgery 1997; 40(5): 944-6.
[http://dx.doi.org/10.1097/00006123-199705000-00012] [PMID: 9149252]

[21] Carrau RL, Jho HD, Ko Y. Transnasal-transsphenoidal endoscopic surgery of the pituitary gland. Laryngoscope 1996; 106(7): 914-8.
[http://dx.doi.org/10.1097/00005537-199607000-00025] [PMID: 8667994]

[22] Jho HD, Carrau RL. Endoscopic endonasal transsphenoidal surgery: experience with 50 patients. J Neurosurg 1997; 87(1): 44-51.
[http://dx.doi.org/10.3171/jns.1997.87.1.0044] [PMID: 9202264]

[23] Badie B, Nguyen P, Preston JK. Endoscopic-guided direct endonasal approach for pituitary surgery. Surg Neurol 2000; 53(2): 168-72.
[http://dx.doi.org/10.1016/S0090-3019(99)00195-0] [PMID: 10713196]

CHAPTER 9

Craniopharyngioma Classification: History and its Merit

Yuntao Lu* and **Jun Pan**

Department of Neurosurgery, Nanfang Neurosurgery Research Institution, Nanfang Hospital, Southern Medical University, 1838 North Guangzhou Avenue, Guangzhou, China

Abstract: The growth pattern of craniopharyngiomas (CP) is yet to be understood due to challenges arising from the diversity of morphological features that exist. This in turn has had implications on the development of safe surgical strategies for management of these lesions. In this chapter, we proposed a morphological classification of CP based on their tumor–membrane relationship, which will contribute to better understanding of CP morphology and prediction of the intraoperative classification. Moreover, based on our studies, the arachnoidal sleeve around the pituitary stalk (ASPS) was noted, and divided the pituitary stalk into four segments. Correspondingly, the growth of CPs was divided into four basic patterns—infra-diaphragmatic (ID), extra-arachnoidal (EA), intra-arachnoidal (IA) and sub-arachnoidal (SA) growth. After analysis of 195 clinical cases of CP, we finally proposed the clinical classification "QST" classification, which detailed the relationship of the surrounding structures to CPs and purports to predict and identify the intraoperative anatomical stratification. It also attempts to help predict the growth patterns of these tumors. Finally, the surgical principle of approach selection for CP was discussed and proposed.

Keywords: ASPS, Classification, Craniopharyngioma, Membrane, Pituiray stalk.

Craniopharyngiomas (CPs) stem from residue of the embryonic canal which stretche from the oropharynx to the suprasellar median eminence and infundibulum. Theoretically, any site along this important axis might serve as the origin. Innumerable CP growth patterns following various locations and diversity of tumor extensions deepen the challenge of understanding intra-operative tumor morphology. Partial tumor resection (PTR) is accepted to avoid the hypothalamus damaged, which was thought to usually accompany gross total tumor removal

* **Corresponding author Yuntao Lu**: Department of Neurosurgery, Nanfang Neurosurgery Research Institution, Nanfang Hospital, Southern Medical University, 1838 North Guangzhou Avenue, Guangzhou, China; Tel/Fax: +8620-61641806; E-mail: lllu2000yun@gmail.com

Songtao Qi (Ed.)

(GTR). But the higher relapse rate of these injurys exhibits an additional conundrum.

Different classification systems [1 - 5] have been created serving for operative planning. A variety of nomenclature is used in the literature regarding CP growth. Some examples including intra or suprasellar, extra or intra ventriculartumors, used by Yasargil *et al.* [6], Wang *et al.* [5, 7], and Steno *et al.* [4]; pre- or postchiasmatic tumor, used by Hoffman [1]; infrachiasmatic tumor, used by Kitano [8]; and pre-infundibular, trans-infundibular, or retro-infundibular tumor, used by Kassam [2] attempted to expound the tumor location followed by facilitating the choice of operative route. Recently a morphological classification of CP was found by us based on the tumor-membrane relationship observed during surgery [9] which provides further understanding of tumor morphology and predicts the stratification during operation, consequently avoiding the injuries of vital nerve tissue.

HITSTORICAL REVIEWS OF CLASSIFICATION

In 1962 the pioneering work of Rougerie divided CPs into five types: intrasellar; intra- and suprasellar and prechiasmatic; retrochiasmatic; huge; and non-typical.

In 1980 Ciric [10] divided CPs into intraventricular; subpial; extrapial and subarachnoidal; intra- and extra-arachnoidal; and extra-arachnoidal (or purely intrasellar) types.

In 1985 Steno *et al.* [11] simply depicted CP growth patterns as classifiable into two types: intra- and suprasellar or purely suprasellar. The latter type was subdivided into intraventricular, extraventricular, and mixed types.

In 1994 Hoffman [1] divided CPs into intrasellar, prechiasmatic, and retrochiasmatic types based simply on the relationship between the tumor and optic chiasm.

In 1995, Samii proposed another classification method in his books. He thought that the degree of vertical CP extension could be divided into five grades. In the horizontalplane, tumors couldgrow anteriorly into the prechiasmatic cistern and subfrontal space, posteriorly into the interpeduncular cisterns and prepontine cisterns, cerebellopontine angle, and foramen magnum, and laterally into the subtemporal space.

In an article published by Samii in 1997 [12] in which he reviewed the surgical treatment of CP, Samii thought that the classification of four major types was the best one includingintrasellar, infundibulum-tuberian, intraventricular, and dumbbell-shaped, as proposed by Fukusima *et al.* [13]. In consideration of tumor involvement, Samii also selected the optic chiasm as a reference point and used the terms retro-, pre-, and subchiasmatic plus intrasellar to describe CPs.

In a landmark report in the CP classification literature from 1990, Yasargil *et al.* [6] reported six types: a) purely intrasellar-infradiaphragmatic, b) intrasellar and suprasellar + infradiaphragmatic and supradiaphragmatic, c) supradiaphragmatic + parachiasmatic + extraventricular, d) intraventricular and extraventricular, e) paraventricular with respect to the third ventricle, and f) purely intraventricular.

In 2004 Pascual *et al.* [14] concluded two diverse topographic entities as either strict or nonstrict intraventricular CP (IVC), according to an extensive review of well-described cases on CP by intraventricular location. In 2008 schematic diagrams [3] were introducedto illustrate in detail the different stratifications of strict and nonstrict IVC. Pascual and colleagues also described the difference between primary IVC, pseudo-intraventricular CP, and secondary IVC.

With the rapid development of endoscopic techniques, a trans-nasal approach-based classification of CP growth proposed by Kassam *et al.* [2]. He divided tumors into four types according to the tumor–infundibulum relationship: Type I, pre-infundibular. The tumor anterior to the infundibulum is visible.and It may stretch superiorly intothe prechiasmatic cistern, and the anterior communicating artery (AcoA) and A2 segment will cover the dome in these cases. The chiasm is often elevated for posteriorly displaced. The basilar artery can be saw posterior to the infundibulum and rarely encroached upon in these cases. The tumor is supportedlaterally by the internal carotid artery (ICA).

Type II, trans-infundibular (extending into the stalk). The tumor is visible conjoint with the substance of the pituitary stalk and expand the stalk from the pituitary gland and hypothalamus. it also can be seen stretching rostrally into the anterior third ventricle (ATV). The inflated stalk contains the tumor which moves retrochiasmatically at the adjacency of the optic nerve and optic tract, promoting the posterior portion of the chiasm and pushing the chiasm forward (prefixed chiasm). Again, the tumor is wraped by ICA and ON/OT bilaterally.

Type III, retro-infundibular which extends behind the pituitary gland and stalk, with two subsections (IIIa, stretching into the third ventricle; and IIIb, stretching into the interpeduncular cistern); and Type IV, which is separated to the third ventricle and/or optic recess and intangible *via* an endonasal approach. The gland is within the sella. the tumor lies in the retro-infundibular space, and the stalk is undergoing thinning and attenuation, causing it difficult to distinguish,. Entering the retroinfundibular retrochiasmatic space allows the tumor expand rostrally to infringe on the ATV (Type IIIa). This type of tumor may also move to caudallyenter the interpeduncular fossa under the mammillary bodies and infringe upon the posterior circulation (Type IIIb). In these cases, the tumor is wraped laterally *via* oculomotor nerve (III N) and posterior communicating artery (PcoA) as it brackets the ICA and posterior carotid artery.

GENERAL CLASSIFICATION AND ITS ADVANTAGES AND SHORTCOMINGS

In the above diverse classifications, several elements such as the location and relationship of CP to pituitary fossa, pituitary stalk (PS), infundibulum, and third ventricle floor (3rd VF), were taken into account. Regarding the tumor's location, a review of these existing reports reveals that the classification systems of CP can be roughly divided into two sorts: (1) Classifying CP with respect to the sella turcica, optic chiasm, and 3rd VF into prechiasmatic, retrochiasmatic, subchiasmatic, and intraventricular CPs, respectively, according to horizontal extension (such as Hoffman [1]); and (2) Classifying CPs into Grade I (intrasellar or infradiaphragmatic), II (occupying the cistern with or without an intrasellar component), III (lower half of the third ventricle), IV (upper half of the third ventricle), and V (reaching the septum pellucidum or lateral ventricles) [12, 15] according to vertical extension (such as Sammi *et al.*).

Nevertheless, in effect, CPs with a various kind of extension patterns may present similar magnetic resonance imaging (MRI) results. Examples likeinfundibulo-tuberal tumors with inferior extensions may violate the intrasellar region, by contrast, infradiaphragmatic tumors extending upword can also displace the 3rd VF. Notably, in a few classifications such as those of Yasargil *et al.* and Pascual, the true tumor growth and the distorted surrounding structures were also considered in addition to the tumor location [6, 14]. These authors had already noted the different interface of the tumor and nervous parenchyma. In particular, Pascual proposed the conception of pseudo- and secondary intraventricular CP, which provided a deep understanding of tubero-infundibular tumors.

However, in clinical, some large tumors with extension to anterior skull base or interpeduncular cistern actually have a relatively restricted basis at the PS, allowing adequate protection during the surgery of total tumor resection. Normal-sized tumors locating entirely within the PS or 3rd VF will give rise to much more challenge as attempting to protect the integrity of normal structures. In consideration of the above-described problems and the confusion regarding the growth pattern of CP, we recently proposed a supplementary classification to the previous systems [1 - 7] according to the tumor–membrane relationship.

ASPS AND FOUR SEGEMENTS OF THE PITUITARY STALK

As we know, CPs are very closely related to the PS. Theoretically, all tumors will contact the PS in different patterns. Meanwhile, the membranous structures surrounding the stalk play an indispensable role in directing the tumor–stalk relationship, although this was ignored by all above-described classifications. During clinical operations, we found that in some cases, diaphragmatic or arachnoid mater enveloped the tumor and provided a separation interface to facilitate safe surgery. The historical study of these membranes and corresponding segmentation of the PS were described with great and meaningful annotation as follows.

Arachnoidal sleeves have been studied more than 300 years since being discovered by Gerardus in 1666 and subsequently named by Frederick in 1692. The detailed anatomy of the subarachnoidal cisterns were described by Yasargil *et al.* in his landmark studies published in 1976 and 1984 [16]. The arachnoid covered the sellar region has garnered particular attention in recent years because of the relevant complexities and important structures. similarly, the cisterns formed by membranes like chiasmatic, carotid, and prepontine cisterns, have been well documented. The chiasmatic cistern located near the PS has traditionally been a acknowledged corridor for utilization during operation. As described by Jian L [17], the chiasmatic membrane is composed of two leaves including suprachiasmatic leaf and basal leaf. The suprachiasmatic leaf extends posterosuperiorly along the superior surface of the optic chiasm. The basal leaf is located under the optic chiasm and diffuse posteriorly against the surface of the diaphragm. it stretchs from the ventral aspect of chiasm to the PS and then onto the surface of diaphragm. Inoue *et al.* firstly proposed the idea on an outer and inner component of arachnoid membrane [18] in their deepening studies of the chiasmatic cistern. This proposal described that the outer component surrounds the entire brain and the inner component divides the subarachnoid space into cisterns. The walls of the chiasmatic cistern are thought to be constituted by two medial carotid membranes, a diencephalic membrane (inner arachnoid) and outer arachnoid staying on the diaphragm, Although all previously published studies has depicted the PS as located within this cistern, the surrounding arachnoid membrane has been correspondingly neglected.

In our study [19], 21 adults and eight fetal cadavers were studied anatomically and histologically. In sagittal sections through the PS, it was observed that the suprasellar arachnoid origining from the basic membrane of arachnoid (BAM) surrounding PS and then constitute an arachnoidal sleeve (ASPS). The ASPS was found to be comprised by two parts: outer layer (fibrous component) and inner layer (trabecular component) (Fig. **1**). The fibrous component covers the tuberculum and diaphragm and courses toward the PS, wrapping the stalk superiorly. The trabecular component lies in the ventral aspect of the optic chiasm and is considered to connect the lamina terminalis and medial carotid membrane. This inner arachnoid wraps the PS inferiorly. Therefore, the PS is well protected by these membranes.

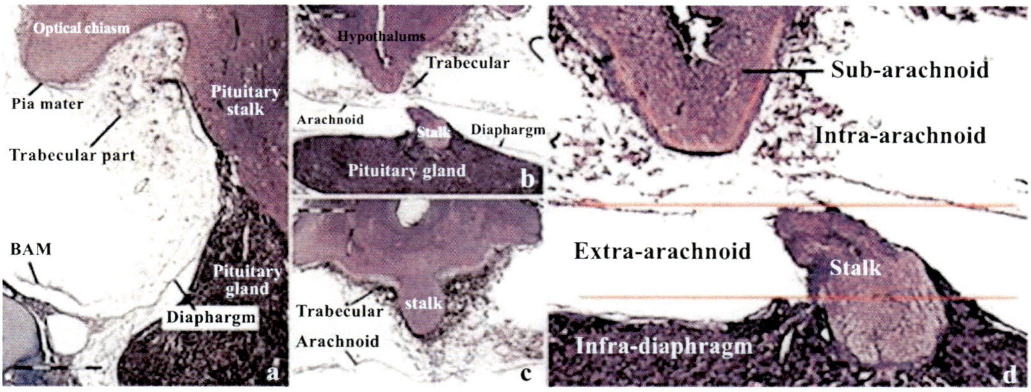

Fig. (1). (Reference from Songtao Qi *et al.* [9]). Sagittal section and coronal section through the pituitary stalk (PS), demonstrating the arachnoidal sleeve (ASPS) and four segmentations of the PS (Masson trichrome stain). (A–C) The suprasellar arachnoid, which is continuous with the basement membrane of the arachnoid (BAM), wraps the PS to form the fibrous component of the ASPS. The ASPS tends to thicken at the ventral aspect of the optic chiasm because of along with reinforcement from the trabecular component,; it also adheres tightly to the pia mater. (D) Amplification view showing the division of whole PS into infradiaphragmatic, extra-arachnoidal, intra-arachnoidal, and subarachnoidal segments.

The ASPS was found to adhere tightly to the pia mater covering the external surface of the optic chiasm in the coronal sections whichpresents a challenge to the histological differentiation of these structures. The distal part of the PS is beneath the ASPS without arachnoidal sleeve envelopment. The whole PS can be divided into four segments: infradiaphragmatic, extra-arachnoidal, intra-arachnoidal, and subarachnoidal from the magnified coronal section depicted in (Fig. **4d**).

TOPOGRAPHIC CLASSIFICATION BASED ON THE RELEVANT PARASELLAR MEMBRANES

The stratification of structures surrounding tumor has been neglected within the above-described existing classification systems . It is highly challenging during the surgery of tumor dissection, especially for an inexperienced neurosurgeon. The interface among the tumor and surrounding structures is always unclear, even in the hands of an expert surgeon. As present study indicated, depending on the arachnoid sleeve envelope, the PS might have variable morphological features [19]. We propose a topographic classification according to the unique relationship of tumor and arachnoid that directly correlates with surgical stratification.This classification can clearly describe the interaction between tumor and surrounding structures for neurosurgeons. Correspondingly, the membranes provide a particular surgical interface when handling each type of tumor growth pattern which in turn directly decides the surgical technique and the feasibility of both PS and 3rd VF preservation.

CP growth patterns are divided into four subtypes based on the locations, relationships with arachnoidal structures, complete analysis of the pre-operative MRI, and intra-operative findings of 195 CPs. The four basic growth patterns are infradiaphragmatic (ID), extra-arachnoidal (EA), intra-arachnoidal (IA), and subarachnoidal (SA; depicted in Fig. (**2**)). The possible original sites of CPs with varying growth patterns are also delineated in this figure.

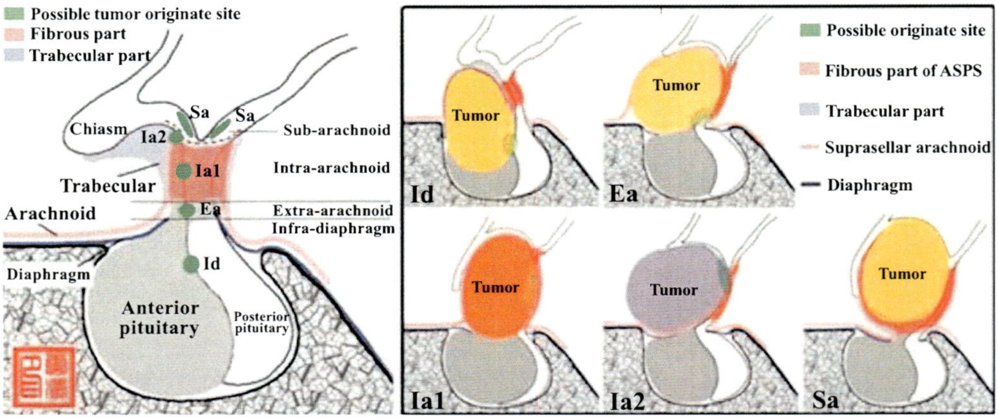

Fig. (2). (Reference from Songtao Qi *et al.* [9]). The four basic craniopharyngioma growth patterns are showed in this schematic diagram . The arachnoid sleeve (ASPS) and four stalk segments shown at left,. Correspondingly, several different possible points of tumor origin indicated as “ID, EA, IA1, IA2, and SA” correspond to the basic tumor growth patterns are shown at right.

ID Pattern

In this subtype, the suprasellar arachnoid crosses beyond the upper surface of the diaphragm. The original site of tumor is most likely under the diaphragm, and the entire tumor is wraped by the dura mater. The optic chiasm and ASPS are shoved superiorly by the tumor. According to the tumor growth orientation and also the tilt angle of pituitary stalk to the dorsum sellae, the pre-chiasmatic space (the first space) can be enlarged or not, which should be evaluated carefully in the MRI scan before surgery.

With ID growth pattern, the tumor is distinctly separated from all suprasellar structures because of tending to be covered by dura mater and arachnoid outside the diaphragm.. Hence, the tumor can be free from the suprasellar neurovascular structures by blunt dissection. However, given the tumor's intrasellar location, the diaphragm must be incised to reveal the tumor. The proximal third of the stalk was always found to be whole with this type of tumor. The fibrous part of stalk was identified posterior to the tumor, and attempts have been paid to preserve it in some cases. Based on tumor location and morphology and the protection provided by diaphragm and suprasellar arachnoid, the trans-sphenoidal (TS) approach might be an applicable corridor treating the tumor with respect to avoiding injury to vital structures (such as the optic chiasm and 3rd VF).

EA Pattern

The site of tumor origin likely locates at the extra-arachnoidal segment of PS. With external growth, the tumor inevitably encroaches into the extremely enlarged first space. The tumor, which lacks a diaphragmatic cover, directly contacts with the suprasellar arachnoid followed by providing an interface at which separating the tumor from optic chiasm and tubero-infundibulum.

As a result of being covered with a relatively compact fibrous arachnoid, the tumor exhibiting EA growth provides a surgical interface among tumor and surrounding structures. Generally speaking, a relatively intact PS is identified posterior to the tumor. The continuity of the 3rd VF–stalk–pituitary gland can be well protected during operation with this type of tumor. The above two types of tumors are considered to originate from the lower part of PS and directly connect with the stalk.

IA Pattern

The tumor, originating from the intra-arachnoidal segment of PS, expands into the ASPS. This pattern can be divided into two subtypes: IA1 and IA2. With IA1, the tumor enlarges the PS because of growing within the fibrous part of ASPS. The diaphragm pushed downwards and the optic chiasm displaced anteriorly result a comparatively small first space. Tumors exhibiting the IA2 growth pattern mainly infringe the trabecular part of ASPS, displacing the suprasellar arachnoid inferiorly and the PS posteriorly. Some tumors will also enlarge first space *via* expanding prechiasmatically.

Tumors exhibiting IA growth present two different patterns. For Pattern IA1, the tumor grows within the fibrous part of the ASPS with a median point of origin, and subsequent growth causes the expansion of PS. on this occasion, although the ASPS can isolate the tumor from surrounding structures, the stalk must be vertically dissected for removing tumor. The other scenario is that the tumor originates in the upper portion. The relatively loose trabecular part of the ASPS yields a tumor that presents as growing outside of the stalk and within the trabeculae (pattern IA2). These tumors can adhere to the different surrounding neurovascular structures, necessitating sharp dissection to free the structures.

SA Pattern

With a probable original site of tubero-infundibulum, these tumors encroach within the 3rd VF and are entirely located within the subarachnoidal space, thus pushing the ASPS inferiorly. These tumors tend to infringe the hypothalamus which often lack of membranous plane for separation.

For the patterns of ID, EA, and IA, the extra-axial approach is the optimal surgical option for avoiding injury to the 3rd VF because these tumors separated from the subarachnoidal area by membranous structures. In contrast, the intra-axial route, either alone or in conjunction with the extra-axial route, is the most appropriate operative approach for tumors exhibiting SA growth since these tumors grow within the 3rd VF without any separation from the arachnoid.

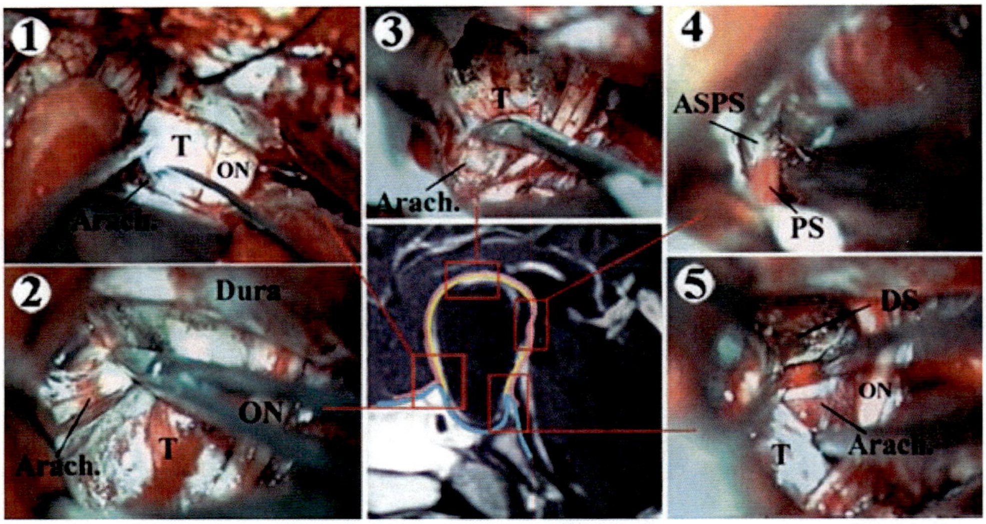

Fig. (3). (Reference from Songtao Qi *et al.* [9]). Infra-diaphragmatic craniopharyngioma (CP) with single ID growth pattern. *Via* presurgical magnetic resonance imaging (sagittal), a cystic CP was found in the intra- and suprasellar region, with enhanced signal in the tumor wall. The diaphragm exhibited an eggshell shape and covered the whole tumor because of the constant pushing from tumor,. The pituitary gland and stalk (PS) are difficult to be clearly identified because of severe sellar involvement. Intra-operative image: a large prechiasmatic space is observed *via* the frontointerhemispheric approach in most tumors of this type (1). Through this space, a smooth tumor boundary (T) appears continuous with the dura mater covering the Sphenoid platform (2). Furthermore, a thin layer of arachnoid (Arach.) covered the tumor surface (2, 3). Behind the tumor, the upper third of the PS, which is wrapped by the arachnoid sleeve, is observed (4, 5); however, the lower two-thirds is seldom clearly identifiable because of extreme tumor expansion. ON, optic nerve, DS, dorsum sellae.

CLINICAL ANALYSIS

195 cases of CPs in our department were used to depict tumorous growth pattern as illustrated in Figs. (**3**, **4**, **5**, **6**, **7**, **8** and **9**) after reviewing pre-operative imaging and intraoperative videos. For distinguishing various structures, individual color codes are used on pre-operative images following: dura mater, blue; diaphragm, yellow; suprasellar arachnoid, pink; and ASPS, pink (fibrous part) and blue (trabecular part).

Infra-Diaphragmatic Tumor

The ID pattern is the basic growth pattern of CP Fig. (**3**). In some cases, however, CP can break through the enlarged diaphragmatic opening and grow extra-arachnoidally, thus exhibiting the ID+EA pattern (Fig. **4**).

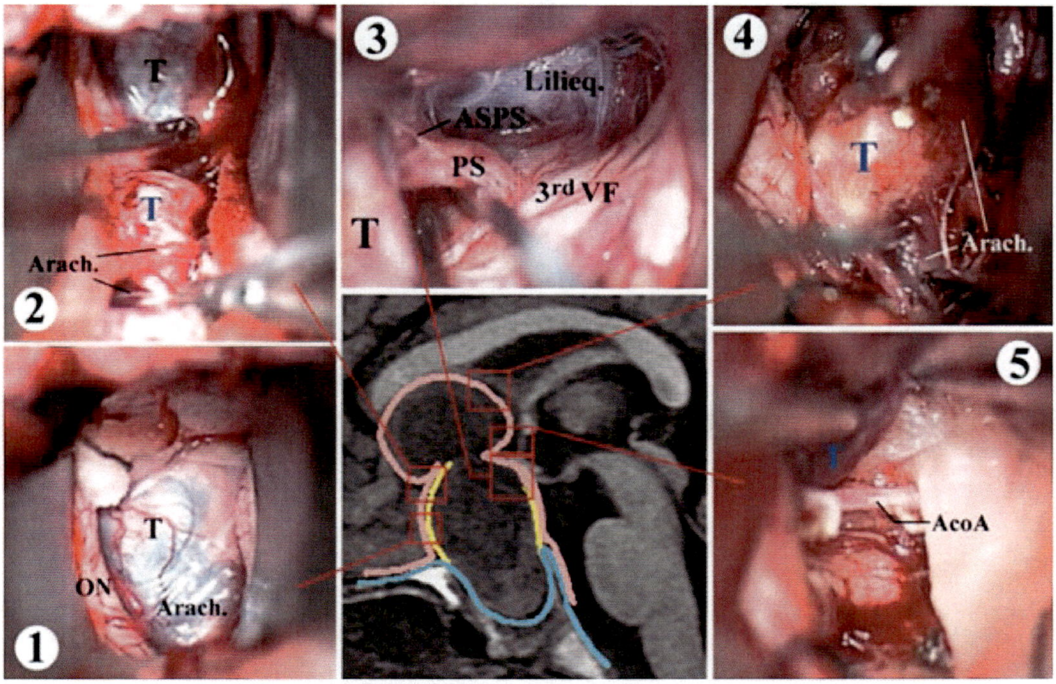

Fig. (4). (Reference from Songtao Qi *et al.* [9]). Infra-diaphragmatic CP with ID+EA pattern. As in the tumor with a single ID pattern (Fig. 6), a smooth tumor (black T) boundary seemed to continue with the dura mater through the enlarged prechiasmatic space covering the Sphenoid platform (1). A layer of arachnoid (Arach.) can be found covering the tumor surface (ID pattern), whereas part of tumor break through the diaphragmatic opening (blue T). the restriction of diaphragmatic opening formed a snowman shape (2) on the preoperative magnetic resonance imaging. In such cases, the part of tumor behind the diaphragm still be covered by arachnoid (EA pattern) (4), which is separated by optic chiasm and anterior communicating artery as indicated in (5). The arachnoid sleeve (ASPS) was found to wrap the pituitary stalk (PS). Simultaneously, the proximal part of the PS and third ventricle floor always remain intact (3). generally, pituitary gland and the distal part of PS are hardly identifiable. ON, optic nerve; Lilieq., Liliequist, membrane.

Suprasellar Extraventricular Tumor

This type of tumor has two distinct basic growth patterns that correspond to either lower or upper origin of PS. A tumor with lower site of origin (extra-arachnoidal segment of the PS) was found to grow under the fibrous arachnoid and the ASPS, so itpresents as the EA pattern (Fig. **5**). On the other hand, a tumor with upper site of beginning (proximal part of the intra-arachnoidal section) grew within the trabecular component of the ASPS and pushed the fibrous arachnoid downwards, thus exhibiting as the IA2 growth pattern (Fig. **6**), the extra-ventricular part of tumor).

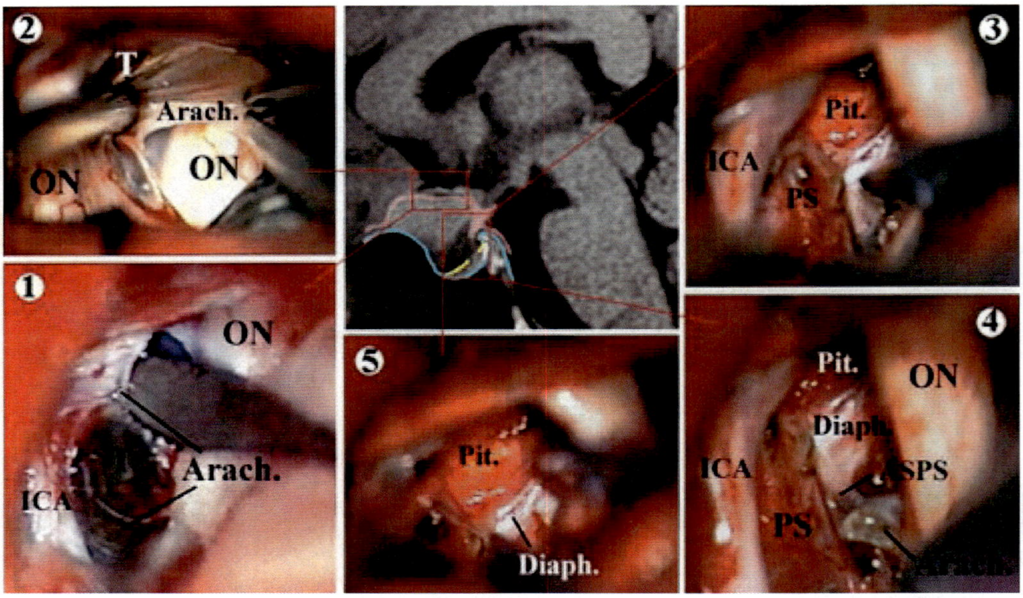

Fig. (5). (Reference from Songtao Qi *et al.* [9]). Extra-ventricular craniopharyngioma with EA growth. An intra- and suprasellar tumor can be identified *via* the presurgical MRI T1-weighted image,. An intact third ventricle floor (3rd VF) and prechiasmatic growth indicate an extraventricular tumor. This tumor grew and protruded outside the pituitary stalk (PS) and arachnoidal cistern. The PS was shoved backwards and the normal pituitary gland, which is covered by the diaphragm, moved at the bottom of the hypophyseal fossa. Intraoperative images: a fibrous arachnoid (Arachnoid.) is observed to cover the tumor surface (T) (2) using a left pterional approach through the inflated first space and blunt dissection can be used to free this type of tumor from the optic nerves and internal carotid artery (1). The downward-displaced diaphragm (Diaph.) and enlarged diaphragmatic opening were observed (3, 5) at the bottom of tumor. A relatively intact PS was found to be surrounded by ASPS, and the ASPS is continuous with the arachnoidal membrane (4). Generally speaking, the integrity of 3rd VF–stalk–pituitary gland (Pit.) can be completely preserved. ON, optic nerve.

Extra- and Intra-Ventricular Tumor

Extra-ventricular tumors with the IA2 pattern may also exhibit subarachnoidal growth (SA pattern) in some cases, thereby exhibiting a combined extra- and intraventricular growth pattern (IA2+SA; Fig. **6**).

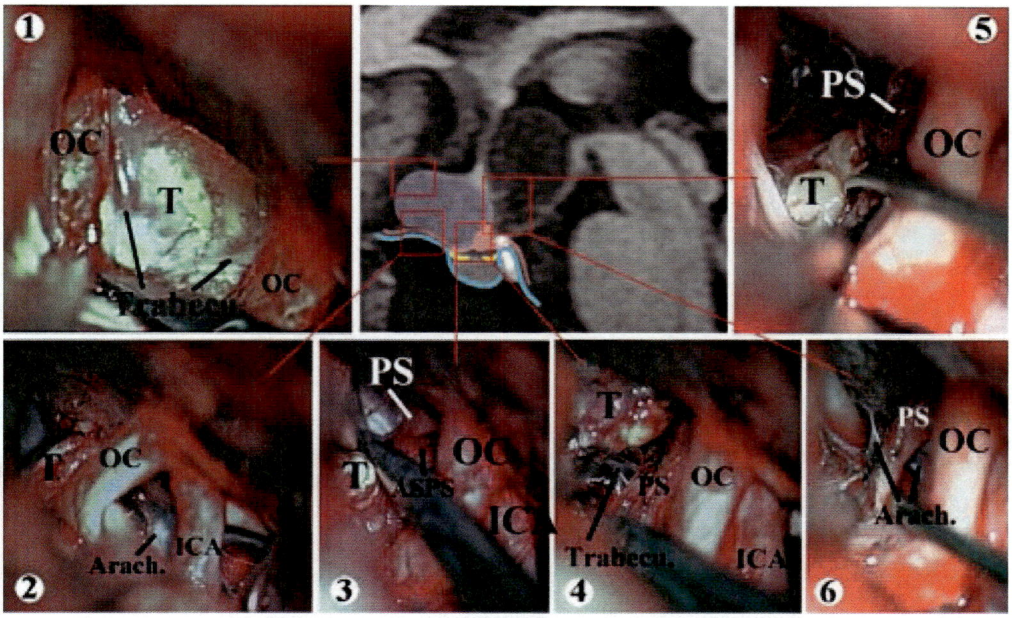

Fig. (6). (Reference from Songtao Qi *et al.* [9]). Extra- and intraventricular (IA2+SA) craniopharyngioma. Using presurgical T1-weighted MRI, prechiasmatic growth and an identifiable pituitary stalk (PS) indicate that the anterior part of tumor grows outside the ventricle (IA2 pattern). The enlarged infundibulum and third ventricle floor (3rd VF) certify the intraventricular part of the tumor (SA pattern). The blue area indicates the trabecular part of arachnoid sleeve (ASPS), which covers the surface of extraventricular tumor. Intraoperative images: A layer of relatively loose membranous trabeculum (Trabecu.) was observed to surround the tumor through the inflated first space. The tumor always tightly adhered to the neurovascular structure even after isolating these trabeculae, which must be freed *via* sharp dissection (1). As is continuous with the ASPS,, a layer of intact fibrous arachnoid is observed beneath the tumor,, which wraps the PS (2, 3). Some trabeculae segment the tumor and nerve tissue near the 3rd VF and at the top of extraventricular tumor(4),. An enlarged 3rd VF can be observed after removing the tumor inside the trabecular part of the ASPS. The intraventricular tumor was exposed after incising the enlarged 3rd VF (5),; no membranous separation was observed between tumor and nervous structures. Continuity of the 3rd VF–stalk–pituitary gland was partly protected as tumor totally be removed (6). ON, optic nerve.

Trans-infundibular Tumor

CPs with a original site in the intra-arachnoidal segment of PS tend to encroach superiorly and inferiorly within the stalk which is wraped by the fibrous part of ASPS (IA1 pattern) and it will cause the stalk to bulge and expand conversely (Fig. **7**). This type of tumor can expand to the subarachnoidal area (SA pattern) and encroach tothe pituitary fossa *via* penetrating through the diaphragm. The intrasellar part of tumor is then covered by diaphragm (ID pattern). So the resulting growth pattern is ID+IA1+SA.

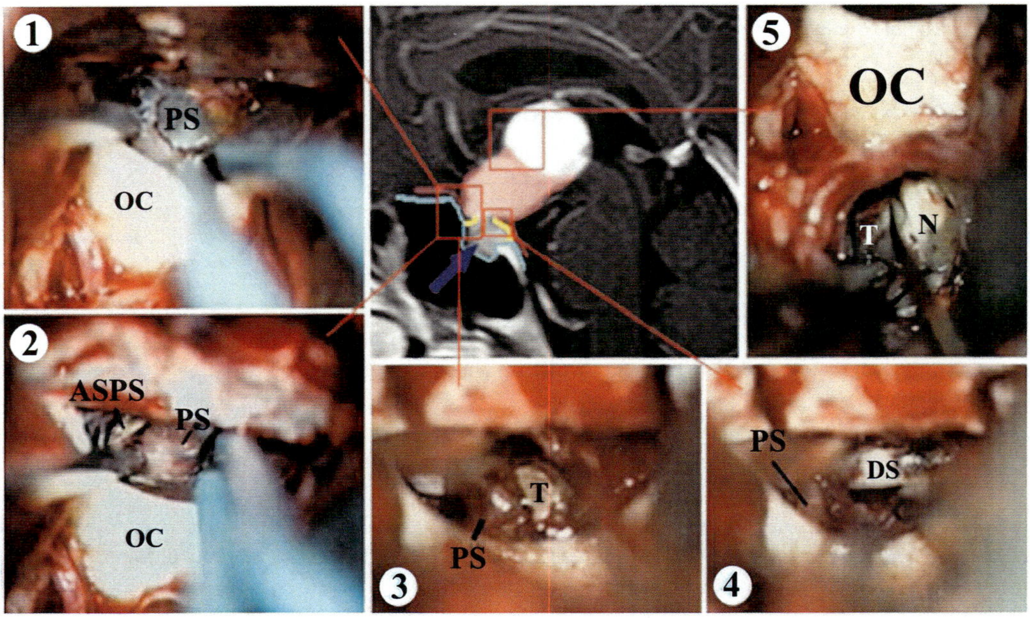

Fig. (7). (Reference from Songtao Qi *et al.* [9]). Trans-infundibular craniopharyngioma with ID+IA1+SA growth pattern. The tumor grew and expanded inside the pituitary stalk (PS) and theparts in the suprasellar and intrasellar (blue arrow) presenting "Mickey Mouse" on the presurgical enhanced magnetic resonance imaging. The diaphragm covers the intrasellar part of tumor(ID pattern) not the suprasellar. The normal pituitary gland is hardly identified. the lower part of suprasellar tumor (IA1) is separated from the surrounding structures because the tumor is wraped by fibrous arachnoid sleeve (ASPS). The upper part of tumor is situated directly inside the third ventricle floor (3rd VF) with no arachnoid-mediated separation (SA). Intra-operative images: An expanded PS was found to be surrounded by ASPS through an almost normal-sized first space, (1, 2). The proximal part of the stalk is expanded in a reverse-umbrella shape. After incising the bulgy PS, the tumor could be exposed inside the pituitary stalk (3) and the diaphragm boundary could be certified (4). The lamina terminalis space could be used to remove intraventricular tumors which was observed to grow inside the 3rd VF without arachnoidal separation. This type of tumor surface (T) is still covered by a thicker nervous tissue layer (N) (5). OC, optic chiasm; DS, dorsum sellae.

Infundibulo-tuberal Tumor

This kind of tumor appears to originate at the subarachnoidal segment of PS and presents an SA growth pattern (Fig. **8**). With subsequent CP growth, there is the consequence of 3rd VF deformation and hydrocephalus secondary to the obstruction of foramen of Monro. In addition to the straightforward SA growth pattern, infundibulo-tuberal CP can also inflate in the fibrous part of ASPS, causing the SA+IA1 growth pattern (Fig. **9**). Given tumors as mentioned above differ from trans-fundibular tumors, the ID pattern is not noted in this subgroup.

Notably, our classification system should not replaces other pre-existing classification systems (*e.g.*, those of Yasargil *et al.*, Hoffman, and Kassam *et al.*)

because of basing on anatomical growth models. Instead, it should be regarded as a supplement to those earlier classification systems in consideration of the complex morphological and clinical features of CP. A description of tumor growth only based on analysis of the membranous structures is inadequate. Following the above analysis of 195 cases of CPs, which were divided into four basic growth patterns as infradiaphragmatic pattern, extraventricular pattern, extra- and intraventricular pattern, tubero-infundibular pattern, and trans-infundibular pattern according to previous classification systems, our classification system allows a further understanding of tumor growth and intraoperative stratification. Even CPs with highly changeful appearances can still be understood according to our classification system.

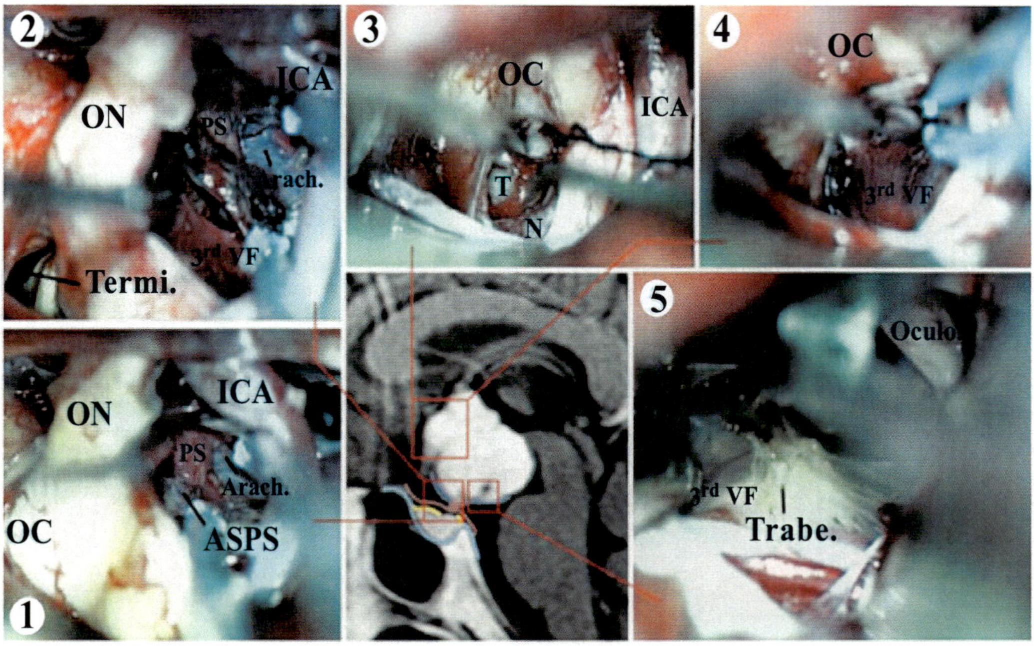

Fig. (8). (Reference from Songtao Qi *et al.* [9]). Infundibulo-tuberal craniopharyngioma with a single SA growth pattern. On preoperative T1-weighted magnetic resonance images, a suprasellar tumor is shown to displace the third ventricle floor (3rd VF). The distal part of pituitary stalk (PS) is found to associate with the normal pituitary gland, which is wraped by arachnoid sleeve (ASPS). The diaphragm which is marked continues to seal the pituitary fossa. The blue area indicates the trabecular part of ASPS, a small first space is observed with most tumors of this type during the surgery (1).The intact distal part of the PS, which is wrapped in a thickened ASPS, is always observed in tumors of this type through the optic-internal carotid artery space (second space) (1). The inflated, bulging ("frog-belly" shaped) 3rd VF is covered with trabeculae (Trabe; 5). The craniopharyngioma (T) contacts the nervous tissue layer (N) directly without membranous isolation (3) through the lamina terminalis opening (Termi.). As tumor is removed, the residual 3rd VF can be certified at one lateral side (4); incision of the 3rd VF can also make it. The integrity of 3rd VF–PS–pituitary gland is partly preserved (2). However, in some cases involving huge calcifications, an extremely thin 3rd VF necessitates disruption of this continuity. ON, optic nerve; OC, optic chiasm.

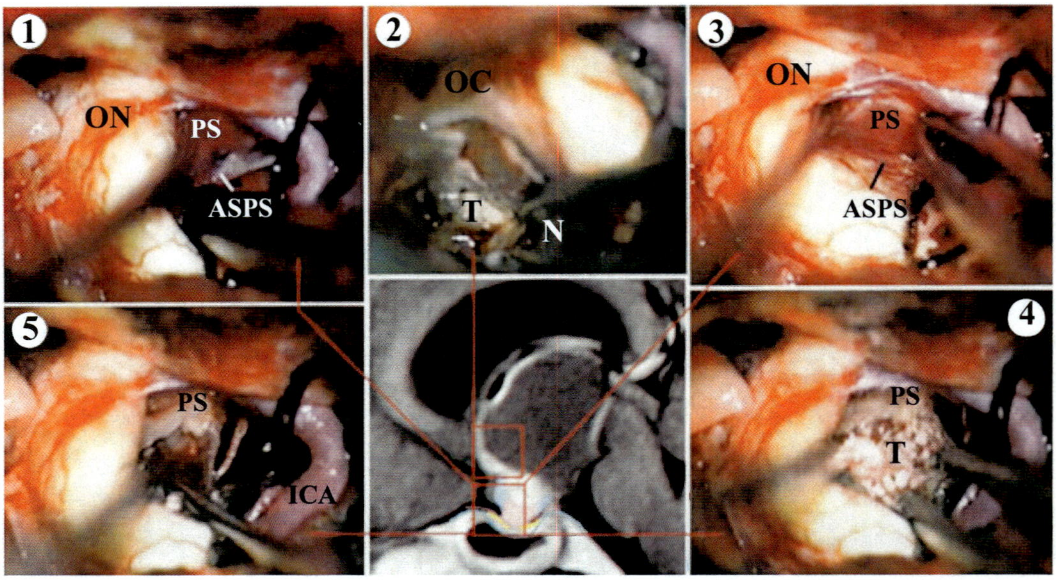

Fig. (9). (Reference from Songtao Qi *et al.* [9]). An infundibulo-tuberal craniopharyngioma (CP) with an IA1+SA growth pattern. On preoperative T1-weighted magnetic resonance imaging (MRI), an intraventricular CP is shown to cause severe hydrocephalus. The diaphragm and normal gland are pushed downwards and located in the bottom of the hypophyseal fossa, causing the sellar involvement on MRI. The tumor expand to the third ventricle floor which is behind the optic chiasm, causing a very small first space. Intraoperative images: The enlarged pituitary stalk (PS) enveloped in the arachnoid sleeve can be certified through the second space (1, 3). Opening the lamina terminalis space was required before removing the intraventricular part of tumor (T), which was found to contact the nervous tissue layer (N) with no membranous isolation (2). Next, a vertical incision in the pituitary stalk was required to expose the tumor (4). After tumor removed, the distal part of pituitary stalk remained intact (5). ON, optical nerve.

Comparison of Cases Between Adults and Children

There are no published data regarding differences in the growth patterns of CPs in adults *versus* children previously. Nevertheless, some patterns could be identified through a review of the literature. Gabriel *et al.* [20] introduced their experience in treating 47 children with CP. The authors divided cases into four types: 14 were purely intrasellar (29.8%), 25 were tubero-infundibular (53.2%), 1 was strictly intraventricular (2%), and 7 were global or giant (14.9%). Lee *et al.* [21] used the Choux–Raybaud [22] classification to distinguish 66 pediatric CPs as purely intrasellar CPs (n = 27, 40.9%) and third ventricular (infundibulum and tuber cinereum) CPs (n = 39, 59.1%) from MRI, computed tomography (CT) and surgical findings. Interestingly, no extraventricular tumors were reported in these cases. All of these data basing on morphological features of tumors in pediatric populations indicate a lack of the extraventricular type among young patients. This finding has been certified in our study too.

From our cohort, 195 cases of CPs were statistically analyzed (Table **1**, locations of tumors with various growth patterns in children and adults). Compared to adults, children with CP showed significantly different growth patterns (p = 0.023) and Infradiaphragmatic CPss were predominantly observed in children too (42% vs. 7.0%, p <0.0001). On the contrary, almost all extraventricular tumors were diagnosed in adult patients (28.1% vs. 3.7%, p <0.0001). But there was no significant difference in the locations of extra- and intraventricular tumors (4.4% vs. 6.2%, p = 0.578) or trans-infundibular tumors (2.6% vs. 1.3%, p = 0.499). Furthermore, with regard to infundibulo-tuberal CPs, although no significant difference found between children and adults (57.9% vs. 46.8%, p = 0.131), tumors with a pure SA pattern were primary in adults (47.4% vs. 30.8%, p = 0.021). A p-value of 0.257, however, manifested a lack of a statistically significant difference in the location of infundibulo-tuberal tumors with the IA+SA pattern between children and adults.

Table 1. Clinical case analysis of 195 cases of craniopharyngioma (CP).

No. of CP with the indicated growth pattern		**Adult***		**Pediatric**		**Total**
		n	**%**	**n**	**%**	
Infradiaphragmatic #	ID Pattern	8	7.0%	25	30.8%	42
	ID+EA Pattern	0	0%	9	11.2%	
Extraventricular ##	EA Pattern	24	21.1%	3	3.7%	35
	IA2 Pattern	8	7.0%	0	0%	
Extra- and intraventricular	IA2+SA Pattern	5	4.4%	5	6.2%	10
Trans-infundibular	ID+IA1+SA Pattern	3	2.6%	1	1.3%	4
Infundibulo-tuberal	SA Pattern	54 Δ	47.4%	25	30.8%	104
	IA1+SA Pattern	12	10.5%	13	16.0%	
Total		**114**		**81**		**195**

p-values were calculated using a two independent sample test (Mann–Whitney Test).
* Significant variation was foundin growth pattern distribution (*vs.* pediatric patients, *p* = 0.023).
# Infra-diaphragmatic CPs were predominantly distributed among pediatric cases (*p* <0.0001).
Extra-ventricular CPs were predominantly found among adult patients (*p* <0.0001).
Δ Infundibulo-tuberal CPs with pure SA pattern were preferentially distributed among adult cases (*p* = 0.021).
ID, infradiaphragmatic; EA, extra-arachnoid; IA, intra-arachnoid; SA, subarachnoid

Following a statistical analysis, only three of the 81 children with CPss (3.7%) were found exhibiting the extraventricular subtype, much lower incidence than the 28.1% (32/114) found in adult patients. In addition, infradiaphragmatic tumors were predominantly found in children (42.0% vs. 7.0%). A review of reports [23 - 26] regarding the early use of TS approach to treat CPs revealed that most of patients were young, with the subdiaphragmatic tumor subtype, although no published literatures have specifically addressed CPss in adults,., Recently, several papers emphasis on adult patients with CPs following the application of endoscopy to supradiaphragmatic TS approach [27 - 31]. In 2010, Jane *et al.* [30] introduced their experience with endoscopy in the treatment of 12 cases of adult CP. These tumors were exclusively suprasellar but nosubdiaphragmatic tumors.

On the other hand, our study exhibited a predominance of the purely SA pattern tumors in adults (47.4% vs. 30.8% in children), although no significant difference was found between adults and children regarding the incidence of tubero-infundibular tumors.. Purely SA pattern tumors originate from the tuber cinereum and infundibulum with a tumor nest in the 3rd VF, itgrows upwards to the ventricular cavity or within the PS but no extension to the extra-ventricular region. These are common features of intraventricular CPs. Agreeing with pre-existing published literature, we found that intraventricular CPs occurred in older patients [3, 14, 32, 33].

In a word, Astatistically significant difference in tumor subtype location between children and adults was revealed in a clinical analysis of our cohort (Table **1**) ($p = 0.023$). These results not only indicate the variations of CP growth patterns basing on age, but also suggest that membranous structures (such as the diaphragm and ASPS) may participate in directing tumor growth.

SURGICAL CLASSIFICATION ("QST" CLASSIFICATION)

The above-described topographical classification was helpful for understanding tumor growth and possible sites of origin and facilitated a better identification of the interface between the tumor and nervous parenchyma. However, this is not so easily used in clinical practice, we also suggest a surgical classification.

The craniopharyngioma was divided into Type Q: Infra-diaphragmatic type, Type S: Supra-sellar extra-ventricular type, and Type T: Tubero-infundibular type (Fig. **13**). According to the extra extension, the Infra-diaphragmatic type of tumors could be further classified as Q1) Purely infra-diaphragmatic, Q2) With supra-sellar extension. S type tumors can be further divided into either prestalk (Between the arachnoidal and ventral aspect chiasma) or, occasionally, retrostalk (Between the ventral aspect of the 3rd VF and Liliequist's membrane) depending on the origin site and direction of tumor expansion (See Chapter 11). Additionally, depending on combined with or without intra-arachnoidal cistern expanding and its directions, the type T of tumors could be further divided into T1) The tubero-infundibular growth without expansion to arachnoidal cistern, T2 and T3) With intra-arachnoidal cistern extension, and T4) With trans-infundibulum expanding.

For subdiaphragmatic CP, "Q" is used as the abbreviation because of morphological reasons. Regarding the morphological features of sub-diaphragmatic CP, the tumor is always round in shape (Fig. (**10**) "Q1") with the PS located at the posterior or posterosuperior end of the tumor. Occasionally, the tumor might be snowman-shaped because of a suprasellar extension with protrusion into the diaphragmatic foramen (Fig. (**13**) "Q2"). The tumor shapes in both of these situations are quite similar to the alphabet letter "Q", with the tail of "Q" representing the residual PS. The abbreviation "S" is used to represent extra-ventricular type because this type of tumor is generally located in suprasellar region and inside the subarachnoid cistern. Third-type CPs always originate from the tubero-infundibular of the PS, with compression of the 3rd VF and occupation of the third ventricular cavity. Although some tumors might expand extensively toward the arachnoid cistern, the site of tumor origin remained in the tubero-infundibular part. Therefore, the alphabet letter "T" was used as the abbreviation for this type of CP.

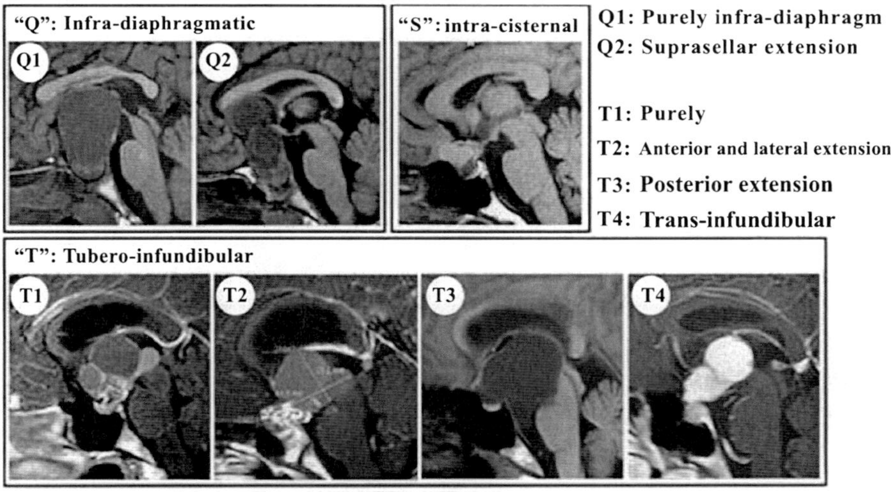

Fig. (10). Surgical classification of craniopharyngioma.

Notably, the terminology of IVC was previously used to describe the tumors that appeared to localize solely inside the third ventricular cavity. Although IVC is also a type of purely tubero-infundibular tumor (Type T1) according to our understanding, this tumor is wraped within the thinning nerve tissue of the 3rd VF and nervous tissue parenchyma. The difference is that IVC grows predominantly upwards into the third ventricle and is covered by extremely thin nervous and ependymal layers. IVC will be described in detail in Chapter 13 of this section.

The origin of tumor and surrounding membranous structure are the bases of QST classification. Identification of different classifications of craniopharyngiomas is essential to selecting the appropriate surgical procedure and can predict operation difficulty and outcome. The main difference is that the origin location of type Q tumor is below the diaphragm, type S tumor is on the extra-arachnoidal and intra-arachnoidal segment of stalk, and type T tumor is at tubero-infundibulum of stalk. Actually, there is a close relationship between the surgical and morphological classifications. The advantage of the surgical classification is that it is based on presurgical images, which are more practical in clinical work; however, the rationale and conception remain based on the morphological classification. This discussion is depicted as follows.

a. Type Q. The Q1 type of tumor with the ID growth pattern is entirely covered by the dura mater and arachnoid, as described previously. However, if a part of tumor protrudes outside diaphragmatic opening and displaces the arachnoid upwards (Type Q2), the tumor's morphological features are described as the ID+EA growth pattern.
b. Type S. Extra-arachnoidal (EA) growth indicates that this type of tumor is separated *via* the arachnoid from the undersurface of the optic chiasm and 3rd VF, except for a pedicle attachment to the pituitary stalk and infundibulum.
c. Type T. Tubero-infundibular CP, the most common subtype, exhibits much more complicated growth patterns. SA growth represents the basic pattern of this type of tumor. The T1 (pure) tumor with only SA growth can grow upwards and occupy the third ventricular cavity. However, in some cases (T2 and T3), the tumor will grow with anterior or posterior protrusion into the trabecular part of the ASPS. The SA+IA2 pattern is used to depict the growth of this tumor type. In type T4 cases, the tumors grow downwards inside the fibrous part of ASPS (IA1 growth) and may even expand into the pituitary fossa (ID growth). Therefore, the growth pattern of T4 is SA+IA1+ID.

The relationship between the tumor and surrounding structures can be predicted with a sufficient understanding of the morphological and surgical classification, even from observations of pre-surgical MRI data. Consequently, an appropriate surgical approach can be selected to utilize the extra-axial or intra-axial corridor and avoid injury to neurovascular structures.

BASIC PRINCIPLES OF OPERATIVE APPROACH SELECTION

Selection of the proper surgical approach according to the tumor growth pattern and surgeon's preference is indispensable to ensuring successful surgical completion. The main elements to consider include the tumor's anatomical location, size, growth direction, and possible relationships with surrounding structures. Additionally, the location of the cystic part of the tumor, calcification shape and, more importantly, the tumor–ventricle relationship should also be emphasized. The basic principle for selecting the corresponding approach is as follows: 1) make the greatest endeavor to reduce surgical injury (*e.g.*, select a unilateral approach); 2) strive to maintain the intactness of normal nervous tissues, especially the infundibulum-pituitary stalk tract; and 3) avoid dissection of functional nervous tissues when exposing the tumor.

Commonly used approaches include the TS approach, unilateral or bilateral subfrontal approach (SF), pterional or fronto-temporal approach (FT), fronto-basal interhemispheric approach (FIH), and trans-callosal approach (TSC).

Common Surgical Approach

1. **Trans-sphenoidal Approach (TS)**. This approach is usually used to treat infradiaphragmatic and extraventricular CPs located mainly within the suprasellar subarachnoidal cistern (Fig. **11**). Inherent advantages of this approach include facilitating the dissection of tumors from the undersurface of the optic chiasm and 3rd VF, which are usually hidden from direct view when using a trans-cranial basal approach, avoiding reclination of the frontal and temporal lobes, particularly manipulating the optic nerves and dissecting of tumors passing between the optic nerve and carotid artery. In contrast to soft adenomas, CPs are firm, calcified and always adhering to adjacent structures. The TS approach to radical CP removal requires extensive exposure of the sellar region, especially the anterior extension of the tuberculum sellae and planum sphenoidale. Pneumatization of the sphenoidal sinus is poorer in young children; drilling of incompletely pneumatized sphenoid sinuses oftenneeded to allow approach to the sellar region. As reported in previous studies [24, 34], drilling of the sphenoid does not limit the TS procedure and should not be accepted as a contraindication to trans-nasal surgery.

More recently, the widespread use of endoscopy in the context of TS surgery has also improved the removal of supradiaphragmatic CPs. The main drawbacks of the TS approach to surgery for CP are 1) the risk of postoperative cerebrospinal fluid (CSF) leakage and meningitis; and 2) further deterioration of anterior pituitary function. Laws *et al.* emphasized that a stricter indication for the TS approach should be used when treating CP patients with normal pituitary function because the TS approach was not reported to be advantageous when compared with the trans-cranial approach in terms of normal hypophyseal function.

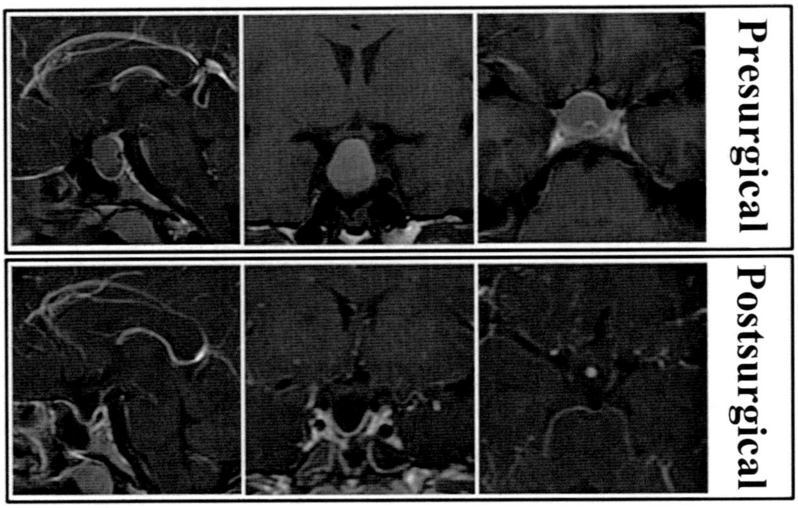

Fig. (11). A purely infradiaphragmatic tumor (Type a1) was treated *via* the trans-sphenoidal approach. On presurgical magnetic resonance images, a significant fissure was found between the tumor and optic chiasm, and the diaphragm and suprasellar arachnoid were shown to separate the two structures. After surgery, the PS was maintained and the CP was completely excised.

Our opinion is that the functions of the adenohypophysis and neurohypophysis are vulnerable in the context of of CP. This vulnerability can be explained by two reasons: 1) tumor pressure always causes the anterior lobe of pituitary gland to localize at the ventral aspect and therefore a vertical incision of the normal pituitary gland is always required to reach dorsal tumors; 2) the distal end of the PS is always scattered and fused with the supraposterior part of the tumor capsule and stretched diaphragm (DS); therefore, total removal of the tumor usually does not permit preservation of the PS.

2. **Pterional Approach.** As proposed by Yasargil *et al*., the pterional approach is the most frequently used approach to treat suprasellar or intra- and suprasellar CP (Fig. **12**). This method introduces the proximal access route to supra- and parasellar regions and uses natural surgical spaces in the sellar region such as the pre-chiasmatic space (first), optic-carotid space (second), carotid-oculomotor space (third), and some expanding spaces such as the lamina terminalis space (fourth) and interspace superior to the fork of the ICA (fifth). Neurosurgeons can reach and expose most of the CP through these surgical spaces.

This approach provides access beneath the arterial ring of Willis and a direct view of the optic nerves and chiasm. Additionally, the pterional approach is better than the SF approach for directly exposing the posterior of the sellae and inter-peduncular or prepontile cistern. Moreover, tumors protruding into the third ventricular space can also be removed through an incision in the lamina terminalis (Fig. **13**).

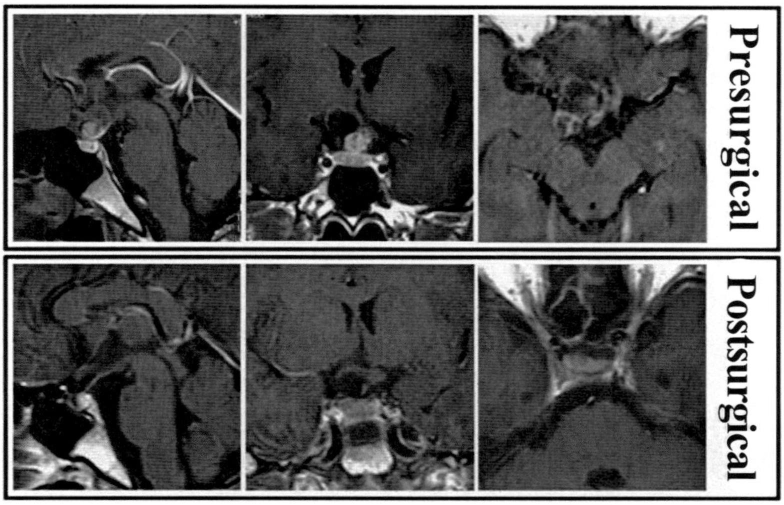

Fig. (12). An extraventricular tumor (Type b) was surgically removed *via* the pterional approach. On presurgical magnetic resonance images, a mixed cystic and solid tumor was identified in the prechiasmatic cistern. The arachnoid still separated the tumor from the pituitary stalk (PS), optic chiasm, and bilateral internal carotid artery. After surgery, the PS and normal pituitary gland were found to remain intact. The tumor was completely removed.

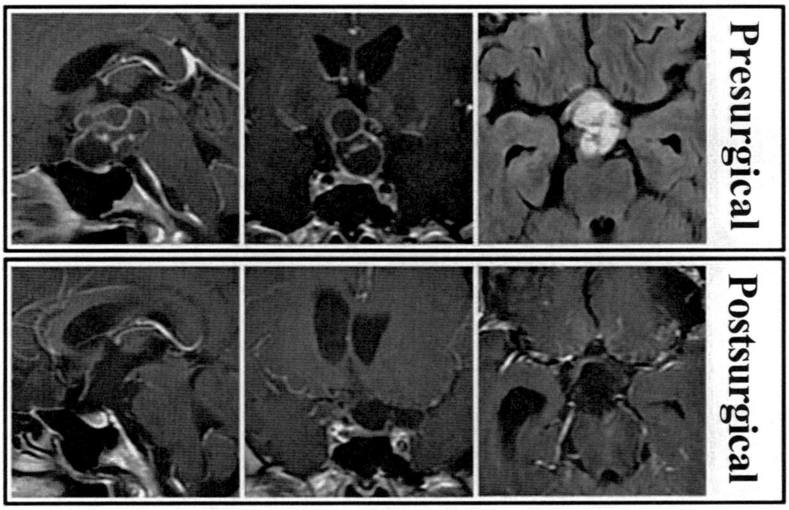

Fig. (13). A tubero-infundibular tumor with anterior extension (Type c2). The pterional approach was selected. First, the suprasellar intracisternal part of the tumor was removed *via* the extra-axial corridor. Next, the lamina terminalis was opened to remove the infundibular tumor, which was inside the nervous tissue parenchyma. After surgery, no residual tumor was found *via* magnetic resonance imaging. However, a defect in the third ventricle floor was found.

The posture and head presentation should be set specifically to provide a better viewing angle according to the corresponding tumor location. Natural gravity is employed to promote frontal lobe falling and avoid retraction injury to the lobe. The entire manipulation is processed inside the subarachnoidal cisterns, and as a result the cranial nerves and vessels can be preserved. Notably, the arachnoidal trabecula will connect with the neurovascular structures, and this should be sharply dissected with microscissors. Rough retraction *via* bipolar electrocautery will cause injury. Regarding the above description, the pterional approach undoubtedly remains the most irreplaceable approach for total tumor removal.

3. **Subfrontal Approach (SF).** Compared to the pterional approach, the SF approach can provide better exposure of the anterior part of the optical pathway and is also a more direct approach to treating IVC. In a review of the previous literature, several articles reported the use of a unilateral SF approach to treat CP. However, according to our experience, this approach will cause more severe retraction of the frontal lobe because of the relatively narrow exposure field and because it avoids opening the cistern of the lateral sulcus to drain the CSF. Meanwhile, in cases with planum sphenoidale obstruction, tumors located beneath the isolateral optical tract and chiasm cannot be exposed and observed directly. Accordingly, the intrasellar part of the tumor must be removed blindly. The unilateral SF approach should undergo more strict selection, especially in cases with small prechiasmatic spaces.

On the other hand, a bilateral SF approach can increase the exposure field of the frontal base *via* the ligation of anterior superior sagittal sinus and can release attachment between the cerebral falx and crista galli. A more direct access to third ventricle through lamina terminalis, interpeduncular cistern, even the upper clivus can be completed while providing a better viewing angle. For cases that expand into the third or even lateral ventricle, this bilateral SF approach can be used together with the interhemispheric approach, which has also been repeatedly described as the fronto-basal interhemispheric approach (FIH). Therefore, the FIH approach is always used for surgical removal of huge retrochiasmatic CPs.

4. **Fronto-basal Interhemispheric Approach (FIH).** Because of the risk of frontal lobe injury as well as several consequent complications such as mental dysfunction or venous return disorder, use of the FIH approach was initially limited. However, in recent decades and with advances in the development of surgical instruments and microscopic illuminating equipment, this approach has been widely used and has been proven an effective and safe approach through which to access the sellar region (Figs. **14**, **15**, **16**).

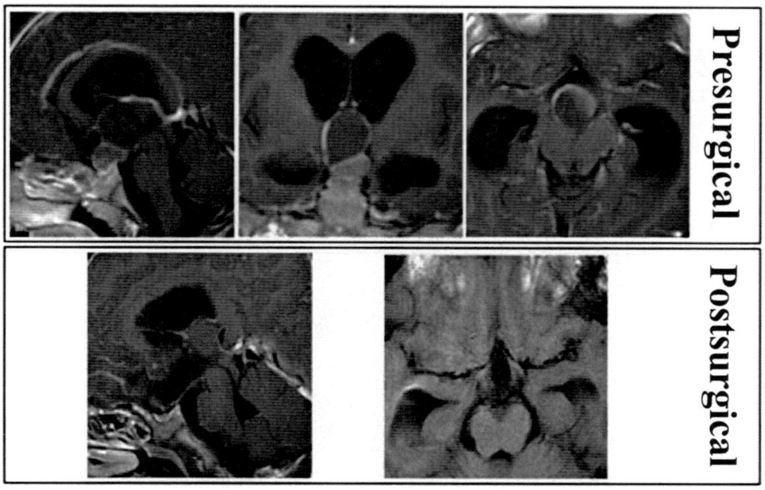

Fig. (14). A tubero-infundibular tumor with extreme third ventricular extension (Type c1) was removed *via* fronto-basal interhemispheric approach. During surgery, trans-terminalis corridor was predominantly used. On postsurgical magnetic resonance images, the third ventricle floor and bilateral walls were found to remain intact.

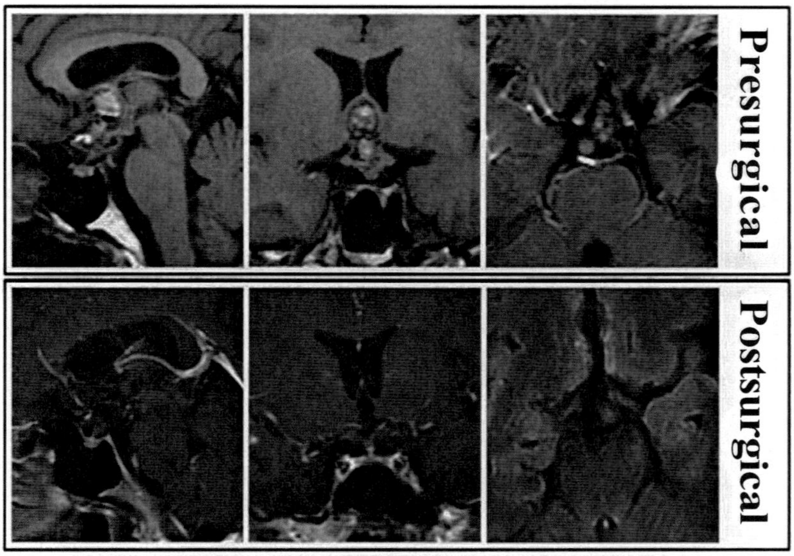

Fig. (15). A purely tubero-infundibular tumor located inside the third ventricle (3rd VF) floor (Type c1). The fronto-basal interhemispheric approach was used to remove the tumor. As indicated by postsurgical magnetic resonance imaging, the pituitary stalk and 3rd VF remained intact.

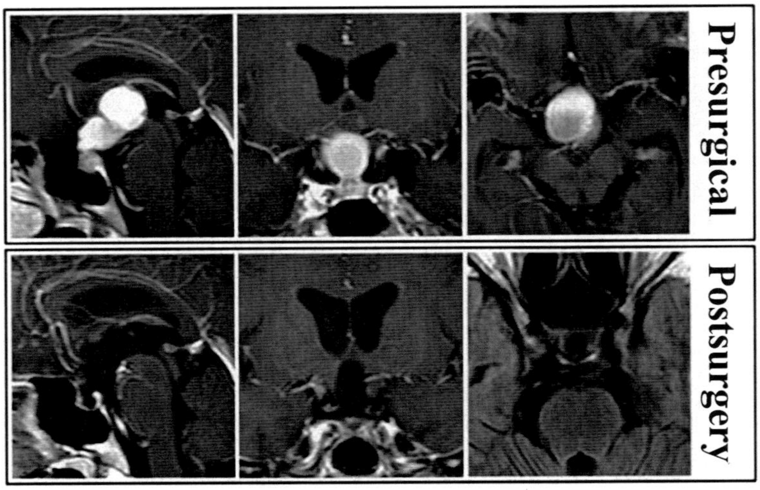

Fig. (16). A trans-infundibular tumor (Type c4) was surgically removed *via* the fronto-basal interhemispheric approach. On postsurgical magnetic resonance images, a defect was found in the third ventricle floor; however, the lateral wall of the third ventricle was maintained.

During craniotomy, the highlighted techniques include the following. 1) The lower margin of the bone flap should be as close to the skull base of anterior cranial fossa as possible. Generally, the frontal sinus is deliberately opened; the mucosa inside the sinus should be carefully removed, followed by bactericidal cleaning to reduce secondary infection. 2) In some cases, part of the posterior wall of frontal sinus have to be drilled to reduce further obstruction and allow direct exposure. 3) The basement of the crista galli should be drilled from the extra-dura in order to safely remove the attached crista galli from the intra-dura. Complete removal of the crista galli provides a sufficient surgical view to the chiasmatic cistern parallel to the skull base. 4) Considerable attempts should be made to reduce olfactory nerve injury when dissecting the arachnoid laying on the anterior skull base to reduce venous bleeding.

In the FIH approach, the primary spaces for manipulation are the prechiasmatic space (first) and terminalis space (fourth). For cystic CPs with large first spaces, intra-cystic decompression will provide sufficient space for manipulation, and most such tumors can be removed solely *via* the first space. On the other hand, for tumors with small first spaces and very short optic nerves, the fourth space is predominantly used. The AcoA complex can be pulled somewhat posteriorly to enlarge the space. For cases with huge calcifications or large tumors with posterior extension, the space behind the AcoA can also be used. If the bilateral A1 and A2 segments of the ACA have large diameters, reputation of the AcoA is feasible, thus producing more space.

Occasionally, a huge tumor might initially prevent exposure of contact between the lateral tumor wall and the ICA and its branches. In this situation, before freeing the tumor from the vascular structures, the cystic fluid should be carefully and patiently drained and intra-tumor deblocking dissection performed to enlarge the surgical space. In the intrasellar part of the tumor, curettement can also be completed if a direct view is available. In most cases, it is not necessary to drill the planum sphenoidale to facilitate manipulation.

Regardless of the type of tumor growth, close adherence of the tumor to the PS or infundibulum is exclusively identified and is also considered the site of tumor origin. The FIH approach provides a straight viewing angle from the infundibulum to the intrasellar region. However, when treating the lateral part of the tumor, the median exposure achieved *via* the FIH approach provides no advantage. Therefore, selection of the FIH approach is inadvisable for cases with a single, lateral extreme extension, even to the middle cranial fossa.

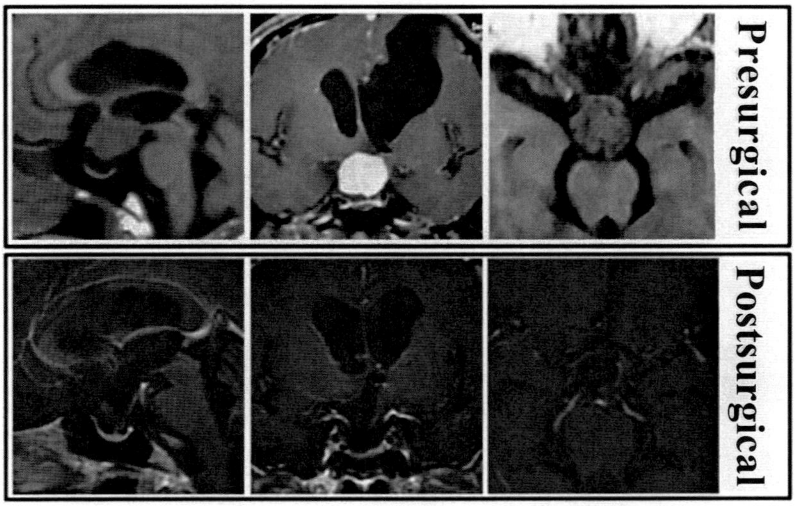

Fig. (17). A patient with a recurrent tumor who had undergone primary surgery *via* the trans-cortex trans-third ventricular approach. We used the primary corridor to access, dissect, and remove the tumor. As indicated *via* postsurgical magnetic resonance imaging, the pituitary stalk and bilateral wall of the third ventricle remained intact.

5. **Trans-third Ventricular Approach.** The trans-callosal approach (TSC) or trans-cortex lateral ventricular approach (TCL) is indicated for tumors located entirely or predominantly within the third ventricle. The incidence of this type of CP is fairly low. Unidentifiable anatomical landmarks make it easy to injure the bilateral fornix and hypothalamus, especially in the presence of hydrocephalus and a huge tumor. Because the basements of most tumors with invasion into the third ventricle are located inferior to the optic chiasm, a long distance is required

to reach the basement *via* the trans-third ventricular approach. The minimal surgical manipulation space available with this approach results in some disadvantages in terms of tumor exposure and removal. Our opinion is that this approach should be used rarely. In a limited number of cases, this approach could be used in combination with other approaches (Fig. **17**).

Approach Selection Based on Surgical Classification

According to the surgical classification of CPs and the anatomical features of these common approaches, we conclude with the following approach selection principle:

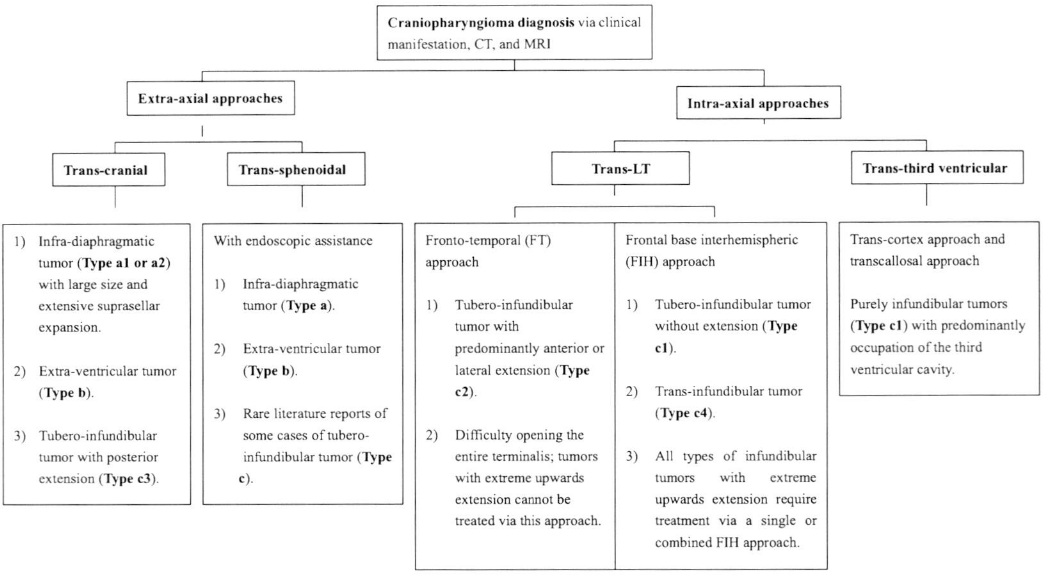

CONFLICT OF INTEREST

The authors (editor) declares no conflict of interest, financial or otherwise.

ACKNOWLEDGEMENTS

Declared none.

REFERENCES

[1] Hoffman HJ. Surgical management of craniopharyngioma. Pediatr Neurosurg 1994; 21 (Suppl. 1): 44-9.
[http://dx.doi.org/10.1159/000120861] [PMID: 7530990]

[2] Kassam AB, Gardner PA, Snyderman CH, Carrau RL, Mintz AH, Prevedello DM. Expanded endonasal approach, a fully endoscopic transnasal approach for the resection of midline suprasellar craniopharyngiomas: a new classification based on the infundibulum. J Neurosurg 2008; 108(4): 715-28.

[http://dx.doi.org/10.3171/JNS/2008/108/4/0715] [PMID: 18377251]

[3] Pascual JM, Carrasco R, Prieto R, Gonzalez-Llanos F, Alvarez F, Roda JM. Craniopharyngioma classification. J Neurosurg 2008; 109(6): 1180-2. [http://dx.doi.org/10.3171/JNS.2008.109.12.1180] [PMID: 19035739]

[4] Steno J, Malácek M, Bízik I. Tumor-third ventricular relationships in supradiaphragmatic craniopharyngiomas: correlation of morphological, magnetic resonance imaging, and operative findings. Neurosurgery 2004; 54(5): 1051-8. [http://dx.doi.org/10.1227/01.NEU.0000120421.11171.61] [PMID: 15113458]

[5] Wang KC, Kim SK, Choe G, Chi JG, Cho BK. Growth patterns of craniopharyngioma in children: role of the diaphragm sellae and its surgical implication. Surg Neurol 2002; 57(1): 25-33. [http://dx.doi.org/10.1016/S0090-3019(01)00657-7] [PMID: 11834269]

[6] Yaşargil MG, Curcic M, Kis M, Siegenthaler G, Teddy PJ, Roth P. Total removal of craniopharyngiomas. Approaches and long-term results in 144 patients. J Neurosurg 1990; 73(1): 3-11. [http://dx.doi.org/10.3171/jns.1990.73.1.0003] [PMID: 2352020]

[7] Wang KC, Hong SH, Kim SK, Cho BK. Origin of craniopharyngiomas: implication on the growth pattern. Childs Nerv Syst 2005; 21(8-9): 628-34. [http://dx.doi.org/10.1007/s00381-005-1203-8] [PMID: 16059733]

[8] Kitano M, Taneda M. Extended transsphenoidal surgery for suprasellar craniopharyngiomas: infrachiasmatic radical resection combined with or without a suprachiasmatic trans-lamina terminalis approach. Surg Neurol 2009; 71(3): 290-8. [http://dx.doi.org/10.1016/j.surneu.2007.11.014] [PMID: 18291485]

[9] Qi S, *et al.* Anatomic relations of the arachnoidea around the pituitary stalk: relevance for surgical removal of craniopharyngiomas. Acta Neurochir (Wien) 2011.

[10] Ciric IS, Cozzens JW. Craniopharyngiomas: transsphenoidal method of approach--for the virtuoso only? Clin Neurosurg 1980; 27: 169-87. [PMID: 7273552]

[11] Steno J. Microsurgical topography of craniopharyngiomas. Acta Neurochir Suppl (Wien) 1985; 35: 94-100. [http://dx.doi.org/10.1007/978-3-7091-8813-2_16] [PMID: 3867266]

[12] Samii M, Tatagiba M. Surgical management of craniopharyngiomas: a review. Neurol Med Chir (Tokyo) 1997; 37(2): 141-9. [http://dx.doi.org/10.2176/nmc.37.141] [PMID: 9059036]

[13] Fukushima T, Hirakawa K, Kimura M, Tomonaga M. Intraventricular craniopharyngioma: its characteristics in magnetic resonance imaging and successful total removal. Surg Neurol 1990; 33(1): 22-7. [http://dx.doi.org/10.1016/0090-3019(90)90220-J] [PMID: 2405528]

[14] Pascual JM, González-Llanos F, Barrios L, Roda JM. Intraventricular craniopharyngiomas: topographical classification and surgical approach selection based on an extensive overview. Acta Neurochir (Wien) 2004; 146(8): 785-802. [http://dx.doi.org/10.1007/s00701-004-0295-3] [PMID: 15254801]

[15] Samii M, Bini W. Surgical treatment of craniopharyngiomas. Zentralbl Neurochir 1991; 52(1): 17-23. [PMID: 1862672]

[16] Yasargil MG, Kasdaglis K, Jain KK, Weber HP. Anatomical observations of the subarachnoid cisterns of the brain during surgery. J Neurosurg 1976; 44(3): 298-302. [http://dx.doi.org/10.3171/jns.1976.44.3.0298] [PMID: 1082498]

[17] Lü J, Zhu XL. Characteristics of distribution and configuration of intracranial arachnoid membranes. Surg Radiol Anat 2005; 27(6): 472-81. [http://dx.doi.org/10.1007/s00276-005-0025-4] [PMID: 16151970]

[18] Inoue K, Seker A, Osawa S, Alencastro LF, Matsushima T, Rhoton AL Jr. Microsurgical and endoscopic anatomy of the supratentorial arachnoidal membranes and cisterns. Neurosurgery 2009; 65(4): 644-64.
[http://dx.doi.org/10.1227/01.NEU.0000351774.81674.32] [PMID: 19834369]

[19] Song-tao Q, Xi-an Z, Hao L, Jun F, Jun P, Yun-tao L. The arachnoid sleeve enveloping the pituitary stalk: anatomical and histologic study. Neurosurgery 2010; 66(3): 585-9.
[http://dx.doi.org/10.1227/01.NEU.0000365371.50165.06] [PMID: 20173553]

[20] Lena G, *et al.* Craniopharyngioma in children: Marseille experience. Child's nervous system: ChNS: Official journal of the International Society for Pediatric Neurosurgery 2005; 21(8-9): 778-84.

[21] Lee Y-Y, Wong TT, Fang YT, Chang KP, Chen YW, Niu DM. Comparison of hypothalamopituitary axis dysfunction of intrasellar and third ventricular craniopharyngiomas in children. Brain Dev 2008; 30(3): 189-94.
[http://dx.doi.org/10.1016/j.braindev.2007.07.011] [PMID: 17870266]

[22] Brunel H, Raybaud C, Peretti-Viton P, *et al.* [Craniopharyngioma in children: MRI study of 43 cases]. Neurochirurgie 2002; 48(4): 309-18. [Craniopharyngioma in children: MRI study of 43 cases]. [PMID: 12407316]

[23] Abe T, Lüdecke DK. Transnasal surgery for infradiaphragmatic craniopharyngiomas in pediatric patients. Neurosurgery 1999; 44(5): 957-64.
[http://dx.doi.org/10.1097/00006123-199905000-00012] [PMID: 10232528]

[24] König A, Lüdecke DK, Herrmann HD. Transnasal surgery in the treatment of craniopharyngiomas. Acta Neurochir (Wien) 1986; 83(1-2): 1-7.
[http://dx.doi.org/10.1007/BF01420500] [PMID: 3799245]

[25] Laws ER Jr. Transsphenoidal microsurgery in the management of craniopharyngioma. J Neurosurg 1980; 52(5): 661-6.
[http://dx.doi.org/10.3171/jns.1980.52.5.0661] [PMID: 7373393]

[26] Laws ER Jr. Transsphenoidal removal of craniopharyngioma. Pediatr Neurosurg 1994; 21 (Suppl. 1): 57-63.
[http://dx.doi.org/10.1159/000120863] [PMID: 7841079]

[27] Campbell PG, McGettigan B, Luginbuhl A, Yadla S, Rosen M, Evans JJ. Endocrinological and ophthalmological consequences of an initial endonasal endoscopic approach for resection of craniopharyngiomas. Neurosurg Focus 2010; 28(4): E8.
[http://dx.doi.org/10.3171/2010.1.FOCUS09292] [PMID: 20367365]

[28] Dusick JR, Esposito F, Kelly DF, *et al.* The extended direct endonasal transsphenoidal approach for nonadenomatous suprasellar tumors. J Neurosurg 2005; 102(5): 832-41.
[http://dx.doi.org/10.3171/jns.2005.102.5.0832] [PMID: 15926706]

[29] Frank G, *et al.* The endoscopic extended transsphenoidal approach for craniopharyngiomas. Neurosurgery 2006; 59(1 Suppl 1): 75-83.

[30] Jane JA Jr, Kiehna E, Payne SC, Early SV, Laws ER Jr. Early outcomes of endoscopic transsphenoidal surgery for adult craniopharyngiomas. Neurosurg Focus 2010; 28(4): E9.
[http://dx.doi.org/10.3171/2010.1.FOCUS09319] [PMID: 20367523]

[31] Jane JA Jr, Prevedello DM, Alden TD, Laws ER Jr. The transsphenoidal resection of pediatric craniopharyngiomas: a case series. J Neurosurg Pediatr 2010; 5(1): 49-60.
[http://dx.doi.org/10.3171/2009.7.PEDS09252] [PMID: 20043736]

[32] Behari S, Banerji D, Mishra A, *et al.* Intrinsic third ventricular craniopharyngiomas: report on six cases and a review of the literature. Surg Neurol 2003; 60(3): 245-52.
[http://dx.doi.org/10.1016/S0090-3019(03)00132-0] [PMID: 12922045]

[33] Ikezaki K, Fujii K, Kishikawa T. Magnetic resonance imaging of an intraventricular

craniopharyngioma. Neuroradiology 1990; 32(3): 247-9.
[http://dx.doi.org/10.1007/BF00589123] [PMID: 2215911]

[34] Knappe UJ, Lüdecke DK. Transnasal microsurgery in children and adolescents with Cushing's disease. Neurosurgery 1996; 39(3): 484-92.
[http://dx.doi.org/10.1227/00006123-199609000-00010] [PMID: 8875478]

CHAPTER 10

Subdiaphragmatic Craniopharyngioma (Type "Q")

Jun Pan*

Department of Neurosurgery, Nanfang Neurosurgery Research Institution, Nanfang Hospital, Southern Medical University, 1838 North Guangzhou Avenue, Guangzhou, China

Abstract: Craniopharyngiomas (CPs) could occurred in anywhere along craniopharyngeal canal. The diverse original points of tumor lead to significant differences in expansion [1]. Although the majority of CPs have a supradiaphragmatic origin (infundibular stalk/pars tuberalis), a number of CPs arise primarily from the subdiaphragmatic space and usually cause marked sellar enlargement before extending intracranially. Several terms, such as "sub- or infradiaphragmatic CP" and "sellar CP" have been coined to describe this type of tumor [2-6]. However, details of the clinical and morphological features of this tumor type were missing from previous literature reports. In this chapter, we focus on CPs that originate from the infradiaphragmatic space (Id-CP) and illustrate the tumor growth patterns, preoperative clinical and radiological features, intraoperative findings, and long-term outcomes.

Keywords: Craniopharyngioma, Pituitary Stalk, Sellar Region, Subdiaphragma.

DEFINITION, INCIDENCE AND TUMOR TOPOGRAPHY

Few previous literature publications have specifically discussed Id-CP. A likely potential reason for this lack of discussion is that in some special cases, a definite site of origin cannot be confirmed because of intra and suprasellar growth along the pituitary stalk (PS). However, in our opinion, this type of growth pattern is rare. The majority of Id-CPs share common morphological features that appear to represent a particular type of tumor. To date, the Id-CP literature is limited to several small case reports [2, 5, 6]. Among 122 cases of CPs (in children and adults) reported by Effenterre and Boch, 37% were considered to be of infradiaphragmatic origin based on the anatomical relationship between the tumor and sella turcica and diaphragma sellae (DS) (purely intrasellar in 4%, intra- and suprasellar transdiaphragmatic in 7% and intra- and suprasellar infradiaphragmatic in 26% of cases) [7]. In the Craniopharyngioma chapter of Oncology of CNS tumors by Effenterre and Boch, they described the similar result [8].

* **Corresponding author Jun Pan**: Department of Neurosurgery, Nanfang Neurosurgery Research Institution, Nanfang Hospital, Southern Medical University, 1838 North Guangzhou Avenue, Guangzhou, China; Tel/Fax: +8620-61641806; E-mail: panjundu@hotmail.com

Songtao Qi (Ed.)

Furthermore, infradiaphragmatic tumors accounted for 40.9% of 66 cases of pediatric CP reported by Lee *et al.* [4].

Interestingly, all of these reports focused on pediatric CP, except for one publication from "World Neurosurgery," which described Id-CP in adult patients. Therefore, it is reasonable to believe that Id-CP is a common "juvenile type" that occurs predominantly in children rather than in adults who have reached puberty. We respectively reviewed 311 cases of CP at our hospital during a recent 16-year period and selected 62 cases (27.4%) with typical Id-CP morphological features. Of these cases, 48 occurred in children (≤16 years), accounting for 52% of pediatric cases in the total sample (48/88), whereas only 14 cases occurred in adults, accounting for 10.2% of adult cases in the total sample (14/138). The contents of this chapter are based on clinical data and a long-term follow-up of these cohort cases. Related clinical issues are discussed along with an analysis involving the previous literature reports.

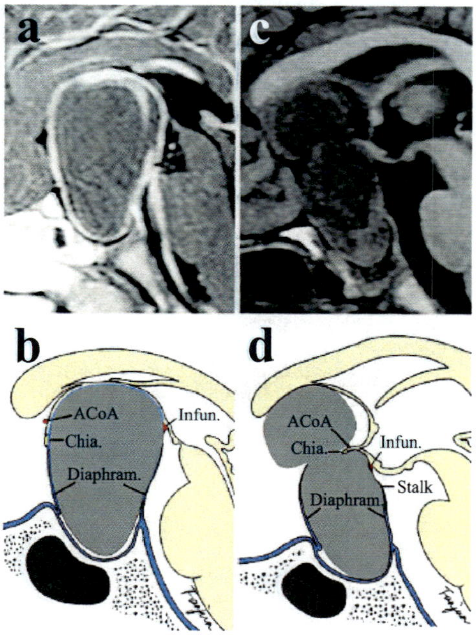

Fig. (1). (Reference from Jun Pan,Songtao Qi *et al.*, Growth patterns of craniopharyngiomas: clinical analysis of 226 patients. Journal of Neurosurgery Pediatrics, 2015:1-16). Sagittal T1-weighted MRIs and schematic drawings demonstrating the typical growth pattern of infradiaphragmatic CP. Growth of tumor cause prominent enlargement of pituitary fossa and a huge, rounded, and uniform extension to suprasellar space. The upper portion of tumor capsule could expanded through the opening of the diaphragm and protruded in front of the ACoA above the chiasm. a and c: preoperative sagittal contrast-enhanced T1-weighted MR imagings showing a 6 years old boy and a 5 -year -old boy with large infradiaphragmatic CP. b and d: schematic drawings showing the displacement of surrounding structures. blue line: diaphragm and sellar floor dura. ACoA: anterior communicating artery; Chia: optic chiasm; diaphragm: diaphragm sellar turcica; infun: infundibulum; stalk: pituitary stalk.

NEUROIMAGING

Id-CPs usually exhibit a more uniform expansion pattern when compared with their suprasellar counterparts. The lobulated tumor shape commonly seen in suprasellar hypothalamic CPs is rare among Id-CPs because of the uniform tumor extension pattern. Id-CPs alwayspresent with prominent enlargement of pituitary fossa and a huge, rounded, and uniform extension to suprasellar space (Fig. **1**). The smaller solid part and calcification are usually located in the enlarged hypophyseal fossa and lower portion of the tumor; rarely, the tumor might be more deeply rooted with infrasellar region involvement includeing pharynx, sphenoid sinus and ethmoid sinus, among others. The larger cystic portion extends to the subchiasmatic space, forcing the optic chiasm upward along with other normal neural structures, which includes the rostral part of corpus callosum and anterior communicating artery (AcoA), in some cases involving large tumors (Fig. **2**). Once in a while, the tumor could stretch upward protruding the diaphragm longitudinally along PS and finally into parenchyma around walls of the third ventricle (Fig. **3**). Sometimes, these tumors may even dilate the PS (Fig. **4**).

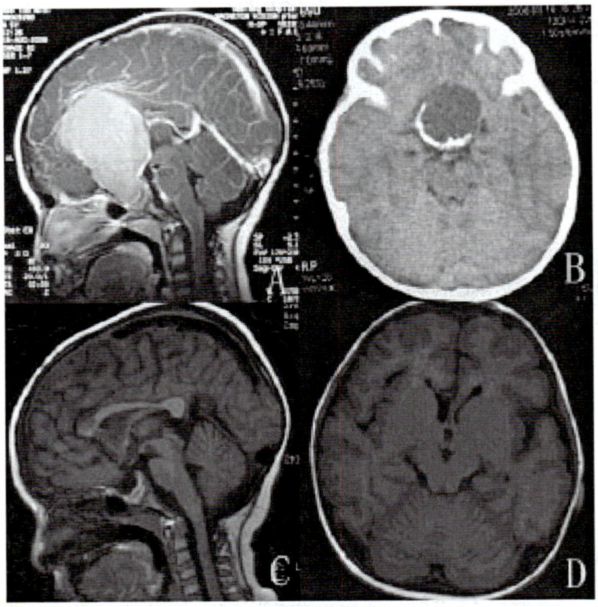

Fig. (2). Sagittal contrast-enhanced T1-weighted MRI and CT scanning before(A and B) and after operation (C and D) in a 5 -year-old boy demonstrating a huge infradiaphragmatic craniopharyngioma. The supra-sellar expansion of tumor capsule caused the optic chiasm upward along with other normal neural structures which includes the rostral part of corpus callosum and anterior communicating artery. Pre-operative CT scan (b) revealed eggshell like calcification along with the supra-sellar tumor capsule. The tumor was totally removed with integrity of third ventricle floor *via* front-basal interhemispheric approach.

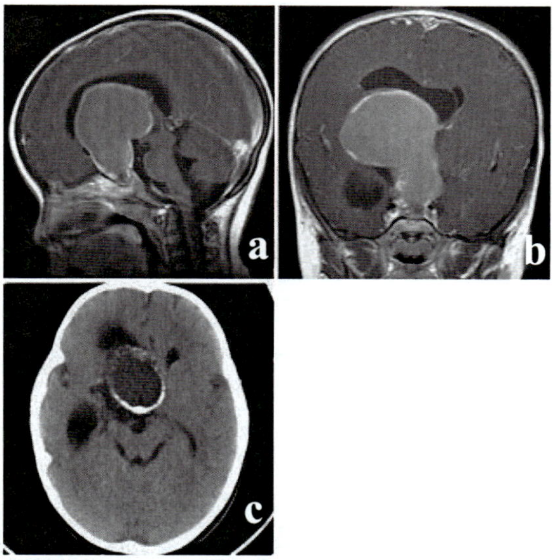

Fig. (3). Sagittal and Coronal contrast-enhanced T1-weighted MRI (a and b) and CT scanning (c) before surgery in a 3-year-old boy demonstrating a huge infradiaphragmatic CP. The tumor expanded upward protruding the diaphragm longitudinally along the PS and eventually grown into parenchyma around the boundarys of third ventricle. Pre-operative CT scan (c) revealed eggshell like calcification along with the supra-sellar tumor capsule. The most possible reason of tumor's expanding pattern is a large, incompetent diaphragm openings.

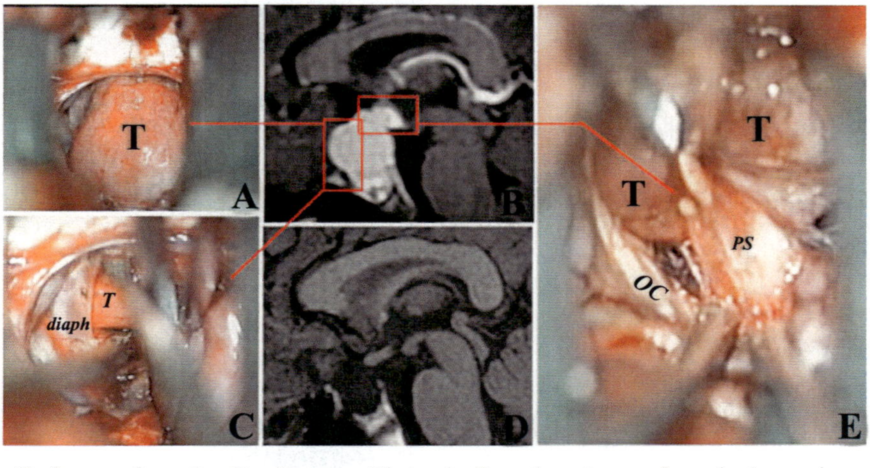

Fig. (4). (Reference from Jun Pan,Songtao Qi *et al.*, Growth patterns of craniopharyngiomas: clinical analysis of 226 patients. Journal of Neurosurgery Pediatrics, 2015:1-16).. Images showing a case of infra-diaphragmatic CP with trans-infundibulum growth in a 9-year-old boy. **A, C**, and **E** showed the various aspects of tumor during operation. The smooth surface of supra-sellar tumor capsule exposed through anterior inter-hemispheric approach (**A**). A clear dissecting plane between the stretched diaphragm and underneath tumor capsule could be traced in order to total removal of the intra-sellar tumor portion (**C**). The suprasellar tumor invaginated into the supra-diaphragmatic segement of PS (**E**). **B and D**: Pre- and Post-operative Sagittal T1-weighted MR images showing the tumor-stalk relationship and total removal of the tumor. diaph: incised diaphragma sellae; OC: optic chiasm; PS:pituitary stalk; T:tumor.

In Id-CP, calcification, which always occurs in CPs, has special morphological features. Normally, calcification is micaceous or eggshell-shaped. The former type is always located at the tumor basement inside the pituitary fossa, whereas the latter type is always distributed along the inner face of the tumor cystic cavity with suprasellar extension (Figs. **2b** and **3c**). In rare cases (usually those with long medical histories and repeated treatment), huge calcifications may also be observed (Fig. **5**). Calcification is thought to be closely related to the tumor itself with respect to biological behavior and medical history (Fig. **6**). In contrast to suprasellar tubero-infundibular CP, it is rare for Id-CP to cause hydrocephalus because of diaphragmatic obstruction. Obstructive hydrocephalus occurs only when the tumor grows upwards and extends towards the third ventricular floor (3rd VF) longitudinally through PS with protrusion through the diaphragmatic foramen (Fig. **7**).

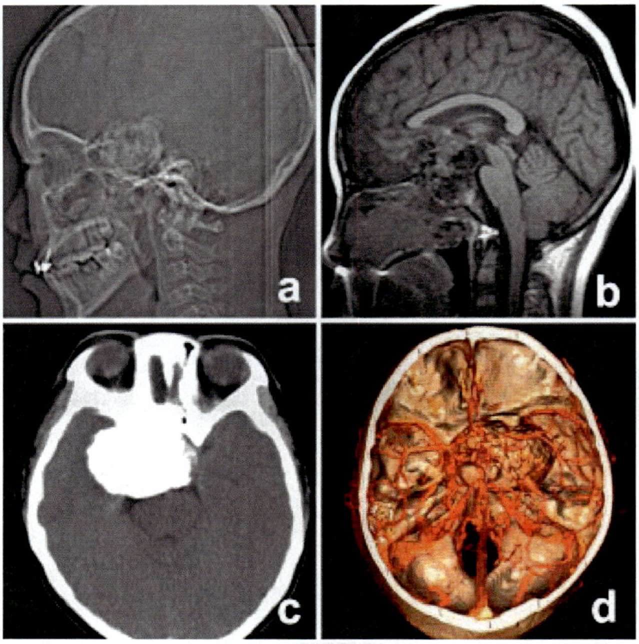

Fig. (5). Presurgical MRI(b) and CT scanning (a, c, d) of a regrowthed tumor in a 19-year-old woman with 10-year history of craniopharyngioma who underwent a surgical excision at the local hospital 8 years before admitted to our institute. CT scanning revealed huge calcification (c); 3-D reconstructed image revealed encasement of main artery by tumor calcification (d), which makes the radical removal of the tumor almost impossible.

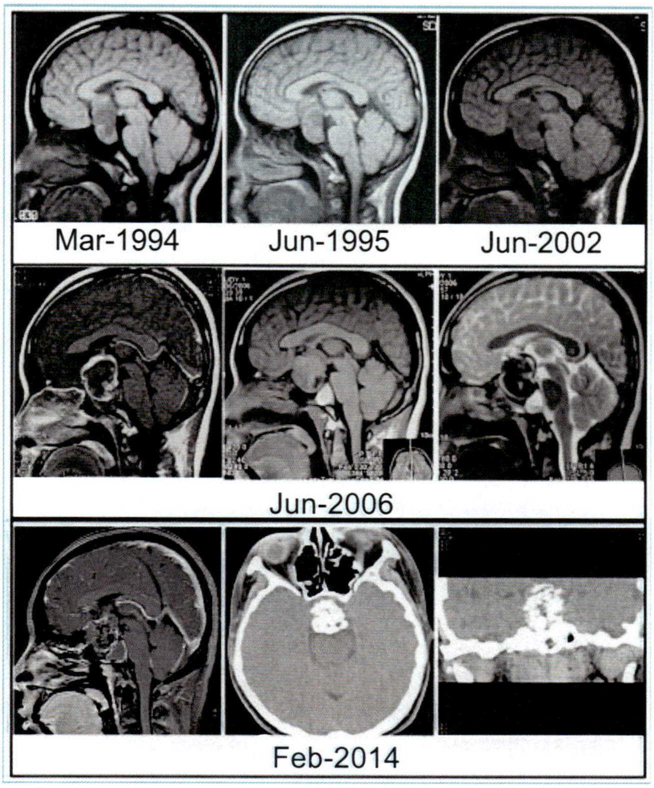

Fig. (6). Serial MR and CT images in a 36-year-old woman carrying craniopharyngioma for 21-year history without surgical intervention. Sagittal T1-weighted MRIs demonstrating the typical growth pattern of an infradiaphragmatic CP in early years. Serial MR and CT images showing the growth of tumor and progressive enlargement of the tumor calcification and the destruction of bone of sella turcica.

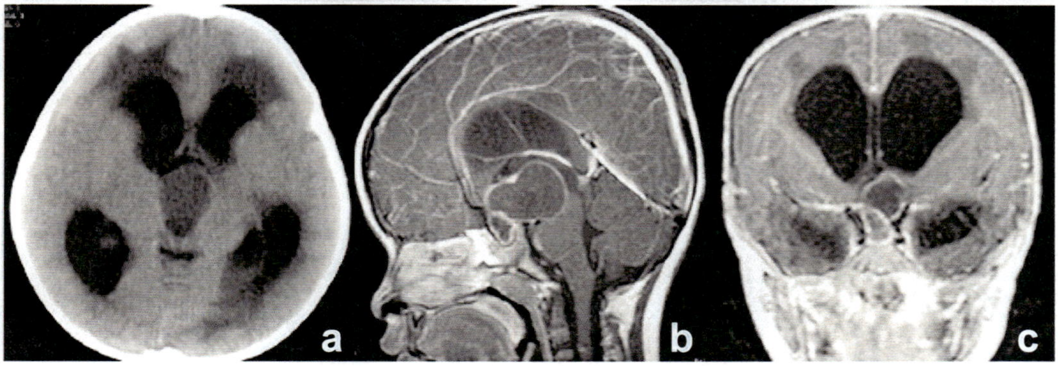

Fig. (7). CT scan and MRI before surgery in a 3-year-old boy who complained about headache, vomit and impaired vision on both eyes. CT scan indicated severe obstructive hydrocephalus (a). Sagittal and Coronal contrast-enhanced T1-weighted MRI (b and c) revealed that the supra-sellar tumor capsule extended mainly in posterosuperior direction into the third ventricle chamber.

MORPHOLOGICAL ANALYSIS OF ID-CP

Juvenile Cases: Pediatric Id-CP cases always present with huge tumors. This can be partially explained by the late diagnoses of hypopituitarism and visual disorders in young patients. On median sagittal magnetic resonance imaging (MRI), the average tumor size in the 48 juvenile cases in our series was 4.39 ± 1.52 cm, which was much larger than the median Id-CP size in adult cases. Regarding anatomical location, our series included one case of totally nasopharyngeal and sphenoid sinus CP without involvement of the suprasellar region Fig. (**8**), four cases of nasopharyngeal CP with involvement of the intra- and suprasellar region Fig. (**9**), six cases of sphenoid or ethmoid sinus intra- and suprasellar CP Fig. (**10**), 31 cases of intra- and suprasellar CP Fig. (**1**), and 5 cases of intra- and suprasellar with trans-infundibular CP (Fig. **11**).

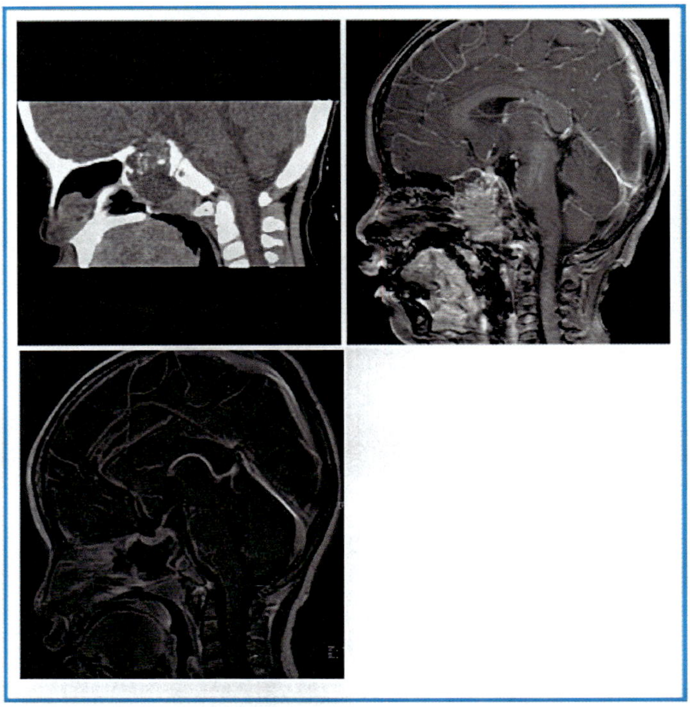

Fig. (8). CT and MR images in a 3-year-old boy who complain about nasal obstruction, protopsis and heterotropia on right eye. CT scan revealed the destruction of sphenoid bone (a). Sagittal contrast-enhanced T1-weighted MRI before operation showed the tumor involved mainly the ethmoid, sphenoid sinus and sella turcica without involving the supra-sellar region (b). Postsurgical Sagittal contrast-enhanced T1-weighted MRI demonstrating the totally removed of the tumor *via* transsphenoidal surgery (**c**).

Adult Cases: Adult Id-CP cases were rare and had an average tumor size of only 2.75 ± 1.09 cm. The anatomical location included six cases of totally intrasellar CP, five cases of intra- and suprasellar CP, and three cases of trans-infundibular

CP causing invagination of the 3rd VF (Fig. **12**). We summarize the differences between Id-CP in pediatric and adult patients, and we observed that in pediatric cases, the distribution of tumor origins was more extensive, ranging from the nasopharynx to the infradiaphragmatic segment of the PS. In contrast, adult Id-CP usually originated from the infradiaphragmatic segment near the diaphragmatic foramen.

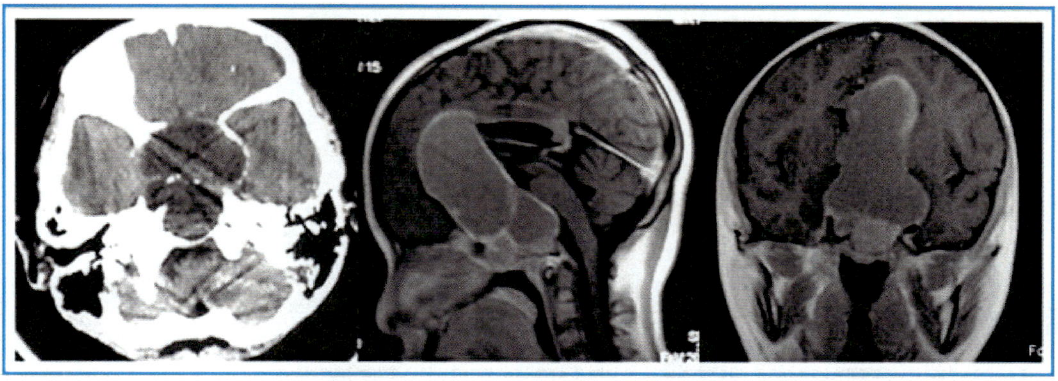

Fig. (9). CT scan (a) and sagittal and Coronal contrast-enhanced T1-weighted MRI (b and c) before operation in a 16-year-old boy showing a huge nasopharynx CP with involvement of intra- supra-sellar region. This kind of CP usually is giant in tumor size involving extensive region from the nasopharynx to the sellar and supra sellar region along the developing path of the craniopharyngeal canal.

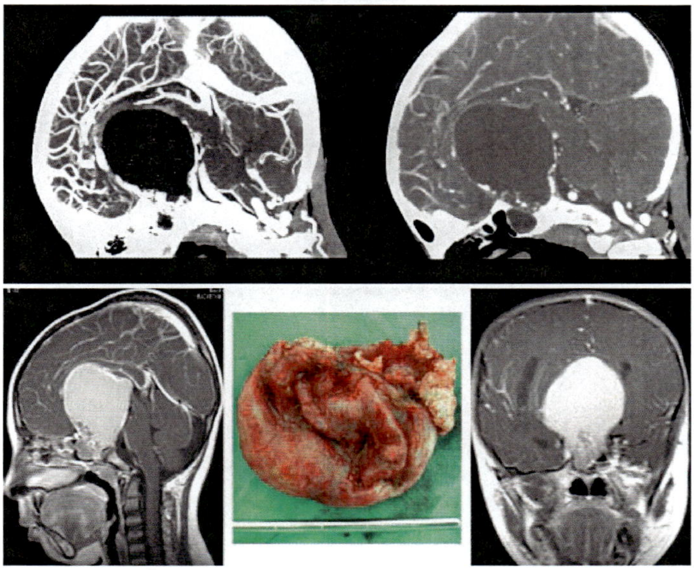

Fig. (10). CT scanning (upper) and Sagittal and Coronal contrast-enhanced T1-weighted MRI (low) before operation in a 8-year-old boy showing a huge infradiaphragmatic CP. This tumor arise from the sphenoid and ethmoidal sinus in involving the intra- and supra-sellar region.

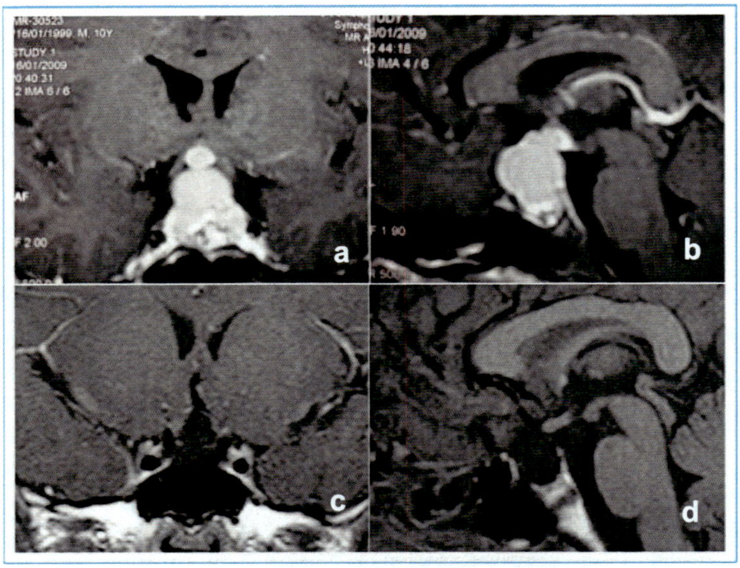

Fig. (11). Sagittal and Coronal contrast-enhanced T1-weighted MRI before (a and b) and after (c and d) operation in a 9-year-old boy showing a infradiaphragmatic CP. The tumor stretched upward protruding diaphragm longitudinally along the PS and coused infundibulum dilated. Postsurgical MRI showed totally removed of CP by a front-basal transhemispheric approach.

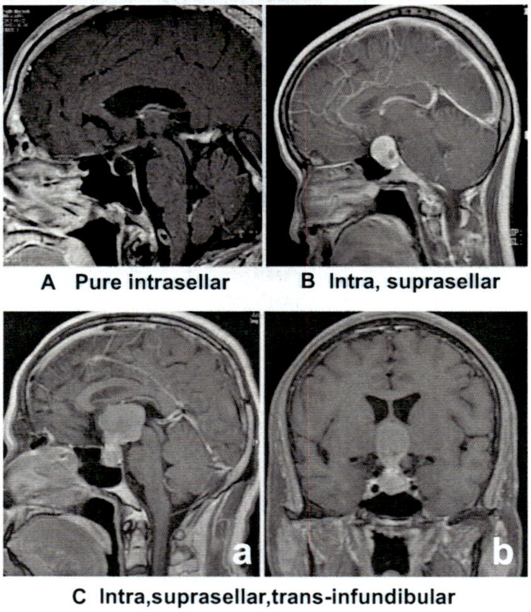

Fig. (12). The common MRI in adults infra-diaphragmatic CPs: A, Sagittal T1-weighted MRIs of a pure intrasellar CP in a 60-year-old man . B, Sagittal T1-weighted MRI demonstrated an intra,suprasellar CPs in a 27-year-old woman; C, Sagittal and Coronal contrast-enhanced T1-weighted MRI (a and b) showed an intra,suprasellar, trans-infundibular CPs of a 43-year-old man.

CLINICAL MANIFESTATION OF ID-CP

The majority of pediatric cases manifested with growth retardation and visual disorders. Although growth retardation occurred in almost all patients, fewer than half presented at our hospital because of this condition, possibly because growth retardation is difficult to evaluate objectively in young children. On the other hand, parental negligence might be another possible reason for the lack of hospital presentation. Ophthalmological detection indicated that a majority of Id-CP patients had severe visual injuries. In our series, more than 50% of cases involved unilateral or bilateral visual defects (*e.g.*, difficulties with counting fingers and light perception or even blindness). This was difficult to detect in younger children, which might explain the severity of the visual defects. In cases involving huge tumors, atypical hypertension symptoms such as headache, nausea, and vomiting were observed in 20% of cases from our series.

At the time of statement, patients with childhood-onset tumors suffered from diverse clinical manifestations. Apart from symptoms related to intracranial hypertension such as nonspecific headaches and vomiting, all patients who presented at our institute had progressive visual deficits as the primary indication for surgery; in agreement with the finding that visual function is usually severely compromised in children with Id-CPs, more than half of our patients stated with unilateral or bilateral blindness, reduced light perception, likely reflecting delayed detection and diagnosis in the pediatric patients. Signs and symptoms associated with endocrinopathy in childhood-onset infra-diaphragmatic tumors usually include growth failure and sexual immaturity in adolescent patients. Preoperative polydipsia and polyuria have also been commonly observed in children suffering from Id-CP; these conditions likely reflect the intimate relationship between the tumor and PS. Neurological symptoms such as hemiplegia, seizures, and cranial nerve paralysis are relatively uncommon and are usually observed in patients with large tumors. In rare cases with nasopharyngeal involvement, patients likely present at the hospital with respiratory tract and nasal cavity obstruction, nasal discharge, and epistaxis. In a case from our series, a 17-year-old patient with extensive involvement of the nasopharynx, sphenoidal sinus, sphenoidal bone body, and intracranial region presented with total blindness, polydipsia, polyuria, growth retardation, nasal obstruction, protopsis, visual disorder, undeveloped secondary sex characters, atresia auris externa, and developmental malformation of the right external ear (Fig. **13**).

On the other hand, symptoms in patients with adult-onset tumors usually include sexual axis dysfunction; menstrual disorders or amenorrhea in women and sexual disorders in men are the most common presenting manifestations. Tumors identified at an early stage are always small in size. Patients might also complain of reduced visual accuracy and visual field injury if the tumor has grown upward to the suprasellar region and displaced the optical chiasm. Normally, symptoms related to visual changes are mild. Nonspecific headache (likely due to the expansion of sella turcica) and visual symptoms depend on the tumor size.

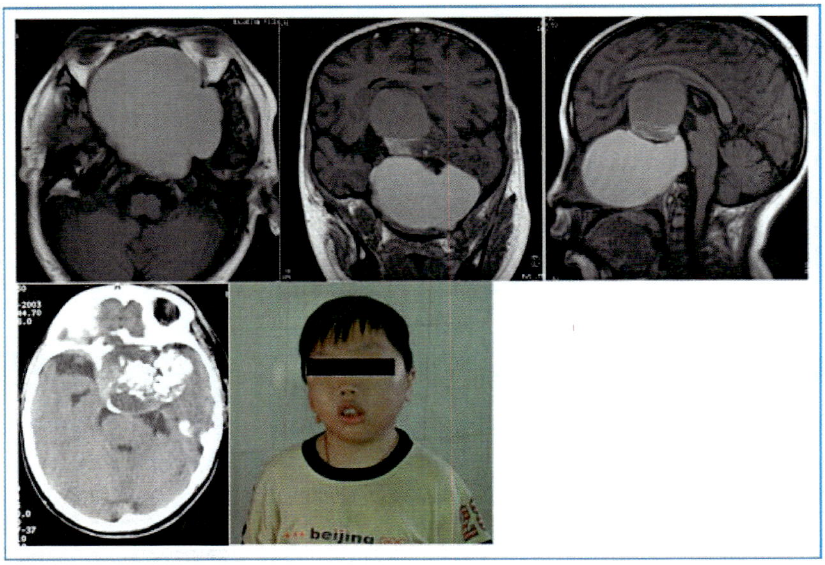

Fig. (13). Axial, Sagittal and Coronal contrast-enhanced T1-weighted MRI (upper row) and CT scanning (low row) and the patient picture before operation in a 17-year-old boy showing a huge nasopharynx CP involving in intra- supra-sellar region. The patient suffered from total blindness, polydipsia polyuria, growth retardation, nasal obstruction, protopsis, visual disorder, undevelopment of secondary sex characters, atresia auris externa and development malformation of right external ear.

ENDOCRNINE EVALUATION

Pituitary function is a critical step curing the childhood CPs. An obvious contradiction in the morbidity of pituitary hormone axis imperfections has been recorded early. Adrenocorticotropic hormone (ACTH) insufficient is introduced in 21–62%, Growth hormone (GH) insufficient in 35–95% of evaluated patients, thyroid-stimulating hormone (TSH) insufficient in 21–42%,, follicle-stimulating hormone (FSH)/luteinizing hormone (LH) insufficient in 38–82%, and diabetes insipidus (DI) in 6–38% [7 - 11]. The discrepancy may be partly attributable to the variations of diagnostic criteria [12]. As shown in our previous study [13], in patients with Id-CP, the pituitary function at statement was more severely compromised, compared to patients with suprasellar 3rd VF tumors. The importance of introducing pituitary impairment associates significantly with tumor size in patients with infra-diaphragmatic, suggesting that the relative effects of tumor bulk on pituitary function are intimately related to tumor location. These results are anastomotic with the anatomy of sellar region.

Our series also indicated that most patients with Id-CP patients had some degree of hypopituitarism. In general, endocrine disorders were more severe among pediatric cases. In our series, more than 40% of pediatric cases presented with panhypopituitarism. All cases had at least single pituitary hypothalamic axis dysfunction. Regarding the hypothalamic axes, 100% of cases presented with GH deficiency and 67% with TSH deficiency. Although polyuria and polydipsia were rare complaints at presentation, careful presurgical detection revealed that more than 70% of pediatric patients suffered from DI. No similar reports were found in a review of previous publications. Poor secondary sexual development was identified in all pubertal cases, and this remained consistent during the follow-up period. In contrast, hypothalamic dysfunction was rare among Id-CP cases, comparing with tubero-infundibular CP cases. Growth retardation and partial hypopituitarism were more common presentations in children and adults, respectively. Among adults, more than half of the patients had normal pituitary function. DI was only observed in one case before surgery. In a few cases wherein the Id-CP grew along the PS and involved the lateral wall of the third ventricle, patients suffered from obesity and DI (Fig. **12**).

SURGICAL AIMS AND STRATEGY

Treatment of Id-CP can be initiated once a diagnosis has been secured. This is done by documenting in an appropriate clinical setting the presence of a tumor mass in the intra- and/or supra-sellar region, related endocrinological abnormalities (usually manifesting as hypopituitarism such as growth failure in younger patients, and menstrual disorder and amenorrhea or impotence in adult patients), and calcification from an imaging study. The aims of Id-CP treatment are multi-faceted, as treatment must address issues related to the tumor mass itself as well as to the endocrinological abnormalities and their resultant systemic effects. Regarding the initial presentation of patients, control of the tumor mass may be paramount, as large tumors can produce mass effects on visual or neurological structures adjacent to the pituitary region that need to be relieved; this is particularly true for pediatric patients, who usually present initially with larger tumors. Treatment also aims to preserve normal pituitary function and cause as few side effects as possible.

In this situation, definition of therapeutic strategies is challenging in all cases of CP, especially with respect to the choice between complete resection and subtotal resection with adjuvant radiotherapy. patients younger than 16 who suffer complete operative resection might receive serious endocrinological sequelae that could lead to phenotypic changes and affect psychological health severely. Fortunately, adult patients can better tolerate these sequelae under the hands of a practised surgeon who possesses sufficient knowledge of surgical anatomy and the experience to know when to stop resection to ensure patient`s safety. Regarding the septation function of the diaphragm and suprasellar arachnoid during Id-CP growth, vital structures such as the hypothalamus and 3rd VF are only compressed and displaced by the tumor. In contrast to suprasellar tubero-infundibular CP, Id-CP has a clear dissection interface at which to separate the tumor from the hypothalamus and optic chiasm. Accordingly, Id-CP is considered a resectable tumor. The surgical aim was gross total tumor removal (GTR) in an attempt to avoid combined radiotherapy and the associated complications. Dissection of the suprasellar part of the tumor includes not only removal of the tumor but also some of the enlarged diaphragm. As we know, a tendency to recur is characteristic of CP and is the ultimate result of any tiny residual tumor. According to our follow-up data, even if intrasurgical findings or postsurgical MRI indicated total tumor removal, CP could still recur during the long-term follow-up. GTR emphasizes removal of the intrasellar tumor. Another difficult surgical issue is how to dissect along the true tumor capsule while preserving the residual pituitary gland and PS.

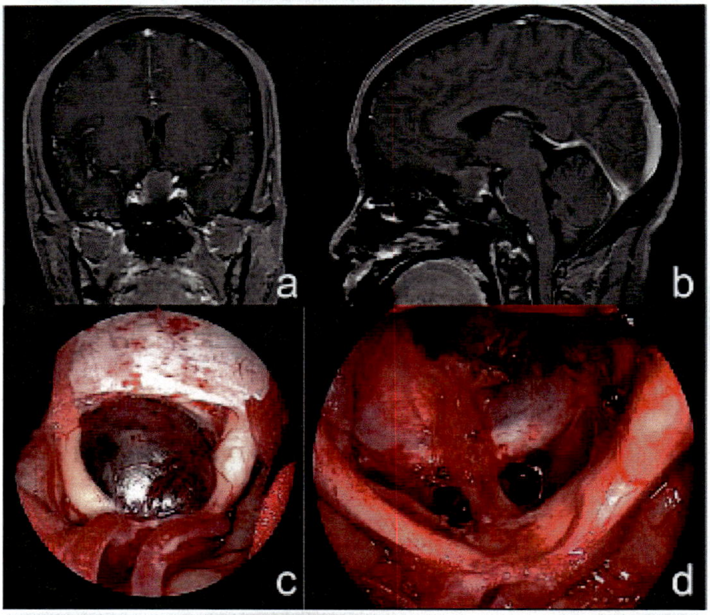

Fig. (14). For a case of Id-IP, we used endoscopy to observe the relationship between tumor with pituitary stalk in operation. The distal segment of the PS inflated into an umbrella shape and the tumor capsule always fuses with the PS.

SPECIAL CONSIDERATION IN THE MANAGEMENT OF ID-CP

Id-CP differs from pituitary adenoma in several aspects: first, there are differences in the topographic relationships between the tumor and pituitary stalk. Adenomas that originate from adenohypophyseal cells compress and displace the PS, which can usually be preserved intact after surgery. However, in cases of Id-CP, the distal segment of the PS always inflates into an umbrella shape and the tumor capsule always fuses with the PS (Fig. **14**). As result, preservation of the PS always leaves residual tumor. Therefore, surgery for Id-CP is more difficult than surgery for adenoma in terms of PS preservation.

Based on the morphological tumor features, we proposed a surgical risk score based on presurgical MRI scan data Fig. (**15**), which might be meaningful for the surgical treatment of Id-CP.

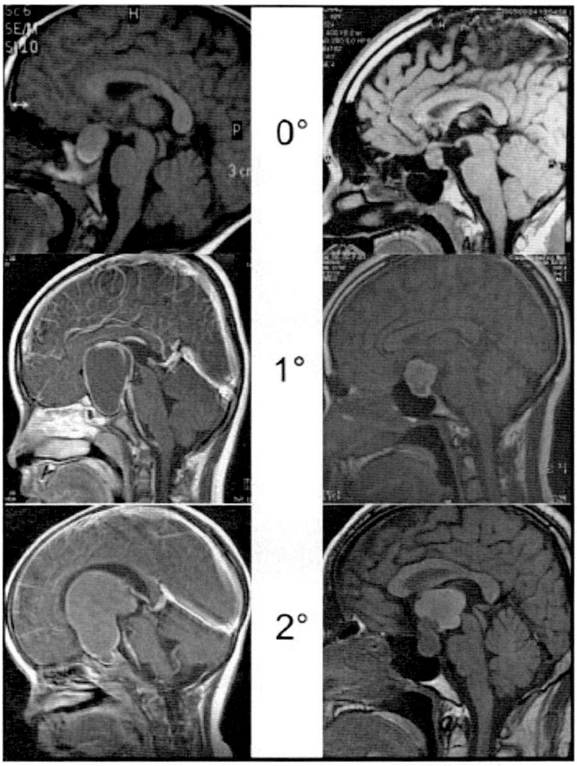

Fig. (15). (Reference from Jun Pan,Songtao Qi *et al.*, Growth patterns of craniopharyngiomas: clinical analysis of 226 patients. Journal of Neurosurgery Pediatrics, 2015:1-16). Criteria of Hypothalamic Involvement Scale based on tumor's growth pattern.

SELECTION OF SURGICAL APPROACH

Id-CPs are considered the optimal tumor type for the trans-sphenoidal approach [9, 14 - 30]. With minimal neurovascular manipulation, this approach allows excellent midline access and visibility of suprasellar region without brain retraction. Up until very recently, the removal of supradiaphragmatic CPs also has been improved *via* thewidespread use of endoscope in trans-sphenoidal surgery [22, 31 - 35].

However, in the previous literature, cases of CP treated *via* trans-sphenoidal approach all involved relatively small (<4 cm) tumors. This led to inherent selection bias during case selection. According to an analysis of the above-described publications, the maximum size of tumors selected for trans-sphenoidal approach was relatively smaller. Among the 168 cases reported by Fahlbusch *et al.*, 31 were treated *via* the trans-sphenoidal approach. Most of these cases involved tumors smaller than 3 cm and only one case involved a tumor larger than 4 cm. Frank *et al.* reported 10 cases of endoscope-assisted trans-sphenoid surgery in which the average tumor size was 2.9 cm. In a similar publication, Abe reported 11 cases of CP with an average tumor diameter of 1.7 cm. According to our opinion and experience, cases of Id-CP usually involve larger tumors and the suprasellar-extending part of the tumor is always larger than the intrasellar part. The minimal tumor diameter in our series was 3 cm. Therefore, there are several difficulties associated with selection of the trans-sphenoidal approach. 1) The suprasellar part of the tumor grows larger in higher locations, which might present a significant challenge to GTR. 2) The cystic walls of suprasellar tumors are always thick, with an eggshell appearance. 3) In some patients, the normal pituitary gland is located beneath the tumor. To reach the tumor, the normal gland might be resected *via* the trans-sphenoidal approach. Therefore, this approach increases the risk of disrupting pituitary function. 4) It is convenient to treat the adherence between the tumor and PS *via* the trans-sphenoidal approach. Meanwhile, only short-term follow-up data are available with respect to use of the endoscope-assisted trans-sphenoidal approach to treat CP; therefore, a longer evaluation time is needed. In pediatric cases, several elements should be considered. 1) In contrast to pituitary adenoma, the cystic walls of CP adhere closely to the bilateral wall of the cavernous sinus (CS) and sellar floor. Therefore, only draining cystic fluid and removing calcification inside the cystic walls will cause a short-term tumor recurrence. However, when dissecting the tumor cystic walls, large amounts of venous bleeding will affect the visual field provided by the trans-sphenoidal approach. 2) It is difficult to identify the normal adenohypophysis. As described previously, the PS alway s inflates and fuses with the tumoral cystic walls; as a result, these tumors are difficult to treat surgically *via* the trans-sphenoidal approach. 3) Id-CP always protrudes into the enlarged diaphragmatic foramen and grows upward to the suprasellar region. As a result, the tumor might envelop vascular structures. 4) A poor pneumatic sphenoid sinus might increase the risk associated with the trans-sphenoid approach. However, the trans-sphenoidal approach is the first option, particularly for adult patients with Id-CP [36], unless the tumor has grown along the PS and caused invagination of the third ventricle.

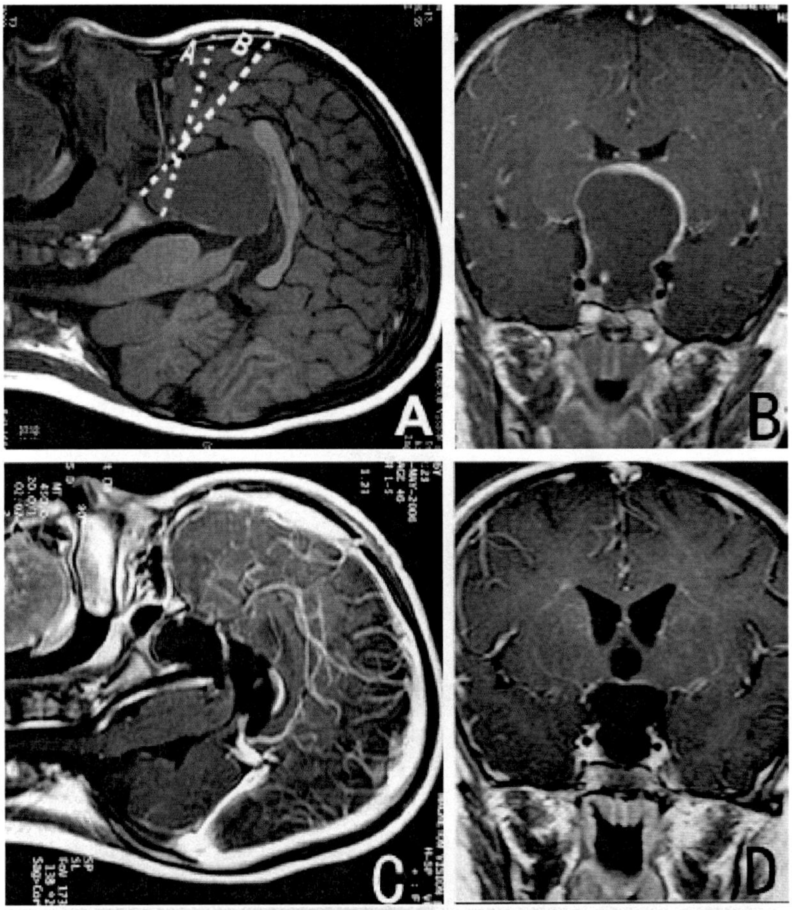

Fig 16. Sagittal and Coronal contrast-enhanced T1-weighted MRI before (a, b) and after (c, d) operstion in a 5-year-old boy showing an intra,suprasellar infra-diaphragmatic CP. The dotted lines on Fig. (A) indicated the superiority of inter- hemispheric approach: line A indicated the surgical view towards the intrasellar tumor portion obtained by standard skull base approaches as the pterional or subfrontal approaches. Line B showed the enhanced direct view within the intrasellar space achieved by a inter-hemispheric trans anterior fissure approach.

Id-CP predominately occurs in children, and the tumor size at presentation is always very large. Therefore, trans-cranial surgery remains the first-choice surgical approach. The frontotemporal and frontobasal interhemispheric approaches are the most frequently used approaches and are selected according to tumor size, calcification features, and extension orientation. According to our experience, the interhemispheric approach was advantageous when the suprasellar tumor cyst reached or even extended beyond the AcoA complex (Fig. **16**). Diaphragmatic septation facilitates separation of the suprasellar cyst from the surrounding structures *via* blunt dissection. The standard frontotemporal craniotomy is extended into the anterior frontal region by 1.5–2 cm from the keyhole being parallel to the superior orbital rim to allow more direct vision of the prechiasmatic space and enlarged pituitary fossa. In the authors' experience, the midline interhemispheric approach is superior to the lateral approach because the former provides direct visualization into the deepened and enlarged pituitary fossa, thus guaranteeing removal of the intrasellar part of the tumor under direct vision. Notably, the intra-axial approach should be abandoned in surgery for Id-CP, regardless of the lateral or median corridor. In rare cases involving an extremely high tumor location with protrusion into the third ventricular wall parenchyma, the lamina terminalis space might be used. In this situation, cotton can be used to help push the tumor capsule into the extra-axial visual field. Intra-axial dissection must be abandoned to avoid injury to the 3rd VF.

SURGICAL TECHNOLOGY AND SKILL

Transsphenoidal Approach

As the growth pattern of Id-CP, the transsphenoidal approach is one of the most important treatment selections. However, as our opinion, the transsphenoidal approach was only used as the supplemental selection in pediatric Id-CP, such as the palliative treatment for residual part of tumor by transcranial approach or the recurrent tumor. As the growth modal of tumor, the transsphenoidal approach for Id-CP is quite different from it's used for pituitary adenomas. The exposure for sellar floor should be more extensive. So strictly speaking, the transsphenoidal approach used for Id-CP is extensive ones. The development of endoscopic techniques was extremely meaningful for promote the usage of this approach to treat the Id-CP.

Trans-cranial Approach

The operative steps involving craniotomy utilized for the removal of Id-CP can be summarized as follows: 1) standardized skull base craniotomy (Frontotemporal craniotomy or frontobasal interhemispheric craniotomy; 2) separation of the tumor from suprasellar structures and the stretched, attenuating DS; 3) rounded incision of the elevated DS; and 4) tumor dissection along the true capsule while attempting to preserve the neurohypophysis and continuity of the PS.

The Relationship Between the Diaphragmatic Sellae and Tumor Fig. (17)

Three growth pattern types have been delineated based on the tumor–DS relationships: 1) intrasuprasellar infradiaphragmatic tumor, wherein the DS has been lifted by the suprasellar portion of the tumor but remains covered above the entire tumor; 2) intra- and suprasellar trans-diaphragmatic tumor, wherein most of the tumor, which involves both sides of the dural leaf, remains covered by the DS, although a part of the tumor could break through the diaphragm; and 3) intra- and suprasellar trans-infundibulum tumor, wherein part of the tumor invaginates into the supradiaphragmatic segment of the PS, resulting in a distended stalk.

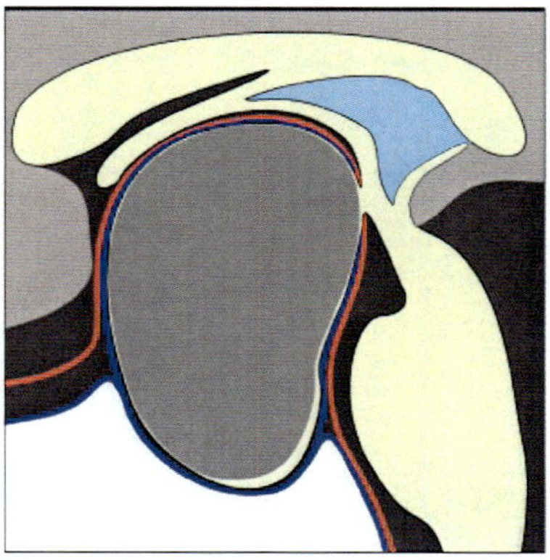

Fig. (17). The relationship between the diaphragmatic sellae and tumor in Id-CP.

Following separation by the DS, the tumor capsule along with the stretched attenuating DS is less adherent to suprasellar structures such as the chiasm, circle of Willis vessels and, more importantly, the 3rd VF. Therefore, tumors can always be freed from these structures with gentle retraction after adequate debulking. In trans-diaphragmatic tumors, the supradiaphragmatic portion of the tumor may encase the branches of the AcoA complex, which require acute dissection (See Chapter 19 of this book, type "Q" cases 2). Nevertheless, the supradiaphragmatic portion of the tumor remains covered by the basal arachnoid membrane above the DS and has a well-defined dissection plane distinct from suprasellar structures such as the PS and 3rd VF. In most recurrent cases, however, more severe adhesions are encountered, especially cases in which Ommaya reservoirs have been implanted; in this scenario, the tube lumen always adheres tightly to the surrounding structures. In the latter two growth pattern types, tumor cell transmigration along the tracts of the previous surgical route and the Ommaya tube can result in ectopic cystic formation, which always compromises radical removal.

Regarding morphological changes in the PS, the proximal part of the PS, which connects to the infundibulum, is always kept intact, whereas its distal end is scattered and fuses with the supraposterior part of the tumor capsule and stretched DS. Rarely, the supradiaphragmatic segment of the PS may become distended due to tumor invagination. The relationship between the tumor and PS presents a challenge during surgery. Most tumors are huge and it is difficult to preserve the

PS, which is inflated and thin. However, preservation of the continuity of the pituitary–hypothalamic axis could provide a morphological basis for the recovery of pituitary function. In our series, pituitary function was recovered to a different degree continuity of the PS was preserved, indicating that this is an important foundation for preservation of continuity.

PATHOLOGICAL DIAGNOSIS

In our series of 62 cases of Id-CP, the pathological results of three cases indicated squamous papillary-type tumors. The remaining cases were of typical adamantinomatous-type CP.

Outcomes and Complications

Surgical Extension

Personal series investigated by senior author included 62 patients with Id-CP. Among these, 48 were children under the age of 17 years at the time of initial surgery. The remaining patients were adults. All 14 cases of adult-onset tumors involved relatively small tumors and achieved GTR either *via* the trans-sphenoidal approach or *via* a standard pterional approach. Of the 48 cases of childhood-onset tumors, standard frontotemporal craniotomy was used in 26 cases involving relatively smaller tumors, while the frontobasal interhemispheric approach was used in the residual 22 cases. Total resection (evidenced by both the surgeon's intra-operative impression and the postoperative MRI) was performed in 41 patients of CPs. The reasons for partial or subtotal resection were extensive cystic involvement of the infrasellar region in five cases and a remaining fragment of the thinning tumor capsule in one recurrent cystic tumor with distant tumoral transformation. It is worth noting that, involving the extent of tumor removal, there was no significant difference between the primary and recurrent cases (5/50 *vs.* 2/12). Although recurrent tumors adhere more tightly to the surrounding structures than do primary CPs, in most cases the suprasellar tumor cysts could be resected safely.

Tumor Recurrence

According to the follow-up of 46 juvenile cases with GTR in our series, the 5- and 10-year progression-free survival (PFS) rates were 87.6% and 79.6%, respectively. Similarly, among cases that achieved GTR *via* the trans-sphenoidal approach (most of which were adults), the 5- and 10-year PFS rates were 87.1% and 76.1%, respectively. There was no pregnant statistical difference between adult and children (log-rank test, $p = 0.719$). Notably, the average time to recurrence after surgery was 4.5 years among cases of Id-CP, which differed considerably from the 2 years reported for cases of suprasellar tubero-infundibular CP. Therefore, long-term follow-up of Id-CP cases, particularly pediatric cases, is very important.

Most Id-CP recurrences occurred inside the pituitary fossa, and therefore intrasellar dissection is indispensable during primary surgery. Most recurrent tumors maintained growth characteristic of Id-CP (See typical Id-CP case 15). Despite suprasellar tumor adherence, surgical interfaces for safe tumor removal could be identified in most recurrent cases. Therefore, a second GTR should also be pursued in most recurrent cases. Strict postsurgical follow-up is necessary to ensure the early observation of recurrent tumors. For localized, recurrent tumors, the trans-sphenoidal approach might provide a good prognosis (See typical Id-CP Case 6). In a few cases, the morphology of the recurrent tumor changed dramatically Fig. (**18**) as a result of trans-infundibular tumor growth. In this scenario, secondary surgery must manipulate the tumor within the vital third ventricular nervous tissue, which significantly increases the risk of hypothalamic complications.

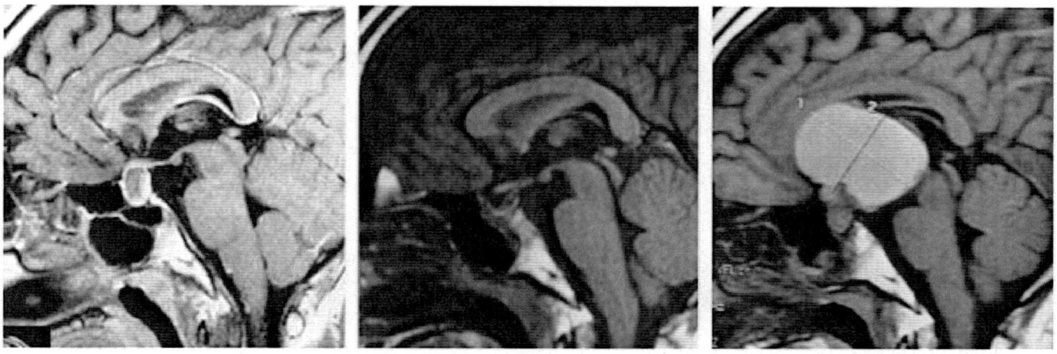

Fig. (18). In a case of recurrent CP, the morphological change of tumor was observed significantly. The tumor growth pattern was changed from sub-diaphragmatic (Type Q) to the tubero-infundibular type (Type T).

Regarding overall survival (OS), our opinion is that the OS rate was higher among Id-CP cases. Most cases could achieve long-term survival with appropriate hormone substitution. Among pediatric patients, the 5-and 10-year OS rates were 95.6% and 89.2% according to the long-term follow-up of our 52 cases of Id-CP, respectively, and the 10-year OS among adult patients was 92.2%.

Visual Outcome

Ophthalmological conditions represent an significant limitation of autonomy in the previous reports. Effenterre and Boch [7, 8] summarized four conclusions after reviewing the literature focused this topic: 1) the severity of preoperative impairment determined the probability of recuperation. The optic atrophy (observed *via* fundoscopy) before surgery conferred the worst prognosis; 2) children are more often attacked than adults. Whereas, at the parallel impairment degree, the prognosis after optic decompression is equal whether the age; 3) Surgery is better than radiotherapy for treatment; and 4) Relapse is often responsible for definitive visual deterioration.

Among the patients in our series, all pediatric patients and six adult patients presented with visual deterioration. Eighteen pediatric cases presented with poor preoperative vision (unilateral or bilateral blindness or affected light perception). After surgery, vision was improved (at least in one eye) or normalized in 62% (eight normalized, 24 improved), unchanged in 25% (13 patients) and worsened in 14% of the patients (seven patients). Vision was normalized in all six adult patients. Of the 18 pediatric cases with poor preoperative vision (19 eyes in total), vision improved in only six patients, remained unchanged in five, and worsened in seven.

Endocrine Sequelae

After surgical resection, the pituitary dysfunction was significant increase in our patient series. Overall, thepituitary function was more severely compromised in children than adults after operation, as nearly half of the pediatric patients suffered from panhypopituitarism during the long-term follow-up study. In contrast, no adult patients experienced panhypopituitarism. Panhypopituitarism was more prevalent in patients with recurrent tumors than in those with primary tumors. And for patients who underwent GTR or subtotal resection, there was no difference in postoperative pituitary function .

Postoperative Hypothalamic Status

Unlike suprasellar 3rd VF CPs, patients with Id-CPs appeared to suffer less hypothalamic dysfunction during follow-up. No patients in our series suffered from morbid obesity or hyperphagia, and apparent obesity occurred only in three pediatric patients during the long-term follow up period. Furthermore, other complications associated with hypothalamic impairment such as emotionally labile behavior, sleep–wake cycle disruption, memory deficits, and thermoregulatory abnormalities were absent in our patients with Id-CP.

SUMMARY AND CONCLUSIONS

Id-CPs represent a specific topographic location and entity that should be distinguished from supradiaphragmatic CPs. The marked sellar enlargement and deepening and the unique rounded symmetrical suprasellar expansion pattern are the major radiological characteristics of this type of tumor. A large size and predominant incidence in children and adolescents are the other two clinical features. Because of diaphragmatic restriction, expansion toward the upper clivus, parasellar region, and middle cranial fossa rarely occurs with this type of tumor. Total tumor removal during primary surgery would most likely achieve good long-term tumor control and the better living quality. Long-term DI and hypopituitarism appeared to be common sequelae among our pediatric patients, who required long-term hormonal supplementation therapy. Hypothalamic dysfunction such as obesity, cognitive deterioration, and behavioral disorders, which are frequently reported with pediatric suprasellar CP following radical removal, were less frequently observed in patients with Id-CP, despite their young ages and the large sizes of tumors from the midline, which are considered predisposing factors for hypothalamic morbidity [36 - 38].

CONFLICT OF INTEREST

The author (editor) declares no conflict of interest, financial or otherwise.

ACKNOWLEDGEMENTS

Declared none

REFERENCES

[1] Qi S, Lu Y, Pan J, Zhang X, Long H, Fan J. Anatomic relations of the arachnoidea around the pituitary stalk: relevance for surgical removal of craniopharyngiomas. Acta Neurochir (Wien) 2011; 153(4): 785-96.
[http://dx.doi.org/10.1007/s00701-010-0940-y] [PMID: 21271263]

[2] Brunel H, Raybaud C, Peretti-Viton P, *et al.* [Craniopharyngioma in children: MRI study of 43 cases]. Neurochirurgie 2002; 48(4): 309-18. [Craniopharyngioma in children: MRI study of 43 cases]. [PMID: 12407316]

[3] Hoffman HJ. Surgical management of craniopharyngioma. Pediatr Neurosurg 1994; 21 (Suppl. 1): 44-9.
[http://dx.doi.org/10.1159/000120861] [PMID: 7530990]

[4] Lee YY, Wong TT, Fang YT, Chang KP, Chen YW, Niu DM. Comparison of hypothalamopituitary axis dysfunction of intrasellar and third ventricular craniopharyngiomas in children. Brain Dev 2008; 30(3): 189-94.
[http://dx.doi.org/10.1016/j.braindev.2007.07.011] [PMID: 17870266]

[5] Wang KC, Hong SH, Kim SK, Cho BK. Origin of craniopharyngiomas: implication on the growth pattern. Childs Nerv Syst 2005; 21(8-9): 628-34.
[http://dx.doi.org/10.1007/s00381-005-1203-8] [PMID: 16059733]

[6] Wang KC, Kim SK, Choe G, Chi JG, Cho BK. Growth patterns of craniopharyngioma in children: role of the diaphragm sellae and its surgical implication. Surg Neurol 2002; 57(1): 25-33.
[http://dx.doi.org/10.1016/S0090-3019(01)00657-7] [PMID: 11834269]

[7] Van Effenterre R, Boch AL. Craniopharyngioma in adults and children: a study of 122 surgical cases. J Neurosurg 2002; 97(1): 3-11.

[http://dx.doi.org/10.3171/jns.2002.97.1.0003] [PMID: 12134929]

[8] Rémy van Effenterre. Anne-Laure Boch. Craniopharyngioma Oncology of CNS Tumors 559-70.

[9] Honegger J, Buchfelder M, Fahlbusch R. Surgical treatment of craniopharyngiomas: endocrinological results. J Neurosurg 1999; 90(2): 251-7.
[http://dx.doi.org/10.3171/jns.1999.90.2.0251] [PMID: 9950495]

[10] DeVile CJ, Grant DB, Hayward RD, Stanhope R. Growth and endocrine sequelae of craniopharyngioma. Arch Dis Child 1996; 75(2): 108-14.
[http://dx.doi.org/10.1136/adc.75.2.108] [PMID: 8869189]

[11] Thomsett MJ, Conte FA, Kaplan SL, Grumbach MM. Endocrine and neurologic outcome in childhood craniopharyngioma: Review of effect of treatment in 42 patients. J Pediatr 1980; 97(5): 728-35.
[http://dx.doi.org/10.1016/S0022-3476(80)80254-X] [PMID: 7431164]

[12] Karavitaki N, Cudlip S, Adams CB, Wass JA. Craniopharyngiomas. Endocr Rev 2006; 27(4): 371-97.
[http://dx.doi.org/10.1210/er.2006-0002] [PMID: 16543382]

[13] Qi S, Pan J, Lu Y, *et al.* The impact of the site of origin and rate of tumour growth on clinical outcome in children with craniopharyngiomas. Clin Endocrinol (Oxf) 2012; 76(1): 103-10.
[http://dx.doi.org/10.1111/j.1365-2265.2011.04172.x] [PMID: 21752042]

[14] Abe T, Lüdecke DK. Transnasal surgery for infradiaphragmatic craniopharyngiomas in pediatric patients. Neurosurgery 1999; 44(5): 957-64.
[http://dx.doi.org/10.1097/00006123-199905000-00012] [PMID: 10232528]

[15] Cavallo LM, Prevedello D, Esposito F, *et al.* The role of the endoscope in the transsphenoidal management of cystic lesions of the sellar region. Neurosurg Rev 2008; 31(1): 55-64.
[http://dx.doi.org/10.1007/s10143-007-0098-0] [PMID: 17922153]

[16] Chakrabarti I, Amar AP, Couldwell W, Weiss MH. Long-term neurological, visual, and endocrine outcomes following transnasal resection of craniopharyngioma. J Neurosurg 2005; 102(4): 650-7.
[http://dx.doi.org/10.3171/jns.2005.102.4.0650] [PMID: 15871507]

[17] Couldwell WT, Weiss MH, Rabb C, Liu JK, Apfelbaum RI, Fukushima T. Variations on the standard transsphenoidal approach to the sellar region, with emphasis on the extended approaches and parasellar approaches: surgical experience in 105 cases. Neurosurgery 2004; 55(3): 539-47.
[http://dx.doi.org/10.1227/01.NEU.0000134287.19377.A2] [PMID: 15335421]

[18] de Divitiis E, Cappabianca P, Cavallo LM, Esposito F, de Divitiis O, Messina A. Extended endoscopic transsphenoidal approach for extrasellar craniopharyngiomas. Neurosurgery 2007; 61(5) (Suppl. 2): 219-27.
[PMID: 18091236]

[19] Dusick JR, Esposito F, Kelly DF, *et al.* The extended direct endonasal transsphenoidal approach for nonadenomatous suprasellar tumors. J Neurosurg 2005; 102(5): 832-41.
[http://dx.doi.org/10.3171/jns.2005.102.5.0832] [PMID: 15926706]

[20] Dusick JR, Fatemi N, Mattozo C, *et al.* Pituitary function after endonasal surgery for nonadenomatous parasellar tumors: Rathke's cleft cysts, craniopharyngiomas, and meningiomas. Surg Neurol 2008; 70(5): 482-90.
[http://dx.doi.org/10.1016/j.surneu.2008.03.027] [PMID: 18482750]

[21] Fahlbusch R, Honegger J, Paulus W, Huk W, Buchfelder M. Surgical treatment of craniopharyngiomas: experience with 168 patients. J Neurosurg 1999; 90(2): 237-50.
[http://dx.doi.org/10.3171/jns.1999.90.2.0237] [PMID: 9950494]

[22] Frank G, *et al.* The endoscopic extended transsphenoidal approach for craniopharyngiomas. Neurosurgery 2006; 59(1 Suppl 1): 75-83.
[http://dx.doi.org/10.1227/01.NEU.0000219897.98238.A3]

[23] Frazier JL, Chaichana K, Jallo GI, Quiñones-Hinojosa A. Combined endoscopic and microscopic

management of pediatric pituitary region tumors through one nostril: technical note with case illustrations. Childs Nerv Syst 2008; 24(12): 1469-78. [http://dx.doi.org/10.1007/s00381-008-0710-9] [PMID: 18769925]

[24] Gardner PA, Prevedello DM, Kassam AB, Snyderman CH, Carrau RL, Mintz AH. The evolution of the endonasal approach for craniopharyngiomas. J Neurosurg 2008; 108(5): 1043-7. [http://dx.doi.org/10.3171/JNS/2008/108/5/1043] [PMID: 18447729]

[25] Kitano M, Taneda M. Extended transsphenoidal surgery for suprasellar craniopharyngiomas: infrachiasmatic radical resection combined with or without a suprachiasmatic trans-lamina terminalis approach. Surg Neurol 2009; 71(3): 290-8. [http://dx.doi.org/10.1016/j.surneu.2007.11.014] [PMID: 18291485]

[26] Laws ER Jr. Transsphenoidal removal of craniopharyngioma. Pediatr Neurosurg 1994; 21 (Suppl. 1): 57-63. [http://dx.doi.org/10.1159/000120863] [PMID: 7841079]

[27] Locatelli D, Levi D, Rampa F, Pezzotta S, Castelnuovo P. Endoscopic approach for the treatment of relapses in cystic craniopharyngiomas. Childs Nerv Syst 2004; 20(11-12): 863-7. [http://dx.doi.org/10.1007/s00381-004-0944-0] [PMID: 15185112]

[28] Maira G, Anile C, Albanese A, Cabezas D, Pardi F, Vignati A. The role of transsphenoidal surgery in the treatment of craniopharyngiomas. J Neurosurg 2004; 100(3): 445-51. [http://dx.doi.org/10.3171/jns.2004.100.3.0445] [PMID: 15035280]

[29] Maira G, Anile C, Rossi GF, Colosimo C. Surgical treatment of craniopharyngiomas: an evaluation of the transsphenoidal and pterional approaches. Neurosurgery 1995; 36(4): 715-24. [http://dx.doi.org/10.1227/00006123-199504000-00012] [PMID: 7596502]

[30] Norris JS, Pavaresh M, Afshar F. Primary transsphenoidal microsurgery in the treatment of craniopharyngiomas. Br J Neurosurg 1998; 12(4): 305-12. [http://dx.doi.org/10.1080/02688699844790] [PMID: 10070421]

[31] Gardner PA, Kassam AB, Snyderman CH, *et al.* Outcomes following endoscopic, expanded endonasal resection of suprasellar craniopharyngiomas: a case series. J Neurosurg 2008; 109(1): 6-16. [http://dx.doi.org/10.3171/JNS/2008/109/7/0006] [PMID: 18590427]

[32] Kassam AB, Gardner PA, Snyderman CH, Carrau RL, Mintz AH, Prevedello DM. Expanded endonasal approach, a fully endoscopic transnasal approach for the resection of midline suprasellar craniopharyngiomas: a new classification based on the infundibulum. J Neurosurg 2008; 108(4): 715-28. [http://dx.doi.org/10.3171/JNS/2008/108/4/0715] [PMID: 18377251]

[33] Laufer I, Anand VK, Schwartz TH. Endoscopic, endonasal extended transsphenoidal, transplanum transtuberculum approach for resection of suprasellar lesions. J Neurosurg 2007; 106(3): 400-6. [http://dx.doi.org/10.3171/jns.2007.106.3.400] [PMID: 17367062]

[34] Laws ER, Kanter AS, Jane JA Jr, Dumont AS. Extended transsphenoidal approach. J Neurosurg 2005; 102(5): 825-7. [http://dx.doi.org/10.3171/jns.2005.102.5.0825] [PMID: 15926704]

[35] Stamm AC, Vellutini E, Harvey RJ, Nogeira JF Jr, Herman DR. Endoscopic transnasal craniotomy and the resection of craniopharyngioma. Laryngoscope 2008; 118(7): 1142-8. [http://dx.doi.org/10.1097/MLG.0b013e318170b5dc] [PMID: 18438262]

[36] De Vile CJ, Grant DB, Kendall BE, *et al.* Management of childhood craniopharyngioma: can the morbidity of radical surgery be predicted? J Neurosurg 1996; 85(1): 73-81. [http://dx.doi.org/10.3171/jns.1996.85.1.0073] [PMID: 8683285]

[37] Loyo-Varela M, Herrada Pineda T. Infradiaphragmatic craniopharyngioma in the adult. World Neurosurg 2014; 81(5-6): 680-2. [http://dx.doi.org/10.1016/j.wneu.2013.03.039] [PMID: 23523679]

[38] Poretti A, Grotzer MA, Ribi K, Schönle E, Boltshauser E. Outcome of craniopharyngioma in children: long-term complications and quality of life. Dev Med Child Neurol 2004; 46(4): 220-9. [http://dx.doi.org/10.1111/j.1469-8749.2004.tb00476.x] [PMID: 15077699]

CHAPTER 11

Subarachnoid Cisternal Craniopharyngioma (Type "S")

Jun Pan[*]

Department of Neurosurgery, Nanfang Neurosurgery Research Institution, Nanfang Hospital, Southern Medical University, 1838 North Guangzhou Avenue, Guangzhou, China

Abstract: In this chapter, we focus on a subgroup of craniopharyngioma (CP) in which the main tumor body is located exclusively in the suprasellar subarachnoid cisternal space around the pituitary stalk (PS) and there is no third ventricle involvement. Notably, the cases of CP reported in this chapter were not clearly defined in previous literature. The main reason for the confusion regarding this type of CP might be the lack of uniform criteria for evaluating the relationship between the tumor and third ventricle walls. The terminology "suprasellar extraventricular CP," which is used in previous literature, might be another term for the cases described in this chapter; however, this term does not truly reflect the tumor origin and location.

Keywords: Craniopharyngioma, Extraventricular, Pituitary stalk, Subarachnoid.

DEFINITION

By retrospectively reviewing the presurgical magnetic resonance imaging (MRI) data and intra-surgical findings from 226 cases of primary CP, the following features of this type of tumor were identified:

1. Tumor dissection occurs entirely inside the subarachnoid cistern space *via* the extra-axial approach.
2. Although the main tumor body is located inside the subarachnoid cistern and around the PS, the site of origin of this type of tumor is at the proximal segment of the stalk and infundibulum.
3. The tumor does not involve the third ventricular walls.
4. According to the relationship between the tumor and suprasellar membranous structures, this type of tumor can be classified as suprasellar, extra-pia mater, and subarachnoid. Therefore, a more precise definition of this type of tumors would be infundibular CP with main growth toward the subarachnoid cistern.

[*] **Corresponding author Jun Pan**: Department of Neurosurgery, Nanfang Neurosurgery Research Institution, Nanfang Hospital, Southern Medical University, 1838 North Guangzhou Avenue, Guangzhou, China; Tel/Fax: +8620-61641806; E-mail: panjundu@hotmail.com

Songtao Qi (Ed.)

No previously available publications have reported the incidence of this type of tumor among all cases of CP. According to a description provided by Steno *et al.* [1], suprasellar extraventricular tumors accounted for approximately one-third of the investigated suprasellar lesions (15/46). However, among the 122 cases of CP reported by Effenterre and Boch [2], extraventricular CP accounted for 92% of the cases. This discrepancy may be partly attributable to the variable diagnostic criteria used to define extraventricular tumors. As our experience by intra-surgical findings, CPs that can be dissected entirely through the suprasellar arachnoid cistern without entering the third ventricular cavity accounted for 42% of all cases (95/226). This incidence rate did not exclude tumors of subdiaphragmatic origin that had protruded to the suprasellar region (48 cases); therefore, if only suprasellar CPs were counted, extraventricular tumors would account for 20.8% of all cases. We specifically describe this type of tumor in this chapter because this type differs considerably from third ventricle floor (3rd VF) CP with respect to surgical strategy, approach selection, and prognosis.

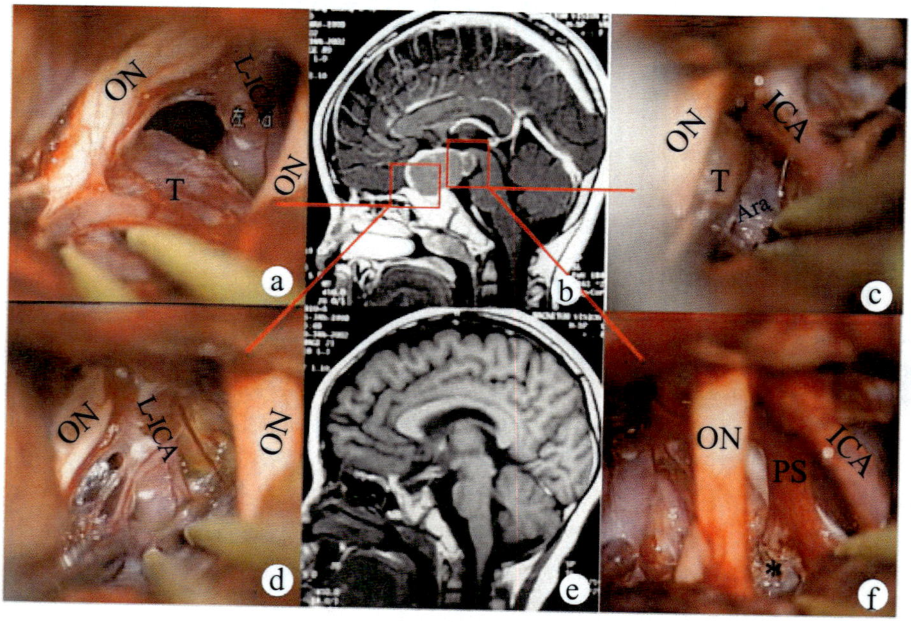

Fig. (1). (Reference from Jun Pan,Songtao Qi *et al.*, Growth patterns of craniopharyngiomas: clinical analysis of 226 patients. Journal of Neurosurgery Pediatrics, 2015:1-16). Pre- and post-operative Sagittal T1-weighted MRIs (b and e) and intra-operative pictures (a,c,d, and f) demonstrating the typical growth pattern of supra-sellar subarachnoid cisternal craniopharyngioma. b: The tumor arise from the pituitary stalk and mainly locating inside the optical chiasm cistern. e: postoperative MRI showed total removal of tumor by right side pterional approach. The tumor was mainly dissected through the pre-chiasm space (a and d). Tumor can be dissected along its own arachnoid dissecting plane, except at the site of tumor origin where the tumor need sharp dissecting (c and f). Note the site of tumor origin after tumor removal (asterisk in Fig. (**f**). **Abbreviations:** Ara: arachnoid around the pituitary stalk. ICA: internal carotid artery; ON: optic nerve; PS: pituitary stalk; T:tumor.

ANATOMICAL LOCATION OF THE TUMOR

This type of tumor can be subdivided into two groups according to the anatomical location: 1) pre-stalk CP mainly located inside the optical chiasm cistern (Figs. **1** and **2**) retro-stalk CP with extension posterior to the interpeduncular cistern and even involvement of the posterior cranial fossa (Fig. **2**). Regarding tumoral extension, after originating from the PS inside the chiasm cistern, the tumor easily extended towards the surrounding cisterns. The primary orientations of the extensions were anterior and posterior. Most CPs of this type are limited to localization inside the optic chiasm cistern; for this reason, a higher incidence of prechiasm tumors *vs.* retrochiasm tumors was reported in a large case-control study [3, 4].

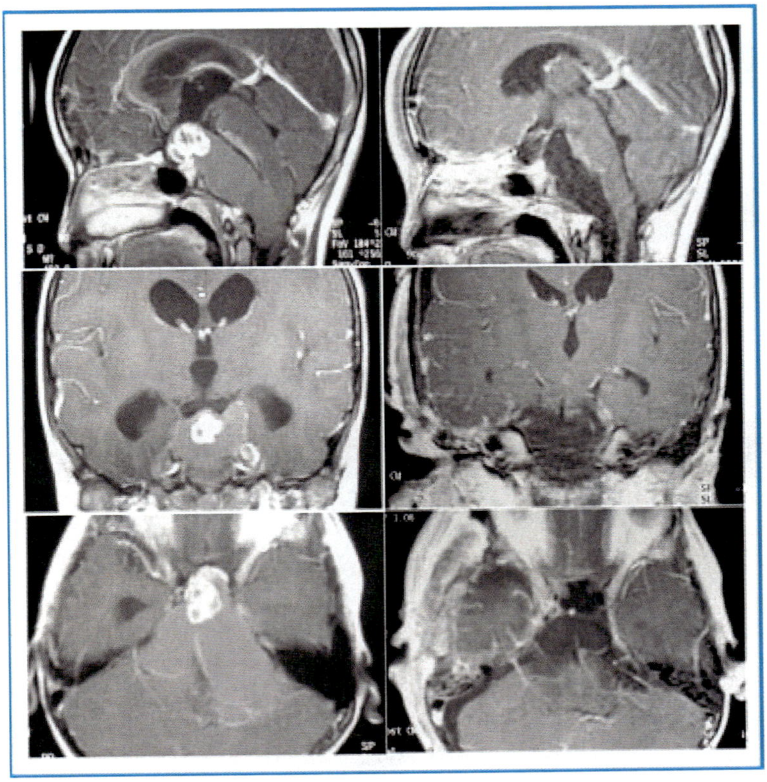

Fig. (2). Pre- (left column) and post-operative (right column) Sagittal-, coronal-, and axial- T1-weighted MRIs demonstrating the typical growth pattern of supra-sellar subarachnoid cisternal craniopharyngioma with retro-clivus expansion. Left column: The tumor arise from the infundibulum region and mainly spreading backwards along the subarachnoid space into the posterior fossa and involved bilateral CPAs. Right column: early postoperative MRIs showed the total removal of the tumor. The detailed intraoperative findings and long-term follow-up result of this patient could be find in the Chapter 19.

The relationship between the tumor and surrounding structures determines some objective rules of extension to the surrounding cisterns. For example, prestalk CP mainly extends forward through the prechiasmatic cistern (Fig. **3**), and further toward the anterior cranial fossa, olfactory cistern/bilateral internal carotid artery (ICA) median or lateral cistern, and even the lateral fissure cistern. This type of tumor can also protrude upward at the anterior border of the chiasm with extension to the terminalis cistern and even expansion into the frontotemporal lobe (Fig. **4**). On the other hand, retrostalk tumors always involve the posterior cranial fossa and extend to the basilar cistern, prepons cistern, and even the inside of the cervical canal (Fig. **5**). Posterior tumor extension may even involve the pineal region by spreading along the para-mesencephalon cistern (Fig. **6**). Although the tumor cystic cavities of retrostalk tumors are always very large, the tumors are in fact located between the posterior third ventricle and diencephalon lobe of Liliequist's membrane. Therefore, surgical dissection along the arachnoid interface to separate the tumor walls is a safe technique that protects the cranial nerves and vascular structures enveloped by the tumor.

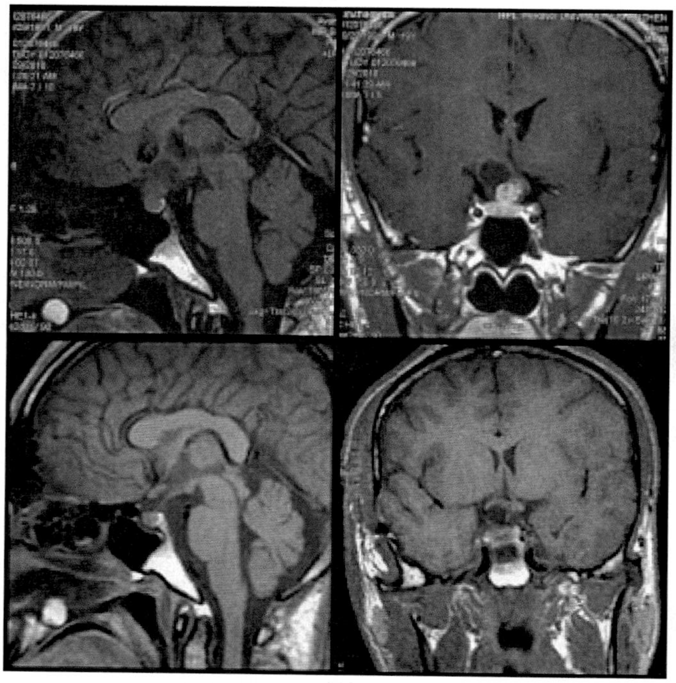

Fig. (3). Pre- (upper row) and post-operative (lower row) Sagittal-,and coronal T1-weighted MRIs demonstrating the typical growth pattern of supra-sellar subarachnoid cisternal craniopharyngioma. Upper row: The tumor arise from the infundibulum region and mainly spreading forwards through pre-chiasmatic cistern. Lower row: postoperative MRIs showed the total removal of the tumor with preservation of the pituitary stalk. The detailed intraoperative findings and long-term follow-up result of this patient could be find in the Chapter 19.

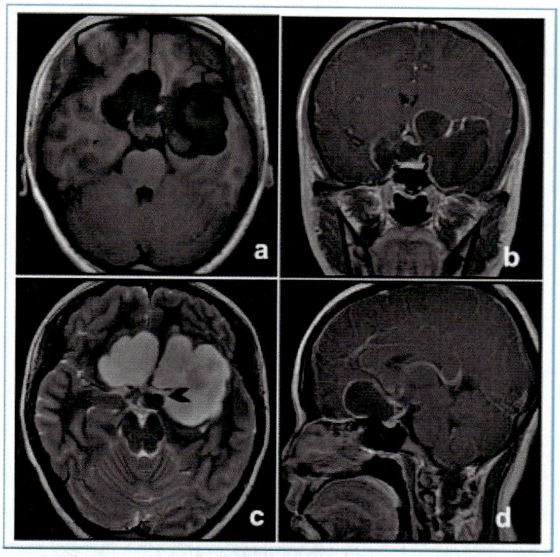

Fig. (4). Pre-operative Sagittal-,and coronal-,and axial T1-, T2-weighted MRIs demonstrating a typical subarachnoid cisternal craniopharyngioma. The tumor arise from the infundibulum region and mainly spreading forwards through pre-chiasmatic cistern into the anterior cranial fossa, lateral fissure cistern and the fronto-temporal lobe. Forked tail arrow on the T2-weighted MR image indicated the coarse calcification at the infundibulum and the pituitary stalk.

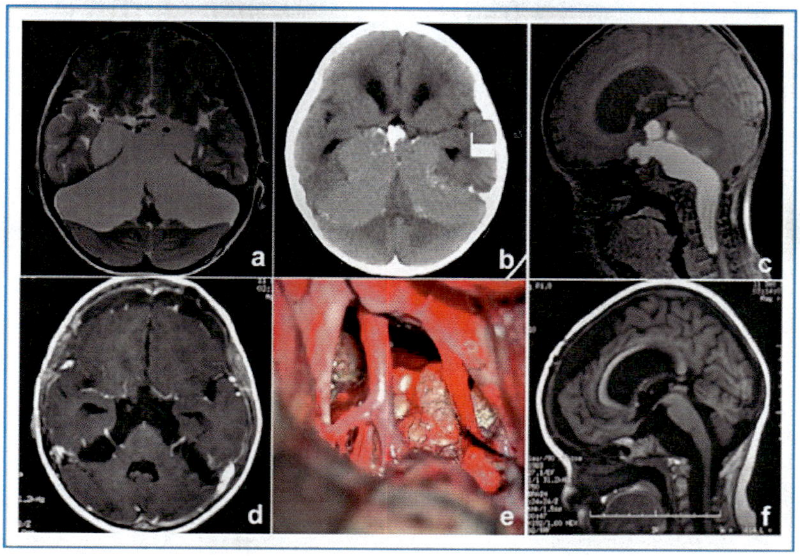

Fig. (5). Pre-operative (a and c) sagittal-,and axial-T1-weighted MRIs demonstrated a huge subarachnoid cisternal craniopharyngioma with retro-clivus expansion. The tumor involved posterior fossa and bilateral CPAs. Pre-operative CT scan showed the calcification of the tumor (b). Post-operative sagittal-,and axial-T--weighted MRIs (d and f) showed total removal of the tumor. Intraoperative picture showed exposure of the tumor through the medial and lateral corridors of ICA, and also the tentorial spaces. The detailed intraoperative findings and long-term follow-up result of this patient could be found in the Chapter 19.

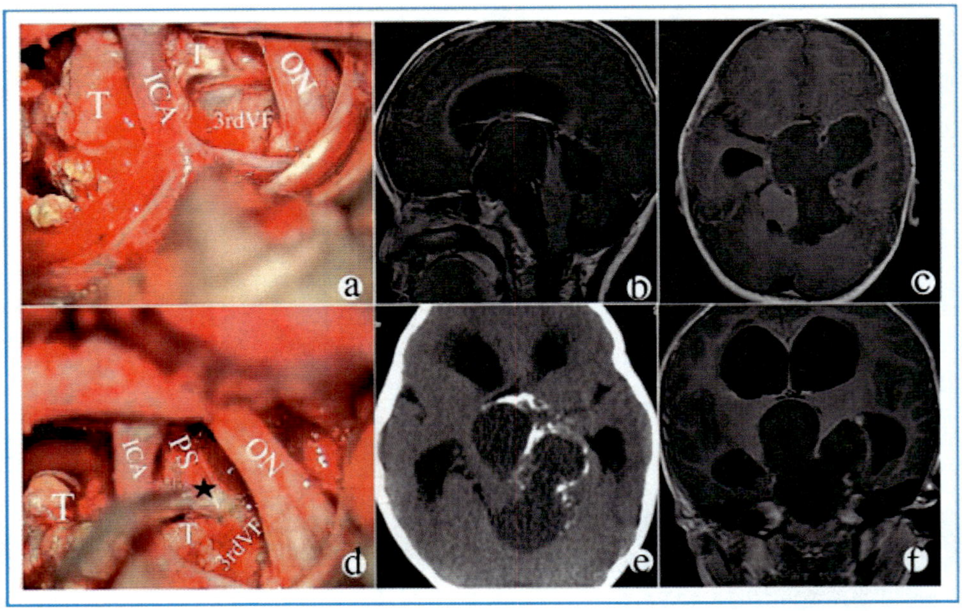

Fig. (6). Preoperative MRI and CT scan (b,c,e and f) and intra-operative pictures (a and d) demonstrating a huge subarachnoid cisternal craniopharyngioma with retro-stalk extension. From the origin site at the chiasmatic cistern around the pituitary stalk, the tumor capsule compress third ventricle floor significantly by extending into the adjacent basal cistern, and finally involved multiple cisterns. The tumor was removed by a left side frontotemporal combined supra- and infratentorial approach. Intra-operative photos showed the various aspects of the tumor: a: the tumor adhered tightly to the third ventricle floor but without infiltrating into it (a). Only at the proximal portion of the pituitary stalk and infundibulum (asterisk in Fig. (d) the tumor has sub-pail relationship with the nerve tissue (d). **Abbreviations:** 3rd VF: third ventricle floor; ICA: internal carotid artery; ON: optic nerve; PS: pituitary stalk; T:tumor.

In the analysis of our series, significant age differences were observed between the two tumor subgroups. The prestalk type predominantly occurred in adult patients; however, the retrostalk type was predominant in pediatric cases. Table X lists results from a statistical analysis of 47 cases of subarachnoid CP that underwent surgery at our department. Among those cases, prestalk tumors occurred in 37 cases, including 34 adult cases (average age, 37.4 years) and three pediatric cases (age, <17 years). In contrast, retrostalk tumors occurred in nine cases, including seven pediatric and two adult cases. The true reason for this difference remains unknown. We cannot give a definite answer with respect to differences in growth patterns between children and adult; however, we believe that the membrane structures around the PS may be partially responsible for directing tumor growth. This phenomenon was observed in a few recurrent tumors in which the membrane structures had been destroyed in the previous surgery and the recurrent tumors exhibited a different growth pattern (Figs. **7-10**). Morphological differences in the PS between adults and children might be another reason.

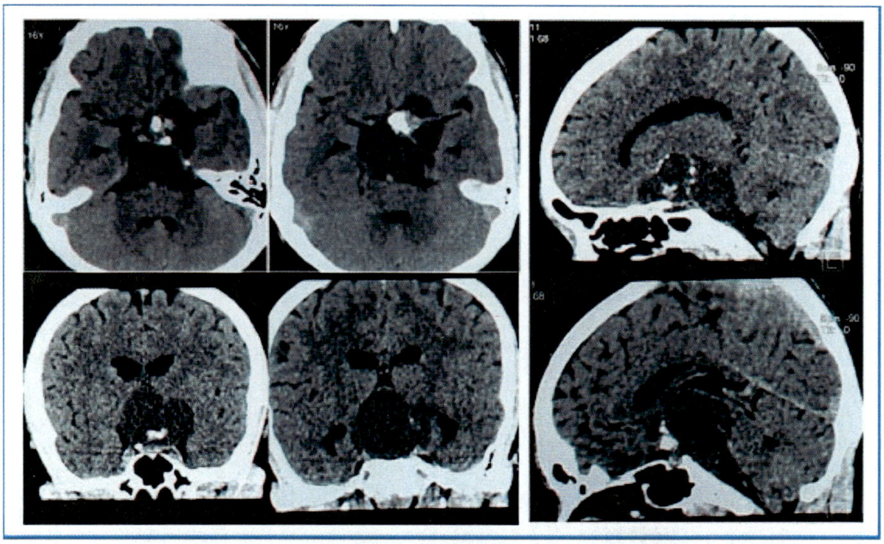

Fig. (7). Preoperative CT scans demonstrated a large retra-clivus extraventricular CP of a 16-year-old boy. The tumor has coarse calcification at the suprasellar cistern.

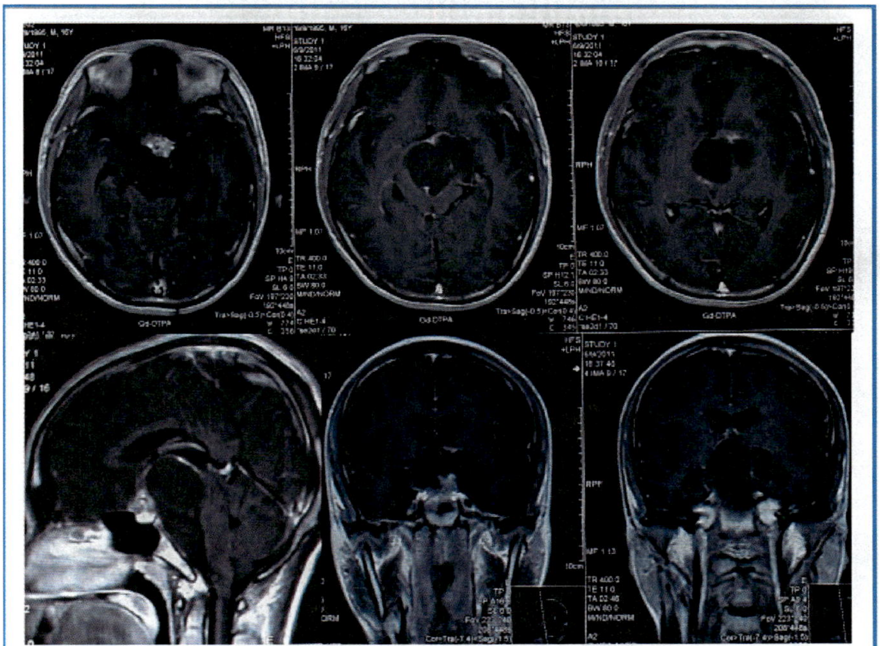

Fig. (8). Preoperative MRIs of the same patient as Fig. (7) showed the detailed tumor's relationship with surrounding structures. The solid tumor part at the suprasellar region with its cystic portion compressed the third ventricle floor significantly.

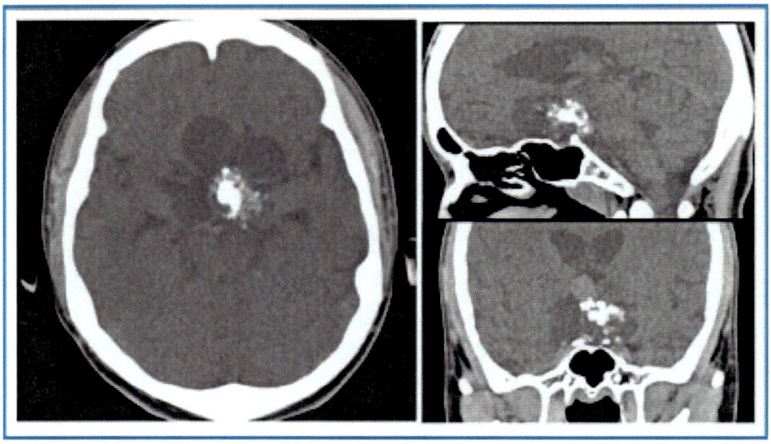

Fig. (9). The patient underwent a subtotal resection of the tumor at the local hospital and his clinical symptoms (visual disturbances and headache) released markedly. And gave replacement therapy for his hypopituitarism. However, after 3 years follow up, the tumor recurred, CT scans obtained before the second operation showed a massive calcification and enlarged lobulated cysts.

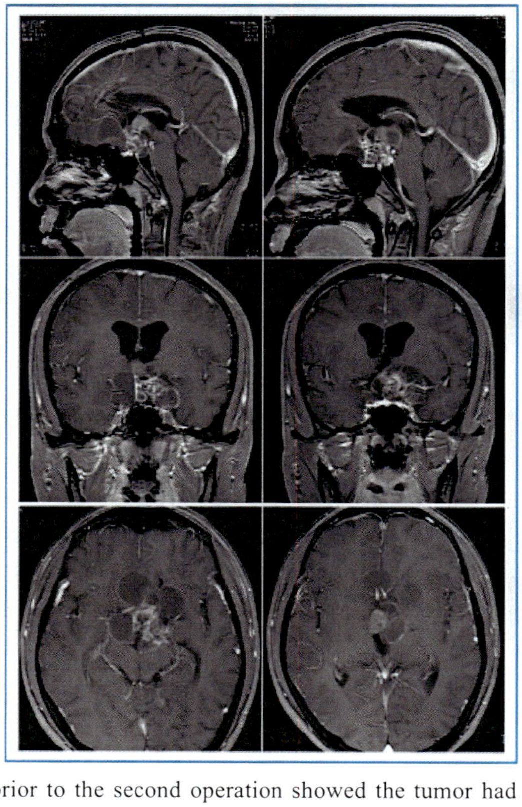

Fig. (10). MR image in prior to the second operation showed the tumor had frank invasion to the third ventricle walls.

NEUROIMAGING OF SUBARACHNOID CPS

On computed tomography (CT) scans, subarachnoid CP is always visible as a mixed-density area in the suprasellar cistern with a low-density cystic extension inside the subarachnoid cistern. In a few cases, huge calcifications occurred at the proximal and infundibular segment of the PS Fig. (**11**), which would present a great surgical challenge. MRI can more clearly reveal the tumor and surrounding involved structures. A multilobular shape is strongly characteristic of tumors of the subarachnoid cistern, in significant contrast to the tubero-infundibular CPs with 3rd VF involvement. Because of the external ventricular growth, hydrocephalus is rarely observed with this type of tumor, except in cases involving huge tumors.

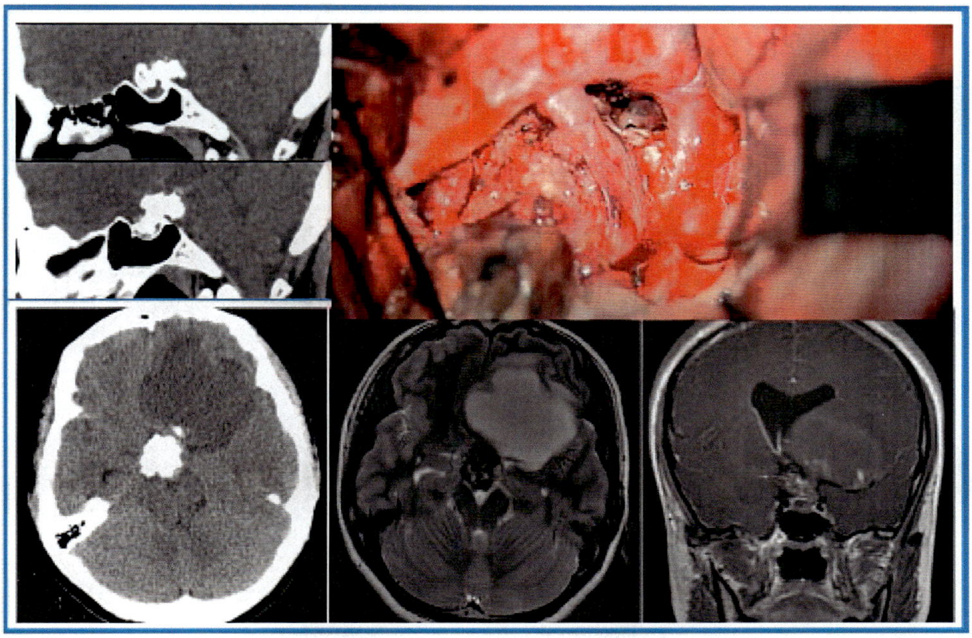

Fig. (11). Preoperative MR, CT images, and intraoperative picture showed the huge calcification encountered in a 30-year-old man. Such a massive calcification hinder from radical removal at surgery.

CLINICAL PRESENTATION OF SUBARACHNOID CPS

The clinical manifestation of subarachnoid CP is closely related to the location of tumor involvement; however, common symptoms of CP such as endocrinological disorders and visual dysfunction are present. If the tumor extends forward to compress the optic chiasm, visual defects might occur, whereas further extension to the anterior cranial fossa might cause olfactory dysfunction. Involvement of the frontotemporal lobe might cause conditions such as mental disorders and epilepsy. Moreover, if the tumor extends toward the posterior cranial fossa, gait disturbances, cranial nerve dysfunction, and physical balance disturbances might manifest. Huge tumors might also cause high intracranial pressure and related symptoms.

SURGICAL CONSIDERATION

The surgical management of subarachnoid CPs has rarely been addressed specifically, likely because these tumors are more accessible than intra-3rd VF tumors. Despite being considered the most resectable tumors, subarachnoid CPs present a neurosurgical challenge because of their various directions of expansion around the PS, as well as the patient's high expectations. Unlike 3rd VF tumors, in which the tumor's internal invagination along hypothalamic structures may impede radical surgery, radical tumor removal is the gold-standard treatment for subarachnoid CP. As the likelihood of total removal is much lower and the complication rate higher during a second operation than during the first operation, the objective of surgical treatment in all cases should be GTR during the first operation.

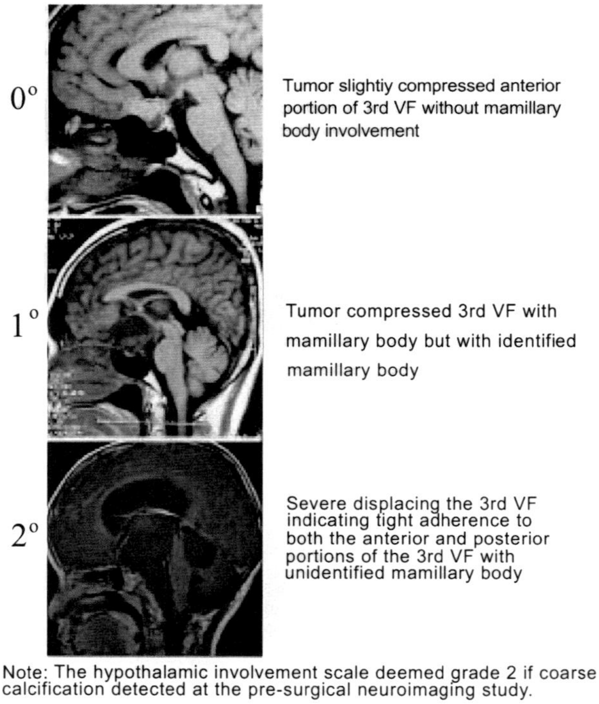

Fig. (12). (Reference from Jun Pan,Songtao Qi et al., Growth patterns of craniopharyngiomas: clinical analysis of 226 patients. Journal of Neurosurgery Pediatrics, 2015:1-16). The degree scores for evaluating the degree of involvement of subarachnoid CP.

SURGICAL DIFFICULTY DEGRADING

Suprasellar subarachnoid CPs can induce various degrees of 3rd VF and hypothalamic involvement. The reason for this variability is mainly the different sites of tumor origin and the relative location of the tumor to the surrounding pituitary sleeve [5]. We proposed a degree of surgical difficulty according to the topographic relationship of the tumor with the arachnoid. This degree was also based on surgical considerations and related to the operative strategy and challenges. Fig. (**12**) and Table **1** showed the degree scores for evaluating the degree of involvement of subarachnoid CP with respect to the hypothalamus in the 226 cases in our personal surgical experience. Notably, when huge calcifications existed at the site of tumor origin, the difficulty score would increase. Our opinion is that the retrostalk type of tumor is associated with more severe hypothalamic involvement than the prestalk type.

Table 1. Criteria of Hypothalamic Involvement Scale based on tumor's growth pattern.

	Grade 0	**Grade 1**	**Grade 2**
Infra-dia CPs	Tumor confined to the intra-sellar space, no hypothalamic involvement; or tumor compressed anterior portion of 3rd VF	The tumor abuting or displacing both the anterior and posterior portions of the hypothalamus	The tumor extremely compressed 3rd VF causing unidentified mamillary body or tumor expanded along the PS involving into the hypothalamus
Supra-sellar cisternal CPs	Tumor slightly compressed anterior portion of 3rd VF without mamillary body involvement	Tumor compressed 3rd VF with mamillary body	Severe displacing the 3rd VF with unidentified mamillary body

SURGICAL APPROACH SELECTION

The prestalk type of subarachnoid CP always grows around the PS. Accordingly, the frontotemporal approach (including pterional, lateral frontal, and subfrontal approaches) could provide sufficient exposure for this type of tumor. During surgery, the pterional bone flap can be extended toward the frontal or temporal bone according to the tumor involvement field. Recently, the extended endoscopic trans-sphenoid approach has been widely used, as this technique allows access to the ventral aspect of the optical chiasm and anterior space of the PS [6]. Surgical manipulation of the subarachnoid CP at the ventral aspect might reduce retraction of the optical chiasm. The disadvantage is a small space for manipulation, which might affect both total tumor removal and PS protection. However, with the rapid development of endoscopic techniques, this approach represents an important research field. For most retrostalk-type cases, we usually use the frontotemporal trans-tentorium approach, as dissection and opening of the tentorium can significantly increase exposure to the CP in the posterior cranial fossa. Other retrostalk-type tumors have been treated *via* the subtemporal and Kawase approaches [7 - 10].

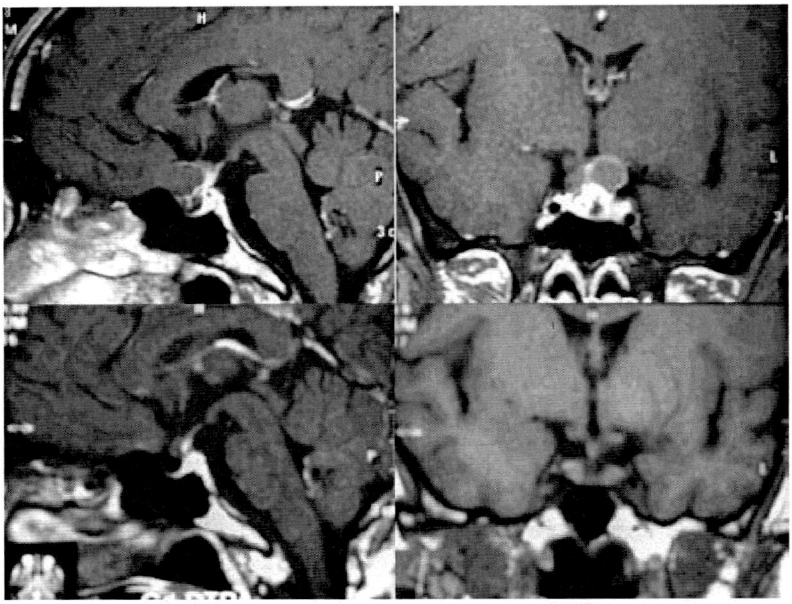

Fig. (13). Sagittal and coronal T1-weighted MRIs before (upper row) and after (lower row) surgery in a 27-year-old women demonstrating the typical growth pattern of supra-sellar subarachnoid cisternal craniopharyngioma. Tumor can be dissected along its own arachnoid dissecting plane from the chiasm, third ventricle floor with preserving the hypothalamic pituitary stalk tract intact. The pituitary function of this patient recovered entirely with resume of the menstrual cycle.

SURGICAL TECHNIQUES

Tumor dissection should proceed strictly along the arachnoid interface. Except for the site of origin at the PS and 3rd VF, it was easy to separate the tumor and suprasellar neurovascular structures, including the circle of Willis arteries, optic chiasm, and oculomotor nerves. In significant contrast to 3rd VF CPs with severe tubero-infundibulum involvement, which might sacrifice PS continuity to ensure tumor total removal, surgery for subarachnoid CP has two key considerations with respect to tumor removal: 1) Attempt to protect continuity to avoid severe injuries to pituitary function injury that would influence the patient's quality of life. Because the tumor originates from the proximal segment of the PS, stalk injury is inevitable during dissection. However, protection of the longitudinal stalk fibers would provide a morphological foundation for the recovery of hypophyseal function during the follow-up period (Fig. **13**). 2) The arterial branches in the PS and optic chiasm should be protected to the extent possible. Blood is usually supplied to subarachnoid CPs *via* the bilateral superior hypophyseal artery, which is also the main supplying artery to the PS and ventral aspect of chiasm. Excessive coagulation might affect the blood supply to the PS and optic chiasm and induce corresponding injuries and symptoms.

Compared with surgery for prestalk CP, there are more challenges associated with surgery for retrostalk CPs with excessive extension at the subarachnoid cistern. First, the site of origin is located at the posterior aspect of the PS and tubero-infundibulum, which is difficult to expose during surgery. Second, because of the excessive extension, severe enveloping and adherence always occur between the tumor cyst and cranial nerves as well as posterior vascular circulation, which might present a significant surgical challenge. The surgical approach must be changed according to the extension area; for this reason, some publications have reported the use of the subtemporal, Kawase, and even Poppen approaches. The key point of these techniques is strict dissection following the arachnoid interface. Theoretically, in cases with posterior and downward extension, Liliequist's membrane forms an interface between the tumor and posterior neurovascular structures. However, because of the extreme compression of the arachnoid membrane, the tumor cyst might envelope these vital structures, resulting in a situation requiring extremely patient dissection. On the other hand, the huge cystic cavity associated with this type of tumor provides an extremely large space for surgical manipulation. Occasionally, the pterional approach with tentorial incision can expose the entire posterior cranial fossa and even the upper cervical area. As described above, at the site of origin, this type of tumor may tightly adhere to the tubero-infundibulum and 3rd VF under the pia mater, which must be dissected sharply. Regarding whether PS continuity preservation can significantly influence endocrinological function, continuity maintenance was determined to be quite important (See typical Sa-CP cases 3).

PROGNOSIS

As hypothalamus–infundibulum–PS continuity can be preserved in most cases of subarachnoid CP, the prognosis of this type of tumor is always good. As summarized the long-term follow-up results from our 47 cases, most patients experienced a long survival, with 5- and 10-year progression-free survival (PFS) of 89.4% and 81.4% respectively, and a 10-year overall survival rate of 94.7%. Within the follow-up period, most patients developed hypopituitarism; however, panhypopituitarism was observed only in 16% of cases, a significantly lower rate than that observed for patients with infradiaphragmatic and tubero-infundibular tumors. Notably, the incidence of cranial nerve injury-related symptoms was higher, at a rate of approximately 30% [11, 12]. However, a statistical analysis of

PFS among patients with and without PS preservation did not identify any significant statistical differences. The results indicated that the growth pattern of the tumor itself might determine whether the PS can be preserved or not. Another noteworthy point was that severe involvement of the 3rd VF and hypothalamus always occurred with recurrences of this type of tumor, especially if GTR was attempted during the primary surgery. This finding might be explained by destruction of the arachnoid membrane around the 3rd VF during primary surgery, which could have facilitated tumor involvement in these structures.

CONFLICT OF INTEREST

The author (editor) declares no conflict of interest, financial or otherwise.

ACKNOWLEDGEMENT

Declared none.

REFERENCES

[1] Steno J, Malácek M, Bízik I. Tumor-third ventricular relationships in supradiaphragmatic craniopharyngiomas: correlation of morphological, magnetic resonance imaging, and operative findings. Neurosurgery 2004; 54(5): 1051-8.
[http://dx.doi.org/10.1227/01.NEU.0000120421.11171.61] [PMID: 15113458]

[2] Van Effenterre R, Boch AL. Craniopharyngioma in adults and children: a study of 122 surgical cases. J Neurosurg 2002; 97(1): 3-11.
[http://dx.doi.org/10.3171/jns.2002.97.1.0003] [PMID: 12134929]

[3] Yaşargil MG, Curcic M, Kis M, Siegenthaler G, Teddy PJ, Roth P. Total removal of craniopharyngiomas. Approaches and long-term results in 144 patients. J Neurosurg 1990; 73(1): 3-11.
[http://dx.doi.org/10.3171/jns.1990.73.1.0003] [PMID: 2352020]

[4] Hoffman HJ. Surgical management of craniopharyngioma. Pediatr Neurosurg 1994; 21 (Suppl. 1): 44-9.
[http://dx.doi.org/10.1159/000120861] [PMID: 7530990]

[5] Qi S, Lu Y, Pan J, Zhang X, Long H, Fan J. Anatomic relations of the arachnoidea around the pituitary stalk: relevance for surgical removal of craniopharyngiomas. Acta Neurochir (Wien) 2011; 153(4): 785-96.
[http://dx.doi.org/10.1007/s00701-010-0940-y] [PMID: 21271263]

[6] Kassam AB, Gardner PA, Snyderman CH, Carrau RL, Mintz AH, Prevedello DM. Expanded endonasal approach, a fully endoscopic transnasal approach for the resection of midline suprasellar craniopharyngiomas: a new classification based on the infundibulum. J Neurosurg 2008; 108(4): 715-28.
[http://dx.doi.org/10.3171/JNS/2008/108/4/0715] [PMID: 18377251]

[7] Al-Mefty O, Ayoubi S, Kadri PA. The petrosal approach for the total removal of giant retrochiasmatic craniopharyngiomas in children. J Neurosurg 2007; 106(2) (Suppl.): 87-92.
[PMID: 17330531]

[8] Klimo P Jr, Browd SR, Pravdenkova S, Couldwell WT, Walker ML, Al-Mefty O. The posterior petrosal approach: technique and applications in pediatric neurosurgery. J Neurosurg Pediatr 2009; 4(4): 353-62.
[http://dx.doi.org/10.3171/2009.4.PEDS08426] [PMID: 19795967]

[9] Kiran NA, Suri A, Kasliwal MK, Garg A, Ahmad FU, Mahapatra AK. Gross total excision of pediatric giant cystic craniopharyngioma with huge retroclival extension to the level of foramen magnum by anterior trans petrous approach: report of two cases and review of literature. Childs Nerv Syst 2008; 24(3): 385-91.
[http://dx.doi.org/10.1007/s00381-007-0522-3] [PMID: 18034348]

[10] Hakuba A, Nishimura S, Inoue Y. Transpetrosal-transtentorial approach and its application in the therapy of retrochiasmatic craniopharyngiomas. Surg Neurol 1985; 24(4): 405-15.
[http://dx.doi.org/10.1016/0090-3019(85)90300-3] [PMID: 4035550]

[11] Connolly ES Jr, Winfree CJ, Carmel PW. Giant posterior fossa cystic craniopharyngiomas presenting with hearing loss. Report of three cases and review of the literature. Surg Neurol 1997; 47(3): 291-9.
[http://dx.doi.org/10.1016/S0090-3019(96)00253-4] [PMID: 9068702]

[12] Bashir EM, Lewis PD, Edwards MR. Posterior fast craniopharyngioma. Br J Neurosurg 1996; 10(6): 613-5.
[http://dx.doi.org/10.1080/02688699646970] [PMID: 9115662]

CHAPTER 12

Suprasellar Infundibulo-Tuberal Craniopharyngioma (Type "T")

Jun Pan*

Department of Neurosurgery, Nanfang Neurosurgery Research Institution, Nanfang Hospital, Southern Medical University, 1838 North Guangzhou Avenue, Guangzhou, China

Abstract: Suprasellar infundibulo-tuberal craniopharyngiomas "Type T" were the most important and difficult tumors with all types of CP, which also the most common type. In this chapter, we focused on the clinical manifestation, growth pattern and prognosis of this type of CP. With summarizing our data and previous literatures review, the advantage of frontobasal interhemispheric approach was depicted emphasizedly. Moreover, by analysis of the relationship between tumor and the third ventricular walls, the defect and merit of transnasal and transcranial approach were discussed as well. Finally, the injury of hypothalamic structures and the psychological evaluation were depicted.

Keywords: Craniopharyngioma, Infundibulum, Suprasellar, Third ventricular floor.

Craniopharyngioma (CP) may involve third ventricular floor (3rd VF) structures. Several terms, such as "retrochiasmatic ventricular CP", "intraventricular CP", or "intra-extraventricular CP", have been used to depict such tumors in previous literature reports [1]. However, some authors have used inaccurate terms such as hypothalamic CP and infundibulum CP. Therefore, a precise definition of this type of CP remained uncertain [2]. Since first discovering CP, some neurosurgeons have been aware that CP always adheres closely to neural tissues at the anterior part of the third ventricle, infundibulum, and tuberalis. These adhesions may be quite strong, rendering it difficult to identify the tumor cystic wall and neural tissue of the 3rd VF [3, 4]. However, the autopsy and intraoperative observations described in several publications [5, 6] there indicated the existence of a safe interface for separation of the tumor from neural tissue. In some places, though, sections of tumor seemed to replace the tuberalis neural

* **Corresponding author Jun Pan:** Department of Neurosurgery, Nanfang Neurosurgery Research Institution, Nanfang Hospital, Southern Medical University, 1838 North Guangzhou Avenue, Guangzhou, China; Tel\Fax: +8620-61641806; E-mail: panjundu@hotmail.com

Songtao Qi (Ed.)

tissue either partly or totally [2, 7]. Radical surgery can also cause injury to the anterior part of the 3rd VF. A diverse range of relationships exists between the tumor and 3rd VF. Accordingly, controversies still surround attempts to classify the above-described tumors into a single type. In this chapter, we summarize the main body of knowledge regarding CPs embedded within the neural tissues of the third ventricular walls and occupying the third ventricular cavity. CPs with the above-mentioned morphological features are classified together for analysis and discussion. The term "infundibulo-tuberal CP" is used to differentiate subarachnoid tumors located within cisterns. For subarachnoid intracistern CPs, an absolute extra-axial approach through the suprasellar cisterns is used for tumor removal. The site of stem-like adherence to neural tissue occurs at the infundibulum of the 3rd VF. However, as depicted in this chapter, the surgical strategy and techniques used to treat infundibulo-tuberal CPs are extremely different.

CPs involving the third ventricle includes lesions that present the utmost difficulty with respect to complete surgical excision because of their intimate anatomical and functional relationships with the hypothalamus. However, larger controversies regarding topography exist. Additionally, the controversy regarding radical gross total tumor removal (GTR) or safe hypothalamic-sparing surgery with radiotherapy also focused on this type of tumor [8, 9]. In this chapter, infundibulo-tuberal CP will be discussed in the context of the tumor's topographical features, relationship between the tumor and 3rd VF, surgical approach selection, and inoperative techniques.

DEFINITION OF "INFUNDIBULO-TUBER CP"

Since the earliest reports, the vague definition of a suprasellar position has been used for CPs to affirm the presumed extraparenchymatous development of these lesions, either from epithelial remnants of the craniopharyngeal duct or, alternatively, from the metaplastic transformation of glandular, adenohypophyseal cells along the pituitary gland stalk (PS) Fig. (**1**) [5]. An accurate description of lesion topography of the lesion is lacking in most articles from the pre-magnetic resonance imaging (MRI) era. In fact, a large percentage of CPs occupy the hypothalamic area at the time of diagnosis, in which three structures are specifically affected by the tumor: the infundibulum, 3rd VF (tuber cinereum), and third ventricle walls (including the fornices and lamina terminalis).

As described above, CPs that involve the 3rd VF and hypothalamus were previously always reported as "intraventricular CPs". This terminology was selected because of the tumor's relationship with the third ventricle in radiological images. This name was easily understood and appeared to reflect the tumor's anatomical location, and therefore was accepted widely. However, some scholars have always questioned the proposed name "intraventricular CPs". As reported by some publications, autopsies of patients with early-stage disease who had not undergone surgery proved that this type of CP replaces part of the neural tissue layer of the 3rd VF. This tumor involvement with and destruction of the hypothalamus might be the major cause of death. Moreover, many scholars have questioned whether an "intraventricular CP" entirely located within the third ventricular cavity actually existed. Pascual *et al.* [10, 11] analyzed previous publications regarding CPs with involvement of the 3rd VF and hypothalamus and subdivided the CPs into two types: strictly intraventricular and not-strictly intraventricular CPs. Pascual *et al.* thought that strictly intraventricular was the purely intraventricular CP type reported in papers; these were rare and occurred frequently among the squamous papillary tumor type. However, a majority of tumors grew around the infundibulo-tuberal center inside the neural tissue of the 3rd VF. The authors defined this type of tumor as "non-strictly intraventricular CP".

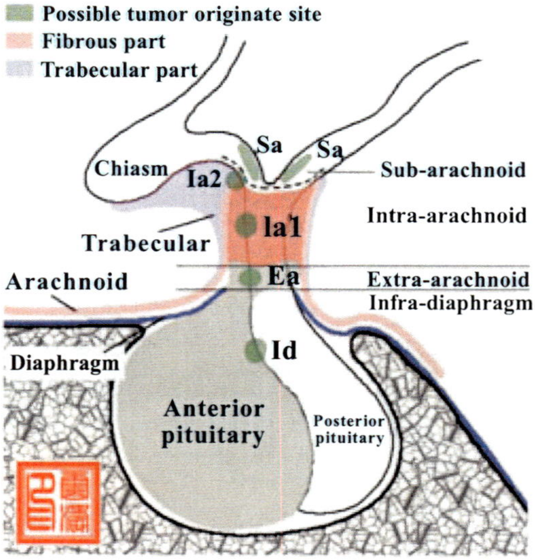

Fig. (1). (Reference from Songtao Qi *et al.*, Anatomic relations of the arachnoidea around the pituitary stalk: relevance for surgical removal of craniopharyngiomas. Acta Neurochir (Wien), 2011.). Schematic drawing of pituitary gland and surrounding arachnoid.

Recently, Qi *et al.* [12] summarized the morphological features of IVC based on their experience with 17 cases of CPs that met the diagnostic criteria of IVC. The authors concluded that intraventricular tumors—even those classed as "strictly IVC" and located purely within the cavity without ependymal or neural tissue covering—still have a pedicle stem closely attached to the 3rd VF. The terms "strictly" or "non-strictly" IVC do not indicate the true growth patterns of CPs located exclusively within the third ventricle cavity, as depicted in previous reports [10, 11]. All IVCs, whether "strictly" or "non-strictly", had a similar site of origin, and the variation observed was the result of differential growth and variable patterns of invasion into surrounding structures. More recently, Pascual *et al.* [10] provided several clinical, neuroradiological, pathological, and surgical evidences and verified the infundibulo-tuberal topography of CPs. Pascual *et al.* thought that an accurate subdivision for this type of tumor, with similar sites of origin but different growth patterns, was meaningful and necessary to prevent any undue injury to vital diencephalon centers. Although the term "infundibulo-tuberal CPs" reflected the tumors' true origination, the flawed nature of this term remained obvious. For example, CPs that originate from the infundibulum might expand downwards to the suprasellar cistern, with the existing connection to neural tissue at the tumoral stem on the infundibular part Fig. (**2**).

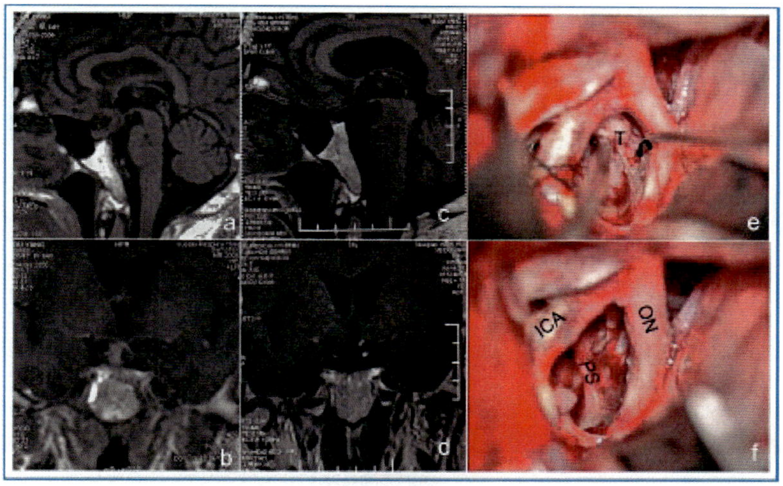

Fig. (2). Pre-, and post-operative MR imaging and intra-operative pictures in a 64-year old man with a subarachnoid cisternal craniopharyngioma. Tumor mainly expand downwards to the suprasellar cistern (left column), the connection with neural tissue exists at the tumoral stem on infundibular part (arrowhead in Fig. (**b**). Post-operative MR image demonstrated total removal of the tumor with a relatively intact third ventricle floor (middle column). Intra-operative Fig. (s showed the tumor-3rd VF relationship (right column). The tumor tightly adhered to the 3rd VF where also thought to be the site of tumor origin (curved arrow in e). The tumor was totally removed with preservation of the pituitary stalk (f). **Abbreviations:** 3rd VF: third ventricle floor; ICA: internal carotid artery; ON: optic nerve; PS: pituitary stalk; T:tumor.

Regarding strictly IVC tumors, this tumor type (which develops mainly in the extraventricular space) shares a common site of origin with infundibulo-tuberal CPs. Therefore, in some cases it is difficult to clearly distinguish infundibulo-tuberal CP and suprasellar cisternal CP. Despite possible defects in the terminology, this classification was beneficial for understanding the relationship between the tumor and third ventricular walls and also for determining the surgical therapeutic strategy. In summary, infundibulo-tuberal CP represents a subtype of tumors with primary subpial development within the 3rd VF.

As depicted in the recent literature, the radiological and surgical evidence for infundibulo-tuberal CPs includes the following: 1) third ventricle involvement by tumors in radiological images. The distal segment of the PS and pituitary gland were not involved. In most cases, a significant downward 3rd VF and patent suprasellar cistern around the PS could be identified on coronal MRI images (Fig. **3**). 2) After tumor removal, the morphology of involved 3rd VF recovered normally in some cases. More commonly, however, the anterior part of the 3rd VF retained a defect (GTR) or residual tumor at the infundibulo-tuberal part (partial and subtotal tumor removal). 3) Intra-operatively, the surgeon cannot observe the tumor directly, although the frog belly-like inflated infundibulo-tuberal part is visible. After GTR, the preserved thin 3rd VF can be observed through the lamina terminalis. 4) Based on autopsy results.

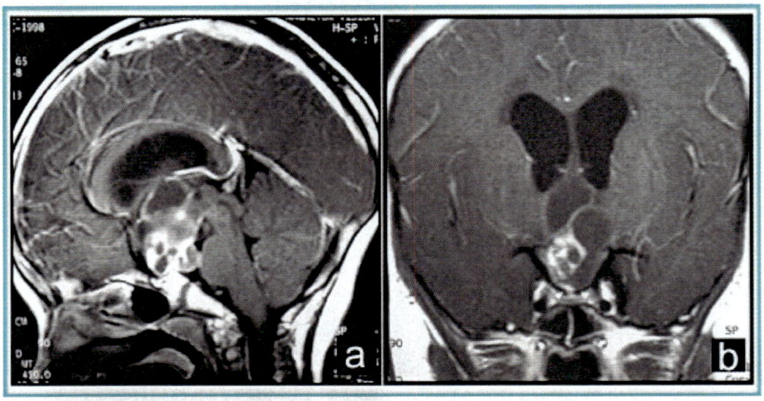

Fig. (3). Sagittal and Coronal contrast-enhanced T1-weighted MRI (**a** and **b**) before surgery in a 3-year-old girl with a typical infundibulo-tuberal CP. Note the significant downwards displacement of 3rd VF and patent suprasellar cistern around the pituitary stalk (white arrow in Fig. (**b**)).

Relationship Between the Tumor and Third Ventricular Floor

The close relationship between the tumor, 3rd VF, and hypothalamus was proven *via* autopsy by the Australian pathologist Erdheim [13]. Using autopsy, several scholars proved that early-stage CPs could replace the neural tissue layer of the 3rd VF at the infundibulo-tuberal part [11]. Through the suprasellar cistern, surgeons can only observe the enlarged and inflated frog belly-like anterior part of the third ventricle Fig. (**4**). This growth pattern is also considered a major reason for the short lifespans of affected patients. The close relationship observed between the tumor and neural tissues of the third ventricular walls challenged traditional ideas about the extra-axial origin of CPs. Moreover, as reviewed by Pascual et al., this variant represents a major topographical category among the enigmatic and complicated growth patterns of CPs, with incidence rates of 42% in the literature and 52% in the authors' own series [2, 10]. As the relationship between an infundibulo-tuberal CP occupying the third ventricle and distorted ventricle boundaries represents a major CP growth pattern, an understanding of this relationship has become of paramount importance. This relationship also directly determines surgical strategies and techniques. In contrast to subdiaphragmatic tumors and some suprasellar extraventricular tumors with upward involvement into the third ventricle and a so-called "pseudo-intraventricular location" (tumors with an apparent third ventricle location that in fact originate from a suprasellar extra-axial position), in the majority cases of infundibulo-tuberal CP, the normal nerve tissues of the third ventricle walls (containing viable hypothalamic tissue) remain in a lower position and attached to the basal tumor pole.

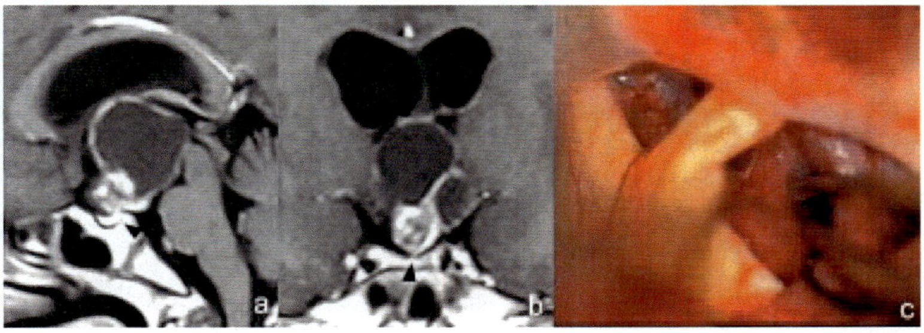

Fig. (4). Sagittal and Coronal contrast-enhanced T1-weighted MRI (a and b) before surgery and intra-operative photo in a 6-year-old girl with a typical infundibulo-tuberal CP. Note the inferiorly compressed pituitary stalk (arrow in Fig. (**a** and **b**)). intra-operative picture showing the enlarged frog-belly-like inflated anterior part of 3rd ventricle (arrow in Fig. (**c**)).

More recent research has proven that these tumors are totally embedded within the neural tissue of the 3rd VF. According to the degree of involvement, there are potentially three different morphological characteristics observed between tumors and third ventricular walls: 1) totally envelopment, in which the upper and lower pole of the tumor are both covered by neural tissue; these tumors usually involve a unilateral ventricular wall (Fig. **5**). 2) Predominant growth toward the third ventricular cavity, with the lower pole of the tumor containing some residual neural tissue of the 3rd VF; CPs with these morphological features have occasionally been described as purely intraventricular CPs in the literature (Fig. **6**). 3) Progressive tumor growth with protrusion out of the neural tissue of the 3rd VF, with ultimate replacement of the 3rd VF by the lesion and subsequent loss of anatomical integrity; as a result, "intra- and extraventricular CPs" are formed. Tumors with invasion to the extra-ventricular region have two significant features: 1) in the majority of cases, the solid tumor and calcification become inflated along the hypothalamic-pituitary axis, causing umbrella-like inflation of the PS and infundibulum (Fig. **7**). 2) The tumor protrudes through the infundibulo-tuberal neural tissue and grows towards the suprasellar arachnoidal cistern (Fig. **8**).

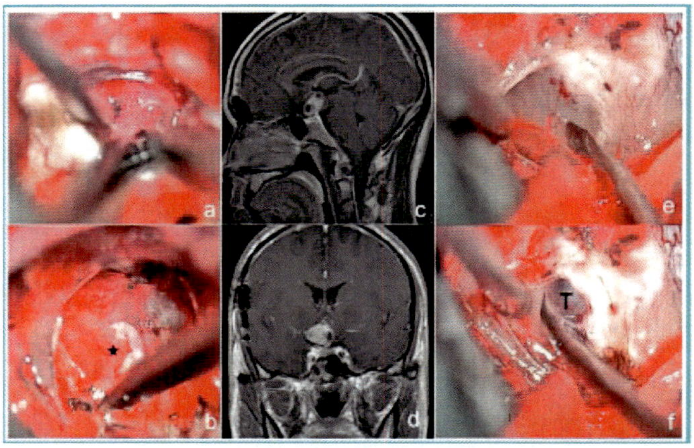

Fig. (5). Sagittal and Coronal contrast-enhanced T1-weighted MRI (**a** and **b**) before surgery in a 29-year-old man with a typical infundibulo-tuberal CP (papillary variant). The tumor located at the anterior portion of the third ventricle, actually embedded within the nerve tissue of right side lateral wall of the third ventricle (**c**, **d**). Intra-operative pictures showing the various aspects of surgery: the pituitary stalk was keep intact and compressed inferior to the tumor (**a**). Opening of the lamina terminalis revealed the bulged nerve tissue of the lateral wall on the right side of the third ventricle (**e**). Tumor (T) was exposed only after the incision of this nerve tissue layer (**f**). The attenuated but uninterrupted 3rd VF after tumor removal (**b**). Note the fold of the 3rd VF (asterisk). The right side lateral wall of the third ventricle was not involved by the tumor.

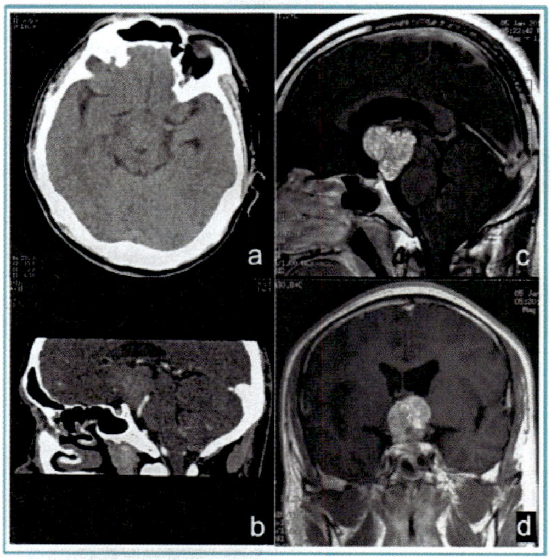

Fig. (6). CT and MR images before surgery in a 46-year-old man with a typical infundibulo-tuberal CP (papillary variant). Axial and sagittal CT scanning revealed a surpasellar solid mass at the surpa-sellar cistern without calcification and cystic formation (**a**,**b**). Sagittal and Coronal contrast-enhanced T1-weighted MRI (**c**,**d**) showed it was a large solid tumor filling up the 3rd ventricular chamber and caused obstructed hydrocephalus.

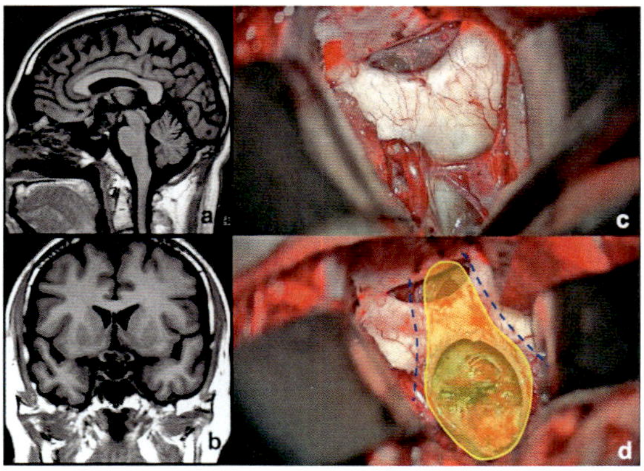

Fig. (7). Preoperative Sagittal and Coronal contrast-enhanced T1-weighted MRI (**a** and **b**) and intra-operative pictures (**c** and **d**) in a 36-year old man with a typical infundibulo-tuberal CP. Tumor mainly expand within the floor of the third ventricle (right column), globe extension of tumor caused universal expansion of the infundibulum and the cisternal course of the pituitary stalk which was outlined in Fig. (**d**) (semitransparent yellow area, dotted blue line indicated the tumor boundary before tumor remove).

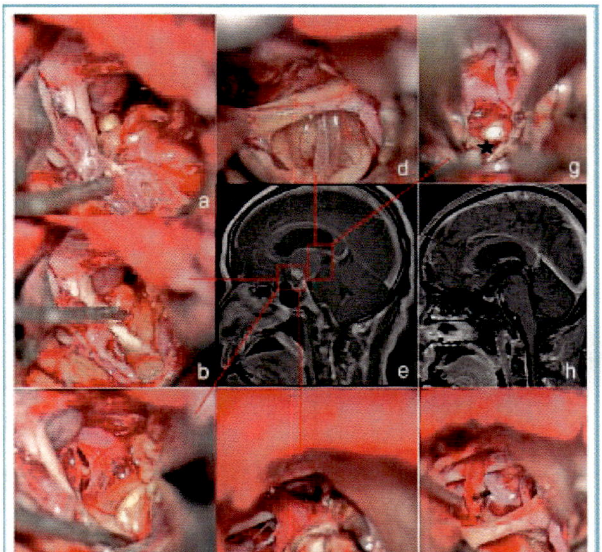

Fig. (8). Pre-and post-operative MRI and intra-operative photos in a 58-year-old man with a typical infundibulo-tuberal CP. Pre-operative sagittal contrast-enhanced T1-weighted MRI showed a lobulated cystic-solid mass at the supra-sellar region (**e**). Intra-operative pictures revealed the growth pattern of the tumor. Being originated from infundibulo-tuberal part of the 3rd VF, the tumor located partially outside and partially inside of the third ventricle cavity. The extra-ventricular part of tumor has arachnoid interface to the chiasm and AcoA (**a**,**b**). The posterosuperior tumor cyst invaginated into the gray matter (tuber cinereum, asterisk in Fig. (**g**) of the floor of the third ventricle (**d**). Note a flying saucer-shaped expansion of tumor through the infundibulo-tuberal region of the 3rd VF (**c**). The involvement pattern of the pituitary stalk was showing in Fig. (**f**). Post-operative sagittal contrast-enhanced T1-weighted MRI (**h**) and intra-operative picture (**i**) showed total removal of the tumor.

DEMOGRAPHIC INCIDENCE

Although the definition of "infundibulo-tuberal CPs" was recently proposed (Infundibulo-tuberal or not strictly intraventricular craniopharyngioma: evidence for a major topographical category *Pascual, Ruth Prieto, Rodrigo Carrasco*), the incidence of such tumors among the total CP population was unknown. Pascual *et al.* respectively analyzed the published literature regarding CP. These authors selected 67 groups and a total of 3571 cases of CPs with complete clinical data. Among these, infundibulo-tuberal CPs accounted for 1494 cases or 42%, including 122 cases that had been proven *via* autopsies of dead patients who had not received surgical treatment. The above evidence eloquently proves that infundibulo-tuberal CP is the major type of CP. We analyzed 226 cases of CP treated *via* primary surgery at our hospital (unpublished data), among which 118 cases (52.2%) met the diagnostic criteria of infundibulo-tuberal CP. The patient age of onset was also not confirmed in the current series. As in most publications, there were no special morphological classifications; additionally, more publications have focused on pediatric patients, and we therefore could not reach an objective conclusion about the different incidence rates among children and adults. However, we remained able to find much useful information in the literature. In general, the incidence of infundibulo-tuberal CP among adults was slightly higher than that among children. Qi *et al.* statistically analyzed 195 cases of primary CPs; among these cases, the infundibular type accounted for 104 cases, including 38 pediatric (47%) and 66 adult cases (58%). The major explanations for the predominance of infundibular CP among adult patients are as follows: 1) infradiaphragmatic CP (Id-CP) predominantly occurs in children [14] and accounts for nearly half of all pediatric cases. On the other hand, Id-CP is rare in adults; and 2) the significant features of third ventricle involvement and squamous papillary CP (SPCP) occurred almost exclusively in adults [15 - 18]. Tumors with these features increased the incidence of infundibulo-tuberal CP among adults. Therefore, this type of CP was the most important tumor type both in adults and children, regardless of other factors.

CLNICAL MANIFESTATION

Similar to previous reports, patients with infundibulo-tuberal CP most frequently present with headaches, nausea/vomiting, visual disturbances, growth failure (in children), and hypogonadism (in adults). Compared with suprasellar extra-ventricular or Id-CP, symptoms such as headache and nausea/vomiting, which reflect a high intracranial pressure (ICP), occur more frequently with infundibulo-tuberal CPs, a finding that might be attributable to tumor-induced hydrocephalus. However, symptoms related to the optical pathway are less frequent.

Regarding pediatric Id-CP and infundibulo-tuberal CP, the hypothalamo-pituitary function at presentation is severely compromised in both topographic variants. However, significant differences in the details remain. In pediatric Id-CP, hypopituitarism is the major clinical manifestation. Significant differences between the two tumor types are evident when evaluating the hypophyseal functional disorder scores [19]. In contrast, hypothalamic disorders cause weight gain, fat or emaciation, and behavioral disturbances more less frequently in Id-CP. The above-mentioned hypothalamic symptoms, if present, appear in almost all cases of infundibulo-tuberal CP before surgery. Interestingly, diabetes insipidus (DI), which represents injury to the posterior lobe of the pituitary gland, occurs more frequently at presentation with Id-CP than with infundibulo-tuberal CP, although there have been no reported statistically significant differences in postsurgical incidence between the two types. The incidence rates of other symptoms such as epilepsy, cranial nerve function, and other rare symptoms also do not significantly differ between the two tumor types.

Compared to extraventricular CPs, mental disturbances (40%), memory dysfunction (33.3%), and somnolence occur more frequently in adults with infundibulo-tuberal CPs; endocrinological function disorder is an exception to this pattern. It should be noted that clinical manifestation data should be interpreted cautiously because they have been extracted from retrospective studies and are not based on specific systematic questionnaires, but rather represent information documented in patients' medical records.

NEUROIMAGING

Currently, useful tools for the neuroradiological characterization of CP include plain skull x-rays, computed tomography (CT), MRI and, occasionally, cerebral angiography. Although plain skull X-ray is rarely used, it remains valuable for observing calcification and sphenoidal bone structures. CT scans are also quite useful for evaluating bone structural changes and calcification. Meanwhile, these scans are also meaningful for diagnosing cystic tumors and hydrocephalus. The calcification shape in infundibulo-tuberal CP is likely piecemeal or coarse. Normally, on CT scans calcification is located inside the suprasellar cisterns. The exact location is at the site of origin around the infundibulo-tuberal part. Calcification can expand along the longitudinal axis of the PS, thus indicating the direction of tumor growth Fig. (**9**). These signs are also useful when determining the surgical strategy. More often, calcification covers the cystic wall in a piecemeal manner. However, in infundibulo-tuberal CPs, eggshell-like calcification is rarely observed, although it is frequently present in Id-CPs. SPCPs are normally solid and predominantly without calcification Fig. (**10**). MRI scans can clearly show the anatomical location of the tumor and its relationships with surrounding structures and accordingly comprise the most important radiological image detection modality.

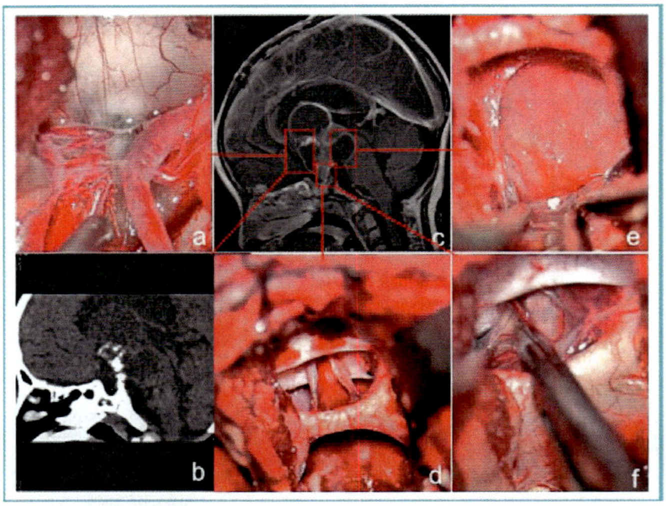

Fig. (9). (Reference from Jun Pan,Songtao Qi *et al.*, Growth patterns of craniopharyngiomas: clinical analysis of 226 patients. Journal of Neurosurgery Pediatrics, 2015:1-16). Pre-operative MRI and intra-operative photos in a 7-year-old boy with a typical infundibulo-tuberal CP. Pre-operative sagittal contrast-enhanced T1-weighted MRI after a flawed surgery through the trans-corpus callosum trans-fornix approach at the local hospital (**c**). The preoperative CT scan showed that the tumor calcification expanded along the longitude axis of pituitary stalk, indicating the involvement of pituitary stalk by tumor (**b**). Intra-operative pictures showing surgical procedure of this patient. The AcoA was divided to enhance the tumor exposure (**a**). After dissecting of the arachnoid enveloping the pituitary stalk, the bulged pituitary stalk was exposed (**f**). Tumor was totally removed by the combination of trans-LT and extra-axial route. The pituitary stalk was vertically split to expose the tumor (**d**). Note the attenuated but uninterrupted 3rd VF after tumor removal (**e**).

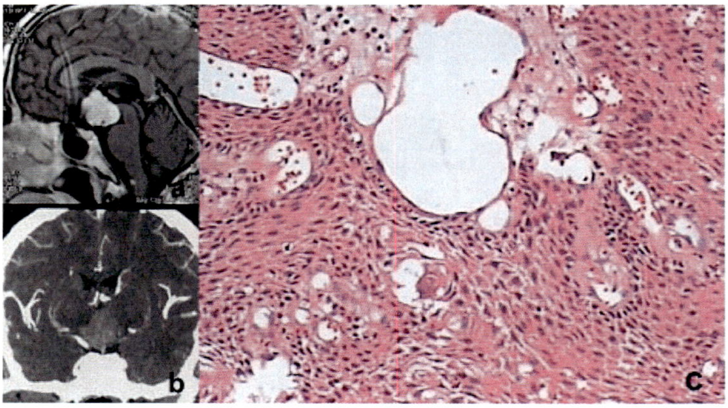

Fig. (10). Pre-operative MRI and CT scan in a 46-year-old nan with a typical Squamous papillary CP. Pre-operative sagittal contrast-enhanced T1-weighted MRI (**a**) showed the tumor was a solid mass with homogeneous enhanced after injection of Gd-DTPA. The preoperative CT scan (**b**) showed that the tumor involved mainly into the third ventricle with a patent spurasellar cistern. Postoperative Pathological study (**c**) demonstrated a typical Squamous papillary CP.

For adamantinomatous CP (ACP), MRI scans of infundibulo-tuberal CPs always reveal a cystic–solid mixed tumor; totally cystic or solid tumors are rare. The tumor parenchyma and/or calcification are always located in the anteroinferior part of the tumor (infundibulo-tuberal part), whereas cysts expand along the neural tissue of the 3rd VF and occupy the third ventricular cavity. Accordingly, a typical tumor is shaped like an upside-down pear Fig. (**11**) with parenchyma and calcification located at the anteroinferior part of the tumor and the cystic cavity at the posterosuperior part. These tumors always grow extensively and cause frog belly-like inflation of the 3rd VF. The distal segmental of the PS is displaced to the anteroinferior part of the tumor. Additionally, some of the tumor might expand beyond the third ventricle. The features of expansion can be summarized into two types: 1) penetration of the pia mater in infundibulo-tuberal part with expansion to the subarachnoid cisterns around pituitary stalk and formation of intra- and extraventricular CPs. In this situation, the tumor always has an irregular and lobular shape (Fig. **8**). 2) Expansion of the infundibular tumor and its calcification along the longitudinal axis of the PS, with possible entry into the intrasellar region along the PS, which might cause dilation of the full-length stalk (Fig. **9**). The predominantly ventricular location of infundibulo-tuberal CP can easily lead to obstructed hydrocephalus as the tumor increases in size.

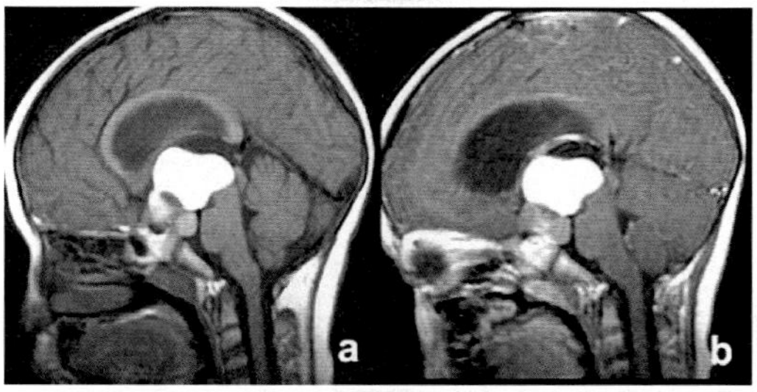

Fig. (11). Sagittal non-contrast (**a**) and contrast-enhanced (**b**) T1-weighted MRI in a 7-year-old girl with a typical infundibulo-tuberal CP. The tumor appeared as an inverted pear-shaped mass with its calcification and solid portions located at the suprasellar infundibulum region, while its cystic part protruded into the third ventricle. The solid part of tumor had an inhomogeneous enhancement after the injection of Gd-DTPA.

Because of tumoral expansion inside the neural tissue of the 3rd VF, most modern MRI scans cannot identify the tumoral cystic wall and neural tissue of the 3rd VF. Although some scholars believe that T2-weighted, heavily T2-weighted, and/or 3D-FIESTA MRI sequences might be useful for differentiating tumors from the neural tissue of the 3rd VF, our opinion is that these identifiable tumors are rare. Such identification is quite difficult for most tumors, especially in cases with tumoral expansion outside of the third ventricular cavity or along the PS.

The growth pattern of SPCP is more uniform than that of ACP. The former type always presents as a solid or predominantly solid tumor. Calcification is rare.

Small tumors are limited to localization at the infundibulo-tuberal part and anterior of the third ventricle (Fig. **12**). However, an enlarged tumor can fill the third ventricular cavity and cause an obstructed hydrocephalus (Fig. **6**). SPCPs always feature a regular and nearly round shape. Features of the third ventricular cavity also limit the tumor shape. SPCP can also undergo cystic changes; however, the cystic shape of these tumors differs considerably from that of ACPs (Fig. **13**).

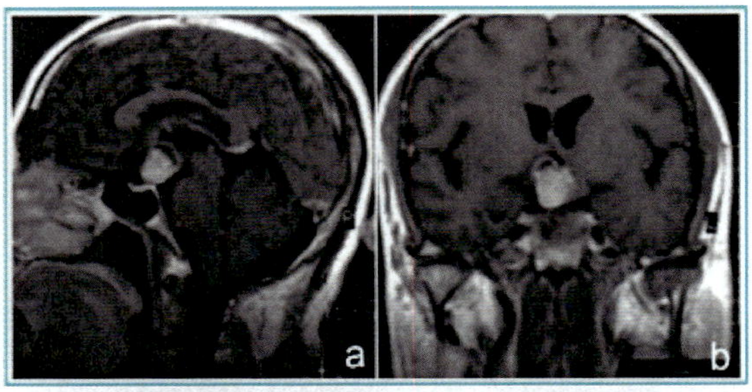

Fig. (12). Sagittal and Coronal contrast-enhanced T1-weighted MRI (**a** and **b**) before surgery in a 42-yea--old man with a typical infundibulo-tuberal CP (papillary variant). The tumor located at the anterior portion of the third ventricle chamber, posterior portion of the third ventricle cavity was unobstructed due to the small size of the tumor.

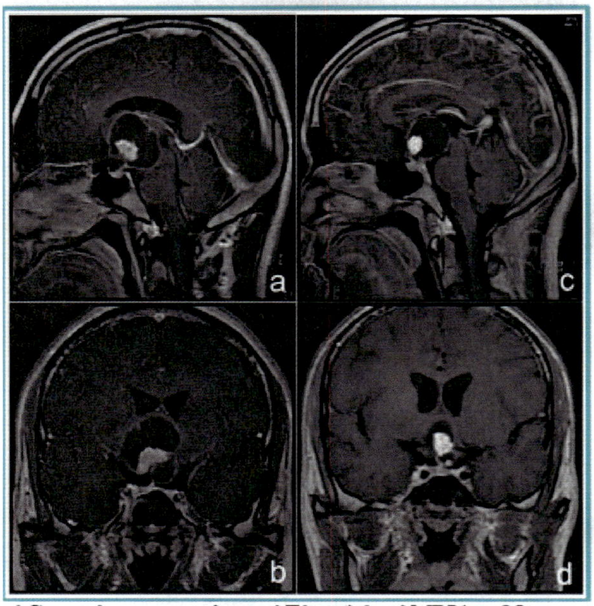

Fig. (13). Pre-operative Sagittal and Coronal contrast-enhanced T1-weighted MRI in a 35-year-old man (left column) and 27-year-old man (right column) demonstrated the typical pattern of cystic formation in Squamous papillary CP with infundibulo-tuberal growth pattern. The solid tumor part locates inside the cystic wall (usually near the infundibular recess) which differed from the lobulated cysts in adamantinomatous variant.

SURGICAL TREATMENT

Overview

Surgical treatment of infundibulo-tuberal CP is a most difficult and important point and is also the area of this field with the greatest controversies. The function of the hypothalamic–infundibular–pituitary axis function is severely damaged. Normally, hypopituitarism caused by adenohypophyseal function injury can be relieved by hormone substitution, which results in the maintenance of a moderate quality of life (QOL). In the literature, although the reported incidence of DI was not high (approximate average = 18%), a majority of cases will be accompanied by postsurgical DI. The above-described endocrinological diseases are constant and may be caused by the CP itself. There is consensus that both are acceptable, whereas severe hypothalamic dysfunction (*e.g.*, obesity, narcolepsy, adipsia, severe behavioral disorders) is not [20]. When determining the surgical strategy, the neurosurgeon will face a dilemma and must attempt to find a balance between GTR to reduce tumor recurrence and subtotal tumor removal to avoid a severe hypothalamic reaction. A great challenge for future studies is the definition of an 'intermediate approach' that uses clear objective criteria to identify the best candidates for a radical *versus* conservative approach.

Evaluation of Surgical Risk

For infundibulo-tuberal tumors, the primary aim of the neurosurgeon should be determination of the degree of tumor involvement in the hypothalamus based on radiological images in order to avoid severe postsurgical hypothalamic injuries induced by intraoperative manipulation. Recently, some scholars have classified subgroups of patients and proposed different treatment strategies according to hypothalamic involvement [20 - 22]. These schemes more suitably account for the gross morphological distortion of the hypothalamus by the CP and the potentially hazardous surgical manipulation of this area. A more tailored surgical strategy for CP management is useful but nevertheless does not provide any clues regarding the actual origin of the lesion nor details of the hypothalamus–CP relationship. Consequently, accurate CP topography and the individual surgical risk associated with radical lesion removal cannot be adequately addressed using these schemes.

In this book, we have morphologically classified CPs according to the site of tumor origin and involved anatomical structures. Id-CP and suprasellar extraventricular CP have been discussed separately. Sainte-Rose *et al.* have subdivided infundibulo-tuberal CPs into two grades according to the degree of hypothalamic involvement. In our clinical practice, further stratification of treatment should be considered in order to focus on this major CP type, and this also proves the graded method to be crude and inapplicable. Presurgical MRI scan-based evaluations of hypothalamic involvement have occasionally been proven incorrect following the morphological recovery of the 3rd VF as determined *via* postsurgical MRI (Fig. **14**). Therefore, it is currently difficult to predict good outcomes based on preoperative imaging features of CPs.

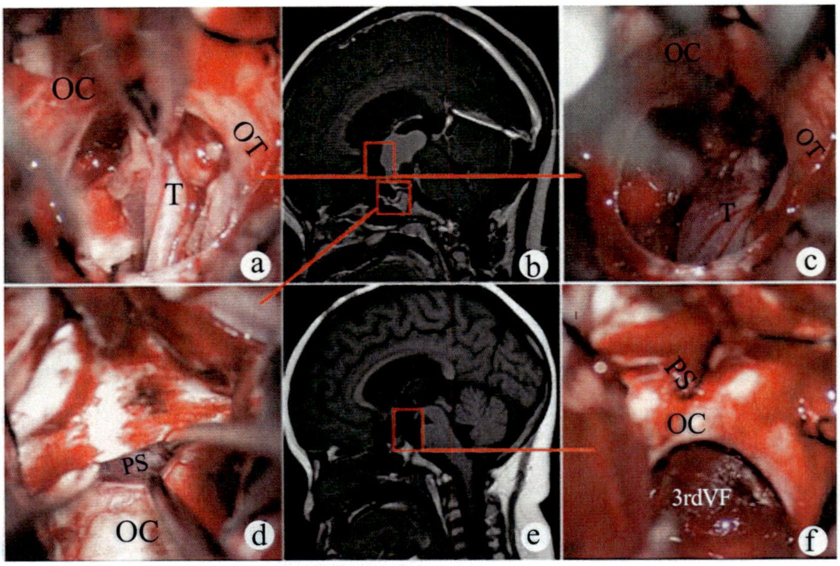

Fig. (14). (Reference from Jun Pan,Songtao Qi *et al.*, Growth patterns of craniopharyngiomas: clinical analysis of 226 patients. Journal of Neurosurgery Pediatrics, 2015:1-16). Pre-, and postoperative MRIs and intra-operative pictures in a 7-year-old boy with a typical infundibulo-tuberal CP. Pre-operative sagittal contrast-enhanced T1-weighted MRI (**b**) showed the tumor had an intimate relationship with the third ventricle (with a involvement grade 2 according to the grading system previously described by Saint-Rose). However, both intraoperative findings and postoperative MR image (**a**,**c**,**d**,**e**,**f**) proved the tinning but intact third ventricle floor with the preservation of the pituitary stalk and infundibulum.

Further evaluation of the resectability of infundibulo-tuberal CPs is needed. Using the grades described by Sainte-Rose et al., several scholars made further classifications based on the presence or absence of a clear interface between the tumor and neural tissue at the posterior part of the 3rd VF. We thought that this classification was meaningful [23]. We summarized a large series of infundibulo-tuberal CP cases with respect to presurgical imaging and intraoperative findings and found the following features to be valuable when assessing the risk of surgically induced hypothalamic injury.

Firstly, based on preoperative neuroimaging: 1) the enlarged PS or calcification with growth along the longitudinal axis of the PS is indicated by MRI or CT scanning, respectively. These signs suggest severe tumor involvement in the infundibulum–pituitary axis; and 2) the residual 3rd VF is identifiable and the tumor is involved in the posterior part of the mammillary body structures.

Secondary, when compared with presurgical MRI scans, we thought that intraoperative findings made by the surgeon were more important. Intraoperative findings supportive of radical removal include the following: 1) after incising the attenuated neural tissue of the 3rd VF *via* the lamina terminalis approach, a clear interface for tumor separation can be identified, especially within the infundibulum recessus at a retrochiasmatic position. 2) When dissecting the tumor, continuity of the hypothalamic–pituitary axis can be partially preserved as predicted. 3) After tumor removal, no or only slight cracked defects are visible in the thin 3rd VF. Among the above three points, a clear dissection plane between the tumor and neural tissue of the third ventricle walls is most important because this clear interface provides a foundation for preserving the 3rd VF and its function. Large defects in the 3rd VF, such as defects at the anterior margin of the mammillary bodies and anterior part of the 3rd VF, discontinuity of the hypothalamic–pituitary axis, and complete exposure of the top of basilar artery (BA) should be avoided if possible during tumor removal. Some authors have thought that postsurgical MRI-detected 3rd VF injury grades correlated positively with hypothalamic obesity during the follow-up period [24, 25]. Postsurgical MRI scans indicated that the 3rd VF injury grade was a predictive factor for the hypothalamic functional status during long-term follow-up. Similar to the grades of presurgical MR-based hypothalamic involvement, an assessment of the degree of injury based on morphological changes on postsurgical images of the 3rd VF might also include some mistakes. For example, 1) after tumor removal, the morphological features of 3rd VF changed insignificantly only in rare cases; in contrast, the 3rd VF in most cases was attenuated by the tumor after radical removal, and this attenuated, distorted 3rd VF could not be truly reflected *via* MRI. 2) CPs have a propensity to recur with an origin from the residual tumor inside the 3rd VF following so-called hypothalamic-spare tumor removal. If left untreated, these recurrences can cause death through their aggressive local behaviors in the critical site of origin. Therefore, continued combined treatments such as resurgery and irradiation remain necessary; however, these treatments will also injure hypothalamic function.

To date, the existence of significant differences in terms of the long-term hypothalamic functional status is widely accepted between patients who have undergone complex treatment regimens (CTrR) comprising multiple subtotal resection surgeries and/or radiotherapy and patients who have undergone only one surgery without radiotherapy. Therefore, the use of multiple treatments is another important predictive factor for hypothalamic dysfunction [26]. After systematic summarization, we propose a four-grade system for evaluating hypothalamic structural injury (Table **1**). Although this grading system is somewhat subjective, as it is based on operational observations, it compensates for the fact that that true degrees of 3rd VF structural injury cannot be reflected by postsurgical MRI because of tumor displacement.

Table 1. Four-grade scoring system for postoperative hypothalamic impairment in infundibulo-tuberal CPs.

Post-op scale	Criteria
Grade I	a thinned intact floor with preservation of infundibulum and stalk
Grade II	a breached floor with a small deficient at the anterior portion of the third ventricle floor with continuity of infundibulum and stalk OR the third ventricle floor occupation with tumor remnants
Grade III	a breached floor with large deficient at the posterior portion of the third ventricle floor with sacrifice of the infundibulum and stalk
Grade IV	wholly deficient (grade V) third ventricle floor with sacrifice of the infundibulum and stalk.

Surgical Approach Selection

Infundibulo-tuberal CPs predominantly occupy the third ventricular cavity; therefore, selection of a surgical approach should consider exposure of the tumor within the third ventricular cavity and infundibulum, which is also the critical site of origin. These lesions are hardly visible through the standard basal approaches—subfrontal or pterional—leading to a high rate of failed surgical procedures. Those classic frontotemporal approaches introduce blind spots with respect to exposure of the posterosuperior portion of the tumor near the third ventricle. In the apparently tumor-free suprasellar space, the lower pole of the CP is the only part observable under the optic chiasm or through the optic-carotid triangle *via* a basal pterional or subfrontal approach. Although the superior space between the bifurcate of the internal carotid artery (ICA) compensates for surgical exposure, the penetrating branches restricts the use of this space. As a result, the above-mentioned classic skull base approach cannot provide satisfactory exposure of most infundibulo-tuberal tumors.

Articles that have addressed infundibulo-tuberal CP have proposed three major surgical corridors:

Superior corridor (trans-callosal trans-ventricular approach): This includes the trans-callosal–interfornix–third ventricular approach and trans-cortical–lateral ventricle–foramen of Monro–third ventricle approach. The surgical procedures associated with approaches through the superior corridor are relatively convenient. Associated hydrocephalus would also facilitate surgical manipulation.

The slightly adherent superior tumor part is first treated, after which the infundibulo-tuberal site of origin is dissected further. However, this type of approach has obvious shortcomings: 1) firstly and importantly, tumor dissection *via* the superior approach begins from the distal and dorsal part of the tumor, whereas the tumor part with the most severe adhesions, which must be dissected under a direct surgical view, is usually hidden in a retrochiasmatic position within the anteroinferior portion of the third ventricle. Additionally, this tumor part is far from the surgeon, thus rendering surgical manipulation quite difficult. 2) The surgical manipulation space was deep and narrow, and the foramen of Monro and fornix limit the exposure. 3) The risk of fornix injury and consequent memory disorders and epilepsy are higher with this approach.

Anterior corridor: This includes the frontotemporal, subfrontal trans-terminalis, and frontobasal interhemispheric trans-terminalis approaches. Infundibulo-tuberal CPs are hardly visible when using standard purely basal approaches—subfrontal or pterional. The lamina terminalis space is used most frequently. The lateral surgical view *via* the frontotemporal trans-terminalis approach introduces a blind spot with respect to tumor dissection within the 3rd VF. In general, the site of tumor origin should be dissected under a direct view; as a result, increasing numbers of recent reports have suggested removing infundibulo-tuberal CPs *via* the frontobasal interhemispheric approach. This middle approach can sufficiently expose the longitudinal axis of the hypothalamic–pituitary structure. Division of the anterior communicating artery (AcoA) in certain cases can further enhance tumor exposure [27]. In our department, this approach was selected for almost all cases of infundibulo-tuberal CPs.

Ventral corridor (Extended trans-sphenoidal approach): Along with the recent development and wide acceptance of endoscopic techniques (*e.g.*, neuro-navigation, high-speed electric drills, extendable micro-instrumentation, endonasal ultrasonic aspiration, reconstructive materials, improved endoscope optics), the expanded endonasal approach (EEA) has made it possible to expose the site of tumor origin from a ventral viewpoint [28, 29]. However, 3rd VF injury is inevitable with this approach, so indications for this approach should be strict.

Surgical Techniques

Techniques of the Trans-terminalis Approach

When removing infundibulo-tuberal CPs *via* the trans-terminalis approach, it is very important to understand the relationship between the tumor and third ventricular walls. The operator should be aware that infundibulo-tuberal CP is an intraparenchymal lesion that should be separated within the neural tissue of the 3rd VF. After exposing the tumor by opening the lamina terminalis, we first enter the squeezed and compressed true third ventricular cavity. Theoretically, two layers should be opened before reaching the tumor wall. These two layers are the ependymal layer and attenuated neural tissue layer of the 3rd VF [7, 12]. A stratified relationship between the tumor and 3rd VF, based on differences in tumor growth, can be observed in some patients (Fig. **15**). In this situation, the intact 3rd VF can be preserved after tumor removal. In the other cases, however, the progressive growth of a CP that originated within the 3rd VF causes stretching and atrophy of this neural tissue. As a result, the infundibulo-tuberal area is progressively replaced by the mass. In this situation, the upward-growing tumor might penetrate the neural tissue to the third ventricular cavity. The externally growing tumor might penetrate the neural tissue layer of the 3rd VF, extend to the suprasellar cistern, and formed intra- and extraventricular tumors. However, even in this situation, the lower pole of the CP remains covered by the pia mater. This histological feature might be the major distinguishing factor between infundibulo-tuberal CP and subarachnoid extrapia mater CP (extraventricular CP). The pioneering neurosurgeon William Sweet advocated the use of the trans-lamina terminalis (trans-LT) approach to remove most adult CPs with an infundibulo-tuberal or predominantly intraventricular location [30 - 32]. Sweet thought that an area of gliosis would form around the CP inside the neural tissue of the 3rd VF. These "unfunctional" areas of gliosis were thought to serve as an interface for dissection between the tumor and vital neural structures. Sweet also thought that defects left in the 3rd VF after total lesion removal did not necessarily mean that hypothalamic injury had occurred but were rather a logical consequence that developed around the lesion origin at the base of the third ventricle. Steno and Alexander Konovalov shared this opinion with Sweet. Through patient autopsies, Steno [5, 6] proved eloquently that through progressive growth, CPs could completely replace the neural tissues of infundibulo-tuberal structures. However, the infundibular structures can be displaced to localize at their equators. Alexander Konovalov further proposed a difference between infundibulo-tuberal CP and purely intraventricular CP. In our experience, CP might have the same site of origin, regardless of the intraventricular or extraventricular status. The degree of tumor invasiveness in the neural tissue of the 3rd VF is determined by the direction and timeline of tumor growth. It is unreasonable to attribute 3rd VF defects solely to the replacement of neural tissue by CPs, because in clinical works even cases with severe CP involvement were rarely accompanied by severe presurgical hypothalamic reactions. Our opinion is that patients who undergo total tumor removal with large 3rd VF defects will suffer from severe hypothalamic symptoms without exception. Therefore, the development of surgical techniques should focus on maximal preservation of the nervous tissue of 3rd VF.

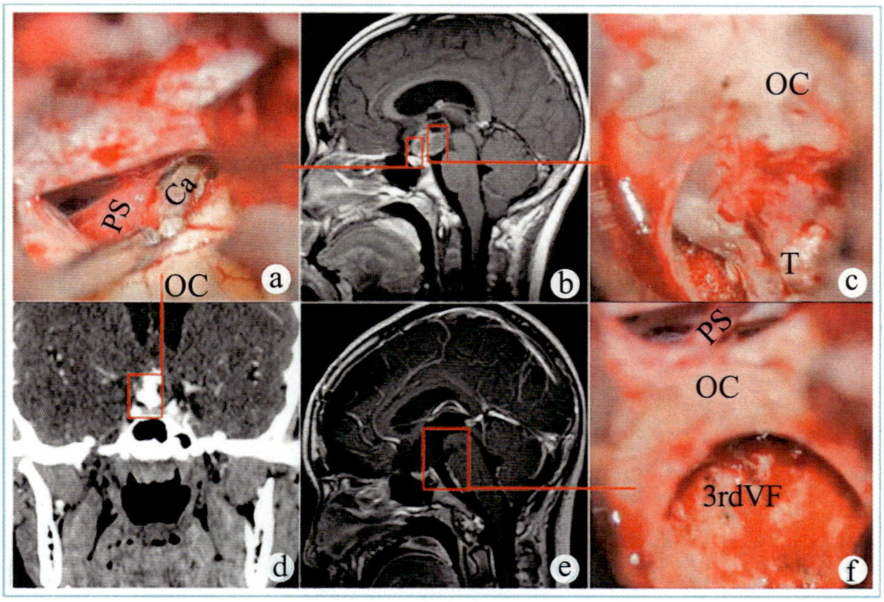

Fig. (15). (Reference from Jun Pan,Songtao Qi *et al.*, Growth patterns of craniopharyngiomas: clinical analysis of 226 patients. Journal of Neurosurgery Pediatrics, 2015:1-16). Pre-and post-operative neuroimaging and intra-operative photos in a 17-year-old man with a typical infundibulo-tuberal CP. Coronal CT scan (**d**) demonstrated the tumor calcification (Ca) at the suprasellar cistern (**d**). Pre-operative sagittal contrast-enhanced T1-weighted MRI showed the tumor located at the anterior portion of the third ventricle (**b**). Intra-operative pictures showed the tumor calcification penetrate nerve tissue of the anterior portion of the third ventricle (**a**). Tumor removal was accomplished through the trans-LT route, tumor encased within the verve tissue of the 3rd VF (**c**). Post-operative sagittal contrast-enhanced T1-weighted MRI (**e**) and intra-operative picture (**f**) showed total removal of the tumor. Note the attenuated but uninterrupted 3rd VF after tumor removal.

AcoA Complex

When removing infundibulo-tuberal CPs *via* the frontobasal interhemispheric approach, an important problem is treatment of the AcoA. The feasibility of interrupting the AcoA was reported in the previous literature [27], but most neurosurgeons might not be willing to permit this type of treatment. Actually, for many infundibulo-tuberal CPs, AcoA division is necessary to facilitate separation of the tumor inside the third ventricular cavity. The following points should be understood when interrupting the AcoA: 1) the surgical aim is radical tumor removal, which is considered feasible; 2) presurgical cerebral angiography (*e.g.*, digital subtraction angiography [DSA] and CT angiography) indicate good development of the bilateral A1 and A2 segments of the anterior carotid artery (ACA); and 3) most importantly, intraoperative observation of the angio-architecture proves the results of presurgical cerebral angiography. The AcoA should also be sufficiently long for coagulation and bipolar interruption. Notably, the penetrated branches of the AcoA should be identified, and injury to these artery branches should be avoided. Following the above indications, we interrupted the AcoA in more than 80 cases of CP and observed no complications related AcoA interruption. Our opinion is that the AcoA angioarchitecture should be understood before surgery for infundibulo-tuberal CPs (Figs. **16** and **17**).

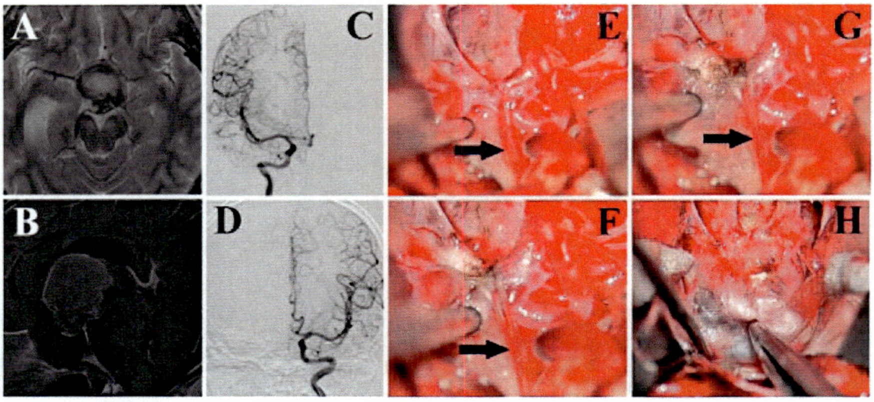

Fig. (16). A cases of craniopharyngioma with type "T" growth pattern, the MRI before surgery indicated that the tumor located suprasellar region. The optic chiasm located prefixed with upwards displacement of bilateral AcoA complex (**A** and **B**). Angiographic images before surgery showed the A1, A2 segment of bilateral ACA developed well (**C** and **D**). In operation, the AcoA complex was separated carefully (**E**), and also its' perforating branches (Black arrow head). With avoiding to injury the branches, the AcoA was coagulated and dissected to provide more exposure of lamina terminalis (**F**-**H**).

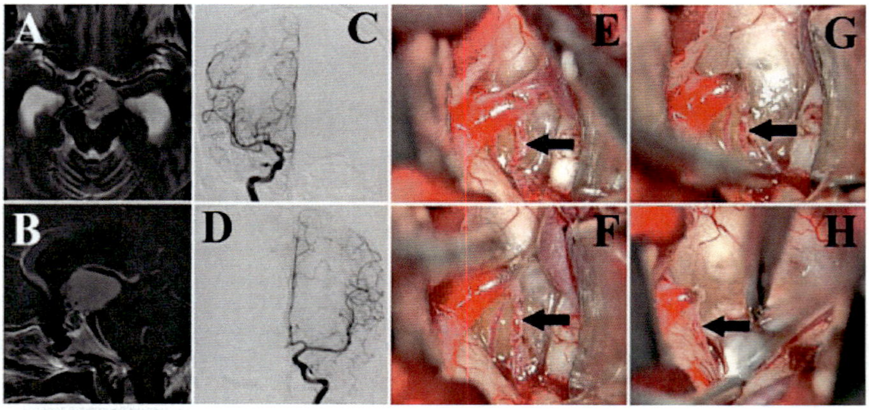

Fig. (17). The second case to illustrate the dissection of AcoA.

PS

PS disposal is the key point in the removal of CPs. This is consistent with protection of the PS and preservation of the infundibulum, which also represents protection of the hypothalamic structures. The degree of tumor involvement is the most important element that influences PS protection. As depicted above, there are three types of features of infundibulo-tuberal CP invasion to the PS: 1) the tumor grows entirely toward the third ventricular cavity (purely intraventricular CP). The infundibular part is compressed and displaced downward, and the suprasellar intracistern segment of the PS remains almost intact. 2) The tumor grew basally around the infundibular stalk, which could be partially protected. 3) The infundibulum and stalk were grossly violated by the tumor and its calcification and became inflated and pocket-shaped. In this situation, continuity of the PS can hardly be protected during radical tumor removal. The three different invasive features lead to three situations of 3rd VF protection. In the first situation, the infundibulum and upper segment of the stalk were thin but could be preserved intact or with only localized small fissure-like defects. Normally, continuity of the hypothalamus–PS–pituitary gland can be maintained. In the second situation, basal growth forms an anatomical foundation for PS preservation. After tumor removal, PS continuity can be maintained. However, in the third situation, which is also most frequent, the tumor not only invades the third ventricular walls but also expands along the infundibular stalk. The stalk fiber becomes inflated into a pocket shape and presents a considerable challenge to stalk protection. During surgical tumor separation, the stalk is always interrupted, leading to significant defects in the anterior part of the 3rd VF and consequent severe hypothalamic reactions.

EVALUATION OF THE EXTENT OF SURGICAL REMOVAL

In early articles, most neurosurgeons evaluated the extent of tumor removal based on surgical records and intraoperative impressions. Later, most scholars thought that postsurgical neuroimaging should provide the main body of evidence for evaluating the extent of removal. CT scans were initially used, followed by MRI. Three-dimensional (3D) MRI significantly increased identification of the third ventricular walls and also increased the evaluation precision. However, even thin-slice and 3D scans might still miss tiny residual tumors. Therefore, these mistakes would be larger when using normal MRI scanning conditions (slice thickness = 5mm). As result, some scholars have proposed that an intraoperative estimation conducted by a surgeon with great CP surgical experience provides the best evaluation of the extent of removal [33]. Although the latter evaluation has not been accepted by the majority of neurosurgeons, in our opinion it remains meaningful. Effenterre and Boch responded to comments about related questions and proposed that among their clinical cases, 15% of all cases of total tumor removal as proven by postsurgical MRI were thought to lack truly total tumor removal based on the surgeon's evaluation. However, among the 32 cases with partial tumor removal based on the surgeon's evaluation, only 10 cases were thought to have residual tumor according to postsurgical MRI and CT scans. In other words, less than one third of subtotal tumor removal cases could be proven by postsurgical neuroimaging. The results of our cases were similar to those reported by Effenterre and Boch. As result, the current objective evaluation for the extent of CP removal should be based on a combination of intraoperative impressions and postsurgical MRI. Notably, the cases reported by Effenterre and Boch were all treated *via* a frontotemporal approach or modified approaches using the lateral corridor. Use of this type of corridor might introduce a surgical blind spot in most cases of infundibulo-tuberal CP, and this might be a major reason for uncertain surgeon-directed evaluations of the extent of removal.

RISK FACTORS FOR RECURRENCE

CP recurs easily and among cases without total tumor removal, the recurrence rate can reach 70–100%. Even among cases of total removal, the rate can reach 20–70%. Different evaluation criteria are responsible for the large variations in reported recurrence rates. The current consensus is that the extent of tumor removal was the most important element that influences tumor recurrence. Gross total tumor removal can significantly reduce the risk of recurrence; for example the 10-year survival rates range from 81.3% to 100% after radiologically confirmed total removal [4, 33, 34], 25% to 86% after subtotal or partial removal [4, 34 - 37], 77% to 100% after partial removal and subsequent radiotherapy [34 - 39], and 81% to 100% after radiotherapy alone [38, 39]. There is also a consensus that cases without total tumor removal will inevitably recur if salvage therapy is not used. Therefore, for cases of infundibulo-tuberal CP, an evaluation of the extent of tumor removal is quite important because this will directly determine whether a patient should undergo additional combined-modality therapy.

In clinical work, some CPs will not recur or will slowly progress for several years or even decades after treatment during the follow-up period. In contrast, tumors may grow rapidly within a short period some other patients. Moreover, there are occasional reports of the malignant transformation CP. These phenomena indicate diversity among tumors with respect to biological features such as CP proliferative activity. However, research focused on these biological features has not yielded consistent results. Some scholars have studied the relationship between the Ki-67 proliferation index and tumor recurrence but received contradictory results. Others have suggested differences between recurrent and nonrecurrent lesions [40], and still others have not reached a similar conclusion [41 - 43].

There have also been no consistent results in terms of an association between patient age and recurrence. Some studies have considered pediatric CP to be more aggressive, whereas others have found that adult tumors are more likely to recur. Additionally, some studies have not found significant differences between the long-term follow-up recurrence rates of children and adults who underwent surgical removal followed or not by irradiation [34]. Following an analysis of 75 pediatric CP cases, De Vile *et al.* [44] determined that an age <5 years was a significant predictive factor for recurrence.

There is also no consistent opinion regarding the relationship between tumoral pathology and recurrence. A few early researchers thought that SPCP would not easily recur and would thus have a better prognosis than ACP [18, 45, 46]. However, several recent studies based on large numbers of cases have indicated that only a few cases of SPCP with stem-like connections to the infundibulo-tuberal part might have an improved prognosis. Patients in this situation had a good prognosis because of the higher GTR rate. Studies involving large numbers of of SPCPs remain lacking, and there might be some degree of overlap between SPCP and transitional-type CP; therefore, differences in the recurrence rates between these two types of pathological tumors remain unconfirmed [15]. We statistically analyzed the long-term follow-up data for 27 cases of SPCP and found no significant differences in the 5- and 10-year progression-free survival rates of patients with SPCP and ACP. Regarding therapeutic methods, most literature supports the use of substitution radiotherapy for significantly reducing tumor recurrences. Current research has focused on reducing irradiation-induced toxicity, especially in younger children. Some scholars have thought that the use of modern high-energy machines and irradiation doses of ≤55 Gy in 1.8-Gy fractions should minimize toxicity.

There have also been no consistent results regarding the influences of the tumor location and radiological features on recurrence [3, 33, 44]. The lesion consistency and location (intrasellar, extrasellar, or both) have no prognostic significance [34, 47, 48]. A few articles reported different recurrence rates for intrasellar-origin and infundibulo-tuberal CPs [19]. Previously, tumors with an intrasellar origin were thought to have a higher GTR rate and corresponding lower recurrence rate when compared with infundibulo-tuberal CPs. However, based on our follow-up results, no significant difference between the two tumoral types was observed in terms of progression-free survival. The influences of tumoral calcification, texture (solid, cystic–solid mixture, and cystic), and hydrocephalus on recurrence have been represented as tumor resectability. Calcification grows quite slowly and may even remain static for several years. However, calcification is also major obstructive element in the context of total tumor removal. On the other hand, although the cystic tumor volume might increase significantly within the short term, the GTR rate of purely cystic tumors is higher than those of cystic–solid mixture and purely solid tumors. Therefore, there are no consistent results regarding the influence of cystic and calcification components on prognosis. Hydrocephalus has always been considered a majorly influential element with respect to total tumor removal and a poor prognosis. Our opinion, given a full understanding of the tumor growth pattern, is that hydrocephalus represents the topographic classification of infundibulo-tuberal CPs and indicates a tumor located in an unresectable location. The impact of hydrocephalus on recurrence may simply reflect the achieved surgical result [4, 19, 44]

PROGNOSIS

CP will cause damage and a decrease in patients' QOL, which is attributed to critical neuronal structure (*e.g.*, hypothalamic, hypophyseal, visual) injuries caused by primary or recurrent tumors as well as various therapeutic interventions. However, statistical patient and survival rate data alone or a grading system that only scores QOL as good, moderate, poor, or death cannot objectively evaluate the patient's QOL. CP involves endocrine, visual, hypothalamic, neurobehavioral, and cognitive sequelae, all of which compromise normal psychosocial integration and influence patients' QOL.

Prognostic Evaluation Methods

Given the low incidence of CPs and different levels of available knowledge and therapy at different centers, it is difficult to objectively evaluate prognosis based on different treatment centers and different methods. Establishment of evaluation criteria is very important, especially for pediatric CP, a very controversial disease. Although many articles in the literature have attempted to assess the functional outcomes and QOL of patients with CP, as yet there is no widely accepted scale for prognostic evaluation. Wen *et al.* proposed a four-tiered outcome scale that combined different domains (Table **2**) [48].

This assessment system includes evaluations of the nervous system, optic accuracy, and pituitary and hypothalamic function. The predominant advantage of this system is its concise nature. However, this scale yields a composite total score that combines deficits in many disparate domains into a single morbidity class. Therefore, it is still generally crude.

Table 2. Wen QOL assessment (Reference from Wen *et al.* [48]).

Class	Criteria
I	Grossly normal & independent
	Mild hormonal disturbances
	Seizures well controlled w/ medication

(Table 2) contd.....

Class	Criteria
II	Independent
	Panhypopituitarism
	Mild-to-moderate visual compromise
	Cranial nerve deficits
	Mild psychological dysfunction
III	Partially dependent
	Serious visual compromise
	Serious neurological deficits (hemiparesis, refractory seizures)
	Learning disabilities or poorly controlled psychological disorders
IV	Entirely dependent on others for self-care

Duff and colleagues [49] proposed dichotomization through an analysis of clinical data from 121 cases. These authors attempted to identify patients who were "well-integrated independent individuals functioning in society" (Table **3**). Patients who failed to satisfy all 8 criteria were considered to have poor outcomes. Such dichotomization, however, causes the loss of a significant amount of functional data and thus limits the completeness of the assessment and the conclusions that can be drawn when comparing treatment modalities.

Table 3. Duff QOL asscessment based on data in the article by Duff *et al.* [49].

Outcome	Criteria
good	Alive at follow-up examination
	No major motor deficit related to op or tumor progression
	Functional vision
	Katz Grade A(able to perform basic ADLs)
	Karmofsky Performance Scale score ≧80
	No more than 1 yr behind in expected school grade
	Employability for adults of working age
	Absence of debilitating psychological or emotional problem
poor	All patients not meeting the "good" criteria

De Vile and colleagues [44] proposed a combined score system Table **4** that includes five domains in the areas of neurological status, vision, pituitary function, hypothalamic function, and educational/occupational status in order to evaluate patients' functional outcomes and QOL. The maximum total score is 15, and a higher score indicates a poorer prognosis. A score of 15 indicates death.

Thompson D *et al.* also proposed that prognostic factors for poor functional outcomes among patients with CP include the following: 1) larger lesion size, 2) hypothalamic tumor involvement, 3) clinical signs of hypothalamic dysfunction (namely obesity), and 4) patient age <5 years. Based on the above factors, the authors proposed an "evidence-based" treatment protocol [50]. Recently, Elliott *et al.* [51] modified the scale proposed by De Vile *et al.* and further proposed a four-tiered Craniopharyngioma Clinical Status Scale (CCSS, Table **5**) that incorporated five domains. This system evaluated patients' functional outcome and QOL in the five domains of neurological, vision, pituitary function, hypothalamic function, and educational/occupational status. Each domain was scored on a scale from 1 to 4 to predict morbidity and offer better counsel to patients, their families, and their primary physicians.

Table 4. De Vilex Morbidity in 75 patients with craniopharyngioma surgery and study assessment (Reference from De Vile *et al.* [44]).

Clinical finding	Morbidity Score assigned
Endocrine	
panhypopituitarism+impaired thirst	3
panhypopituitarism	2
Partial anterior pituitary deficiency±DI	1
No pituitary deficit	0
Vision	
VA≤6/60 both eyes	3
VA 6/18~6/60 or blind in one eye	2
VA 6/9~6/18 in one or both eyes	1
Normal vision	0
Neurology	
Severe motor disorder ± epilepsy	3
Mild-to moderate motor disorder ± epilepsy	2
Signs only; no seizures	1
Normal neurology	0
Education	
Severe learning difficulties ± severe behavioral problems	3
moderate(IQ:71-79)	2
mild(IQ:80-89)	1
normal(IQ>90)	0

(Table 4) contd.....

Clinical finding	Morbidity Score assigned
Hypothalamic	
Severe hypothalamic syndrome	3
moderate	2
mild	1
normal	0
Death	15

DI=diabetes insipidus; IQ=intelligence quotient

Table 5. A four-tiered Craniopharyngioma Clinical Status Scale (Reference from Elliott *et al.* [51]).

Domain & Score	Criteria
N-CCSS	
1	no deficits or seizures
2	mild deficits (cranial nerve palsy, well-controlled seizures)
3	moderate deficits (mild hemiparesis w/ independent ambulation, moderately controlled seizures)
4	severe deficits (moderate-to-severe hemiparesis, major stroke, significant abulia, or lethargy)
V-CCSS	
1	normal VA & VFs
2	mild acuity deficits or field cut
3	unilat blindness, homonymous hemianopia, or bitemporal hemianopia
4	bilat blindness or nearly functional blindness
P-CCSS	
1	normal anterior & posterior pituitary function
2	mild anterior pituitary dysfunction (1 or 2 hormone supplements)
3	DI w/ or w/o mild anterior pituitary dysfunction (1 or 2 hormone supplements)
4	DI & panhypopituitarism
H-CCSS*	
1	normal hypothalamic function
2	postop obesity (BMI >+2 SD), lack of behavioral/psychological symptoms
3	obesity (BMI >+2 SD) w/ hyperphagia, or memory disturbance or BMI >+3 SD w/o frank hyperphagia behaviors
4	extreme obesity (BMI >+4 SD) & hyperphagia, behavioral disturbances (such as rage episodes), & disturbances of thermoregulation, sleep-wake cycles, or memory
E-CCSS	
1	excellent academic performance &/or occupational success
2	good academic performance at grade level &/or maintaining employment†
3	behind in grade academically, requires significant tutoring, or inability to maintain consistent employment‡
4	completely dependent on others for self-care (cannot perform ADLs), IQ <80, severe cognitive deficits

* Modified version of scale proposed by De Vile et al.[12]

† Meeting or exceeding developmental milestones for preschool-aged children.

‡ Not meeting age-appropriate developmental milestones for preschool-aged children.

Formal neuropsychological testing should theoretically be able to evaluate the patient's all-around cognitive, attention, memory, and task-specific performance skills. However, this type of testing always deviates from the patient's true performance in school or at work. A summary by Elliott *et al.* observed that more than one third of patients had good real-life performance despite receiving multi-domain-based scores <50%. Some scholars evaluated the "ecological validity" of formal neuropsychological testing in cranial trauma patients [52 - 54]. These scholars came to the same conclusions. Therefore, it is quite difficult to process neuropsychological testing in some cases of CP, and the results are always difficult to explain.

In summary, for infundibulo-tuberal CPs with hypothalamic structural involvement, an evaluation of patients' functional outcomes and QOL is actually comprehensive. It might be easier to maintain an objective evaluation for optic, pituitary, and hypothalamic function as well as nervous system complications. However, neuropsychological testing for cognition, memory, study, and work abilities might be difficult, especially for younger children.

Endocrine

Almost all studies observed nearly universal endocrinopathy subsequent to treatment. Compared to the preoperative baseline status, a significant increase in pituitary dysfunction occurred after surgery. The literature reports individual hormone deficit frequencies ranging from 88% to 100% for growth hormone (GH), 80% to 95% for follicle-stimulating hormone (FSH)/luteinizing hormone (LH), 55% to 88% for adrenocorticotropic hormone (ACTH), 39% to 95% for thyroid-stimulating hormone (TSH), and 25% to 86% for antidiuretic hormone (ADH) [3, 34, 38, 55 - 58]. As we noted above, the incidence of presurgical pituitary function deficiency was lower among cases of infundibulo-tuberal CP than among cases of subdiaphragmatic CP. However, a significantly greater decline in post-resection pituitary function occurred in the former group when compared with the latter group.

In agreement with De Vile and colleagues [44], we found that DI, especially in the setting of impaired thirst (adipsia), is more persistently disabling and burdensome to patients and families when compared with anterior pituitary dysfunction. Therefore, doctors should communicate with patients' families before surgery about the occurrence of hypopituitarism and DI after surgery, as supplementary treatment might be required throughout the remainder of the patients' lives. Patients, families, and primary physicians should be counseled on the very high likelihood of postoperative hypopituitarism and DI.

The phenomenon of growth without GH has been reported in some children with CP who have exhibited normal or even accelerated linear growth despite an untreated GH deficiency [58, 59]. In our opinion, nearly all pediatric cases involving the above phenomenon occurred in patients with infundibulo-tuberal CPs, which might be related to obesity and high serum insulin levels in children. The pathophysiological mechanism of this phenomenon remains unclear.

Hypothalamus

The risk of hypothalamic dysfunction and its sequelae was another main point of contention. A hypothalamic evaluation is also important when treating infundibulo-tuberal CPs. Hypothalamic dysfunction includes a constellation of disturbances such as obesity, hyperphagia, memory deficits, thermoregulatory abnormalities, emotionally labile behavior, and sleep–wake cycle disruption [8, 20, 44, 60 - 62]. When compared with universal endocrinopathy subsequent to treatment, hypothalamic function deterioration is less dramatic and there is a consensus that hypopituitarism and DI are consistent and may be caused by the tumor itself, whereas hypothalamic function dysfunction is not. Although infundibulo-tuberal CPs all involve the third ventricular walls and hypothalamic structures, manifestations of hypothalamic disturbances at diagnosis are relatively rare when compared with the high rate of pituitary dysfunction at presentation. Therefore, the risks and consequences of hypothalamic dysfunction likely correlate with the surgical manipulations, extent of resection, or follow-up interventions. According to current opinion, the elements related to significant postsurgical hypothalamic morbidity include: 1) a young age (<5 years) [44, 63]; 2) manifestations of hypothalamic disturbance at diagnosis [44]; 3) a tumor height greater than 3.5 cm from the midline [44]; 4) hypothalamic invasion [63, 64]; 5) attempts to remove adherent tumor from the hypothalamic region [44]; and 6) multiple operations to treat recurrences [63]. Irradiation-induced hypothalamic dysfunction correlates predominantly with the dosage. In general, radiation doses >51 Gy toward hypothalamic structures are thought to correlate with significant hypothalamic morbidity (234). Obesity has not been evaluated in a standard manner in most publications, although the total incidence has always exceeded 50% [4, 20, 33, 44, 49, 56, 65 - 67]. In a German multicenter retrospective study conducted by Muller *et al.* [68], the incidence of obesity was 44% among 185 children with CP. For infundibulo-tuberal CPs, the presentation of postsurgical obesity and weight gain is more common. In a series of 226 cases of primary CP in our department (including both pediatric and adult cases), the long-term follow-up data indicated that the incidence of obesity according to the De Vile hypothalamic status scale grades 3 and 4 was 12.6% (19.1% among pediatric patients and 8.5% among adults) and, notably, the incidence of obesity among tubero-infundibular CPs was 42% (44% among pediatric patients and 12.6%

among adults). Pure weight gain and obesity were acceptable, but severe obesity always occurred concomitantly with emotionally labile behavior, social function deficits, and emotional reactivity, which seriously influence the patient's QOL. Meanwhile, during the long-term follow-up, the rate of death related to cardiovascular incidents and obstructive sleep apnea was significantly higher among patients with obesity than among the normal population.

Visual

Evaluations of optic symptoms such as visual accuracy and the visual field are relatively objective. However, the detection process is difficult in younger children. In contrast to pituitary and hypothalamic function, which generally decrease after surgery, significant improvements in vision are usually observed after surgery. Several points regarding visual pathway impairment by CP should be noted: 1) apart from compression, impairment of the optical pathway by infundibulo-tuberal CPs differs from that caused by pituitary adenoma and includes adherence and invasion. Large infundibulo-tuberal CPs always compress the optic chiasm and nerves, and it is inevitable that the visual pathway will be affected by the tumor removal procedure. The improved relief of optic impairment *via* the trans-sphenoidal approach relative to the trans-cranial approach, as reported in the literature, might associate with the tumor growth pattern rather than the surgical corridor. 2) In contrast to subdiaphragmatic CP, infundibulo-tuberal CP is considered unsuitable for surgery *via* the trans-sphenoidal approach. In the literature, severe visual disorders after surgery occurred in approximately 10–30% of all cases. The main elements influencing visual disorder relief included: 1) the visual accuracy and field status before surgery, as the probability of recuperation depends on the severity of preoperative visual pathway impairment. Optic atrophy (observed *via* fundoscopy) carries the worst prognosis [33]. 2) The patient's therapeutic history: compared with patients undergoing one surgery (single Surg), those undergoing CTrR, irradiation, and intra-cystic irradiation were more likely to suffer visual disorders during a long-term follow-up [26]. 3) Tumor recurrences were often responsible for definitive visual aggravation. 4) The influences of surgery and irradiation on visual accuracy and the optic field remain controversial. We agree with the points made by Effenterre and Boch [33]. Surgery conducted by a well-experienced neurosurgeon offers better results than radiotherapy. Some scholars believe that the patient's age is another element that influences postsurgery visual accuracy relief, as children are often more strongly affected than adults. In our opinion, presurgical visual disorders are more severe in young children than in adults. A possible reason for this difference might include the difficulty of diagnosing early-stage visual disorders in children. Furthermore, according to our clinical cases, pediatric patients always have larger tumors than do adult patients. On the other hand, almost half of all pediatric CP cases were of the subdiaphragmatic type. As we described above, this type of CP is always complicated by presurgical severe visual disorders. For infundibulo-tuberal CPs at the same impairment level, the prognosis after optic decompression is the same at every age. We observed no significant differences between children and adults with respect to visual disorder relief.

Neuropsychological and Cognitive/Functional Outcome

In CP cases, neuropsychological detection is the most difficult prognostic evaluation especially among pediatric patients. As we summarized above, formal neuropsychological testing usually differs from true presentations in life and work. Elliott *et al.* thought that patients' current levels of success and achievement should be the ultimate measure of good functional outcomes. Diverse evaluation methods have been used to assess neuropsychological and cognitive function. Among those methods, the patient's academic and work performances were considered most important. Duff *et al.* [49] reported a long-term follow-up (average = 10 years) of 121 cases of CP. The functional outcomes were poor for 40% of the patients, according to criteria based on motor deficits, vision, dependence for activities of daily living, and the Karnofsky Performance Scale (assesses the ability to perform normal activities and active work, the need for assistance, school and work statuses, and debilitating psychological or emotional problems). In another article, Effenterre and Boch report 122 cases of CP treated mainly with surgery; after a 7-year follow-up, 16% of adult and 26% of pediatric patients did not achieve independent living with respect to social integration and normal professional, occupational, or educational status [33]. Pereira reported 54 cases with or without additional treatment and found that after a 10-year follow-up, 47% of cases suffered psychosocial impairment as evaluated according to independent living, social integration, professional occupation, and school performance. An additional 49% had neurological morbidity, defined as the presence of any of the following: concentration problems, personality changes, short-term memory loss, anosmia, or epilepsy [69]. De Vile *et al.* [44], in a series of 75 children who underwent surgical resection followed or not by irradiation, demonstrated that after a mean follow-up period of 6.4 years, 40% of the patients had intelligence quotient scores <80 and 23% had severe motor disorders either with or without epilepsy. Karavitaki *et al.* [34], in a series of 121 patients treated *via* surgery with or without radiotherapy, one fourth of the adults and children were unable to work in their previous occupation or had a lower than expected school status, respectively. The following prognostic factors for a poor functional outcome in CP patients are currently under discussion in the literature: 1) larger lesion size; 2) hypothalamic tumor involvement; 3) clinical signs of hypothalamic dysfunction (namely obesity); and 4) patient age <5 years.

It is quite difficult to evaluate the influences of different treatment strategy on the functional outcomes of patients. CPs are tumors that exhibit various growth patterns. Also, significant differences exist between children and adult regarding growth patterns [19]. Therefore, clinical cases series from different centers feature extreme diversity with respect to tumor type compositions, a factor that makes it difficult to compare different data sets. Meanwhile, the experience of the neurosurgeon [70], recurrences, and subsequent therapeutic interventions also contribute to the final results. Given the above diversity, some publications believe that GTR is associated with poorer postoperative functional outcomes relative to irradiation alone or minimal surgery [71], whereas others consider conservative surgery with adjuvant irradiation to provide the most consistent results with respect to returning to school and employment or tertiary educational achievement [35]. However, the results of Duff [49] indicate that GTR is associated with a better clinical outcome. Finally, some scholars have found no significant differences in neuropsychological and cognitive function among patients treated *via* GTR, partial resection, or partial resection combined with radiotherapy [34, 44].

Our opinion is that the treatment strategy should be selected based on tumor resectability. To date, no single classification can encompass all CP growth patterns. Surprisingly, few literature reports have compared the postoperative neuropsychological and cognitive functions in patients with different CP growth patterns. Based on our clinical data, we observed that postoperative neuropsychological and cognitive function deterioration were normally accompanied by a severe hypothalamic reaction. Infundibulo-tuberal CPs are more likely to be accompanied by psychological or emotional problems after radical tumor removal [19]. Interestingly, the results published by Elliott *et al.* [51] indicated a lack of significant difference in the incidence of good pre- and postoperative functional statuses between patients with pre- and retrochiasmatic tumors.

CONFLICT OF INTEREST

The author (editor) declares no conflict of interest, financial or otherwise.

ACKNOWLEDGEMENTS

Declared none.

REFERENCES

[1] Hoffman HJ. Surgical management of craniopharyngioma. Pediatr Neurosurg 1994; 21 (Suppl. 1): 44-9.
[http://dx.doi.org/10.1159/000120861] [PMID: 7530990]

[2] Pascual JM, Prieto R, Carrasco R. Infundibulo-tuberal or not strictly intraventricular

craniopharyngioma: evidence for a major topographical category. Acta Neurochir (Wien) 2011; 153(12): 2403-25.
[http://dx.doi.org/10.1007/s00701-011-1149-4] [PMID: 21918833]

[3] Yaşargil MG, Curcic M, Kis M, Siegenthaler G, Teddy PJ, Roth P. Total removal of craniopharyngiomas. Approaches and long-term results in 144 patients. J Neurosurg 1990; 73(1): 3-11.
[http://dx.doi.org/10.3171/jns.1990.73.1.0003] [PMID: 2352020]

[4] Fahlbusch R, Honegger J, Paulus W, Huk W, Buchfelder M. Surgical treatment of craniopharyngiomas: experience with 168 patients. J Neurosurg 1999; 90(2): 237-50.
[http://dx.doi.org/10.3171/jns.1999.90.2.0237] [PMID: 9950494]

[5] Steno J. Microsurgical topography of craniopharyngiomas. Acta Neurochir Suppl (Wien) 1985; 35: 94-100.
[http://dx.doi.org/10.1007/978-3-7091-8813-2_16] [PMID: 3867266]

[6] Steno J, Malácek M, Bízik I. Tumor-third ventricular relationships in supradiaphragmatic craniopharyngiomas: correlation of morphological, magnetic resonance imaging, and operative findings. Neurosurgery 2004; 54(5): 1051-8.
[http://dx.doi.org/10.1227/01.NEU.0000120421.11171.61] [PMID: 15113458]

[7] Pascual JM, Prieto R, Dufourny IC, Simoes RG, Carrasco R. Hypothalamus-referenced classification for craniopharyngiomas: evidence provided by the endoscopic endonasal approach. Neurosurg Rev 2013; 36(2): 337-9.
[http://dx.doi.org/10.1007/s10143-012-0439-5] [PMID: 23242508]

[8] Sainte-Rose C, Puget S, Wray A, *et al.* Craniopharyngioma: the pendulum of surgical management. Childs Nerv Syst 2005; 21(8-9): 691-5.
[http://dx.doi.org/10.1007/s00381-005-1209-2] [PMID: 16078079]

[9] Karavitaki N, Cudlip S, Adams CB, Wass JA. Craniopharyngiomas. Endocr Rev 2006; 27(4): 371-97.
[http://dx.doi.org/10.1210/er.2006-0002] [PMID: 16543382]

[10] Pascual JM, González-Llanos F, Barrios L, Roda JM. Intraventricular craniopharyngiomas: topographical classification and surgical approach selection based on an extensive overview. Acta Neurochir (Wien) 2004; 146(8): 785-802.
[http://dx.doi.org/10.1007/s00701-004-0295-3] [PMID: 15254801]

[11] Pascual JM, Carrasco R, Prieto R, Gonzalez-Llanos F, Alvarez F, Roda JM. Craniopharyngioma classification. J Neurosurg 2008; 109(6): 1180-2.
[http://dx.doi.org/10.3171/JNS.2008.109.12.1180] [PMID: 19035739]

[12] Pan J, Qi S, Lu Y, *et al.* Intraventricular craniopharyngioma: morphological analysis and outcome evaluation of 17 cases. Acta Neurochir (Wien) 2011; 153(4): 773-84.
[http://dx.doi.org/10.1007/s00701-010-0938-5] [PMID: 21271265]

[13] Über J, E. Hypophysengangsgeschwulste und Hirmcholesteatome. Sitzungsb Kais Akad Wissen Math Naturw Klin 1904; 113: 537-726.

[14] Songtao Q, *et al.* IDH mutations predict longer survival and response to temozolomide in secondary glioblastoma. Cancer Sci 2011.
[PMID: 22034964]

[15] Crotty TB, Scheithauer BW, Young WF Jr, *et al.* Papillary craniopharyngioma: a clinicopathological study of 48 cases. J Neurosurg 1995; 83(2): 206-14.
[http://dx.doi.org/10.3171/jns.1995.83.2.0206] [PMID: 7616262]

[16] Eldevik OP, Blaivas M, Gabrielsen TO, Hald JK, Chandler WF. Craniopharyngioma: radiologic and histologic findings and recurrence. AJNR Am J Neuroradiol 1996; 17(8): 1427-39.
[PMID: 8883637]

[17] Weiner HL, Wisoff JH, Rosenberg ME, *et al.* Craniopharyngiomas: a clinicopathological analysis of factors predictive of recurrence and functional outcome. Neurosurgery 1994; 35(6): 1001-10.

[http://dx.doi.org/10.1227/00006123-199412000-00001] [PMID: 7885544]

[18] Adamson TE, Wiestler OD, Kleihues P, Yaşargil MG. Correlation of clinical and pathological features in surgically treated craniopharyngiomas. J Neurosurg 1990; 73(1): 12-7. [http://dx.doi.org/10.3171/jns.1990.73.1.0012] [PMID: 2352012]

[19] Qi S, Pan J, Lu Y, *et al.* The impact of the site of origin and rate of tumour growth on clinical outcome in children with craniopharyngiomas. Clin Endocrinol (Oxf) 2012; 76(1): 103-10. [http://dx.doi.org/10.1111/j.1365-2265.2011.04172.x] [PMID: 21752042]

[20] Puget S, Garnett M, Wray A, *et al.* Pediatric craniopharyngiomas: classification and treatment according to the degree of hypothalamic involvement. J Neurosurg 2007; 106(1) (Suppl.): 3-12. [PMID: 17233305]

[21] Lopez-Serna R, Gómez-Amador JL, Barges-Coll J, *et al.* Treatment of craniopharyngioma in adults: systematic analysis of a 25-year experience. Arch Med Res 2012; 43(5): 347-55. [http://dx.doi.org/10.1016/j.arcmed.2012.06.009] [PMID: 22824214]

[22] Mallucci C, Pizer B, Blair J, *et al.* Management of craniopharyngioma: the Liverpool experience following the introduction of the CCLG guidelines. Introducing a new risk assessment grading system. Childs Nerv Syst 2012; 28(8): 1181-92. [http://dx.doi.org/10.1007/s00381-012-1787-8] [PMID: 22570168]

[23] Van Gompel JJ, Nippoldt TB, Higgins DM, Meyer FB. Magnetic resonance imaging-graded hypothalamic compression in surgically treated adult craniopharyngiomas determining postoperative obesity. Neurosurg Focus 2010; 28(4): E3. [http://dx.doi.org/10.3171/2010.1.FOCUS09303] [PMID: 20367360]

[24] de Vile CJ, Grant DB, Hayward RD, Kendall BE, Neville BG, Stanhope R. Obesity in childhood craniopharyngioma: relation to post-operative hypothalamic damage shown by magnetic resonance imaging. J Clin Endocrinol Metab 1996; 81(7): 2734-7. [PMID: 8675604]

[25] Müller HL, Gebhardt U, Teske C, *et al.* Study Committee of KRANIOPHARYNGEOM 2000. Post-operative hypothalamic lesions and obesity in childhood craniopharyngioma: results of the multinational prospective trial KRANIOPHARYNGEOM 2000 after 3-year follow-up. Eur J Endocrinol 2011; 165(1): 17-24. [http://dx.doi.org/10.1530/EJE-11-0158] [PMID: 21490122]

[26] Yuen KC, Koltowska-Häggström M, Cook DM, *et al.* Primary treatment regimen and diabetes insipidus as predictors of health outcomes in adults with childhood-onset craniopharyngioma. J Clin Endocrinol Metab 2014; 99(4): 1227-35. [http://dx.doi.org/10.1210/jc.2013-3631] [PMID: 24476077]

[27] Shibuya M, Takayasu M, Suzuki Y, Saito K, Sugita K. Bifrontal basal interhemispheric approach to craniopharyngioma resection with or without division of the anterior communicating artery. J Neurosurg 1996; 84(6): 951-6. [http://dx.doi.org/10.3171/jns.1996.84.6.0951] [PMID: 8847589]

[28] Kassam AB, Gardner PA, Snyderman CH, Carrau RL, Mintz AH, Prevedello DM. Expanded endonasal approach, a fully endoscopic transnasal approach for the resection of midline suprasellar craniopharyngiomas: a new classification based on the infundibulum. J Neurosurg 2008; 108(4): 715-28. [http://dx.doi.org/10.3171/JNS/2008/108/4/0715] [PMID: 18377251]

[29] Frank G, *et al.* The endoscopic extended transsphenoidal approach for craniopharyngiomas. Neurosurgery 2006; 59(1 Suppl 1): 75-83. [http://dx.doi.org/10.1227/01.NEU.0000219897.98238.A3]

[30] Sweet WH. Radical surgical treatment of craniopharyngioma. Clin Neurosurg 1976; 23: 52-79. [PMID: 975700]

[31] Sweet WH. History of surgery for craniopharyngiomas. Pediatr Neurosurg 1994; 21 (Suppl. 1): 28-38. [http://dx.doi.org/10.1159/000120859] [PMID: 7841076]

[32] Sweet WH. Recurrent craniopharyngiomas: therapeutic alternatives. Clin Neurosurg 1980; 27: 206-29. [PMID: 7273555]

[33] Van Effenterre R, Boch AL. Craniopharyngioma in adults and children: a study of 122 surgical cases. J Neurosurg 2002; 97(1): 3-11. [http://dx.doi.org/10.3171/jns.2002.97.1.0003] [PMID: 12134929]

[34] Karavitaki N, Brufani C, Warner JT, *et al.* Craniopharyngiomas in children and adults: systematic analysis of 121 cases with long-term follow-up. Clin Endocrinol (Oxf) 2005; 62(4): 397-409. [http://dx.doi.org/10.1111/j.1365-2265.2005.02231.x] [PMID: 15807869]

[35] Graham PH, Gattamaneni HR, Birch JM. Paediatric craniopharyngiomas: a regional review. Br J Neurosurg 1992; 6(3): 187-93. [http://dx.doi.org/10.3109/02688699209002926] [PMID: 1632917]

[36] Carmel PW, Antunes JL, Chang CH. Craniopharyngiomas in children. Neurosurgery 1982; 11(3): 382-9. [http://dx.doi.org/10.1227/00006123-198209000-00008] [PMID: 7133354]

[37] Manaka S, Teramoto A, Takakura K. The efficacy of radiotherapy for craniopharyngioma. J Neurosurg 1985; 62(5): 648-56. [http://dx.doi.org/10.3171/jns.1985.62.5.0648] [PMID: 3989587]

[38] Rajan B, Ashley S, Gorman C, *et al.* Craniopharyngioma--a long-term results following limited surgery and radiotherapy. Radiother Oncol 1993; 26(1): 1-10. [http://dx.doi.org/10.1016/0167-8140(93)90019-5] [PMID: 8438080]

[39] Hetelekidis S, Barnes PD, Tao ML, *et al.* 20-year experience in childhood craniopharyngioma. Int J Radiat Oncol Biol Phys 1993; 27(2): 189-95. [http://dx.doi.org/10.1016/0360-3016(93)90227-M] [PMID: 8407391]

[40] Nishi T, Kuratsu J, Takeshima H, Saito Y, Kochi M, Ushio Y. Prognostic significance of the MIB-1 labeling index for patient with craniopharyngioma. Int J Mol Med 1999; 3(2): 157-61. [PMID: 9917523]

[41] Duò D, Gasverde S, Benech F, Zenga F, Giordana MT. MIB-1 immunoreactivity in craniopharyngiomas: a clinico-pathological analysis. Clin Neuropathol 2003; 22(5): 229-34. [PMID: 14531547]

[42] Raghavan R, Dickey WT Jr, Margraf LR, *et al.* Proliferative activity in craniopharyngiomas: clinicopathological correlations in adults and children. Surg Neurol 2000; 54(3): 241-7. [http://dx.doi.org/10.1016/S0090-3019(00)00298-6] [PMID: 11118571]

[43] Losa M, Vimercati A, Acerno S, *et al.* Correlation between clinical characteristics and proliferative activity in patients with craniopharyngioma. J Neurol Neurosurg Psychiatry 2004; 75(6): 889-92. [http://dx.doi.org/10.1136/jnnp.2003.012781] [PMID: 15146007]

[44] De Vile CJ, Grant DB, Kendall BE, *et al.* Management of childhood craniopharyngioma: can the morbidity of radical surgery be predicted? J Neurosurg 1996; 85(1): 73-81. [http://dx.doi.org/10.3171/jns.1996.85.1.0073] [PMID: 8683285]

[45] Kahn EA, Gosch HH, Seeger JF, Hicks SP. Forty-five years experience with the craniopharyngiomas. Surg Neurol 1973; 1(1): 5-12. [PMID: 4544703]

[46] Szeifert GT, Sipos L, Horváth M, *et al.* Pathological characteristics of surgically removed craniopharyngiomas: analysis of 131 cases. Acta Neurochir (Wien) 1993; 124(2-4): 139-43. [http://dx.doi.org/10.1007/BF01401137] [PMID: 7508161]

[47] Petito CK, DeGirolami U, Earle KM. Craniopharyngiomas: a clinical and pathological review. Cancer

1976; 37(4): 1944-52.
[http://dx.doi.org/10.1002/1097-0142(197604)37:4<1944::AID-CNCR2820370446>3.0.CO;2-#] [PMID: 1260697]

[48] Wen BC, Hussey DH, Staples J, *et al.* A comparison of the roles of surgery and radiation therapy in the management of craniopharyngiomas. Int J Radiat Oncol Biol Phys 1989; 16(1): 17-24. [http://dx.doi.org/10.1016/0360-3016(89)90005-9] [PMID: 2912938]

[49] Duff J, Meyer FB, Ilstrup DM, Laws ER Jr, Schleck CD, Scheithauer BW. Long-term outcomes for surgically resected craniopharyngiomas. Neurosurgery 2000; 46(2): 291-302. [http://dx.doi.org/10.1097/00006123-200002000-00007] [PMID: 10690718]

[50] Thompson D, Phipps K, Hayward R. Craniopharyngioma in childhood: our evidence-based approach to management. Childs Nerv Syst 2005; 21(8-9): 660-8. [http://dx.doi.org/10.1007/s00381-005-1210-9] [PMID: 15959733]

[51] Elliott RE, Sands SA, Strom RG, Wisoff JH. Craniopharyngioma Clinical Status Scale: a standardized metric of preoperative function and posttreatment outcome. Neurosurg Focus 2010; 28(4): E2. [http://dx.doi.org/10.3171/2010.2.FOCUS09304] [PMID: 20367359]

[52] LeBlanc JM, Hayden ME, Paulman RG. A comparison of neuropsychological and situational assessment for predicting employability after closed head injury. J Head Trauma Rehabil 2000; 15(4): 1022-40.
[http://dx.doi.org/10.1097/00001199-200008000-00005] [PMID: 10876173]

[53] Sbordone RJ. Limitations of neuropsychological testing to predict the cognitive and behavioral functioning of persons with brain injury in real-world settings. NeuroRehabilitation 2001; 16(4): 199-201.
[PMID: 11790904]

[54] Silver CH. Ecological validity of neuropsychological assessment in childhood traumatic brain injury. J Head Trauma Rehabil 2000; 15(4): 973-88.
[http://dx.doi.org/10.1097/00001199-200008000-00002] [PMID: 10876170]

[55] Honegger J, Buchfelder M, Fahlbusch R. Surgical treatment of craniopharyngiomas: endocrinological results. J Neurosurg 1999; 90(2): 251-7.
[http://dx.doi.org/10.3171/jns.1999.90.2.0251] [PMID: 9950495]

[56] Hoffman HJ, De Silva M, Humphreys RP, Drake JM, Smith ML, Blaser SI. Aggressive surgical management of craniopharyngiomas in children. J Neurosurg 1992; 76(1): 47-52.
[http://dx.doi.org/10.3171/jns.1992.76.1.0047] [PMID: 1727168]

[57] Lyen KR, Grant DB. Endocrine function, morbidity, and mortality after surgery for craniopharyngioma. Arch Dis Child 1982; 57(11): 837-41.
[http://dx.doi.org/10.1136/adc.57.11.837] [PMID: 6293388]

[58] DeVile CJ, Grant DB, Hayward RD, Stanhope R. Growth and endocrine sequelae of craniopharyngioma. Arch Dis Child 1996; 75(2): 108-14.
[http://dx.doi.org/10.1136/adc.75.2.108] [PMID: 8869189]

[59] Bucher H, Zapf J, Torresani T, Prader A, Froesch ER, Illig R. Insulin-like growth factors I and II, prolactin, and insulin in 19 growth hormone-deficient children with excessive, normal, or decreased longitudinal growth after operation for craniopharyngioma. N Engl J Med 1983; 309(19): 1142-6.
[http://dx.doi.org/10.1056/NEJM198311103091902] [PMID: 6353237]

[60] Hayward R. The present and future management of childhood craniopharyngioma. Childs Nerv Syst 1999; 15(11-12): 764-9.
[http://dx.doi.org/10.1007/s003810050468] [PMID: 10603020]

[61] Meuric S, Brauner R, Trivin C, Souberbielle JC, Zerah M, Sainte-Rose C. Influence of tumor location on the presentation and evolution of craniopharyngiomas. J Neurosurg 2005; 103(5) (Suppl.): 421-6. [PMID: 16302613]

[62] Pierre-Kahn A, Recassens C, Pinto G, *et al.* Social and psycho-intellectual outcome following radical removal of craniopharyngiomas in childhood. A prospective series. Childs Nerv Syst 2005; 21(8-9): 817-24.
[http://dx.doi.org/10.1007/s00381-005-1205-6] [PMID: 16049724]

[63] Poretti A, Grotzer MA, Ribi K, Schönle E, Boltshauser E. Outcome of craniopharyngioma in children: long-term complications and quality of life. Dev Med Child Neurol 2004; 46(4): 220-9.
[http://dx.doi.org/10.1111/j.1469-8749.2004.tb00476.x] [PMID: 15077699]

[64] Müller HL, Emser A, Faldum A, *et al.* Longitudinal study on growth and body mass index before and after diagnosis of childhood craniopharyngioma. J Clin Endocrinol Metab 2004; 89(7): 3298-305.
[http://dx.doi.org/10.1210/jc.2003-031751] [PMID: 15240606]

[65] Caldarelli M, Massimi L, Tamburrini G, Cappa M, Di Rocco C. Long-term results of the surgical treatment of craniopharyngioma: the experience at the Policlinico Gemelli, Catholic University, Rome. Childs Nerv Syst 2005; 21(8-9): 747-57.
[http://dx.doi.org/10.1007/s00381-005-1186-5] [PMID: 15995885]

[66] Dhellemmes P, Vinchon M. Radical resection for craniopharyngiomas in children: surgical technique and clinical results. J Pediatr Endocrinol Metab 2006; 19 (Suppl. 1): 329-35.
[PMID: 16700308]

[67] Kalapurakal JA, Goldman S, Hsieh YC, Tomita T, Marymont MH. Clinical outcome in children with craniopharyngioma treated with primary surgery and radiotherapy deferred until relapse. Med Pediatr Oncol 2003; 40(4): 214-8.
[http://dx.doi.org/10.1002/mpo.10247] [PMID: 12555247]

[68] Müller HL, Bueb K, Bartels U, *et al.* Obesity after childhood craniopharyngioma--German multicenter study on pre-operative risk factors and quality of life. Klin Padiatr 2001; 213(4): 244-9.
[http://dx.doi.org/10.1055/s-2001-16855] [PMID: 11528558]

[69] Pereira AM, Schmid EM, Schutte PJ, *et al.* High prevalence of long-term cardiovascular, neurological and psychosocial morbidity after treatment for craniopharyngioma. Clin Endocrinol (Oxf) 2005; 62(2): 197-204.
[http://dx.doi.org/10.1111/j.1365-2265.2004.02196.x] [PMID: 15670196]

[70] Sanford RA. Craniopharyngioma: results of survey of the American Society of Pediatric Neurosurgery. Pediatr Neurosurg 1994; 21 (Suppl. 1): 39-43.
[http://dx.doi.org/10.1159/000120860] [PMID: 7841077]

[71] Cavazzuti V, Fischer EG, Welch K, Belli JA, Winston KR. Neurological and psychophysiological sequelae following different treatments of craniopharyngioma in children. J Neurosurg 1983; 59(3): 409-17.
[http://dx.doi.org/10.3171/jns.1983.59.3.0409] [PMID: 6886754]

CHAPTER 13

Intraventricular Craniopharyngioma?

Jun Pan* and **Yuntao Lu**

Department of Neurosurgery, Nanfang Neurosurgery Research Institution, Nanfang Hospital, Southern Medical University, 1838 North Guangzhou Avenue, Guangzhou, China

Abstract: As we known, adamantinomatous craniopharyngioma (ACP) is thought to originate from residual Rathke's pouch cells along the long axis from nasopharynx to infundibulum [1, 2]. However, the squamous papillary subtype of CP (SPCP) is believed to occur throught squamous metaplasia in the pars tuberalis [2, 3]. In consideration of these inferences, the neural parenchymal layer of third ventricular floor (3rd VF) should locate above the CP, separate both the tumor and third ventricular chamber. However, the first study conducted by Dubos *et al.* in 1953 extensively reported the tumors completely located inside the third ventricle cavity by autopsy or intraoperative finding [4-13]. Because of this topographical location, the theory of CP origin has been challenged and much more neurosurgeons are interested in pursuing the true morphological characteristics and diagnostic criteria of these tumors [9, 14]. In this chapter, we firstly reviewed the definition of the intraventricular CP in several publications. Then based on our histological and clinical study, the true morphology of intraventricular CP was proposed. The related approach selection and surgical skills was also depicted.

Keywords: Craniopharyngioma, Intraventricular, Third ventricular floor.

INTRAVENTRICULAR CP (*IVC*) DEFINITION

IVC refers to those craniopharyngioma located completely in the third ventricle. According to the literature reviewing, most diagnosis of IVCs was based on preoperative magnetic resonance imaging (MRI). The intraventricular tumor location determined diagnostic proof [6, 7, 9, 15, 16]. The criteria for IVC diagnosis in the previous literature included [5, 6, 17]: 1) Normal pituitary stalk, 2) absence of sellar abnormality on presurgical MRI images(PS), and 3) a patent suprasellar cistern (Fig. **1**).

As the matter of fact, the terminology of "pure" or "strict" IVC in the literature a lso indicated some primary perplexity about the topographic relationship

* **Corresponding author Jun Pan**: Department of Neurosurgery, Nanfang Neurosurgery Research Institution, Nanfang Hospital, Southern Medical University, 1838 North Guangzhou Avenue, Guangzhou, China; Tel\Fax: +8620-61641806; E-mail: panjundu@hotmail.com

Songtao Qi (Ed.)

between 3rd VF and IVC, In 2004, Pascual [18] concluded two disparate topographic entities, and proposed strictly or nonstrictly IVC following an extensive review of CPs with intraventricular location, . Our understanding of IVC has been helped much by this concept . As our opinion, three criterias should be used to identify a "strict" IVC. These were a pre-, intra-, and postoperatively identifiably intact 3rd VF. Our reported schematic drawings [19] illustrated in detail the different stratification of strict and nonstrict IVCs. We considerd the theoretically topographical relationships between tumor and 3rd VF were described as follows:

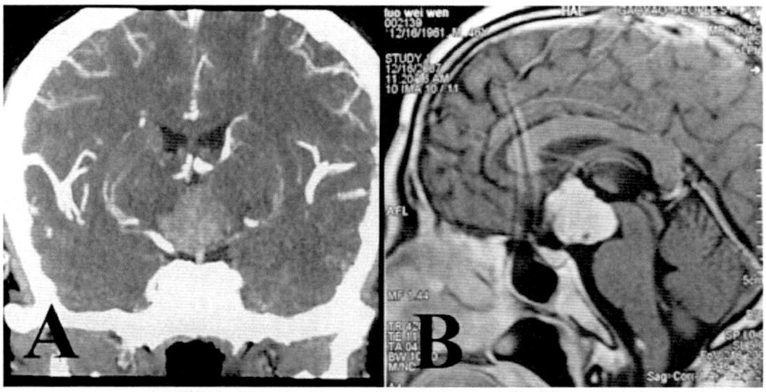

Fig. (1). Presurgical computed tomography (Left: Coronal) and magnetic resonance imaging scans (Right: Sagittal) of a 45-year-old male patient that satisfied the traditional radiological criteria for intraventricular craniopharyngioma diagnosis.

1. Suprasellar tumor that pushes the intact 3rd VF upward (pseudointraventricular CP);
2. Suprasellar mass that protrudes the 3rd VF and enters the third ventricle cavity (secondarily ICP);
3. Intraventricular mass within the third ventricle cavity and 3rd VF, the latter of which is replaced by tumor (nonstrictly IVC); and
4. Intraventricular mass exclusively located in the third ventricle cavity with an intact floor lying below its inferior surface (strictly IVC).

As Pascual indicated, 3rd VF intactness is essential for the diagnosis of true IVC [5, 18], he also illustrated that the prognosis of "strictly IVC" (sIVC) subtype was better then the other. In our recent article (Qi *et al.*) [19], we have summarized the morphological features of IVC based on 17 cases of CP that met the diagnostic criteria of IVC. We concluded that IVC, even those classified as "strictly IVC" and located completely inside the cavity with no significant ependymal or neural tissue coverage, still closely adhered to the 3rd VF by a pedicle stem. As depicted in previous reports, the terms "strictly" or "nonstrictly" IVC do not refer to the true growth patterns of CPs located completely within the third ventricle cavity

[18, 19]. All IVCs have a similar site of origin, whether "strictly" or "nonstrictly", and the observed variations come from differential growth and variable patterns of invasion into adjacent structures.

EMBRYONIC THEORY OF IVC ORIGIN

As mentioned above, CPs with an exclusive intraventricular location challenge the theory of CP origin, as there is no obvious access of ascent from Rathke's pouch-derived epithelial cells to third ventricle cavity. Rush *et al.* [20] believed that these intraventricular tumors might result from the upward growth of squamous cell nests which come from the 3rd VF near tuber cinereum. Konovalov *et al.* [21] demonstrated microscopic areas of the tumor glial capsule in the boundary of anterior part of third ventricle. Finally, Ciric and Cozzens suggested the following hypothesis regarding the development of IVCs: IVCs come from resting epithelial cells (remnants of Rathke's pouch) and are observed within the neuroectoderm of developing cerebral vesicle. This happens as the pars tuberalis attacts with the diencephalic infundibular evagination, and before the pia mater covers the basal brain surface [22]. As they constantly, grow, some tumors would be weak, and finally protrude from the ependymal layer to simulate a so-called intrinsic IVC, which remains covered by a negligible ependymal cellular layer (Type I in Fig. (**2**)). Other tumors may fill the third ventricle chamber cavity but remain implanted within the thinning neural tissue layer of the 3rd VF (Type II in Fig. **2**).

DEMOGRAPHY, INCIDENCE AND CLINICAL PRESENTATION

IVCs tend to occur in older patients [15]. As indicated in the previous literature, IVCs rarely occur in pediatric patients. After retrospectively reviewing our 195 cases of CP, including 81 pediatric cases (<17 years), only two were considered IVC according to the radiological criteria.

Regarding the pathological features, SPCP was predominant, suggesting a predilection of SPCPs for the third ventricle. In our cohort of 19 cases of SPCPs, six had intraventricular locations (31.6%).

Given the relatively rare incidence of these tumors, the true mobidity of IVC has not been adequately studied, so, the existing case series are accordingly small in number. Mori *et al.* [23] found tumors separated in the third ventricle in six of 155 cases. Sweet [24] introduced similar intra-surgical evidence from two cases. In 1990, Yasargil *et al.* [25] reviewed 144 patients who had suffered microsurgical removal and noted six patients in whom the tumors were confined to the ventricle with few hypothalamic adhesions. The incidence of IVC has ranged from 0.7 to 11% [26, 27] of all CPs in the previous literature. After reviewing 195 cases of primary CP, we identified 17 cases of IVC that accounted for 8.7% of all CPs.

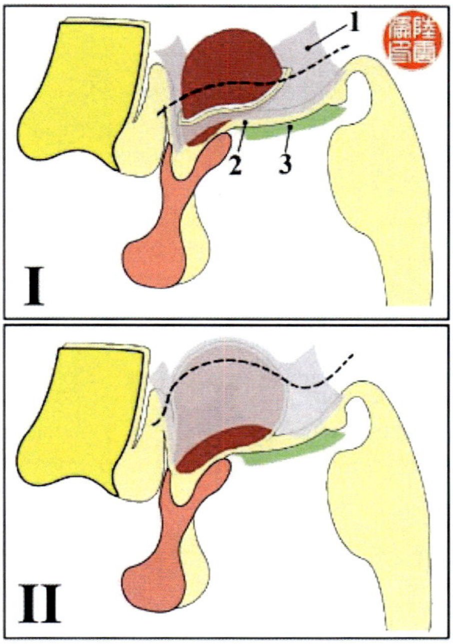

Fig. (2). (Reference from Pan Jun *et al.* [19]). Intraventricular craniopharyngioma stratification. **Type I:** Tumor protrusion into the third ventricular cavity with a negligible ependymal cellular layer (1) and nervous layer (2) covering; **Type II:** Tumor localization inside the ventricular floor with a significant ependymal cellular layer and nervous layer covering the surface of tumor. Both types of tumors are located inside the pia mater layer (3).

The clinical presentation of IVC differs from that of the more common sellar and suprasellar variety. Given to eventual obstructive hydrocephalus, patients with IVC present with headache and increased intracranial pressure rather than primary visual deterioration [28]. Suprasellar CP usually present visual symptoms and signs (28.5%) and endocrine dysfunction (27.5%). Basing on an comprehensive review of well-described cases of CPs with an intraventricular location, Pascual [18] summarized that these symptoms are not very frequent with IVC, while others like mental disturbances (40%), memory dysfunction (33.3%), somnolence (29.5%), and gait disturbances (17%), which do not commonly present with CP, are commonly reported in studies of IVC.

Among the 17 cases of IVC in our cohort, 64.7% (11/17) presented with increased intracranial pressure, and 47.1% (8/17) had cognitive disturbances (disorientation, confusion, apathy, delirium, and memory disturbances). Notably, visual deficits (47.1%, 8/17) and diabetes insipidus (DI) (17.6% 3/17) occurred at a lower incidence in these patients than among those with suprasellar CP [29 - 31]. Somnolence was observed in 17.6% (3/17) of IVC cases, and the most common etiology was hydrocephalus secondary to tumor. Growth retardation was recorded in both pediatric cases, and one of them was more complicated because of the additional symptom of epilepsy.

NEUROIMAGING

Migliori and colleagues [32] differentiate an IVC from a suprasellar tumor according to the radiologic criteria that invaginates the 3rd VF as follows: a coronal computed tomography (CT) or coronal or sagittal MRI scan should definitely reveal an integrated 3rd VF, normal PS, patent suprasellar cistern, and absence of sellar abnormality. Recently, as Qi *et al.* pointed out, preoperative MRI does not correlate directly with the relationship between tumor and 3rd VF. Identification of the 3rd VF *via* preoperative MRI not always indicate a completely intraventricular tumor. Intraventricular tumors, even those classed as "strictly IVC" and located completely within the cavity without ependymal or neural tissue coverage, still feature a pedicle stem closely adhered to the 3rd VF. Only intraoperatively observed and histologically confirmed anatomical stratifications form the foundation for the distinction between "strictly" and "nonstrictly" IVC (rather than pre-, intra-, or postoperative inspection of 3rd VF preservation).

The prevalence of calcification and cystic IVC tumors in the images was reported in several papers, although the results vary widely. The main reason for this variability is the different pathological constituent ratios of the tumors. Because SPCP rarely presents with calcification and cystic tumor, some authors commented that IVC appears as a solid mass without calcification. According to our experience, both ACP and SPCP may be intraventricular, and SPCP may also be accompanied by cystic changes (Fig. **3**). Moreover, the frequency of calcification in our cohort was 52.9% (9/17). Therefore, our opinion is that calcification and cystic change remain among the radiological features of IVC that should be addressed before surgery.

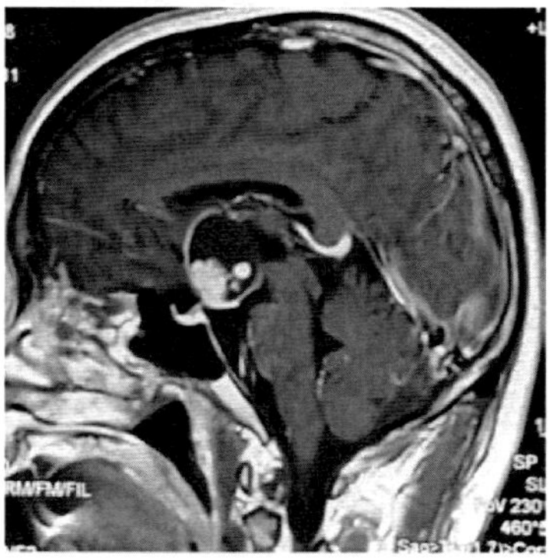

Fig. (3). Pre-operative magnetic resonance imaging revealed intratumoral cyst formation in a 41-year-old male patient. Post-operative pathological study affirmed a typical squamous papillary craniopharyngioma.

SURGICAL REMOVAL OF IVCS

Surgical Strategy

Surgical IVC resection faces with key problems refering to deep localization, the risk of damage to the hypothalamic structures and optic pathways. Pascual reported that overall outcome of IVC was better than that of suprasellar CP with third ventricle involvement. We agree with his comments and also think that radical IVC removal should be advocated because of the high likelihood of a more safe total removal.

Stratification of the 3rd VF and its Relationship with CP

During surgery, the relationship between the tumor and 3rd VF is quite important, a point that was ignored in previous literature reports. According to the traditional conception of IVC, the tumor should be located solely inside the ventricular cavity, and therefore the vital nervous tissue of the ventricular floor should be located entirely underneath the tumor. However, many reports described partial tumor removal because of tumor adherence to the 3rd VF. Because of these differences in adherence, Pascual summarized and divided IVCs into two groups: "strictly" and "nonstrictly" IVC. In our further study, as proposed by Qi et al, the IVC–3rd VF relationship was considered according to three different morphological types:

(a) pedicle affiliation: the tumor is only affiliated to the anterior part of 3rd VF at the infundibulum, the boundary and posterior part of 3rd VF remain intact without adherence, and the 3rd VF remains intact after total tumor resection; (b) wide adherence with a dissectible tumor boundary: although can be safely dissected from the parenchyma, the tumor forms a wide adherence to the third ventricle wall allowing adequate debulking followed by tracing of the tumor capsule, and the integrity of 3rd VF can be protected after total tumor resection but with membranous recession; and (c) wide tight attachment: given to the tumor tightly adhered to the wall, dissection of the tumor from the 3rd VF is quite difficult that necessitate a sacrifice of the parenchyma to complete the removal.

Additionally, a histological analysis revealed two tumor stratification types among IVC:

1. Tumors intruding into the third ventricular cavity with negligible ependymal and nerve tissue layer.
2. Tumors covered by intermittent ependymal cells and a thin nerve tissue layer.

Among 17 cases of IVC in our cohort, only two were found to have tumors purely located within the ventricle cavity without nerve tissue layer coverage. In the majority of cases, tumors actually grew inside the nerve tissue layer parenchyma. During surgery, the tumor capsule was dissected and removed from the surrounding gliosis layer.

Approach Selection

Given their location, IVCs should be resected *via* the approaches used to access other primary intraventricular tumors. The surgical approach can be divided into two types according to the different usage of the surgical space:

1. Frontal–basal interhemispheric trans-terminal approach. This approach, which is essentially a skull base approach, offering the shortest distance to third ventricle and is the most commonly used approach. Utilization of the trans-lamina terminalis (trans-LT) approach places the columns of fornix, tuber cinereum, optic pathway, supraoptic nuclei, and organ vasculosum at risk on account of retraction injury or perforation damage [33, 34].
2. Trans-callosal approach, including interfornical exposure [35, 36], and entrance through the foramen of Monro. The trans-cortical route to the lateral ventricles could also be utilized to approach these craniopharyngiomas [4, 10, 12, 13, 17, 19, 20, 28, 30, 37 - 41]. However, as cortical incision inclines the patient towards edema and seizures, the above approaches were abolished in stages during the epoch of modern neurosurgery. The interhemispheric trans-callosal approach to the third ventricle is endurable and easy to operate, whereas, the distance involved is greater than that of the basic approaches. Damage to the columns of fornix may result in memory deficits, and injury to the veins of the superficial or deep venous systems may lead to venous infarction.

In a few case reports, the inferior occipital splenium of the corpus callosum was selected to treat IVCs with posterior locations in a manner similar to the Poppen approach. However, this approach is seldom used in clinical practice because of the complex deep venous system, approach procedure, and high prevalence of complications.

The trans-LT route is often used to resect IVCs [7, 17, 27, 34, 40, 42 - 44]. This approach can offer a direct permission to the anterior part of third ventricle, where the tumor adheres in the tuber cinereum region. The LT is enterable either along the medial part of frontotemporal approach (including some enlarged approaches with removal of the orbital roof and anterior clinoid process) [25, 45, 46] or *via* an anterior interhemispheric approach [25, 30, 34, 41, 47 - 51]. The lateral approach provides oblique angle to view the LT, which increases difficulty to observe the posterior part of third ventricle. And finally makes it difficult to open the entire

LT. So, providing tumors with broad and tight adhere to the third ventricle wall and/or floor, dissecting the tumor *via* the lateral approach cannot be easy and safe because of the less exposure for the posterior part of third ventricle. On the other aspect, the anterior interhemispheric approach, provides a appropriate view of entire LT. Tumors can be resected either through the space anterior to the anterior communicating artery (AcoA) or, more often, through the bilateral A2 space in cases where the AcoA locates close to the optic chiasm. If the AcoA limits the operative exposure, it can be safely dissected in some cases [49, 50]. Following the tumor boundary through a relatively narrow space like LT sometimes cause extreme difficulties. Internal decompression either by the piecemeal extirpation of solid tumor parts or aspirating cystic components can enlarge the space and thus facilitate removal of the tumor from the third ventricle margins.

Anatomic basis of the ventricle floor and walls and the infundibulum is of most importance during tumor resection. The irregular pattern of adherence among the tumor, 3rd VF, and walls needs special attention. This pattern play a vital role when surgeon makes decision about the possible extent of tumoral resection and predicts the feasibility of preserving the 3rd VF and hypothalamic structures [18]. After opening the LT, a precise inspection of the superior aspect of tumor surface is needed immediately to identify whether the tumor possesses a nerve tissue layer. surgeon should always keep in mind that in the majority of cases the tumor capsule is dissected and removed from the adjacent layer of gliosis, except for a few tumors that shows growth pattern "a". This neuroglial layer, which intervenes between tumor and viable hypothalamic nuclei, may provide a safe dissection area [52] through which total lesion resection can be manipulated in most cases. However, there are dense adhesions that make it impossible for surgeon to follow along a clear plane of cleavage without leading to severe damage to viable neural tissues in some cases.

CASE PRESENTATION

Case No. 1 (Male Patient, 46 Years Old)

Clinical Manifestation

The patient complained of intermittent fever of 10 months' duration, with the highest body temperature reaching 39.4°C. The patient also experienced thirst and polydipsia for 1 month and drank approximately 4000–5000 ml water per day. Other symptoms included a 10-day history of lethargy, disorientation, and confusion.

Physical Examination

No significant abnormalities were found during a fundus examination. The body mass index (BMI) was 22.1, within the normal range of reference values for Chinese adult men.

Chemical Examination

A normal blood and urine routine analysis revealed low plasma thyroxine and free T4 levels; a low progesterone level was revealed through endocrinological detection. An insulin stimulation test for cortisol and growth hormone (GH) revealed subnormal responses.

Neuroimaging Study

A suprasellar isodense neoplasm without calcification and cystic formation occupied the third ventricular cavity as indicated by presurgical CT (Fig. **4**). The tumor size was $4 \times 3.3 \times 3.7$ cm^3. The pituitary stalk could be identified clearly in the coronal CT scan (Fig. **1**). Uniform lesion enhancement was detected *via* enhanced CT. Slight ventricle enlargement was accompanied by obstructive hydrocephalus.

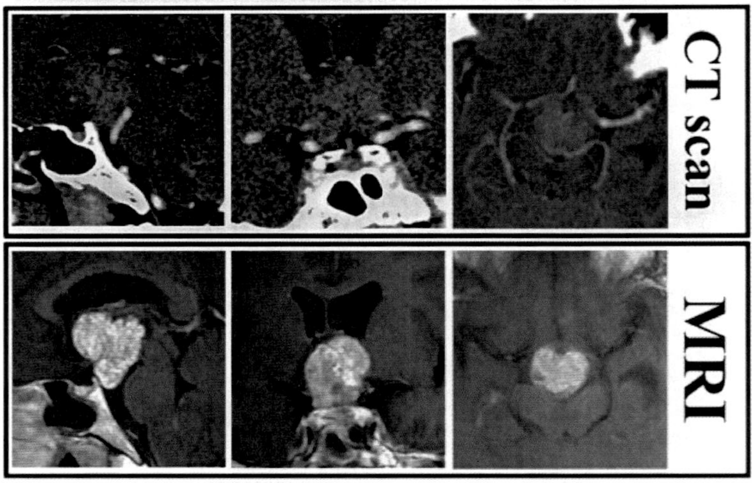

Fig. (4). Presurgical computed tomography and magnetic resonance imaging data from Case 1.

Conventional MRI

A purely solid mass was found within the third ventricle cavity. A normal PS, absence of sellar abnormality, and patent suprasellar cistern were also identified *via* preoperative MRI. A full-length PS was identifiable in the suprasellar cistern

(Fig. **4**). Contrast enhancement of the neoplasm was visible with Gd-DTPA MRI.

Surgery

General Considerations

1. Tumor location: entirely within the third ventricular cavity.
2. Surgical and topographical tumor classifications: tubero-infundibular tumor (Type c1) and subarachnoidal tumor (Type Sa).
3. Relationship to the AcoA: the AcoA complex was pushed downward and anteriorly.
4. Surgical excision should be the first-line therapy. A frontobasal interhemispheric (FIH) approach was finally selected to reach the lesion.

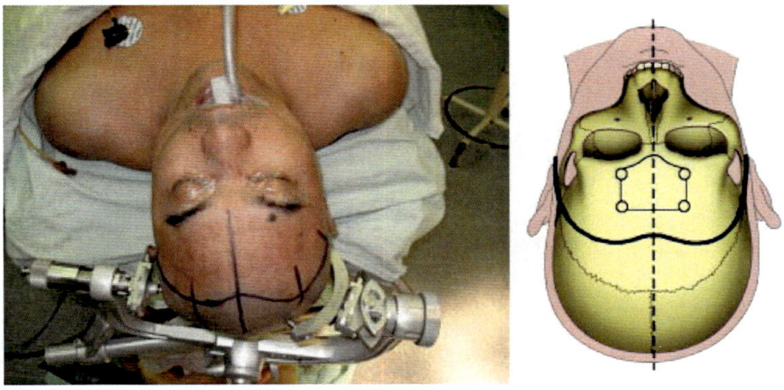

Fig. (5). Illustration of the operating position and incision *via* the frontobasal intrahemispheric approach.

Operative Findings

1. *Craniotomy:* A coronal incision was made, and the skin flap was turned over to the nasal side (Fig. **5**). A forehead periosteal square was maintained for further frontal sinus repair. The bone flap extended beyond the median line, and the lowest margin remained as close as possible to the base of the anterior cranial fossa. The mucosa inside the frontal sinus was removed carefully after completing the bone window opening. The bone was removed from the posterior sinus wall and drilled to provide more exposure. Bone wax with antibiotic powder was then used to completely fill the sinus cavity, thus reducing the risk of intracranial infection. A curved incision near the skull base was made to open the bilateral dura mater next to the superior sagittal sinus. Next, the anterior part of superior sagittal sinus was ligated, followed by the dissection of the cerebral falx. The dura flap was turned over rewards.
2. *Dissection of the Interhemispheric Fissure:* A self-retaining retractor was used to retract the bilateral frontal lobe. Along the inter-hemispheric corridor, the

bilateral frontal lobes were separated and the CSF was drained to the extent possible. Fronto-interhemispheric fissure dissection is occasionally much more complex than dissection with the lateral trans-sylvian approach, especially in patients with increased intracranial pressure. Continuous drainage of lumbar CSF during dissection is a valid method of releasing this pressure. The planum sphenoidale, optic chiasm, and cisterna lamina terminalis were exposed stepwise with the tumbling of the frontal lobe.

3. *Tumor Exposure:* The AcoA complex obstructed exposure of the entire lamina terminalis, as did the two sidewise dragging of the frontal lobe. The AcoA was interrupted after carefully evaluating its angioarchitecture. After vertical incising the ballooning lamina terminalis, thetop surface of the tumor was carefully checked. A small amount of CSF was encountered in the small potential third ventricular cavity. The tumor seemed to be oriented within the ventricular cavity and was covered by a negligibly thin membrane-like layer (Fig. **6**). However, this membrane layer was present as shown in (Fig. **6F**).
4. *Tumor Removal:* Internal decompression by extirpating the piecemeal of the solid parts of tumor helped to expand the space, thus facilitating tumor dissection from the third ventricle margins. The tumor had only developed a pedicle attachment to the anterior part of 3rd VF at the infundibulum, whereas the boundary and posterior part of the 3rd VF remained intact with no adherence (Fig. **4**). The tumor was removed in a piecemeal manner and the 3rd VF was properly persevered after total tumor resection, though there was some attenuation at the adherent infundibular site (Fig. **7**).

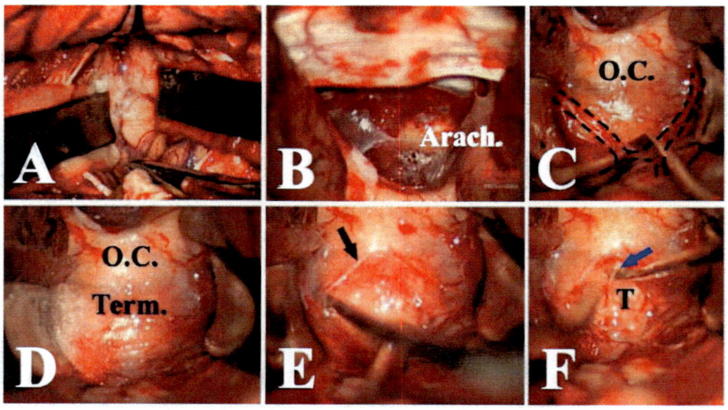

Fig. (6). Tumor exposure *via* the frontobasal interhemispheric approach. **A:** The bilateral frontal lobes and hemispheric fissure were shown after completing the craniotomy. **B:** Through the prechiasmatic space, only suprasellar arachnoid (Arach.) layers were found to envelope the pituitary stalk. No tumor was found. **C:** The tumor was observed through the semitransparent lamina terminalis. The anterior communicating artery (AcoA; indicated by dotted line) covered superior surface of the terminalis and obstructed tumor removal. **D:** The AcoA was dissected to sufficiently expose the tumor. **E.** The terminalis membrane (*black arrow*) was dissected and lifted. **F:** The second membranous layer (*blue arrow*) was found to cover the tumor surface and was thought to comprise extremely inflated nervous and ependymal layers. **O.C.,** Optic chiasm; **T,** Tumor.

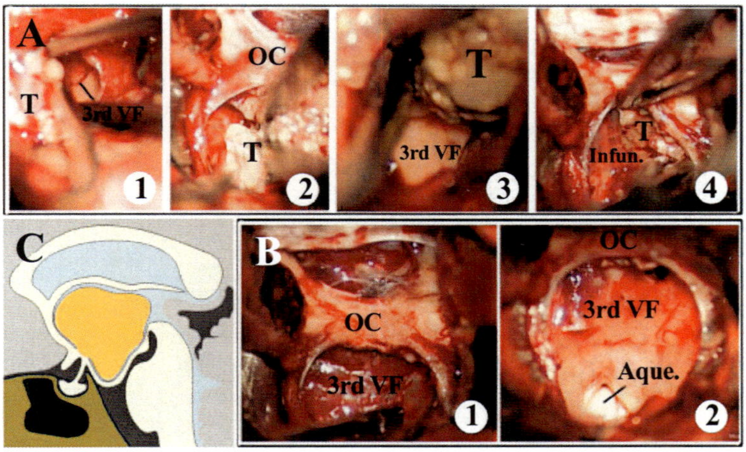

Fig. (7). (Reference from Pan, J., *et al.* [19]). Exposure and removal of the tumor. **A:** It can be certified that there is a vital bilateral interface between the tumor and third ventricular walls on the posterior side (①②③). On the pedicle side (④), the tumor adhered tightly to the tubero-infundibular part. **B:** Following tumor removal, an intact third ventricular floor (3rd VF) and bilateral walls were observed through the opened lamina terminalis (① and ②). The midbrain aqueduct was also observed (②). **C:** A schematic diagram of tumor growth pattern "a". Cerebrospinal fluid is indicated in blue. The tumors is completely located in the ventricular cavity with only one pedicle connected to the 3rd VF. Besides, a potential ventricular space is recorded among the tumor and ventricular walls. **OC,** optical chiasm; **T,** tumor; **Infun.,** infundibulum, **Aque.,** aqueduct of midbrain.

Pathology Study

Typical SPCP was identified on the pathological slides (Fig. **8**). After bluntly separating the tumor from a very thin secondary membrane-like layer, a square of the tumor mass was dissected from the top for histological testing and IVC stratification. As indicated in Fig. (**8**), the tumor was covered with a negligible and extremely thin nervous and ependymal layer and was classified as Type I stratification.

Postoperative Course

Postoperatively, the patient suffered mild, transient DI. The symptoms were relieved by fluid and electrolyte replacement. Endocrinological testing detected low levels of plasma thyroxine, testosterone, and progesterone suggestive of hypopituitarism. Other complications like somnolence, hydrocephalus, and cognitive disturbances suffered similar resolution.

A half-year after surgery, follow-up data revealed improving hypopituitarism with normal levels of plasma thyroxine and free T4. The patient's sexual function had also improved significantly according to the patient. Otherwise, he suffered from moderate weight gain, with an increase in BMI to 28.1 at 3 months post-operatively, although this decreased gradually thereafter.

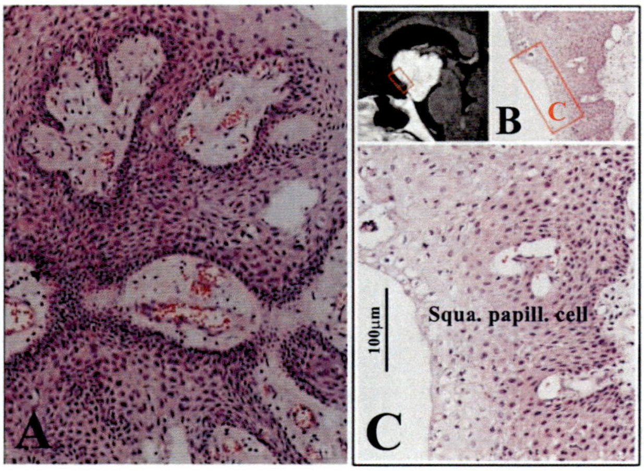

Fig. (8). (Reference from Pan, J., *et al.* [19]). Type I stratification of an IVC. The red square on the presurgical magnetic resonance image indicates the location of tumor specimen (hematoxylin and eosin staining). After peeling back the secondary membranous layer, the tumor mass was subjected to histological detection. **A:** Macroview of the tumor mass (40× magnification); the red-square area is magnified in the Fig. (B; **B (400×):** The smooth outer tumor surface with a typical cover of stratified squamous epithelium can be certified. **Squa.-paplill. Cell,** squamous-papillary cell.

A postoperative MRI study after 3 months showed total tumor removal and adequately maintained 3rd VF thickness (Fig. **9**).

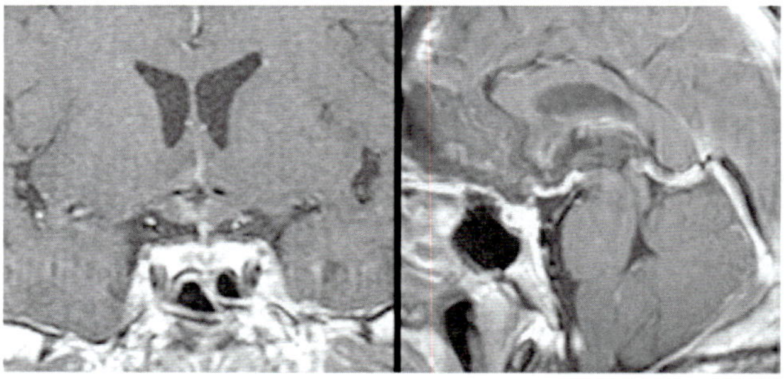

Fig. (9). Postsurgical magnetic resonance imaging indicated total tumor removal. The pituitary stalk and third ventricular floor remained intact.

Case No. 2 (Boy, 7 Years Old)

Clinical Manifestation

The patient complained of headache with gradually increasing severity of 2 weeks' duration, accompanied by a 1-week history of vomiting, thirst, and polydipsia. The volume of drinking water consumed daily by the patient was approximately 2000–3000 ml.

Physical Examination

The patient presented with growth retardation (body height = 125 mm) and mild weight gain (BMI index = 23.1, within the normal range of reference values for Chinese boys). No other abnormalities were observed. A fundus examination revealed bilateral optic atrophy.

Chemical Examination

The routine blood and urine analysis results were normal. Slightly increased plasma prolactin (PRL) levels were detected *via* endocrinological testing; other plasma hormones levels were normal. An insulin stimulation test for cortisol and GH revealed a subnormal GH response and normal cortisol response.

Neuroimaging Study

A cranial CT scan indicated a suprasellar cystic lesion without calcification. MRI (Fig. **11**) revealed a tumor that occupied the third ventricular cavity. The cystic fluid was hyperintense and hypointense in T2- and T1-weighted images, respectively. A patent suprasellar cistern, normal PS, and absence of sellar abnormalities were observed on preoperative MR images. A full-length PS was identifiable in the suprasellar cistern (Fig. **10**). Significant contrast enhancement of the neoplasm was observed with Gd-DTPA MRI. The supratentorial ventricle enlarged slightly with obstructive hydrocephalus.

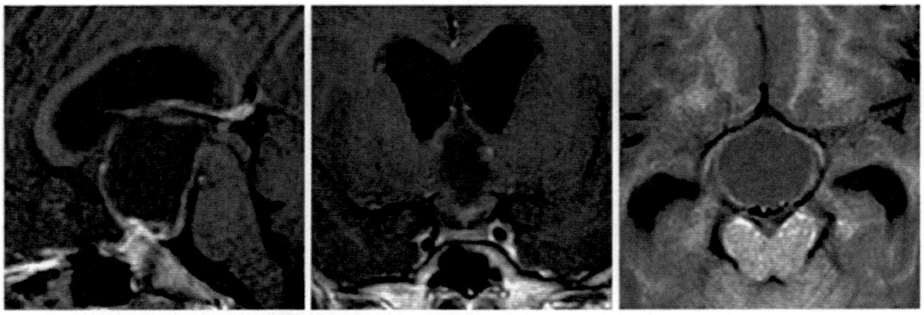

Fig. (10). Presurgical magnetic resonance imaging indicated the cystic tumor occupied the third ventricular cavity. The full-length pituitary stalk was identifiable.

Surgery

General Considerations

1. A predominantly cystic tumor located entirely within the third ventricular cavity.

2. Surgical and topographical tumor classification: tubero-infundibular tumor (Type c1) and subarachnoidal tumor (Type Sa).
3. Relationship with the AcoA: the AcoA complex was pushed downward and anteriorly, causing a fairly small prechiasmatic space that could not be used.
4. Significant enhancement of the tumor cystic wall suggested the strong possibility of a tumor margin with tight adhesions to the third ventricular walls.
5. It was impossible to use the trans-callosal and extra-axial approaches to dissect these adhesions under direct surgical exposure. The frontobasal interhemispheric trans-LT approach was selected to reach the lesion.

Operative Findings

1. *Craniotomy:* The craniotomy procedure was similar to that in Case 1. Craniotomy was more convenient because of the poor frontal sinus pneumatization in the pediatric patient.
2. *Dissection of the Interhemispheric Fissure:* A self-retaining retractor was used to retract the bilateral frontal lobe, similar to Case 1. Notably, brain tissue is more fragile in children than in adults, so sufficient CSF drainage was necessary. The other procedures were the same as in Case 1. The planum sphenoidale, optic chiasm, and cisterna lamina terminalis were exposed in a stepwise manner following the tumbling of the frontal lobe.
3. *Tumor Exposure:* The optic chiasm and AcoA complex were squeezed dorsally toward the tuberculum sellae (Fig. **11A**). Therefore, the AcoA complex obstructed exposure of the entire lamina terminalis and the two sidewise dragging of the frontal lobe. The AcoA was interrupted after careful analysis of its angioarchitecture (Fig. **11A**). After vertically incising the ballooned lamina terminalis, the upper tumor surface was carefully inspected. A small amount of CSF was encountered in the small potential third ventricular cavity. The tumor seemed to be located within the ventricular cavity and was covered by an unidentifiable, extremely thin, membrane-like layer (Fig. **11C**).
4. *Tumor Removal:* Internal decompression *via* piecemeal extirpation of the solid tumor sections provided space in which to help removing tumor from the third ventricle boundary. The tumor had only developed a pedicle attachment to the anterior part of 3rd VF at the infundibulum, while the walls and posterior part of the 3rd VF remained intact with no adhesions (Fig. **11B**). The tumor was removed in a piecemeal manner and the 3rd VF was properly persevered after total tumor resection, although there was some attenuation at the adherent site of the infundibulum (Fig. **11B**).

Pathology Study

Typical ACP was diagnosed from the pathological slides. Hematoxylin and eosin (H.E.) staining of a square histological specimen from the tumor roof showed that the tumor remained wrapped by a thin layer of neural tissue. Ependymal cells were recorded in some areas. Typically, the cystic wall of the IVC contained an outer gliosis layer and an inner adamantinomatous cell layer (Fig. **12**). The tumor was classified as Type II IVC.

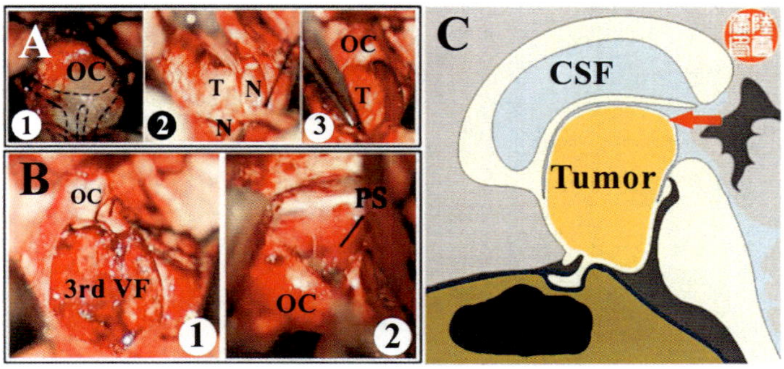

Fig. (11). (Reference from Pan, J., *et al.* [19]). A**:** Intrasurgical findings. Upon exposing the lamina terminalis, the tumor was observed behind interrupted anterior communicating artery (dotted line indicates the artery's original location) (1). A well-defined interface among tumor and third ventricular walls can be followed along the tumor capsule despite extensive adherence to nervous layer (2). During the process of tumor removal, the pedicle side of tumor was observed to cling tightly to the third ventricle floor (3); **B:** Following tumor resection, the integrity of the 3rd VF can be preserved although its intactness was damaged due to the broad adherence. The PS remained intact, as observed across the prechiasmatic space; **C:** A schematic diagram of the tumor growth pattern "b" (blue area: CSF). The tumor was located inside the ventricular floor parenchyma with a wide basis and remained wrapped by a thin nervous layer, as directed by the red arrow. **OC,** optical chiasm; **T,** Tumor; **N,** nervous layer of the 3rd VF; **PS,** pituitary stalk.

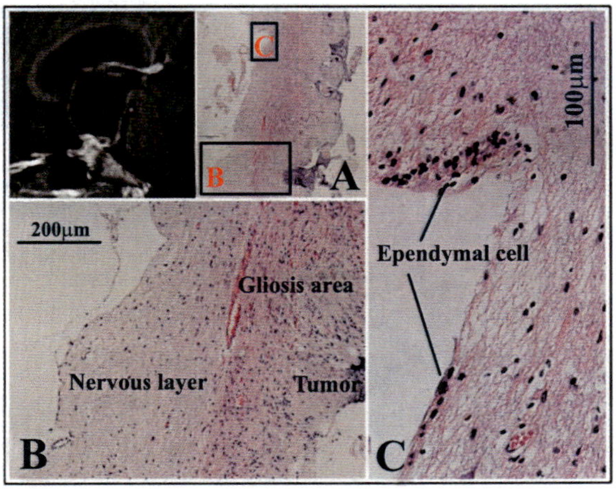

Fig. (12). (Reference from Pan, J., *et al.* [19]). Type II stratification of an intraventricular tumor. On the presurgical magnetic resonance image, the red square indicates the location of the tumor specimen (hematoxylin and eosin staining). **A:** Macroview of the tumor mass (40×); the red-square area in magnified in **B** and **C**. **B:** a thin nervous layer was observed covering the upside of the tumor cystic wall (200×). In addition, two different histological layers could be certified in the cystic wall: the outer gliosis area and inner adamantinomatous cell layer. **C**:Several cuboid epithelial cells can be observed to cover the outer surface of the nervous layer in some areas; these were considered ependymal cells (400×).

Postoperative Course

Postoperatively, the patient suffered mild transient DI, which was palliated by fluid and electrolyte replacement. Endocrinological testing revealed slightly low levels of plasma thyroxine, testosterone, and progesterone, suggesting hypopituitarism. Other complications like headache and hydrocephalus resolved in a parallel manner as described for Case 1.

At 1 year after surgery, the patient's pituitary function had improved. The levels of plasma thyroxine and free T4 recovered. However, the levels of testosterone and progesterone remained low. His BMI index was 25.2 at the last follow-up.

A postoperative MRI study indicated total tumor removal with proper 3rd VF preservation (Fig. **13**).

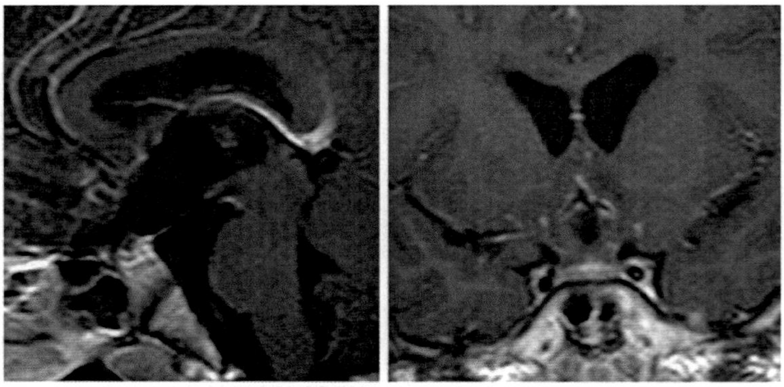

Fig. (13). Postsurgical magnetic resonance indicated total tumor removal. The pituitary stalk and third ventricular floor remained intact.

Case No. 3 (Woman, 50 Years Old, Recurrent Case)

Clinical Manifestation

The patient complained of CP recurrence after undergoing primary surgery and radiotherapy 9 and 4 years earlier, respectively. She had suffered three seizures as well as severe dizziness and mental disorders in the previous 6 months. Nine years ago, she had undergone the tumor removal *via* the trans-callosal approach after presenting with dizziness and a mental disorder. Four years ago, she had undergone conformal modulating radiotherapy after a tumor recurrence was identified on follow-up MRI. Her visual acuity decreased after radiotherapy. Two weeks before admission to our department, MRI again detected a tumor recurrence.

Physical Examination

The patient exhibited lethargy, slow reactivity, and personality changes. A fundus examination indicated bilateral optic atrophy. Her BMI index was 22.1, within the normal range of reference values for Chinese adult women.

Chemical Examination

No significant abnormalities were found in a routine blood and urine analysis. Low levels of plasma thyroxine and free T4 and a low progesterone level were detected in an endocrinological examination. The insulin stimulation test for cortisol and GH revealed subnormal responses.

Neuroimaging Study

A plain CT scan confirmed a recurrent tumor at the anterior part of third ventricle. The anterior horn of left lateral ventricle was enlarged. Additionally, a local brain tissue defect from the previous surgery was observed. The tumor size was 2.4 × 2.3 × 1.9 cm^3 with uniform enhancement (Fig. **14**). Conventional MRI indicated a purely solid mass located at the anterior part of the third ventricle cavity. A patent suprasellar cistern, normal PS, and absence of sellar abnormalities were identifiable on the presurgical MR images Fig. (**14**), and uniform enhancement was observed with Gd-DTPA MRI.

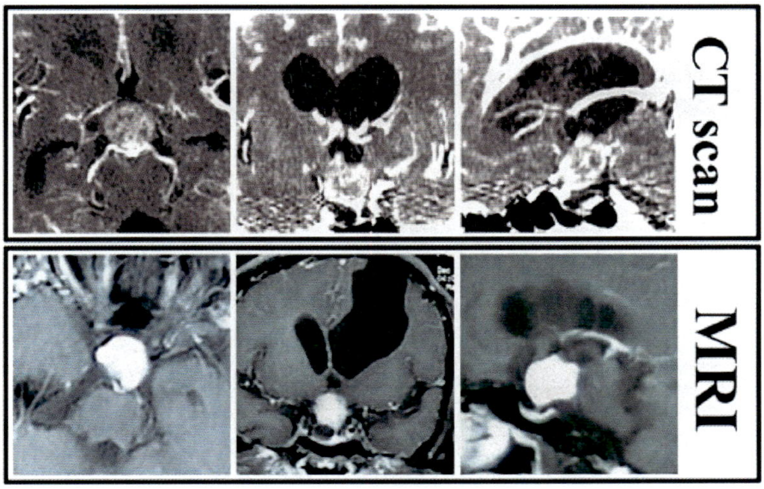

Fig. (14). Presurgical computed tomography and magnetic resonance images. A recurrent tumor was found inside the third ventricular cavity. A patent suprasellar cistern and intact PS were observed. The left side of the lateral ventricle had been opened during the primary surgery.

Surgery

General Considerations

1. A solid predominated tumor located purely in the third ventricular cavity with origination from the tubero-infundibulum.
2. Surgical and topographical tumor classification: tubero-infundibular tumor (Type c1) and subarachnoidal tumor (Type Sa).
3. Small tumor size and significant enlargement of the bilateral ventricles and foramen of Monro.
4. The trans-callosal approach was selected to reach the lesion.

Operative Findings

1. *Craniotomy:* As indicated in Fig. (**15**), a bone flap was opened on the left side of the frontal bone around the coronal suture and beyond the median line. The dura mater was subsequently dissected and turned over with the basement on the superior sagittal sinus.
2. *Tumor Exposure and Removal:* The tumor was exposed *via* the enlarged foramen of Monro (Fig. **16**). The tumor adhered tightly to the anterior part of 3rd VF at the infundibulum, where sharp dissection was necessary. Separation of the tumor from the lateral wall of third ventricle caused a neuroparenchymal defect at the tubero-infundibulum. The structures inside the suprasellar cistern were observed through this defect. The tumor was removed in a piecemeal manner. The 3rd VF developed a local defect at the adherent site of infundibulum (Fig. **16**).

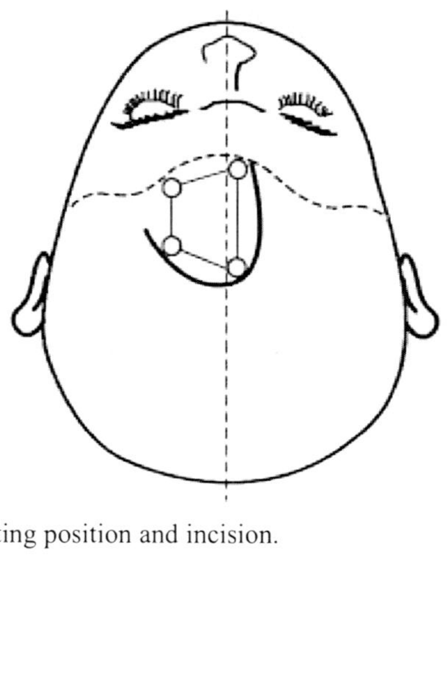

Fig. (15). Illustration of the operating position and incision.

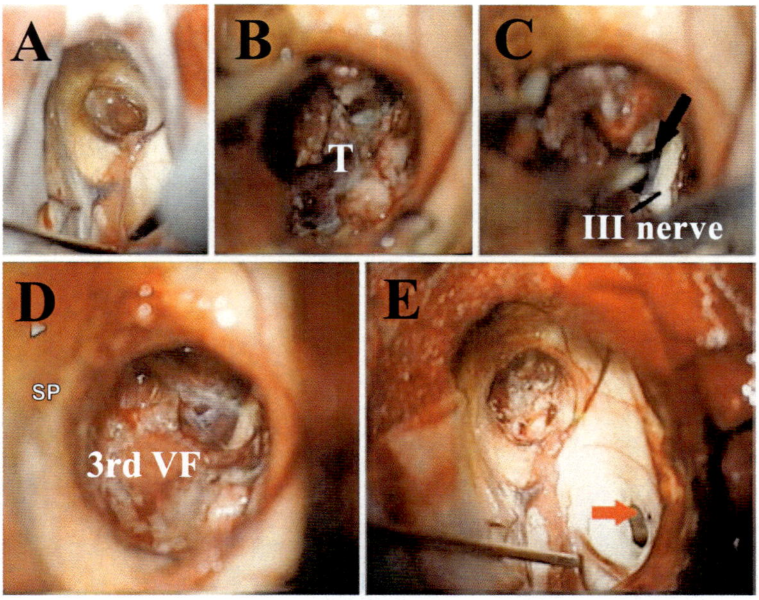

Fig. (16). Exposure and removal of the tumor. **A:** After the craniotomy, the tumor in the third ventricular cavity was observed through the foramen of Monro. **B:** Under microscopic amplification, the tumor (***T***) was found to adhere tightly to the lateral wall of the ventricle during the separation procedure. **C:** A defect was made in the lateral wall, through which the right side of the oculomotor nerve was identified. **D:** The entire tubero-infundibulum structure was exposed after total tumor removal. **E:** Before completing the operation, a septum pellucidum fistulization (***red arrow***) was performed to reduce the possibility of hydrocephalus.

Pathology Study

A typical SPCP was diagnosed from the pathological slides (Fig. **17**).

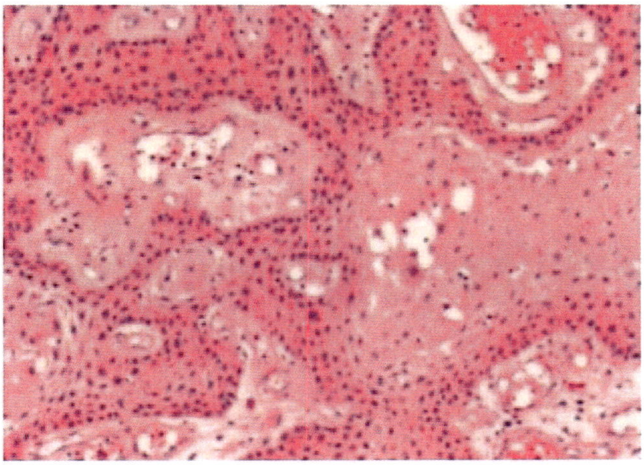

Fig. (17). The pathological analysis revealed a typical squamous-papillary craniopharyngioma.

Postoperative Course

Postoperatively, the patient suffered moderate DI. The symptoms were palliated after fluid and electrolyte replacement therapy. Endocrinological testing revealed slightly low levels of plasma thyroxine, testosterone, and progesterone.

Four years after surgery, the patient still suffered from hypopituitarism. The DI was controlled in stages. No significant weight gain was observed, and her BMI was 22.

An MRI evaluation conducted 4 years postoperatively indicated total tumor removal without recurrence. The PS and left side of the ventricular wall had been maintained (Fig. **18**).

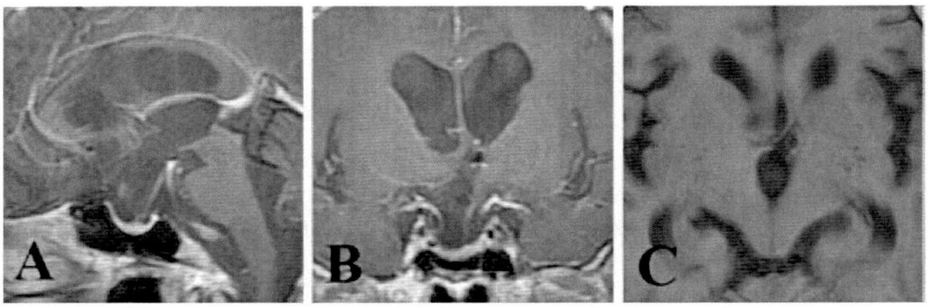

Fig. (18). Postsurgical MRI after 4 years indicated total tumor removal without recurrence. The pituitary stalk and left side of the ventricular wall remained intact.

Case No. 4 (Man, 45 Years Old)

Clinical Manifestation

The patient complained of a 1-year history of sexual disorder and visual disturbance, polydipsia, and polyuria of 2 weeks' duration. The above symptoms had become aggravated during the previous 3 days. The patient consumed approximately 2000–3000 ml of water each day.

Physical Examination

No significant physical abnormalities were observed. The binocular vision had decreased significantly. The patient's BMI index was 24.2, within the normal range of reference values for Chinese adult men.

Chemical Examination

No significant abnormalities were identified in a routine blood and urine analysis. An endocrinological examination indicated roughly normal pituitary function.

Neuroimaging Study

A plain CT scan revealed an isodense tumor located at the suprasellar cistern with occupation of the anterior part of the third ventricle but no calcification or cystic formation. The tumor size was $3.0 \times 2.8 \times 3.2$ cm^3 with uniform enhancement during an enhanced scan (Fig. **19**). The PS was clearly identifiable on coronal CT images. A normal-sized supratentorial ventricular cavity was observed. Conventional MRI indicated a purely solid mass located at the anterior part of the third ventricle cavity. A patent suprasellar cistern, normal PS, and absence of sellar abnormalities were identifiable on the presurgical MR images Fig. (**19**), and uniform Gd-DTPA enhancement was observed. No obstructive hydrocephalus was found.

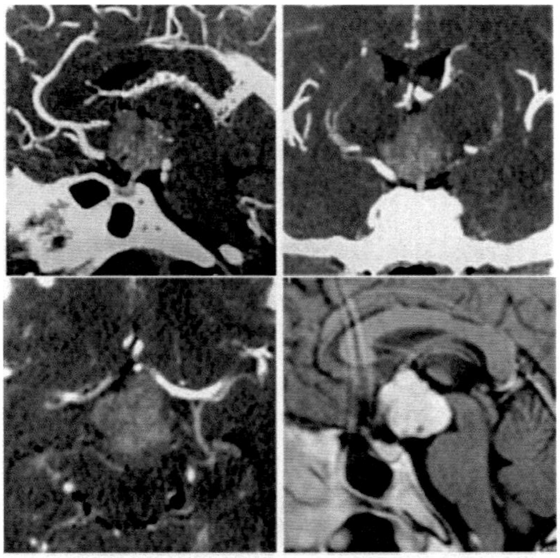

Fig. (19). Presurgical neuroimaging data of the patient. The tumor was located in the anterior part of the third ventricular cavity and had originated from the tubero-infundibulum. The pituitary stalk and a patent suprasellar cistern were identified. No significant hydrocephalus was observed.

Surgery

General Considerations

1. A observably solid tumor located entirely within the third ventricular cavity and originating from the tubero-infundibulum.
2. Surgical and topographical tumor classification: tubero-infundibular tumor (Type c1) and subarachnoidal tumor (Type Sa).
3. A small-sized tumor without significant superior extension.
4. The frontotemporal approach was selected. The lamina terminalis was accessed through the medial aspect of the frontotemporal approach (Fig. **20**).

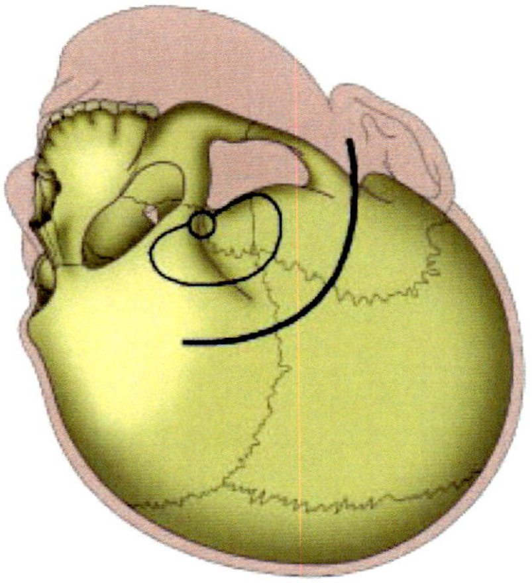

Fig. (20). Illustration of the operating position and incision.

Operative Findings

1. *Craniotomy:* The right-side frontotemporal bone flap was made according to the traditional pterional approach and with extension to the frontal side in order to use more of the space beneath the frontal lobe. The lateral sphenoidal crest was drilled. The dura mater was opened in a curved manner around the crest and turned over in a downward direction.
2. *Tumor Exposure:* Dissection of the lateral fissure and drainage of the CSF as the routine procedures. After sufficient retraction of the brain lobes, the self-retaining retractor was used to lift the frontal lobe and then reached the chiasmatic cistern. Through the surgical spaces median and lateral of the ICA, the third ventricular floor was found being frog belly-like-inflated (Fig. **21**). No tumor was found protruding into the subarachnoidal cistern. The pituitary stalk had a normal morphology.
3. *Opening of the Lamina Terminalis:* While dissecting arachnoids between the foundation of the frontal lobe and optic chiasm, the terminalis cistern was exposed in stages from the medial aspect of the frontotemporal approach. After opening the terminalis membrane, a thin layer of nervous tissue remained over tumor surface. The tumor appeared to be located within the thinning and stretched neural tissue layer of the 3rd VF (Fig. **21**).
4. *Tumor Removal:* The second and fourth surgical spaces were used to remove the tumor. A vertical incision was performed to open the tubero-infundibulum. Internal decompression *via* piecemeal extirpation of the solid tumor parts provided space to promote tumor resection from third ventricle margins. The tumor had adhered tightly to the anterior part of the 3rd VF at the infundibulum (Fig. **22**). The tumor was removed in a piecemeal manner. The 3rd VF developed a local defect at the site of adhesion.

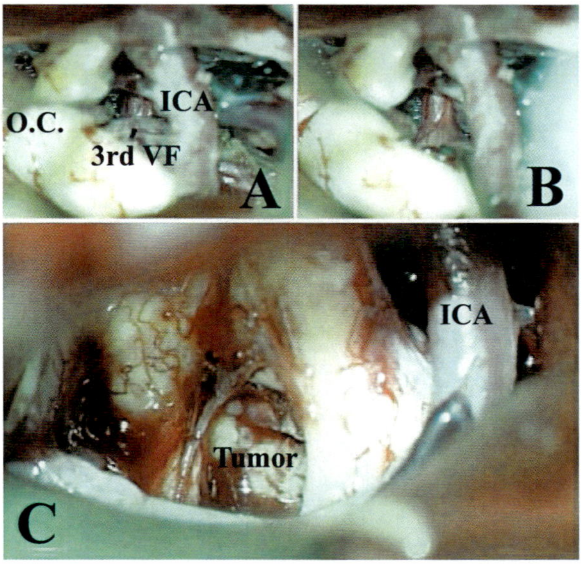

Fig. (21). Tumor exposure. **A:** Through the second space, the tubero-infundibulum, with frog belly-like inflation, was observed. No tumor had protruded into the suprasellar cistern. **B:** The pituitary stalk was fully intact. **C:** Upon opening the terminalis membrane, the tumor was exposed and remained covered by a thin layer of nervous tissue.

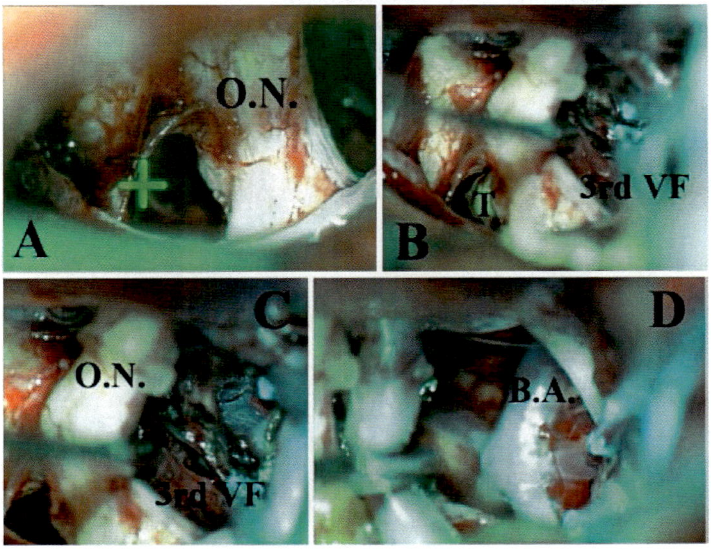

Fig. (22). Total tumor removal was achieved *via* the second and fourth spaces. **A:** The lamina terminalis space (fourth space) was used to remove part of the tumor. **B:** A vertical incision was made at the third ventricular floor (3rd VF). **C:** As the tumor be totally removed, a defect in the 3rd VF was revealed. The suprasellar arachnoid was also observed. **D:** Through the third surgical space between the internal carotid artery and oculomotor nerve, the basal artery, bilateral superior cerebellar artery, and posterior cerebral artery were observed.

Pathology Study

A typical SPCP was confirmed from the pathological slides (Fig. **23**).

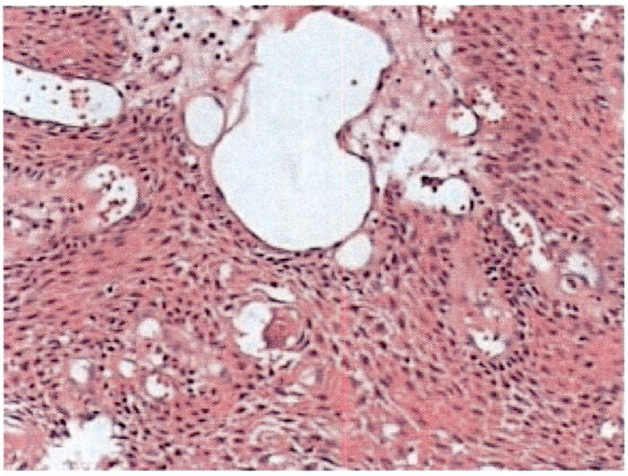

Fig. (23). A typical squamous papillary craniopharyngioma was confirmed using the pathological slides.

Postoperative Course

Postoperatively, the patient suffered from moderate DI. The symptoms were palliated *via* fluid and electrolyte replacement therapy. Endocrinological testing revealed low levels of plasma thyroxine, testosterone, and progesterone.

Six months after surgery, the patient still exhibited hypopituitarism. No significant improvements were observed in sexual function. An antidiuretic was used intermittently to control DI. The patient suffered from moderate weight gain, and his BMI had increased to 26.4 at 6 months postoperatively.

A postoperative MRI study conducted after 2 years revealed total tumor removal and adequate 3rd VF thickness (Fig. **24**).

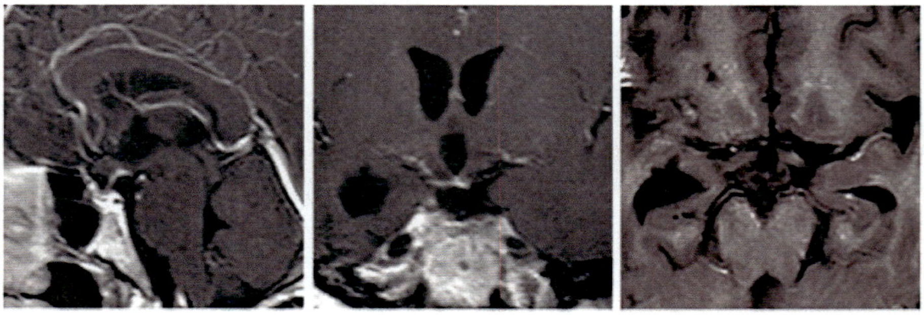

Fig. (24). Total tumor removal was proven by magnetic resonance imaging (MRI) 2 years after surgery. MRI also revealed an intact pituitary stalk.

CONFLICT OF INTEREST

The authors (editor) declares no conflict of interest, financial or otherwise.

ACKNOWLEDGEMENTS

Declared none.

REFERENCES

[1] Hoffman HJ. Surgical management of craniopharyngioma. Pediatr Neurosurg 1994; 21 (Suppl. 1): 44-9.
[http://dx.doi.org/10.1159/000120861] [PMID: 7530990]

[2] Prabhu VC, Brown HG. The pathogenesis of craniopharyngiomas. Childs Nerv Syst 2005; 21(8-9): 622-7.
[http://dx.doi.org/10.1007/s00381-005-1190-9] [PMID: 15965669]

[3] Miller DC. Pathology of craniopharyngiomas: clinical import of pathological findings. Pediatr Neurosurg 1994; 21 (Suppl. 1): 11-7.
[http://dx.doi.org/10.1159/000120855] [PMID: 7841069]

[4] Lobos EI, Freed CG, Ashe SM. An intrinsic tumor of the third ventricle. J Neuropathol Exp Neurol 1953; 12(3): 232-43.
[http://dx.doi.org/10.1097/00005072-195307000-00003] [PMID: 13061971]

[5] Behari S, Banerji D, Mishra A, *et al.* Intrinsic third ventricular craniopharyngiomas: report on six cases and a review of the literature. Surg Neurol 2003; 60(3): 245-52.
[http://dx.doi.org/10.1016/S0090-3019(03)00132-0] [PMID: 12922045]

[6] Cashion EL, Young JM. Intraventricular craniopharyngioma. Report of two cases. J Neurosurg 1971; 34(1): 84-7.
[http://dx.doi.org/10.3171/jns.1971.34.1.0084] [PMID: 5539648]

[7] Chin HW. Adult intraventricular craniopharyngioma. Strahlentherapie 1983; 159(4): 214-6.
[PMID: 6857734]

[8] Cohen-Gadol AA, Geryk B, Binder DK, Tubbs RS. Conquering the third ventricular chamber. J Neurosurg 2009; 111(3): 590-9.
[http://dx.doi.org/10.3171/2008.9.17664] [PMID: 19361257]

[9] Fukushima T, Hirakawa K, Kimura M, Tomonaga M. Intraventricular craniopharyngioma: its characteristics in magnetic resonance imaging and successful total removal. Surg Neurol 1990; 33(1): 22-7.
[http://dx.doi.org/10.1016/0090-3019(90)90220-J] [PMID: 2405528]

[10] Iwasaki K, Kondo A, Takahashi JB, Yamanobe K. Intraventricular craniopharyngioma: report of two cases and review of the literature. Surg Neurol 1992; 38(4): 294-301.
[http://dx.doi.org/10.1016/0090-3019(92)90045-O] [PMID: 1440221]

[11] King TT. Removal of intraventricular craniopharyngiomas through the lamina terminalis. Acta Neurochir (Wien) 1979; 45(3-4): 277-86.
[http://dx.doi.org/10.1007/BF01769141] [PMID: 425858]

[12] Lanzieri CF, Sacher M, Som PM. CT changes in the septum pellucidum associated with intraventricular craniopharyngiomas. J Comput Assist Tomogr 1985; 9(3): 507-10.
[http://dx.doi.org/10.1097/00004728-198505000-00018] [PMID: 3989048]

[13] Pascual JM, Prieto R, Navas M, Carrasco R. Conquest of third ventricle craniopharyngiomas. J Neurosurg 2010; 112(5): 1156-61.

[http://dx.doi.org/10.3171/2009.8.JNS091094] [PMID: 20345221]

[14] Ferrara M, Bizzozero L, D'Angelo V, Corona C, Fiumara E. Intraventricular craniopharyngioma. Clinical and surgical considerations. J Neurosurg Sci 1989; 33(2): 161-4. [PMID: 2795188]

[15] Ikezaki K, Fujii K, Kishikawa T. Magnetic resonance imaging of an intraventricular craniopharyngioma. Neuroradiology 1990; 32(3): 247-9. [http://dx.doi.org/10.1007/BF00589123] [PMID: 2215911]

[16] Sacher M, Gottesman RI, Rothman AS, Rosenblum BR, Handler MS. Magnetic resonance imaging and computed tomography of an intraventricular craniopharyngioma. Clin Imaging 1990; 14(2): 116-9. [http://dx.doi.org/10.1016/0899-7071(90)90005-V] [PMID: 2372728]

[17] Fujitsu K, Sekino T, Sakata K, Kawasaki T. Basal interfalcine approach through a frontal sinusotomy with vein and nerve preservation. Technical note. J Neurosurg 1994; 80(3): 575-9. [http://dx.doi.org/10.3171/jns.1994.80.3.0575] [PMID: 8113875]

[18] Pascual JM, González-Llanos F, Barrios L, Roda JM. Intraventricular craniopharyngiomas: topographical classification and surgical approach selection based on an extensive overview. Acta Neurochir (Wien) 2004; 146(8): 785-802. [http://dx.doi.org/10.1007/s00701-004-0295-3] [PMID: 15254801]

[19] Pan J, Qi S, Lu Y, *et al.* Intraventricular craniopharyngioma: morphological analysis and outcome evaluation of 17 cases. Acta Neurochir (Wien) 2011; 153(4): 773-84. [http://dx.doi.org/10.1007/s00701-010-0938-5] [PMID: 21271265]

[20] Rush JL, Kusske JA, De Feo DR, Pribram HW. Intraventricular craniopharyngioma. Neurology 1975; 25(11): 1094-6. [http://dx.doi.org/10.1212/WNL.25.11.1094] [PMID: 1237829]

[21] Konovalov AN, *et al.* raniopharyngiomas with unusual topography and associated with vascular pathology. Acta neurochirurgica 1988; 53(1-2): 53-68.

[22] Ciric IS, Cozzens JW. Craniopharyngiomas: transsphenoidal method of approach--for the virtuoso only? Clin Neurosurg 1980; 27: 169-87. [PMID: 7273552]

[23] Mori K, Handa H, Murata T, Ishikawa M, Takeuchi J, Osaka K. Craniopharyngiomas with unusual topography and associated with vascular pathology. Acta Neurochir (Wien) 1980; 53(1-2): 53-68. [http://dx.doi.org/10.1007/BF02074521] [PMID: 7435282]

[24] Schmidek HH, Sweet WH. Operative neurosurgical techniques: indications, methods, and results. New York: Grune & Stratton 1982.

[25] Yaşargil MG, Curcic M, Kis M, Siegenthaler G, Teddy PJ, Roth P. Total removal of craniopharyngiomas. Approaches and long-term results in 144 patients. J Neurosurg 1990; 73(1): 3-11. [http://dx.doi.org/10.3171/jns.1990.73.1.0003] [PMID: 2352020]

[26] Sipos L, Vajda J. Craniopharyngioma of the third ventricle. Acta Neurochir (Wien) 1997; 139(1): 92-3. [http://dx.doi.org/10.1007/BF01850877] [PMID: 9059721]

[27] Maira G, Anile C, Rossi GF, Colosimo C. Surgical treatment of craniopharyngiomas: an evaluation of the transsphenoidal and pterional approaches. Neurosurgery 1995; 36(4): 715-24. [http://dx.doi.org/10.1227/00006123-199504000-00012] [PMID: 7596502]

[28] Barreca T, Perria C, Francaviglia N, Rolandi E. Evaluation of anterior pituitary function in adult patients with craniopharyngiomas. Acta Neurochir (Wien) 1984; 71(3-4): 263-72. [http://dx.doi.org/10.1007/BF01401321] [PMID: 6430039]

[29] Adamson TE, Wiestler OD, Kleihues P, Yaşargil MG. Correlation of clinical and pathological features

in surgically treated craniopharyngiomas. J Neurosurg 1990; 73(1): 12-7. [http://dx.doi.org/10.3171/jns.1990.73.1.0012] [PMID: 2352012]

[30] Fahlbusch R, Honegger J, Paulus W, Huk W, Buchfelder M. Surgical treatment of craniopharyngiomas: experience with 168 patients. J Neurosurg 1999; 90(2): 237-50. [http://dx.doi.org/10.3171/jns.1999.90.2.0237] [PMID: 9950494]

[31] Samii M, Bini W. Surgical treatment of craniopharyngiomas. Zentralbl Neurochir 1991; 52(1): 17-23. [PMID: 1862672]

[32] Migliore A, Calzolari F, Marzola A, Ghadirpour R, Migliore MM. Intrinsic III ventricle craniopharyngioma. Childs Nerv Syst 1992; 8(1): 56-8. [http://dx.doi.org/10.1007/BF00316565] [PMID: 1576611]

[33] de Divitiis O, Angileri FF, d'Avella D, Tschabitscher M, Tomasello F. Microsurgical anatomic features of the lamina terminalis. Neurosurgery 2002; 50(3): 563-9. [PMID: 11841725]

[34] Maira G, Anile C, Colosimo C, Cabezas D. Craniopharyngiomas of the third ventricle: trans-lamina terminalis approach. Neurosurgery 2000; 47(4): 857-63. [http://dx.doi.org/10.1097/00006123-200010000-00014] [PMID: 11014425]

[35] Apuzzo M. Transcallosal interfornicial exposure of lesions of the third ventricle. In: Schmidek HH, Sweet WH, Eds. Operative neurosurgical techniques. 2nd ed. New York: Grune and Stratton 1988; Vol. 1: pp. 389-95.

[36] Maira G, Anile C, Colosimo C, Cabezas D. Craniopharyngiomas of the third ventricle: trans-lamina terminalis approach. Neurosurgery 2000; 47(4): 857-63. [http://dx.doi.org/10.1097/00006123-200010000-00014] [PMID: 11014425]

[37] Kubota T, Fujii H, Ikeda K, Ito H, Yamamoto S, Nakanishi I. [A case of intraventricular craniopharyngioma with subarachnoid hemorrhage (author's transl)]. No Shinkei Geka 1980; 8(5): 495-501. [A case of intraventricular craniopharyngioma with subarachnoid hemorrhage (author's transl)]. [PMID: 7383266]

[38] Matthews FD. Intraventricular craniopharyngioma. AJNR Am J Neuroradiol 1983; 4(4): 984-5. [PMID: 6410885]

[39] Namba S, Tsuboi M. Craniopharyngioma in the third ventricle. No To Shinkei 1977; 29(8): 865-9. [PMID: 907760]

[40] Suzuki J, Katakura R, Mori T. Interhemispheric approach through the lamina terminalis to tumors of the anterior part of the third ventricle. Surg Neurol 1984; 22(2): 157-63. [http://dx.doi.org/10.1016/0090-3019(84)90044-2] [PMID: 6740479]

[41] Patterson RH Jr, Danylevich A. Surgical removal of craniopharyngiomas by the transcranial approach through the lamina terminalis and sphenoid sinus. Neurosurgery 1980; 7(2): 111-7. [http://dx.doi.org/10.1227/00006123-198008000-00001] [PMID: 7422106]

[42] Goldstein SJ, Wilson DD, Young AB, Guidry GJ. Craniopharyngioma intrinsic to the third ventricle. Surg Neurol 1983; 20(3): 249-53. [http://dx.doi.org/10.1016/0090-3019(83)90062-9] [PMID: 6879427]

[43] Rhoton AL Jr, Yamamoto I, Peace DA. Microsurgery of the third ventricle: Part 2. Operative approaches. Neurosurgery 1981; 8(3): 357-73. [http://dx.doi.org/10.1227/00006123-198103000-00007] [PMID: 7242884]

[44] Steno J, Malácek M, Bízik I. Tumor-third ventricular relationships in supradiaphragmatic craniopharyngiomas: correlation of morphological, magnetic resonance imaging, and operative findings. Neurosurgery 2004; 54(5): 1051-8. [http://dx.doi.org/10.1227/01.NEU.0000120421.11171.61] [PMID: 15113458]

[45] Jr Rhoton AL. I.Y.,Operative approaches to the third ventricle. In: Wilkins RS, Rengachary SS, Eds. Neurosurgery. 2nd ed. New York: McGraw- Hill 1996; Vol. 1: pp. 1435-49.

[46] Samii M. Technical aspects of excision of giant basal tumors with third ventricular involvement. In: Appuzo ML, Ed. Surgery of the third ventricle. Baltimore: Williams and Wilkins 1987; pp. 684-97.

[47] Dehdashti AR, de Tribolet N. Frontobasal interhemispheric trans-lamina terminalis approach for suprasellar lesions. Neurosurgery 2008; 62(6) (Suppl. 3): 1233-9. [PMID: 18695544]

[48] Hoffman HJ, De Silva M, Humphreys RP, Drake JM, Smith ML, Blaser SI. Aggressive surgical management of craniopharyngiomas in children. J Neurosurg 1992; 76(1): 47-52. [http://dx.doi.org/10.3171/jns.1992.76.1.0047] [PMID: 1727168]

[49] Shibuya M, Takayasu M, Suzuki Y, Saito K, Sugita K. Bifrontal basal interhemispheric approach to craniopharyngioma resection with or without division of the anterior communicating artery. J Neurosurg 1996; 84(6): 951-6. [http://dx.doi.org/10.3171/jns.1996.84.6.0951] [PMID: 8847589]

[50] Shirane R, Ching-Chan S, Kusaka Y, Jokura H, Yoshimoto T. Surgical outcomes in 31 patients with craniopharyngiomas extending outside the suprasellar cistern: an evaluation of the frontobasal interhemispheric approach. J Neurosurg 2002; 96(4): 704-12. [http://dx.doi.org/10.3171/jns.2002.96.4.0704] [PMID: 11990811]

[51] Van Effenterre R, Boch A-L. Craniopharyngioma in adults and children: a study of 122 surgical cases. J Neurosurg 2002; 97(1): 3-11. [http://dx.doi.org/10.3171/jns.2002.97.1.0003] [PMID: 12134929]

[52] Sweet WH. Radical surgical treatment of craniopharyngioma. Clin Neurosurg 1976; 23: 52-79. [PMID: 975700]

CHAPTER 14

Infra-sellar and Nasopharyngeal Craniopharyngioma

Jun Pan*

Department of Neurosurgery, Nanfang Hospital, Southern Medical University, #1838, North Guangzhou Avenue, Guangzhou, China

Abstract: The infra-sellar and nasopharyngeal craniopharyngiomas (CPs) were the special type, which predominantly presented in the children. In this chapter, we briefly depicted the clinical features of this type of tumor. Patients suffered with this type of CP were rarely more than 16 years old. The pathology was all adamantous tumor. As concerned to the clinical manifestation, except the pituitarism, growth retardation, and optical pathway injury, the pediatric patients always suffered with rhinocleisis, homorrhinia and airway obstruction. As extensive involvement, it was quite difficult to radical remove the tumor. As the result, tumor recurrent caused poor quality of life. Until now, the best treatment strategy was still missing.

Keywords: Craniopharyngioma, Intrasellar, Naso-pharyngeal.

INTRODUCTION

Theoretically, craniopharyngioma (CP) can originate from anywhere along the residual embryonic craniopharyngeal canal. As a result, although CPs are normally located in the sellar region, ectopic tumors occur frequently [1 - 27]. Among these, CPs with infrasellar and nasopharyngeal localization exhibit notable special features with respect to clinical manifestations and responses to radiology and treatment. The term "IS-CP" indicates that the main body of the CP is located in an area of the infrasellar region, such as the sphenoid sinus, ethmoid sinus, maxillary sinus, nasopharynx, nasal cavity, clivus, cavernous sinus, or orbital cavity. Differences in the involved regions and structures result in different clinical manifestations. Meanwhile, IS-CP may affect multiple intracranial structures, such as the sella turcica and suprasellar arachnoid cistern. A review of the literature revealed several relevant case reports. The age range of the affected patients was 20–30 years. Fujimoto *et al.* [9] subdivided IS-CPs into three types

* **Corresponding author Jun Pan:** Department of Neurosurgery, Nanfang Hospital, Southern Medical University, #1838, North Guangzhou Avenue, Guangzhou, China; Tel/Fax: +8620-61641806; E-mail: panjundu@hotmail.com

according to the region of involvement Fig. (**1**): Type I, CP with purely nasopharyngeal involvement; Type II, CP with infrasellar region but sella turcica involvement; and Type III, CP with both infrasellar region and sella turcica involvement; the third type could be further divided into type IIIa (no sellar floor dura penetration) and type IIIb (with sellar floor dura penetration into the intracranial region). The growth and expansion of type III CP remains controversial. It also remains unknown whether this type is infrasellar CP with extracranial expansion or nasopharyngeal CP with intracranial extension.

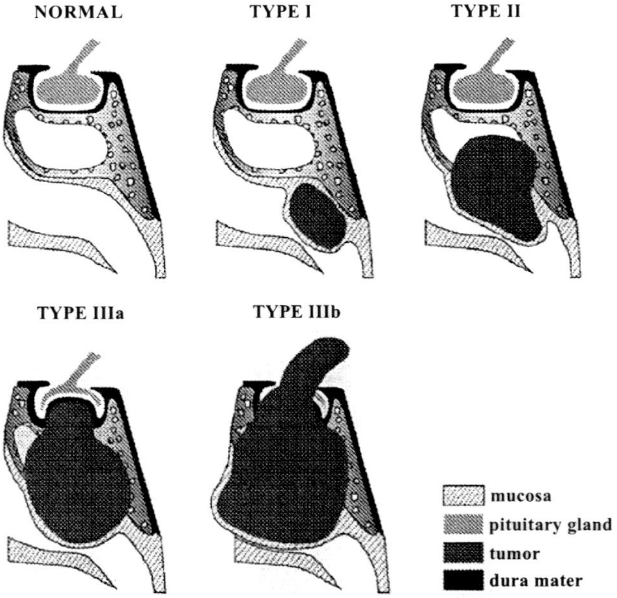

Fig. (1). (Reference from Fujimoto *et al.* [9]). Fujimoto *et al.* subdivided IS-CPs into three types according to the region of involvement: Type I, CP with purely nasopharyngeal involvement; Type II, CP with infrasellar region but sella turcica involvement; and Type III, CP with both infrasellar region and sella turcica involvement; the third type could be further divided into type IIIa (no sellar floor dura penetration) and type IIIb (with sellar floor dura penetration into the intracranial region).

The CP with involvement of the infrasellar region is the rare subtype of craniopharyngioma, which almost happened in children without exclusion. The pediatric patients always had a relative longer medical history, so some scholars thought this type of tumor as embryonic genetic CP. They also thought that the tumoral growth always accompanied with the development of pituitary gland. Because of the involvement of tumor to the pituitary gland happened in the very beginning, the patients always had severely hypopituitarism, such as growth retardation, and the nondevelopment of the secondary sexual characters, *et al.* On the other hand, because of the major tumoral body locating in infrasellar region with less involvement to the suprasellar structures, the tumor size was always huge.

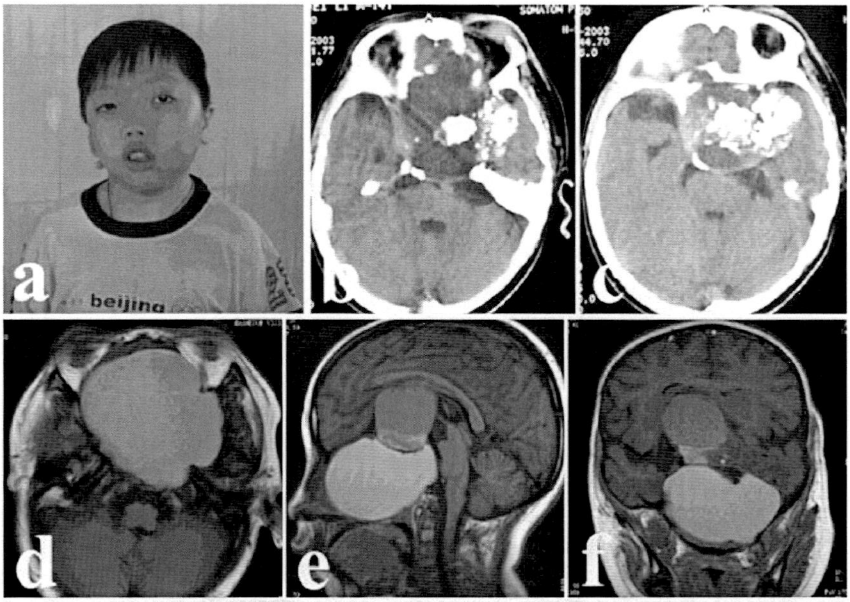

Fig. (2). A case of IS-CP with involvement of the sella turcica, nasopharynx, ethmoidal sinus, orbital cavity, suprasellar region, and even the third ventricular cavity.

CLINICAL MANIFESTATION

The clinical manifestation of infrasellar CPs is quite complicated and is dependent on the region of involvement. Common symptoms include nasal obstruction, epistaxis, headache, decreased optical accuracy, endocrinological disorders, abnormal facial sensation, protopsis, and eye movement disorders. Normally, CP does not cause symptoms such as nasal obstruction, epistaxis, anosphrasia, protopsis, ocular hypertelorism, and cerebrospinal fluid (CSF) leakage. The presenting symptom of diplopia always indicates IS-CP involvement in the middle cranial fossa or orbital cavity. However, visual impairment, visual field defects, and endocrinological dysfunction are among the presenting symptoms indicating sella turcica and suprasellar involvement. Anosphrasia may occur with CPs that involve the ethmoidal region and anterior cranial fossa. Tumor protrusion into the orbital cavity may cause ocular hypertelorism and protopsis. A large tumor with extensive involvement will induce a more complicated clinical manifestation. For example, the author previously encountered a case of IS-CP with involvement of the sella turcica, nasopharynx, ethmoidal sinus, orbital cavity, suprasellar region, and even the third ventricular cavity (Fig. **2**). This patient presented with visual disturbances, panhypopituitarism, nasal obstruction, and ocular hypertelorism of the right eye, right ankylotia, and right auricle developmental disorder.

DIAGNOSIS AND DIFFERENTIAL DIAGNOSIS

During presurgical computed tomography and magnetic resonance imaging evaluations, IS-CPs usually present common features of typical CP such as calcifications and cysts. It is easy to diagnose tumors with not only infrasellar region but also intracranial involvement. However, predominantly solid CPs require differential diagnosis from the following lesions: nasopharyngeal carcinoma, squamous carcinoma, adenoid carcinoma, rhabdomyosarcoma, papillary epithelioma, glioma in nasal cavity, lymphoma, nasosinusitis, childhood angiofibroma, chordoma, and granuloma. Cystic IS-CP requires differential diagnosis from hygroma of the paranasal sinus.

SURGICAL TREATMENT

Surgical removal and fluid drainage should be considered the primary approach for IS-CP treatment. Treatment approach should be selected according to the involved location(s), tumor size, and tumor texture (*e.g.*, predominantly solid or cystic). The trans-nasal or trans-oral approach is always selected when treating CPs with purely nasopharyngeal and paranasal sinus involvement. However, these tumors are often very large, and it is likely that neither approach provides sufficient exposure.

Dissection *via* the external nasal or trans-sphenoid approach with nasal septum resection could provide a larger surgical manipulation space, and this approach is always used to treat type II and III IS-CP. However, a combined trans-sphenoid and trans-cranial approach is suitable for treating type III tumors with significant intracranial extension. In recent years, following the dramatic progress in the field of endoscopic techniques, the trans-sphenoidal approach has become the most useful approach for IS-CP surgery. However, total tumor removal remains quite difficult for large CPs with extensive infrasellar region involvement. In some cases, subtotal tumor removal with sufficient drainage of fluid to the nasal cavity provides an alternative. Radiation therapy, although effective, has limited applications and can cause mental development disorders; these disadvantages might restrict the use of radiation therapy, especially in young children.

CONFLICT OF INTEREST

The author (editor) declares no conflict of interest, financial or otherwise.

ACKNOWLEDGEMENTS

Declared none.

REFERENCES

[1] Akimura T, Kameda H, Abiko S, Aoki H, Kido T. Infrasellar craniopharyngioma. Neuroradiology 1989; 31(2): 180-3. [http://dx.doi.org/10.1007/BF00698851] [PMID: 2747897]

[2] Benitez WI, Sartor KJ, Angtuaco EJ. Craniopharyngioma presenting as a nasopharyngeal mass: CT and MR findings. J Comput Assist Tomogr 1988; 12(6): 1068-72. [http://dx.doi.org/10.1097/00004728-198811000-00034] [PMID: 3183117]

[3] Buhl R, Nabavi A, Fritsch M, Mehdorn HM. Nasopharyngeal extension of a craniopharyngioma in a 4 year old girl. Acta Neurochir (Wien) 2001; 143(12): 1283-5. [http://dx.doi.org/10.1007/s007010100026] [PMID: 11810394]

[4] Byrne MN, Sessions DG. Nasopharyngeal craniopharyngioma. Case report and literature review. Ann Otol Rhinol Laryngol 1990; 99(8): 633-9. [http://dx.doi.org/10.1177/000348949009900809] [PMID: 2200325]

[5] Chakrabarty A, Mitchell P, Bridges LR. Craniopharyngioma invading the nasal and paranasal spaces, and presenting as nasal obstruction. Br J Neurosurg 1998; 12(4): 361-3. [http://dx.doi.org/10.1080/02688699844907] [PMID: 10070432]

[6] Chen CJ. Suprasellar and infrasellar craniopharyngioma with a persistent craniopharyngeal canal: case report and review of the literature. Neuroradiology 2001; 43(9): 760-2. [http://dx.doi.org/10.1007/s002340100581] [PMID: 11594427]

[7] Cooper PR, Ransohoff J. Craniopharyngioma originating in the sphenoid bone. Case report. J Neurosurg 1972; 36(1): 102-6. [http://dx.doi.org/10.3171/jns.1972.36.1.0102] [PMID: 5007266]

[8] Falavigna A, Kraemer JL. Infrasellar craniopharyngioma: case report. Arq Neuropsiquiatr 2001; 59(2-B): 424-30. [http://dx.doi.org/10.1590/S0004-282X2001000300022] [PMID: 11460192]

[9] Fujimoto Y, Matsushita H, Velasco O, Rosemberg S, Plese JP, Marino R Jr. Craniopharyngioma involving the infrasellar region: a case report and review of the literature. Pediatr Neurosurg 2002; 37(4): 210-6. [http://dx.doi.org/10.1159/000065396] [PMID: 12372916]

[10] Fujitani K, Hakuba A, Kojima S, Mishima Y, Tsujimoto T, Nishimura S. Craniopharyngioma, originating in the sphenoid sinus, extending into the nasal cavity (author's transl). No Shinkei Geka 1979; 7(2): 181-6. [PMID: 424066]

[11] Graziani N, Donnet A, Bugha TN, Dufour H, Figarella-Branger D, Grisoli F. Ectopic basisphenoidal craniopharyngioma: case report and review of the literature. Neurosurgery 1994; 34(2): 346-9. [http://dx.doi.org/10.1227/00006123-199402000-00019] [PMID: 8177397]

[12] Hamberger CA, Hammer G, Norlen G, Sjogren B. Surgical treatment of craniopharyngioma; radical removal by the transantrosphenoidal approach. Acta Otolaryngol 1960; 52: 285-92. [http://dx.doi.org/10.3109/00016486009123151] [PMID: 13710959]

[13] Hillman TH, Peyster RG, Hoover ED, Nair S, Finkelstein SD. Infrasellar craniopharyngioma: CT and MR studies. J Comput Assist Tomogr 1988; 12(4): 702-4. [http://dx.doi.org/10.1097/00004728-198807000-00044] [PMID: 3392286]

[14] Illum P, Elbrond O, Nehen AM. Surgical treatment of nasophrayngeal craniopharyngioma. Radical removal by the transpalatal approach. J Laryngol Otol 1977; 91(3): 227-33. [http://dx.doi.org/10.1017/S0022215100083602] [PMID: 850102]

[15] Jiang RS, Wu CY, Jan YJ, Hsu CY. Primary ethmoid sinus craniopharyngioma: a case report. J Laryngol Otol 1998; 112(4): 403-5. [http://dx.doi.org/10.1017/S0022215100140599] [PMID: 9659511]

[16] Kanungo N, Just N, Black M, Mohr G, Glikstein R, Rochon L. Nasopharyngeal craniopharyngioma in an unusual location. AJNR Am J Neuroradiol 1995; 16(6): 1372-4. [PMID: 7677045]

[17] Lewin R, Ruffolo E, Saraceno C. Craniopharyngioma arising in the pharyngeal hypophysis. South Med J 1984; 77(12): 1519-23. [http://dx.doi.org/10.1097/00007611-198412000-00011] [PMID: 6505761]

[18] Maier HC. Craniopharyngioma with erosion and drainage into the nasopharynx. An autobiographical case report. J Neurosurg 1985; 62(1): 132-4. [http://dx.doi.org/10.3171/jns.1985.62.1.0132] [PMID: 3964844]

[19] Maiuri F, Corriero G, Elefante R, Cirillo S, Giamundo A. Craniopharyngioma of the cranial base and nasopharynx. Surg Neurol 1987; 27(2): 191-4. [http://dx.doi.org/10.1016/0090-3019(87)90295-3] [PMID: 3810450]

[20] Majlessi H, Shariat AS, Katirai A. Nasopharyngeal craniopharyngioma. Case report. J Neurosurg 1978; 49(1): 119-20. [http://dx.doi.org/10.3171/jns.1978.49.1.0119] [PMID: 660256]

[21] Mozota Ortiz JR, Medina Sola JJ, Aguado Martínez F, Alfaro García J, Hueto Prado J. [Craniopharyngioma of the cavum: report of a case]. Acta Otorrinolaringol Esp 1988; 39(2): 119-21. [Craniopharyngioma of the cavum: report of a case]. [PMID: 3078882]

[22] Mukada K, Mori S, Matsumura S, Uozumi T, Goishi J. Infrasellar craniopharyngioma. Surg Neurol 1984; 21(6): 565-71. [http://dx.doi.org/10.1016/0090-3019(84)90271-4] [PMID: 6719329]

[23] Pharaboz C, Merran S, Cordoliani Y, Rizzoli P. Rhinopharyngeal craniopharyngioma. CT X-ray and MRI aspects. J Radiol 1989; 70(10): 573-5. [PMID: 2593112]

[24] Pheline C, Jamois Y, Engel P, Leguyarder B, Penot JC. One case of atypical craniopharyngioma located in sphenoïdal body and operated first by nasal then by maxillary sinus route (author's transl). Neurochirurgie 1981; 27(4): 221-4. [PMID: 7322257]

[25] Podoshin L, Rolan L, Altman MM, Peyser E. 'Pharyngeal' craniopharyngioma. J Laryngol Otol 1970; 84(1): 93-9. [http://dx.doi.org/10.1017/S0022215100071681] [PMID: 5504064]

[26] Prasad U, Kwi NK. Nasopharyngeal craniopharyngioma. J Laryngol Otol 1975; 89(4): 445-52. [http://dx.doi.org/10.1017/S0022215100080579] [PMID: 1127337]

[27] Sener RN. Giant craniopharyngioma extending to the anterior cranial fossa and nasopharynx. AJR Am J Roentgenol 1994; 162(2): 441-2. [http://dx.doi.org/10.2214/ajr.162.2.8310943] [PMID: 8310943]

CHAPTER 15

Surgical Treatment of Recurrent Craniopharyngioma

Jun Pan*

Department of Neurosurgery, Nanfang Hospital of Southern Medical University, 1838 North Guangzhou Avenue, Guangzhou, China

Abstract: Any neurosurgeon can't avoid the tumor recurrence within the treatment of craniopharyngiomas. In this chapter, we focused on the description of the clinical manifestation, surgical strategy and prognosis of recurrent CP. Especially, the growth pattern of recurrent tumor as compared to the primary morphological features was emphasized and discussed. The influences of the first surgery or treatment strategy (pallilate or radical) were proposed based on the clinical casese analysis. As our opinion, the recurrent CP can be divided into 1) Intrasellar recurrence of Infra-diaphgragmatic tumor, and 2) Suprasellar infundibulo-tuberal recurrence. Correspondingly, the different treatment strategies were also summarized. We thought for intrasellar recurrent, more radical surgery should be taken. While for the infundibulo-tuberal recurrence casued by palliative first surgery, more radical surgery was still the first choise. However, if radical total removal was selected in the first surgery, the repeated operation must be paid more attention.

Keywords: Craniopharyngioma, Surgical treatment, Tumor recurrent.

INTRODUCTION

Craniopharyngioma (CP) tends to recur [1 - 7]. Among patients without gross total tumor removal (GTR) who fail to undergo substitute irradiation therapy, the tumor recurrence rate can reach 25–100% within a 10-year follow-up period [8 - 10]. Even among neuroradiologically confirmed GTR cases, the recurrence rate remains 0–62% during a 10-year follow-up period [3, 8 - 16]. Although postsurgical irradiation can significantly reduce the tumor recurrence rate, the incidence can still reach 10–63% during a 10-years follow-up period [3, 8 - 18]. Recurrence is therefore the major risk associated with CP evolution. Accordingly, tumor recurrence is an inevitable problem for neurosurgeons.

* **Corresponding author Jun Pan**: Department of Neurosurgery, Nanfang Hospital of Southern Medical University, 1838 North Guangzhou Avenue, Guangzhou, China; Tel/Fax: +8620-61641806; E-mail: panjundu@hotmail.com

CP recurrence occurs in two situations: A) recurrence after GTR as prove by neuroradiology and B) recurrence or regrowth after partial or subtotal removal. In fact, most circumstances do not represent the true relapse but the evolution of tumor fragments left during the primary surgery on account of a blind spot in the operating field or microscopic invasion of the third ventricle wall nervous tissues [11, 19 - 23].

As CP is a slowly growing tumor, a effective evaluation of the recurrence risk requires a long follow-up period,. Although recurrence is believed occur within the first 3 years after surgery, as reported in several articles from the literature [1, 3, 6, 8, 11, 12, 17, 24 - 27], long-term tumor recurrence was also reported [28, 29]. In general, the following elements were reported to correlate with the time of recurrence: 1) extent of surgical removal during the previous surgery: GTR cases will normally exhibit a long time interval before tumor recurrence, whereas partial cases will show recurrence within a shorter time period. 2) Features of the tumor itself: cystic tumors always recur and grow rapidly within a short time period, whereas solid tumors grow and recur slowly. 3) The primary tumor growth pattern: Normally, sub-diaphragmatic tumor recurrences are asymptomatic during the early stage and must be identified by surveillance magnetic resonance imaging (MRI). However, infundibulo-tuberal CP recurrences can be identified during the early stage because of presenting clinical manifestations. 4) Finally, it is likely that only a few tumors are accompanied with malignant transformation, a phenomenon that occurs frequently in repeat-recurrent cases, especially those that have undergone repeated radiotherapy. Malignant CPs always grows rapidly after surgery. Therefore, regular intermittent monitoring after surgery for CP is unconditionally important. Generally, a minimum 5-year follow-up study should be conducted, and a follow-up of >10 years would provide better reassurance to the patient.

RECURRENCE PATTERNS OF CPS

Difficulties associated with secondary surgery because of scarring and adhesions from the previous operation or radiotherapy are always emphasized for recurrent CPs. However, the growth patterns of recurrent tumor seldom have been depicted specifically. However, a better understanding of the tumor growth patterns is very important when determining the surgical strategy for recurrent CP and whether substitution radiotherapy is needed.

CPs have differing sites of origin and growth patterns and, as a result, recurrent CPs also exhibit various growth patterns. In general, recurrent tumors are thought to originate from small islets of CP cells in the gliotic brain surrounding to the tumor. For infundibulo-tuberal CPs, tumor recurrences likely originate from residual tumor cells in the infundibulo-tuberal region. However, according to our therapeutic experiences with more than 300 cases of CP, recurrences can be subdivided into two types according to site: intrasellar recurrence and suprasellar third ventricle floor (3rd VF) recurrence. The former type always occurs in cases of subdiaphragmatic CP, whereas the latter occurs in cases of suprasellar infundibulo-tuberal CP. Distant CP recurrence occurs occasionally but is rare [30 - 33].

Recurrence of Subdiaphragmatic CP

Almost all recurrences of subdiaphragmatic CPs originate from the intrasellar region (Figs. **1-3**). In most cases, the recurrent tumor maintains the growth features of the primary CP. The relationship between the tumor, suprasellar 3rd VF, and optical chiasm involves compression rather than invasion. Despite stronger adhesions between the recurrent tumor and neural tissue, a resectable membranous interface can be used to dissect the tumor. In a few cases, significant changes in the recurrent tumor growth pattern are observed, such as extreme upward growth without diaphragmatic obstruction Fig. (**4**) or growth along the longitudinal axis of the PS followed by invagination into the 3rd VF; these changes present great challenges for resurgery (Fig. **5**).

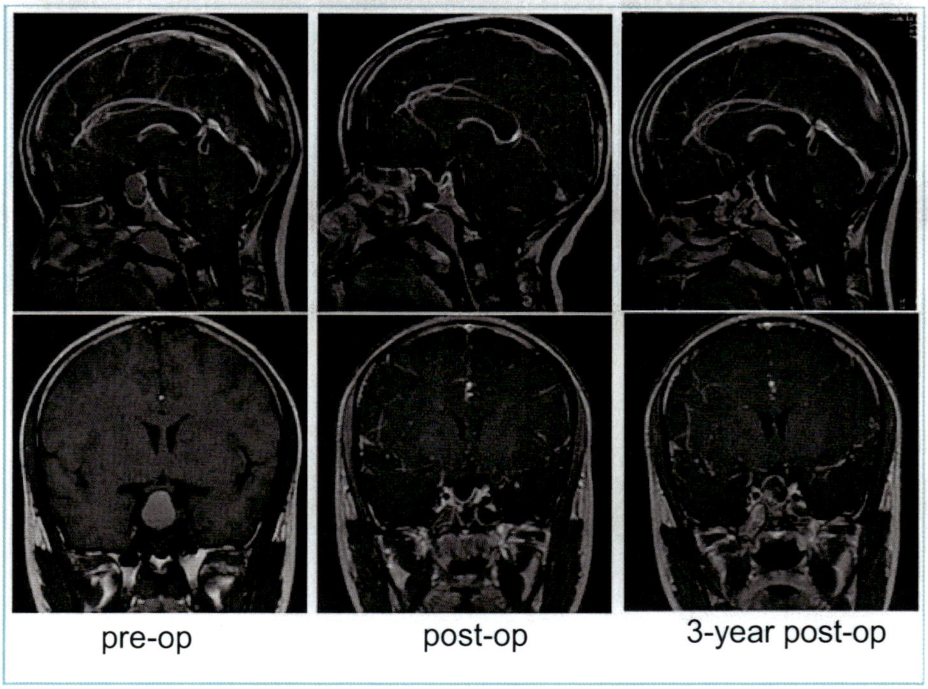

Fig. (1). A recurrent Id-CP case, the intrasellar recurrence was the most growth pattern of Id-CP.

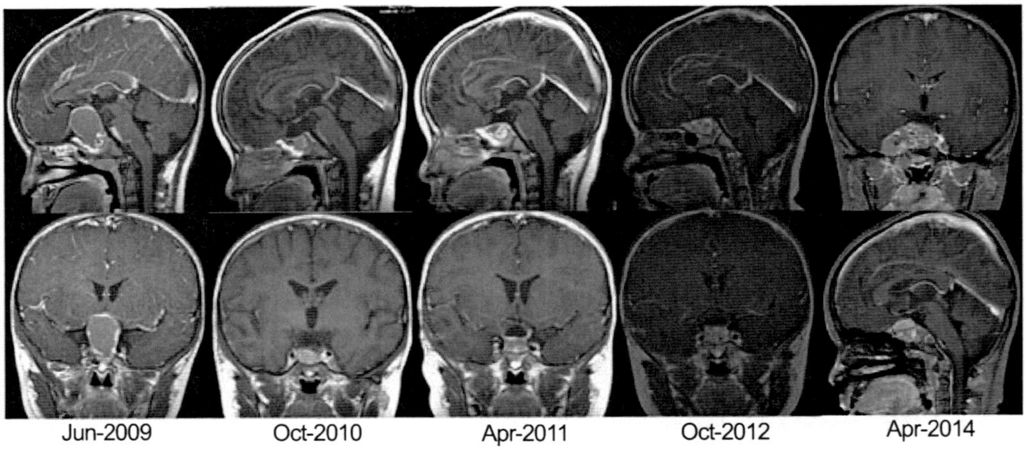

Fig. (2). Second recurrence case of Id-CP, the recurrence tumor involved the right side of cavernous sinus.

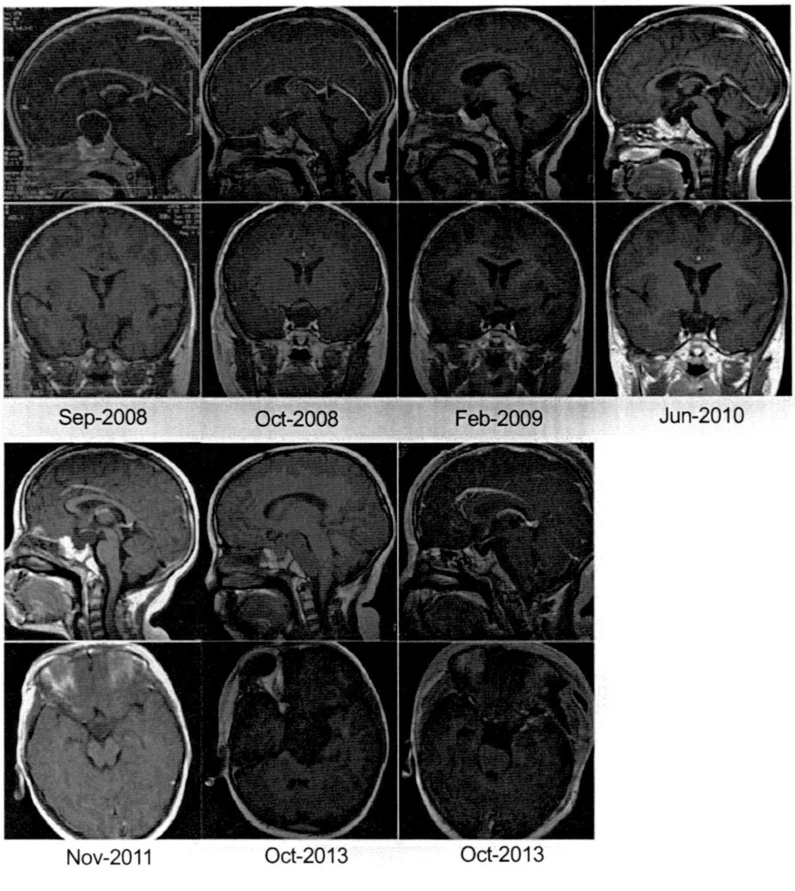

Fig. (3). A third recurrent case of Id-CP, the intrasellar recurrent tumor protruded to the prepontile cistern.

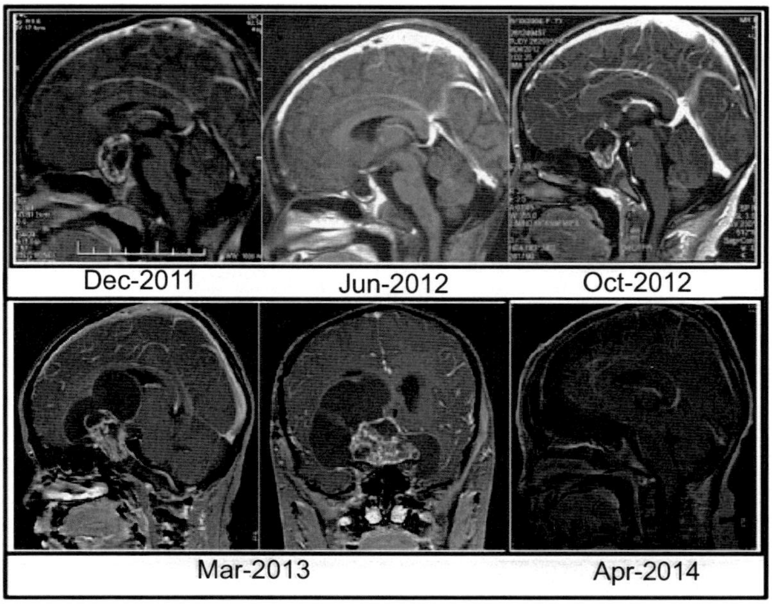

Fig. (4). In a recurrent case of Id-CP, the recurrence tumor expanded extremely upward without diaphragmatic obstruction.

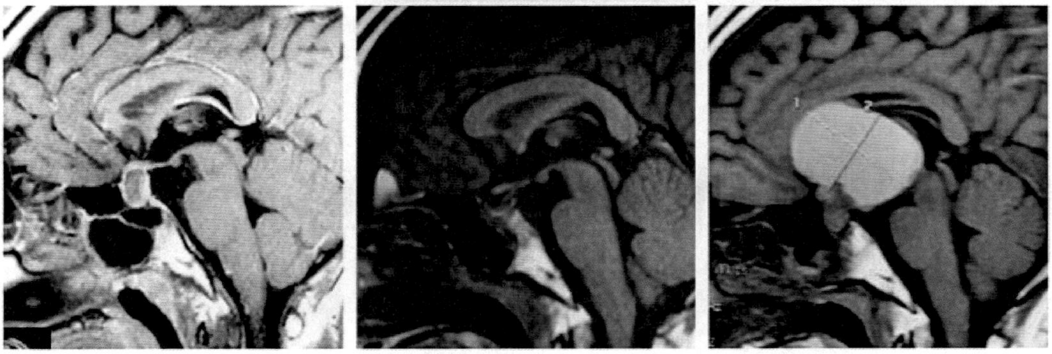

Fig. (5). The recurrent tumor grows along the longitudinal axis of the PS followed by invagination into the 3rd VF.

Recurrence of Suprasellar 3rd VF Tumors

In significant contrast to subdiaphragmatic tumors, recurrences from suprasellar third ventricular wall tumors are always located in the infundibulo-tuberal area Fig. (**6**); however, this area cannot be easily and directly exposed because of obstruction of the optical chiasm. Therefore, patients treated for tumors located inside the third ventricular walls should be subjected to close surveillance in order to provide proper treatment as early as possible.

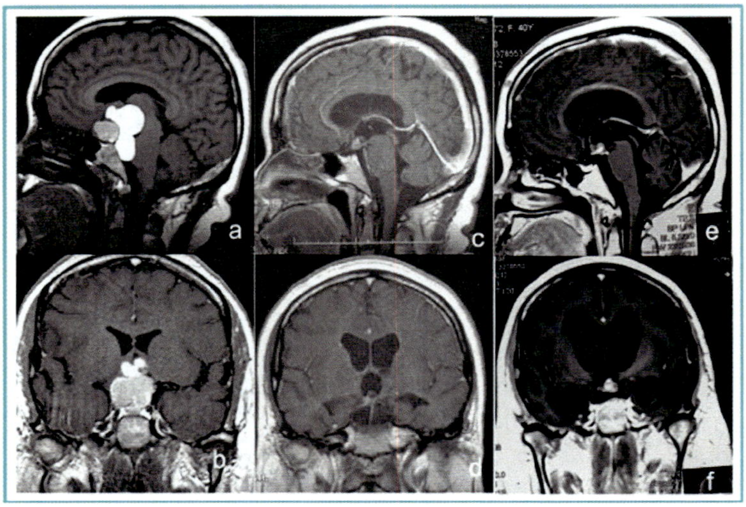

Fig. (6). The recurrences from suprasellar third ventricular wall tumors are always located in the infundibulo-tuberal area.

CLINICAL CHARACTERISTICS OF RECURRENT CPS

Regarding clinical manifestations, recurrent CPs always accompany significant endocrinological disorders. The reported incidence of hypopituitarism was significantly higher among cases of recurrent tumors than among cases of primary tumors [34]. Similar findings were also observed with respect to visual disorders [35]. The frequency of diabetes insipidus (DI) exceeded 80% in most of the reported studies. The majority of cases affected by DI developed permanent insipidus. Therefore, during secondary surgery, more attention should be given to the avoidance of severe complications that would strongly influence the patient's quality of life, such as hypothalamic reactions and neural dysfunction (*e.g.*, visual accuracy, motion, epilepsy, and coma). Regarding surgery, tumoral scarring and adhesions from previous operations or radiotherapy are frequently encountered during surgery for recurrent CPs. It is therefore more difficult in such cases to protect the visual pathway, PS, and third ventricular walls. Additionally, patients who suffer with long-term endocrinological and hypothalamic dysfunction have a lower tolerance for resurgery.

THERAPEUTIC STRTEGY FOR RECURRENT CP

Treatment for recurrent CP should be individualized. Elements that influence to the selection of a therapeutic strategy include the following:

1. During primary surgery, if only palliative surgery such as partial tumor

removal, cystic fluid drainage, or hydrocephalus relief was performed, the surgical strategy for a recurrent tumor should be similar to that for the primary tumor. Except for adhesions in the surgical corridor that might introduce difficulties during secondary surgery, manipulation of the site of tumor origin and key points should be similar to that of the primary tumor.

2. In contrast, if the primary surgery aimed to achieve GTR, the location and growth pattern of the recurrent tumor are more important. For intrasellar recurrences of subdiaphragmatic CP, GTR might be difficult only if the tumor causes extensive involvement of the nasopharynx, sphenoid sinus, and ethmoid sinus among others. Regarding tumor recurrence, the aim of secondary surgery should be GTR. In such cases, secondary surgery can be more radical. Moreover, active volume-reduction surgery could provide an opportunity for radiotherapy. However, for recurrent tumors that originate from the suprasellar infundibulo-tuberal area, the surgical aim should be more conservative because after primary radical tumor removal, this location of this type of recurrent tumor is always near vital structures. Currently, we consider radiotherapy an selective treatment at this stage; this treatment yields favourable results in the most cases with fewer risks than radical surgery. Fortunately, stringent postsurgical MRI evaluation allows the identification of small recurrent tumors during the follow-up period. Patients with CP might not require volume-reduction surgery and can be directly treated *via* stereotactic radiation (*e.g.*, X-knife or Gamma knife). However, the curative effects should be summarized further.
3. Apart from the two above-described important elements, the general condition and endocrinological status should also be considered, along with the patient's and family's tolerance and willingness.

Surgical Techniques for Recurrent CPs

1. The growth pattern of primary CP should be carefully observed and analyzed. In general, recurrent tumors maintain most morphological features of the primary tumor. However, in rare cases, the relationship between tumor and surrounding structures, especially the membranous structures surrounding the tumor, might change significantly.
2. Before secondary surgery, changes in the anatomical relationship between the tumor and suprasellar arachnoidal structures caused by primary surgery and the extent of tumor removal should be sufficiently predicted and understood; this is helpful when selecting the surgical approach and intraoperative manipulations. We will provide further detailed demonstrations in the Chapter 19.
3. If the growth pattern has changed significantly, the surgeon should sufficiently predict potential difficulties that might occur during surgery for temporal

regulation of the surgical strategy. For cases where radiotherapy has been administered, strong adhesions should also be identified before surgery. For cases where Ommaya reservoir placement has been performed, drainage tube removal might be extremely difficult, especially if the tumor or its calcification has grown through the pores of the tube.

4. When selecting the secondary surgical approach, it is necessary to select an anatomical corridor without involvement due to the previous surgery, such as a contralateral craniotomy or an interhemispheric approach if a lateral fissure approach was used in the previous surgery. Attempt early identification of the optic nerves and PS (if preserved during the previous surgery) as anatomical markers. More importantly, the third ventricular walls should be preserved to the extent possible. As in primary surgery, it might be reasonable to scarify the PS and adenohypophysis; however, the third ventricular walls and optical pathway should be preserved to the extent possible.

Altogether, when considering the treatment of recurrent CPs, the surgeon should consider the primary tumor growth patterns, nature of previous interventions, recurrence patterns, and severity of clinical scenario. Control of additional local failure should be individualized. The modalities include cyst-controlling procedures, alternatives to surgical debulking (significant solid life-threatening component), Gamma knife radiosurgery, and systemic chemotherapy (*e.g.*, α-interferon). The selection of different treatment methods requires a comprehensive consideration of all above-described elements.

PROGNOSIS OF RECURRENT CPS

As reported in the literature, the mortality and complication frequencies were significantly higher with recurrent CPs than with primary tumors. Indeed, when compared with that of primary surgery [8, 10, 12], the total removal success rate decreases dramatically (0–25%) in such cases and is accompanied by increased perioperative morbidity [6, 7, 10] and mortality (10.5–24%) [7, 8], demonstrating that palliative surgery is the most realistic target for many recurrent lesions. A study published by Elliott [36] indicated that tumor recurrence was the only predictive factor of a lower long-term survival rate. The related analysis also indicated that the overall and progression-free survival rates dropped significantly among patients with recurrent tumors during a long-term follow-up. According to our clinical data, the recurrent CP growth pattern and nature of the previous interventions might play more important roles. Among patients who had undergone palliative primary surgery or for whom radical total tumor removal might still have been possible, no statistical difference was found between the GTR rates of patients with recurrent and primary CPs. Moreover, secondary surgery did not significantly increase the mortality and complication frequency rates. However, among patients with recurrent CPs in vital locations such as the infundibulo-tuberal area or third ventricular walls, the secondary surgery GTR rate decreases dramatically. According to the literature, the recurrent CP GTR rate was 0–25%, much lower than that of primary tumors. Moreover, reoperation likely caused severe hypothalamic dysfunction, which in turn increased the incidence of mortality and complications. For recurrent CP cases, it might be reasonable to consider alternative therapeutic methods. Unfortunately however, the clinical results associated with the available therapeutic methods for recurrent CP have been unsatisfactory.

Given the difficulty associated with resurgery for recurrences and the associated morbidity and mortality rates, at this stage we currently consider radiotherapy to be an elective treatment that yields good results in the most cases with fewer risks than radical surgery. While the tumor volume is still small and does not need additional surgical debulking, strict radiological follow-up, which is made possible by modern imaging tools, can inspect most relapses. Radiosurgery may be promising, although further evaluation is still required.

Scarring and adhesions from previous surgery or radiotherapy could decrease the probability of successful excision, so, control the recurrence of tumors is still a difficult mission . As we mentioned in the beginning of this section, in such cases, the incidence of total tumor resection drops dramatically (0–25%) and the perioperative morbidity and mortality increased significantly (10.5–24%) [6, 7, 10]. The possitive impact of radiotherapy (preceded or not by a second surgery) for recurrent lesions have been clearly illustrated; in a series of 25 patients suffered irradiation therapy (19 of whom suffered a second surgical procedure before radiotherapy), the 10-year progression-free survival rate from the time of the first recurrence was 72% [37]. Remarkably, the consequence was not affected by the achievement of a second surgery or not (10-year progression-free survival rates among patients subjected or not to salvage surgery were 80 and 69%, respectively) [37]. There was also no obvious difference in tumor control between patients whoreceive adjuvant radiotherapy after primary operation and those receiving radiotherapy for relapses [37]; the authors proposed that radiotherapy might be equally effective for the primary presentation and at the time of relapse although the two therapy groups might not be comparable as far as tumor aggressiveness. Stripp *et al.* [16], after studying a series of 22 children and adolescents undergone radiotherapy for relapses, found an actuarial 10-year local control rate of 83%. Kalapurakal *et al.* [15], in a series of 14 children with relapse tumors, reported 5-year second relapse-free survival rates of 100% among those offered radiotherapy and 0% among those treated with operation alone. Finally, in a group of 19 subjects with relapses, Karavitaki *et al.* [8] introduced obvious differences in the 2.5-year local control rates after partial resection (50%), radiotherapy alone (83%), or partial resection followed by radiotherapy (100%).

Recurrent lesions with significant cystic components that can`t be total extirpated may be treated *via* repetitive aspirations through an indwelling Ommaya reservoir apparatus [38]. Either the establishment of a permanent communication between the cyst and sphenoid sinus for continuous drainage or ventriculocisternal cystostomy (allows spontaneous dilution of cyst contents in the CSF)may be palliative [39]. These procedures carry the risks of aseptic meningitis, CSF fistulae, and ascending infections although they are less invasive [39].

Therapeutic schemes with respect to recurrent disease rely on the nature of previous interventions and the severity of clinical scenario. For recurrent lesions not previously subjected to irradiation, radiotherapy seems effective. Given the high morbidity and mortality that accompany repeat operations, this choice is only suggested for cases with severe pressure effects.

schemes regarding the control of additional local failures are individualized and include the systemic chemotherapy, alternatives of Gamma knife radiosurgery, cyst-controlling procedures, and surgical debulking (for significant solid life-threatening components).

CONFLICT OF INTEREST

The author (editor) declares no conflict of interest, financial or otherwise.

ACKNOWLEDGEMENTS

Declared none.

REFERENCES

[1] Hoffman HJ, De Silva M, Humphreys RP, Drake JM, Smith ML, Blaser SI. Aggressive surgical management of craniopharyngiomas in children. J Neurosurg 1992; 76(1): 47-52. [http://dx.doi.org/10.3171/jns.1992.76.1.0047] [PMID: 1727168]

[2] Katz EL. Late results of radical excision of craniopharyngiomas in children. J Neurosurg 1975; 42(1): 86-93. [http://dx.doi.org/10.3171/jns.1975.42.1.0086] [PMID: 1110394]

[3] Kim SK, Wang KC, Shin SH, Choe G, Chi JG, Cho BK. Radical excision of pediatric craniopharyngioma: recurrence pattern and prognostic factors. Childs Nerv Syst 2001; 17(9): 531-6. [http://dx.doi.org/10.1007/s003810100458] [PMID: 11585327]

[4] Ohmori K, Collins J, Fukushima T. Craniopharyngiomas in children. Pediatr Neurosurg 2007; 43(4): 265-78. [http://dx.doi.org/10.1159/000103306] [PMID: 17627142]

[5] Tomita T, McLone DG. Radical resections of childhood craniopharyngiomas. Pediatr Neurosurg 1993; 19(1): 6-14. [http://dx.doi.org/10.1159/000120693] [PMID: 8422329]

[6] Wisoff JH. Surgical management of recurrent craniopharyngiomas. Pediatr Neurosurg 1994; 21 (Suppl. 1): 108-13.
[http://dx.doi.org/10.1159/000120871] [PMID: 7841068]

[7] Yaşargil MG, Curcic M, Kis M, Siegenthaler G, Teddy PJ, Roth P. Total removal of craniopharyngiomas. Approaches and long-term results in 144 patients. J Neurosurg 1990; 73(1): 3-11.
[http://dx.doi.org/10.3171/jns.1990.73.1.0003] [PMID: 2352020]

[8] Karavitaki N, Brufani C, Warner JT, *et al.* Craniopharyngiomas in children and adults: systematic analysis of 121 cases with long-term follow-up. Clin Endocrinol (Oxf) 2005; 62(4): 397-409.
[http://dx.doi.org/10.1111/j.1365-2265.2005.02231.x] [PMID: 15807869]

[9] Duff J, Meyer FB, Ilstrup DM, Laws ER Jr, Schleck CD, Scheithauer BW. Long-term outcomes for surgically resected craniopharyngiomas. Neurosurgery 2000; 46(2): 291-302.
[http://dx.doi.org/10.1097/00006123-200002000-00007] [PMID: 10690718]

[10] Fahlbusch R, Honegger J, Paulus W, Huk W, Buchfelder M. Surgical treatment of craniopharyngiomas: experience with 168 patients. J Neurosurg 1999; 90(2): 237-50.
[http://dx.doi.org/10.3171/jns.1999.90.2.0237] [PMID: 9950494]

[11] Weiner HL, Wisoff JH, Rosenberg ME, *et al.* Craniopharyngiomas: a clinicopathological analysis of factors predictive of recurrence and functional outcome. Neurosurgery 1994; 35(6): 1001-10.
[http://dx.doi.org/10.1227/00006123-199412000-00001] [PMID: 7885544]

[12] Van Effenterre R, Boch AL. Craniopharyngioma in adults and children: a study of 122 surgical cases. J Neurosurg 2002; 97(1): 3-11.
[http://dx.doi.org/10.3171/jns.2002.97.1.0003] [PMID: 12134929]

[13] De Vile CJ, Grant DB, Kendall BE, *et al.* Management of childhood craniopharyngioma: can the morbidity of radical surgery be predicted? J Neurosurg 1996; 85(1): 73-81.
[http://dx.doi.org/10.3171/jns.1996.85.1.0073] [PMID: 8683285]

[14] Maira G, Anile C, Rossi GF, Colosimo C. Surgical treatment of craniopharyngiomas: an evaluation of the transsphenoidal and pterional approaches. Neurosurgery 1995; 36(4): 715-24.
[http://dx.doi.org/10.1227/00006123-199504000-00012] [PMID: 7596502]

[15] Kalapurakal JA, Goldman S, Hsieh YC, Tomita T, Marymont MH. Clinical outcome in children with craniopharyngioma treated with primary surgery and radiotherapy deferred until relapse. Med Pediatr Oncol 2003; 40(4): 214-8.
[http://dx.doi.org/10.1002/mpo.10247] [PMID: 12555247]

[16] Stripp DC, Maity A, Janss AJ, *et al.* Surgery with or without radiation therapy in the management of craniopharyngiomas in children and young adults. Int J Radiat Oncol Biol Phys 2004; 58(3): 714-20.
[http://dx.doi.org/10.1016/S0360-3016(03)01570-0] [PMID: 14967425]

[17] Rajan B, Ashley S, Gorman C, *et al.* Craniopharyngioma--a long-term results following limited surgery and radiotherapy. Radiother Oncol 1993; 26(1): 1-10.
[http://dx.doi.org/10.1016/0167-8140(93)90019-5] [PMID: 8438080]

[18] Hetelekidis S, Barnes PD, Tao ML, *et al.* 20-year experience in childhood craniopharyngioma. Int J Radiat Oncol Biol Phys 1993; 27(2): 189-95.
[http://dx.doi.org/10.1016/0360-3016(93)90227-M] [PMID: 8407391]

[19] Amacher AL. Craniopharyngioma: the controversy regarding radiotherapy. Childs Brain 1980; 6(2): 57-64.
[PMID: 7353444]

[20] Carmel PW, Antunes JL, Chang CH. Craniopharyngiomas in children. Neurosurgery 1982; 11(3): 382-9.
[http://dx.doi.org/10.1227/00006123-198209000-00008] [PMID: 7133354]

[21] Crotty TB, Scheithauer BW, Young WF Jr, *et al.* Papillary craniopharyngioma: a clinicopathological

study of 48 cases. J Neurosurg 1995; 83(2): 206-14.
[http://dx.doi.org/10.3171/jns.1995.83.2.0206] [PMID: 7616262]

[22] Sweet WH. Radical surgical treatment of craniopharyngioma. Clin Neurosurg 1976; 23: 52-79. [PMID: 975700]

[23] Villarejo FJ. Recurrence in craniopharyngiomas. Neurochirurgia (Stuttg) 1982; 25(2): 73-4. [PMID: 7110495]

[24] Fisher PG, Jenab J, Gopldthwaite PT, *et al.* Outcomes and failure patterns in childhood craniopharyngiomas. Childs Nerv Syst 1998; 14(10): 558-63. [http://dx.doi.org/10.1007/s003810050272] [PMID: 9840379]

[25] Habrand JL, Ganry O, Couanet D, *et al.* The role of radiation therapy in the management of craniopharyngioma: a 25-year experience and review of the literature. Int J Radiat Oncol Biol Phys 1999; 44(2): 255-63. [http://dx.doi.org/10.1016/S0360-3016(99)00030-9] [PMID: 10760417]

[26] Hoff JT, Patterson RH Jr. Craniopharyngiomas in children and adults. J Neurosurg 1972; 36(3): 299-302. [http://dx.doi.org/10.3171/jns.1972.36.3.0299] [PMID: 5059968]

[27] Khafaga Y, Jenkin D, Kanaan I, Hassounah M, Al Shabanah M, Gray A. Craniopharyngioma in children. Int J Radiat Oncol Biol Phys 1998; 42(3): 601-6. [http://dx.doi.org/10.1016/S0360-3016(98)00257-0] [PMID: 9806520]

[28] Keohane C, Hally M, Ryder DQ, Buckley TF. Late recurrence of craniopharyngioma in the cerebellopontine angle in a fertile woman. J Neurol Neurosurg Psychiatry 1994; 57(7): 873-4. [http://dx.doi.org/10.1136/jnnp.57.7.873] [PMID: 8021691]

[29] Kahn EA, Gosch HH, Seeger JF, Hicks SP. Forty-five years experience with the craniopharyngiomas. Surg Neurol 1973; 1(1): 5-12. [PMID: 4544703]

[30] Barloon TJ, Yuh WT, Sato Y, Sickels WJ. Frontal lobe implantation of craniopharyngioma by repeated needle aspirations. AJNR Am J Neuroradiol 1988; 9(2): 406-7. [PMID: 3128093]

[31] Malik JM, Cosgrove GR, VandenBerg SR. Remote recurrence of craniopharyngioma in the epidural space. Case report. J Neurosurg 1992; 77(5): 804-7. [http://dx.doi.org/10.3171/jns.1992.77.5.0804] [PMID: 1403127]

[32] Gupta K, Kuhn MJ, Shevlin DW, Wacaser LE. Metastatic craniopharyngioma. AJNR Am J Neuroradiol 1999; 20(6): 1059-60. [PMID: 10445444]

[33] Ito M, Jamshidi J, Yamanaka K. Does craniopharyngioma metastasize? Case report and review of the literature. Neurosurgery 2001; 48(4): 933-5. [PMID: 11322455]

[34] Karavitaki N, Cudlip S, Adams CB, Wass JA. Craniopharyngiomas. Endocr Rev 2006; 27(4): 371-97. [http://dx.doi.org/10.1210/er.2006-0002] [PMID: 16543382]

[35] Yuen KC, Kołtowska-Häggström M, Cook DM, *et al.* Primary treatment regimen and diabetes insipidus as predictors of health outcomes in adults with childhood-onset craniopharyngioma. J Clin Endocrinol Metab 2014; 99(4): 1227-35. [http://dx.doi.org/10.1210/jc.2013-3631] [PMID: 24476077]

[36] Elliott RE, Sands SA, Strom RG, Wisoff JH. Craniopharyngioma Clinical Status Scale: a standardized metric of preoperative function and posttreatment outcome. Neurosurg Focus 2010; 28(4): E2. [http://dx.doi.org/10.3171/2010.2.FOCUS09304] [PMID: 20367359]

[37] Jose CC, Rajan B, Ashley S, Marsh H, Brada M. Radiotherapy for the treatment of recurrent

craniopharyngioma. Clin Oncol (R Coll Radiol) 1992; 4(5): 287-9.
[http://dx.doi.org/10.1016/S0936-6555(05)81101-X] [PMID: 1390343]

[38] Gutin PH, Klemme WM, Lagger RL, MacKay AR, Pitts LH, Hosobuchi Y. Management of the unresectable cystic craniopharyngioma by aspiration through an Ommaya reservoir drainage system. J Neurosurg 1980; 52(1): 36-40.
[http://dx.doi.org/10.3171/jns.1980.52.1.0036] [PMID: 7350278]

[39] Spaziante R, Irace C, De Divitiis E. Brachytherapy of cystic craniopharyngiomas. J Neurosurg 1993; 79(6): 966-7.
[PMID: 8246069]

CHAPTER 16

Hypopituitarism in Craniopharyngioma

Chun-ling Ye[1,*] and **Jun-xiang Peng**[2]

[1] *College of Pharmacy, Ji'nan University, 601 Western Huangpu Avenue, Guangzhou, China*

[2] *Department of Neurosurgery, Nanfang Neurosurgery Research Institution, Nanfang Hospital, Southern Medical University, 1838 North Guangzhou Avenue, Guangzhou, China*

Abstract: Endocrine dysfunction is a common complication of craniopharyngiomas due to tumor location and the growth pattern. How to diagnose hypopituitarism and implement reasonable hormone replacement therapy, promote the recovery of endocrine function after operation is still a puzzle need to be solved urgently. The purpose of the present chapter is to summarize data on endocrinological evaluation in these patients, discuss clinical characters, and elaborate the growth features of childhood craniopharyngiomas. To understand the hypopituitarism patterns and its influencing factors of patients with craniopharyngioma has important effect on improving the prognosis and long-term quality of life.

Keywords: Craniopharyngioma, Endocrinology evaluation, Hormone, Hypopituitarism.

Craniopharyngioma (CP) accounts for approximately 3% of all intracranial tumors and up to 10% of childhood brain tumors [1]. CP usually grows along the craniopharyngeal canal and presents in the sellar or suprasellar region. Given the proximity of CP to the hormone-producing cells of the hypothalamus and pituitary gland, most patients harboring CP exhibit significant hypopituitarism that either the production or secretion of one or more hormones were insufficient for physiological needs [2, 3]. The order of diminished hormonal reserve function was as follows: growth hormone (GH)/insulin-like growth factor I (IGF-1) axis, gonadal axis, thyroid axis, and adrenocorticotropic hormone (ACTH) axis. The incidence of other pituitary hormone deficits before surgery has been summarized from the previous reports [2 - 4] as 40% for gonadotropin insufficiency, 25% for TSH and ACTH insufficiency, 9-17% for ADH insufficiency and 20% for raised serum prolactin.

* **Corresponding author Chun-ling Ye**: College of Pharmacy, Ji'nan University, 601, Western Huangpu Avenue, Guangzhou, China; Tel\Fax: +8620-61641812; E-mail: yechunling2005@163.com

Songtao Qi (Ed.)

Clinical manifestations of hypopituitarism can vary greatly according to the hormonal affected axis, individual clinical status, and pituitary hormone levels. One feature of biochemical testing for hypopituitarism is insufficient target gland secretion with normal or increasing the individuals' needs. In particular, diagnosis is usually established by provocative testing. Hypothalamic or pituitary illness arising from hypopituitarism is usually associated with different degree of increased prolactin (PRL) or diabetes insipidus (DI) [4 - 7]. In some patients with CP, the functions of some glands may recover after surgery to provide sufficient hormones for physiological needs. The thyroid and ACTH axes are regarded as the most likely to recover; however, the likelihood of GH/IGF-1 axis recovery is almost nonexistent. The ability to reserve pituitary function lies on the accessibility, aggressiveness, size of the tumor; skill of the neurosurgery; and selected operative approach. After surgery, all patients should require an perfect endocrine assessment of pituitary function to avoid undetected deficits in pituitary function. Published reports had indicated that hormone levels should stabilize within 3 months after surgery and would not restore after 1 year.

Hypopituitarism can be asymptomatic presentation and indicated only by hormone measurement, or its clinical symptom might be acute and severe, necessitating hospital admission and intensive care treatment [8, 9]. The symptoms of hypopituitarism are usually nonspecific including fatigue, lack of energy, social isolation, depression, poor concentration, and reduced physical capacity. Other nonspecific signs include general central adiposity, reduced lean tissue mass, and reduced bone mineral density accompany with unfavorable biochemical changes such as hyperlipidemia and glucose intolerance [10]. Treatment for hypopituitarism should comprise individually tailored hormone replacement according to age, sex, hormonal affected levels, and degree of insufficiency, among other related factors. Doses should meet the individuals' needs and mimic physiological rhythm secretion, but overdoses must be avoided to reduce side effects [11, 12]. Before hormone replacement, an completed endocrine assessment of anterior and posterior pituitary function should be needed to determine the drug types and doses. Because the relationships among these hormones are such complex as their effects impact and influence each other. For instance, when the thyroid and ACTH axes functions are recover, the posterior pituitary hormone levels may be considered as insufficient. In addition, patients' pituitary functions have the opportunity for restoration after operation. In general, dose adjustments, timely assessments of symptom and pituitary hormone levels play important roles in hypopituitarism treatment.

LABORATORY EXAMINATION METHODS OF PITUITARY HORMONES

CP can lead to individual hormonal dysfunction and corresponding clinical manifestations. However, the diagnostic assessment of pituitary dysfunction has not yet been standardized.

In general, a combination of peripherally and inappropriately low (below the upper level of the reference range) hypothalamus-pituitary hormone levels indicates hypopituitarism. However, basal concentrations alone might be not distinctive and precise because of the pulsatile, circadian, or situational secretion with various hormones [8, 10]. In fact, the diagnosis of hypopituitarism mostly depends on the outcome of appropriate biochemical test regarding a patient in whom clinical findings have raised the suspicion of hormone insufficiency. The clinical manifestations of hypopituarism in adults are often subcliniacl and potentially, with symptoms that overlap both other clinical medical conditions; consequently, the diagnosis is frequently delayed unless the investigating physician pays enough attention to suspiciousness for a possible underlying endocrine cause [13 - 15].

Basal Anterior Pituitary Hormone Assays

To gain the most information and data about each axis from a basic blood endocrine test, the basal concentrations of both the pituitary and target hormones should be assayed, including luteinizing hormone (LH), follicle-stimulating hormone (FSH), and estradiol or testosterone (09:00 h), as well as TSH, free thyroxine (FT4), ACTH, cortisol (09:00 h), and PRL. Baseline IGF-1, testosterone, and cortisol levels should be measured at 09:00 h because this is the time of peak circadian secretion. Most reference ranges have been set using 9:00 am criterion, it is easier and more efficient to interpret and compare results taken at the same time.

Dynamic Tests of Anterior Pituitary Function

The above-described basal hormone assays provide important information and data, particularly when the tumor is appropriately elevated alone with a low target hormone level which indicate primary target organ failure. The condition is much more complex and intricacy when either a low target hormone level is found in conjunction with inappropriately low ralated pituitary hormone level or when ongoing monitoring is required for patients with known hypothalamus-pituitary hormone insufficient. In these cases, dynamic testing is required to quantify the pituitary reserve more accurately.

Assessing the Hypothalamic–Pituitary–Adrenal (HPA) Axis

In most cases, hypocortisolism develops gradually and carelessly, the clinical manifests are often nonspecific symptoms and signs such as nausea, vomiting, abdominal pain, loss of energy, fatigue, fever, and impaired alertness, as well as hypoglycemia after prolonged fasting. An 09:00h cortisol level of <3.6 mg/dl (<100 nmol/L) is generally adequate to diagnose adrenal insufficiency, whereas a level of ≥18. 1 mg /dl (≥500 nmol/L) is indicative of adequate ACTH reserves [16 - 18]. If the measured data lies between these upper and lower thresholds, a provocative testing is needed. In fact, approximately one quarter of all such patients need to be spared such testing. The insulin tolerance test (ITT), which was originally described in the 1960s [19], is still suggested as the gold standard for dynamic testing of the entire HPA and GH axes in patients harboring CP.

If the required peak cortisol level (normal range: 18.1–21. 0 mg /dl [500– 580 nmol /L]) is achieved during ITT, the patient is cosidered to have sufficient ACTH reserves to mount an adequate response to hypoglycemia. The contraindacations of ITT are epilepsy, ischemic heart disease, and postcraniotomy, and the majority of endocrinologists would not recommend it in above 70 years old patients. Despite the potential hazards, the complication rate of this test can remains very low when conducted by experienced clinician.

Assessing the Hypothalamic–Pituitary–Adrenal (HPA) Axis

The clinical presentation of central hypothyroidism resembles as primary hypothyroidism because of the direct loss of thyroid gland hormone. Current testing methods generally enable to make the diagnosis by measuring the basal thyroid-stimulating hormone (TSH) and FT4 levels. Serum FT4 is essential if the patient is pregnant or taking oral estrogen, Serum FT4 is of great concern for those who under going pregnant or taking oral estrogen, regard the increasing in thyroid hormone-binding globulin [20, 21].

Diagnosis for primary of secondary hypothyroidism commonly through a basic assessment of TSH and thyroxine, including free or total. Because deficiency of TSH is more sensitive and specificity concerning of symptom and sign, it is unnecessary to use the throtropin-releasing hormone (TRH) test (assessment of TSH response to the intravenous administration TRH) [23, 24].

Assessing Growth Hormone Reserve

Human body normally pulse secreted GH at night during sleep, hypoglycemia or exercise state will affect GH release. IGF-1, GH ramification, can mediates many GH progress, also can influence GH secretion and inhibit GH release at upstream (pituitary and hypothalamic level). A single serum GH assessment is not adequate for GH deficiency (GHD), for its pulsatile secreted pattern and its extremely low serum concentration between pulses making difficult for common assays [25 - 31]. In addition, diagnosis of GHD can not through single serum IGF-1 assessment also, as the level may still be normal even if GHD is getting worse [32].

Therefore, GH and IGF-1 assessment can not be separated on this concern. Approximately 30% of patient with GHD would be missed at single criterion for diagnosis, for which of them are at normal IGF-1 level. A provocative testing to assess GH can be subdivided into two classification, one is physiological methods another is pharmacological agent method, both of them can stimulate GH release [25, 33 - 38]. The ITT is still considered as the gold standard for valuating serum GH level. A GH peak <3ug/L provides very strong evidence for GHD, while a value > 5μg/L essentially rules it out [39 - 41].

Assessing the Pituitary–gonadal Axis

Serum testosterone levels vary according to a physiological rhythm and are highest in the early morning. Free, active testosterone only accounts for approximately 1–2% of the total testosterone level, as most total testosterone is bound to albumin and to sex hormone-binding globulin (SHBG). Usually, measurements of baseline testosterone or estradiol and LH, FSH, are efficient to diagnose hypogonadism. Ideally measurement for estradiol is at the period of follicular phase of the menstrual cycle, and testosterone is at 09:00 h of the day [35].

Both sex steroids and SHBG level should be measured to precise determine the amount of biologically active hormone. Women whose menstruate are regular can not be define as a gonadotropin deficient, although their menstruation may clearly be anovulatory. Ovulation can be easy assessed by measuring the progesterone level on day 21 of the menstrual cycle.

A gonadotropin-releasing hormone (GnRH) test can be performed to facilitate the difficult distinction between a constitutional delay of puberty and secondary hypogonadism while considering the normal values for the patient's age and pubertal stage. But this test generally be limit applied in scientific study, nor clinical yet [37].

Posterior Pituitary Assessment

A completed assessment of ACTH reserve and initiation of glucocorticoid replacement are vital before formally posterior pituitary function evaluation as cortisol is required for kidneys to generate and excrete abnormal water load; therefore, symptom of diabetes insipidus may be concealed in patient coexisted with steroid deficencies.

Diagnostic code of central diabetes insipidus (CDI), often caused by vasopressin deficiency, should be included basic clues as below, Low paired plasma and urine osmolalities, in combination with high daily urine output, and disorder of hydroelectrolyte balance. However, patient with nephrogenic DI or primary polydipsia also can result in DI, a formal water deprivation test may be required to excluded those less clear–cut cases [11, 42]. The protocol of water deprivation test has been published before, generally, the responses of urine output and osmolality to a period of fluid restriction followed by a particular dose of exogenous vasopressin are required detected. Plasma osmolalities and serial weights are also need considered. These tests should be performed by experience doctors to protect patients from dangerous caused by dehydration, meanwhile ensure its efficiency.

With more precise methods provided for measurement of endogenous vasopressin nowadays, diagnosis of DI become more easily. However, these are not in wide use at present. In current clinical practice, the performance of pituitary dynamic tests is still erratic [36]. Pitfalls, should be avoided. Include false-positive and false-negative results, the former often result in unnecessary and costly hormone supplementation meanwhile the later lead to the inadequate replacement of essential hormones. There are no any published guidelines in this field, nowadays, with the sole exception of guidelines for the diagnosis of GHD.

CLINICAL MANIFESTATION OF PANHYPOPITUITARISM

Given the hypothalamus and pituitary gland damaged by adjacent tumor, most patients with CP exhibit endocrine dysfunction [42]. In the1970s, two large series reported that about 15% of children had endocrine problems at presentation. Although those studies have demonstrated short stature as a presenting complaint in only 7% of children with CP, exceed 50-86% of patients under studied are found. The majority of these persons underwent subnormal growth rates, one quarter of them are obese, and the majority of the adolescents exhibit pubertal delay at the time of clinical assessment [43 - 45].

Recent molecular studies have made the better comprehend of the pathogenesis of hypopituitarism caused by CP. Anterior pituitary hormone synthesis and secretion are regulated *via* the release and inhibition of hypothalamus hormones including TRH, GnRH, GRIH and CRH. As if hypothalamic hormones and their pituitary receptors genes encoding progress emerge inactivating or loss-of-function mutations, selective or isolated deficiencies will appeared in downstream pituitary hormone. Insufficient of two or more anterior pituitary hormones can also occur, leading to multiple pituitary hormone deficiency (MPHD) [46, 47].

In most patients with CP, hypopituitarism may presents in a long period of time before the tumor diagnosis is made. After treatment with surgery, endocrine problems become a major factor affecting morbidity and mortality. Tomlinson *et al.* [7] studied the association between mortality and hypopituitarism in children CP, which showed that CP caused 10-fold greater mortality rates than other causes of hypopituitarism did. This excess mortality may be due to hypothalamic damage and metabolic dysregulation. Even if normal hormone levels appeared in short time period after treatment, hormone deficiencies may also develop over the years, it is made sense for patient with CP be followed up and monitored closely.

Table 1. Signs and Symptoms of Hypopituitarism in Craniopharyngioma.

Hormone deficiency	Clinical features
ACTH	Chronic: fatigue, pallor, anorexia, weight loss, hypoglycemia, and hyponatremia Acute: weakness, dizziness, nausea, vomiting, circulatory collapse, fever, shock Children: delayed puberty, failure to thrive
TSH	Tiredness, cold intolerance, constipation, hair loss, hoarseness, weight gain, dry skin and hair, constipation, muscle weakness, and cognitive slowing Children: retarded development, growth retardation
GH	Increased fatigue, and increased cardiovascular risk, impaired psychological well-being, reduced lean body mass, Decreased muscle strength and exercise capacity, visceral obesity, fatigue, decreased quality of life, impairment of attention and memory Children: growth retardation
LH and FSH	Women: oligoamenorrhea, loss of libido, dyspareunia, infertility Men: loss of libido, impaired sexual function, mood impairment, loss of facial, scrotal, loss of secondary sexual characteristics and trunk hair Children: delayed puberty
Vasopressin	Polydipsia, polyuria, and nocturia
PRL	Failure of lactation

ACTH, adrenocorticotropic hormone; TSH, thyroid-stimulating hormone; GH, growth hormone; LH, luteinizing hormone; FSH, follicle-stimulating hormone; PRL, prolactin.

ENDOCRINOLOGICAL EVALUATION BEFORE AND AFTER SURGERY

Secretion of anterior pituitary hormones (LH, FSH, PRL, GH, ACTH, and TSH) are under controlled by multiple hypothalamic hormones through complicated mechanism. Vary degrees of hypopituitarism in CP patients are present at diagnosis time or may occur after the operation and/or radiotherapy. Accurate pituitary functional evaluations are essential requirement for diagnosis and monitor of treatment effect. Part of pituitary hormones insufficient can be detected using single blood samples (*e.g.*, TSH together with FT4), whereas others with complicated circadian or pulsatile secretion patterns require dynamic stimulation detections (*e.g.*, ACTH). There are still controversial in the best methods to diagnosis the deficiency of ACTH and GH [18].

It is necessary to assess CP patients' pituitary hormones level at the initial diagnosis to clear and definite the need for hormonal replacement before tumor treatments. A suitable set of endocrinological tests including serum electrolytes, cortisol (at 08.00–09.00 h), FT4, TSH, prolactin, estradiol /testosterone, LH, FSH, and IGF-1 will satisfy the need. ITT should be performed when the serum cortisol level is > 450 nmol/l or GH deficiency is suspected. However, if subjecting the patient to a pre-operative ITT is considered excessively, SST should be used to define baseline function of HPA axis [11, 35, 41].

The using of glucocorticoids in patients undergoing pituitary surgery is decided by the results of pre-operative screening tests. If the preoperative basal cortisol/ITT results are subnormal, hydrocortisone replacement (10–20 mg daily) is required with an increase to cover surgery and the first 48 h postoperatively. A standard perioperative regimen comprises 50– 100 mg hydrocortisone during the induction of anesthesia, 50– 100 mg per 12 h for the first day, 30–80 mg per 12 h for the second day, and then a return to regular dose is depended on the clinical progress and manifestation. For patients that preoperative basal cortisol <100 nmol/L, replacement therapy of steroids should be lasted until the time of definitive testing at 4–6 weeks postoperation. In patients who preoperative basal cortisol >450 nmol/l and/or have a normal SST result, perioperative replacement is also necessary, particularly if a selective adenomectomy is found to be possible; the basal cortisol condition should be assessed every 3–5 days after surgery.

Vasopressin should be used in the patients who have pre-operative DI, and last until the early postoperative period, usually parenterally for the first day or two. Surgical intervention may be responsible for DI and occurred intra-operation or post-operation. Clinical and biochemical vigilance with close cooperation between the anesthetic, endocrine, and surgical teams is mandatory.

Glucocorticoid replacement therapy should be given after the surgery of CP in order to avoid undetected hypoadrenalism, and the therapy should last until postsurgical ACTH deficit, while other pituitary hormones can be excluded. Endocrine assessment should be performed routinely in CP patients, for the glucocorticoid insufficient can be life threatening, hormones replacement should carry out as soon as possible. Thyroid hormone replacement with L-thyroxine is also necessary if hypothyroidism is identified. Because thyroid hormone substitution can increase the glucocorticoid metabolism rate, which can lead to an adrenal crisis, therefore, L-thyroxine should be implemented after hydrocortisone relpacement initiation.

Female sex hormone substitution can rescue the libido, well being, and bone mass to normal level. Many studies in non-hypopituitary post-menopausal patients who received sex hormone replacement showed a higher incidence of cardiovascular and neoplastic diseases among these patients. Therefore, cessation of sex hormone replacement in hypogonadal women after menopause is recommended in published reports. In addition, testosterone substitution in hypogonadal men has been found to rescue bone and muscle mass, sexual function, and hematocrit to normal level. GH substitution treatment can enhance the body composition, lipid variables, and the quality of life. GHD has been assumed to lead to the excess cardiovascular.

Mortality observed with hypopituitarism, although other factors such as cranial radiation, surgery, and other biochemical deficiencies also play important roles. Some studies reported that GH replacement therapy can improve cognitive function, while other hormones have no such effect. Findings of long-term studies, moreover, showed that GH substitution did not increase overall incidence of malignant disease and/or tumor recurrence. However, the sample sizes of these studies are insufficient for a final conclusion, and surveys regarding tumor growth are ongoing.

Follow-up

Once the hypopituitarism has been diagnosed, adequate corresponding hormonal replacement should be carried on as well as regular hormones monitor. After the initial titration phase, 6–12-month intervals are usually recommended. Regular ophthalmological controls and magnetic resonance imaging (MRI) are needed in this period. An initial post-surgery endocrine hormones assessment should be performed during the rehabilitation phase (3-6 months after resection) [11, 36]. The assessment should be reexamination constantly during the chronic phase (approximately 1 year after surgery), as pituitary dysfunction can retort after this phase but new deficiencies may occasionally occur.

Once hypopituitarism was clear and definite, adequate hypothalamus and pituitary hormone replacement can improve the quality of life markedly, decline the morbidity and mortality at the same time, Research revealed that patients who did not undergo endocrine assessment previously are at increased risk for hypopituitarism. The individuals should be actively screened for the disorder. However, for the patients with hypopituitarism, the dose of hormones replacement and the detection time of related treatment are remain unanswered and require further research.

TREATMENT

Treatment of hypopituitarism must consider all cause as well as commencing and optimizing appropriate hormone replacement therapy. Determining the etiology of the pituitary problems will facilitate treatment of the underlying condition. Options may include the use of medical treatments, surgical intervention, and so on [14].

Hormone Replacement Therapy

Treatment regimens generally involving the replace of the target hormones, and components come from the pituitary or hypothalamus are less mentioned. In patients harboring CP, GH, thyroid hormone, cortisol and ADH had been used and mentioned routinely. However, treatment of infertility caused by hypogonadotropic hypogonadism, particularly patients durning their period of duration, should not be overlook [15, 37].

ACTH Deficiency

There is no report on ACTH level measurement in previous literature. The ACTH level was usually responded by serum Cortisol [15]. In our study the postoperative ACTH level was much lower compare with preoperative condition. Some studies [16, 17] had demonstrated that the endocrine abnormalities in CP were due to the impairment of the hypothalamus and/or tumor mass effect on hypophysioportal system. It is believed that direct damage to the pituitary gland, the pituitary portal system and the hypothalamus also responsible for endocrine dysfunction. Therefore the decline of plasma ACTH level ACTH postopsrative probably arose from the injury of both the hypothalamus and the pituitary gland. Furthermore, the assessment of ACTH releasing hormone may help elucidate the cause of ACTH deficiency after tumor resection.

Hydrocortisoneis the most generally accepted glucocorticoid for replacement treatment because it can replaces the deficient target hormone directly and easy to monitor in serum or urine [15, 19]. Alternatives including cortisone acetate and prednisolone and dexamethasone. Cortisone acetate is metabolized firstly to cortisol to exert the glucocorticoid effect. Therefore, its onset of action is later than hydrocortisone which has largely replaced cortisone acetate as the drug of choice. The currently recommended replacement regimen is 10 mg of hydrocortisone upon waking, 5 mg at lunch time, and 5 mg during the early evening. Clearly, patients are heterogeneous, therefore, regimens of hydrocortisone replacement require significant adjustments for individual patients, rely on clinical symptoms and the serum or urine hormone monitor results [17].

TSH Deficiency

Theoretically, the incidence of pre/post-operativeTSH deficiency was 24%-58% and 10%-85% correspondingly [20], The result accordance with the change of thyroid function described above. Patients with hypothalamic pituitary disorder also had a blunted TSH surge [21]. The incidence of hypothyroidism in patients treated with surgery or surgery combination with radiotherapy was reported range from 29% to 85%. Thyroid hormone levels are observed especially closely in kids less than 2 years old since hypothyroidism may contribute to impede mental development.

Thyroxine replacement is the preferred for the treatment of both primary and secondary hypothyroidism, with the average dose of 25– 100ug/day for patients with total deficiency. The starting dose can be 25mg /day, followed 25- mg increments according to the FT4 level that reexamination each four weeks [20, 21]. For patients with serious hypothyroidism, lower starting doses of 25mg can be applied. Triiodothyronine is seldom superior, considering the faster onset of action and shorter half-life, but thyroxine is regularly proper. In primary hypothyroidism, TSH is a sensitive index that can guide precise replacement; but in secondary hypothyroidism, serum TSH level may be low, normal, or even slightly raised. Most endocrinologists are meant for a replacement dose of thyroxine that contributes to hypothyroidism patients and FT4 levels on the upper end of the normal reference range. Steroid dose must to be enough for the patients who receive the replacement treatment, thyroxine is prior to steroid if possible; otherwise, a potentially hypoadrenal crisis may be precipitated [23, 24].

LH/FSH Deficiency

Gonadotropin deficiency and its related symptom are the most common clinical phenotype in adult craniopharyngiomas. Almost all the adolescents may have complaints of delayed puberty. Levels of gonadotropin and estrogen (girls) and testosterone (boys) are prepubertal. The sex steroids (especially estrogen in both sexes) result in the closure of the growth centers of the bones.

The probable complications of estrogen therapy in postmenopausal female had been well informed and may lead to the resistant of treatment. It is essential that each case must be thought over individually and guided well to make a wise choice as the serious long-run results of estrogen deficiency obviously surpass the side effects of such therapy, especially in young female. Many young female prefer the combined of oral contraceptive pill because it is more acceptable among their fellows [43 - 45]. Besides, ransdermal HRT preparations are also available. The transdermal preparations have an advantage over oral estrogen preparations for having no effect on cortisol-binding globulin and, as a result, the result of hydrocortisone replacement monitor won't be disturbed. Androgen replacement in male often starts through intramuscular depot testosterone injections. Trough and/or peak levels are supervised, and the adjusting of the dose or dose interval is used to achieve the optimal treatment effect.

Testosterone Cipionate or Testosterone Enanthate Replacement

The long-acting forms are provided in doses of 250-300 mg for young male and 200-250 mg for the older ones and are administered intramuscularly(IM) in the gluteal muscle every 2 or 3weeks. Short-acting forms are available but need to inject 2 or 3 times every week. Oral preparations are ineffective, very high dose is required, and may carry increased risks. A transdermal system is available and its use is increasing. These forms must be applied daily in scrotal skin. A new transdermal system allowing chest placement is now available and may be used more frequently in the future [43, 45].

Replacement Therapy for LH and FSH Deficiency (women)

Oral conjugated estrogens comprise the most commonly used form estrogen. For patients with an intact uterus, Premarin is administered at 0.625 mg/day for days 1–25; Provera at 5 mg/day is added from days 16-25. From days 25-31, both medications are stopped to allow withdrawal bleeding. If the patient does not have an intact uterus, Premarin at 0.625 mg is given daily on a continuous schedule [45].

GH Deficiency

Among all hormone deficiencies, GHD is the most common with the incidence of 75% of children craniopharyngioma. Although up to 86% of the patients have growth deceleration, it is mostly neglected, causing a delayed diagnosis of craniopharyngioma. Although a great number of children craniopharyngioma have growth retardation, excessive growth has hardly been stated at any presentation. About 90% of the childhood patients show postoperative growth deceleration.

Compared with the previously accepted doctrine, evidence accumulated during the final few decades of the last century to show that GH may play an important part in adulthood. During the 1990s, the availability of recombinant GH, which has eliminated the risks associated with human cadaver -derived GH, has allowed many adult patients with serious GH deficiency to receive proper replacement therapy. GH is administered as a daily subcutaneous injection *via* a pen device mastered quickly by most patients [27, 29, 30].

GH treatment is commenced at a low dose that is titrated up slowly on the basis of clinical and biochemical (IGF-1) parameters. Persuasive evidence has associated GH replacement in GH-deficient adults with very effective. An increase in lean body mass together with a reduction in fat mass and resultant increase in exercise tolerance is observed in patients receiving treatment. GH therapy has also been associated with an improved lipid profile and with long-run improvements in bone mineral density in patients at risk for osteoporosis.

The maximum dose for children receiving GH replacement therapy is 0.1 mg/kg and given subcutaneously (SC) or IM 3 times per week or 0.3 mg/ kg once per week. Notably, both pretreatment and periodic electrolyte levels should be monitored, especially blood urea nitrogen (BUN) and creatinine for increased protein synthesis, glucose for insulin resistance, and alkaline phosphatase as a measure of bone growth. Patients who receive both glucocorticoid and GH replacement should be observed closely. Coordination of medications is essential to avoid inhibitory influences on growth [30].

Adult GH replacement therapy should start at small doses, such as 0.15-0.3 mg (1 mg = 3 iu) injected SC. The advised sex- and age-based dose references are as follows: young men: 0.2 mg/day; young women: 0.3 mg/day; and elderly: 0.1 mg/day. However, the specific dose should be individualized while considering the patient's age, gender, and estrogen levels, and after a period of time the treatment can be adjusted according to the clinical response, drug side effects, and IGF-1 level [27].

Vasopressin Deficiency

Vasopressin hyposecretion from the posterior pituitary gland results in partial or complete cranial DI. Desmopressin, a synthetic analogue of arginine vasopressin, is the replacement drug with oral, intranasal, and parenteral dosage forms. Desmopressin should start at a low dose and gradually titrated up according to the degree of polyuria. Monitoring of paired urine and plasma osmolalities, urea and electrolyte levels, and fluid balance is vital, especially during the early period and when regulating the dose [36].

THE FUTURE

Based on our analyses, endocrinopathy is a common iatrogenic complication of treatment of craniopharyngiomas with either surgical resection or radiosurgery, however it is not unexpectedly higher in surgical cases.Further effort should be invested to monitor and maintain the normal hormones level, hence improve the quality of patients' life.

With the maturing of the concept of saddle membrane structures, and the deeper understanding in the origin and growth pattern of craniopharyngioma, total excision of the tumor has become possible relying on the modern microsurgical techniques. But how to implement reasonable hormone replacement therapy, and promote the recovery of adult endocrine function after operation is still a puzzle need to be solved urgently for neurosurgeons, endocrinologists, obstetrician and gynecologist.

Hypopituitarism Patterns of Adult Craniopharyngioma

To understand the hypopituitarism patterns and its influencing factors of adult patients with craniopharyngioma has important effect on improving the prognosis and long-term quality of life. In this large cohort of adult patients with craniopharyngiomas, we aimed to evaluate the association between tumor growth pattern and hypopituitarism patterns, the endocrine hormones changing is recorded to find out the pattern of hypopituitarism pre- and post-operation. 153 adult patients with craniopharyngioma who underwent primary surgery in our department from January 2006 to December 2011 were enrolled in this study. All pathological material, medical records of these patients were reviewed. The diagnosis of CP was confirmed by histological study. The average age of patients (78 male, 75 female) was 40.25 ± 14.20 years at the time of surgery (Range from 18 to 72 years). All of the clinical, radiological and surgical data were recorded detailed.

Tumor size was calculated as the maximum measurable dimension in the MRI and classified as small (≤2cm), moderate (2cm<--≤4cm), large (4cm<--≤6cm), and huge (>6cm). All 153 patients in this series underwent surgical resection with the aim of total tumor removal.

Accordingly CPs originating along the developing path of the stalk may manifest different topographic relations with these membrane structures [49]. With comprehensive considerations of pre-surgical MR imaging, intra-operative findings, and tumor's most possible originating site, the tumors were classified into 3 subtypes as depicted in the Fig. (**1**): Type Q: Infra-diaphragmatic, Type S: Supra-diaphragmatic inter-arachnoid extra-ventricular, and Type T: Supra-diaphragmatic infundibulo- tuberal. This topographical classification scheme highlights the original site of tumor and the relationship between tumor and the supra-sellar membrane structures.

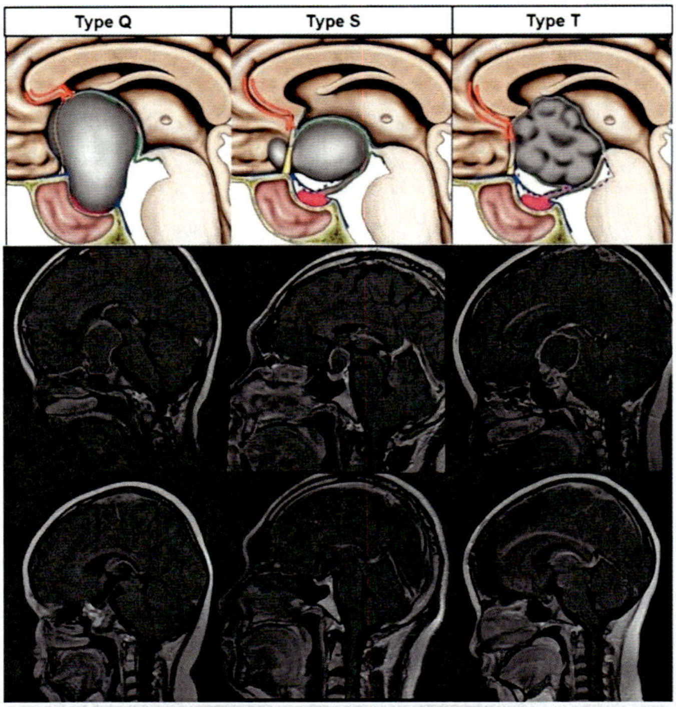

Fig. (1). The schematic diagram and magnetic resonance images show the growth patterns of craniopharyngioma.

Endocrinological Assessment

All of the patients had signed an informed consent form and carried out insulin provocative test one week before the operation. The morning fasting venous blood of all subjects were obtained to detect plasma thyrotropin(TSH), free thyroxine(FT4, FT3), cortisol(Cor), total testosterone (TESTO), follicle stimulating hormone(FSH), luteinizing hormone(LH) and prolactin(PRL), thyroid function tests, growth hormone (GH) and insulin-like growth factor-1 (IGF-1) three days before the operation. And reexamination for those hormones is taken in first, second and third weeks after the operation.

Hypopituitarism was defined as partial or complete loss of hypothalamic-pituitary axes [51]. Growth hormone deficiency (GHD) was diagnosed on the basis of low serum IGF-1 levels or insulin tolerance test (ITT)(GH peak<5ug/L) [52]. Gonadotrophin deficiency was defined as low or inappropriately normal FSH and LH levels with low TESTO levels [6]. Central hypothyroidism was defined as low or inappropriately normal TSH levels in the presence of low free T4 (FT4) levels [53]. ACTH deficiency was defined by a peak cortisol value after provocative testing (insulin hypoglycaemia test, glucagons or short synacthen test) of <18 ng/ml or a baseline plasma cortisol level of <3 ng/ml; GH deficiency was defined by a peak value after effective stimulation in an insulin stimulation test of <5 ng/ml [54].

Endocrine Characteristics Before and After Operation

Preoperative Endocrine

Preoperatively patients (77.1%) had one or more pituitary hormones dysfunction, including 27 cases of patients with panhypopituitarism, 90 patients had partial hypopituitarism. The incidence of thyroxine deficiency (HPT) 39.2% (60/153), adrenal cortex hormone deficiency (HPA) 31.4% (48/453), gonadal hormone deficiency (HPG) 62.7% (96/153), growth hormone deficiency (GHD) 47.1% (72/153), preoperative diabetes insipidus (DI) incidence rate was 28.8% (44/153). Hypopituitarism frequency goes from high to low is: HPG>GHD>HPT>HPA>DI. To compare with the endocrine change before and after surgery in 146 cases who had been followed up for more than a year by repeated measures analysis of variance, we suggest that there is an significant increasing trend for GH, Cor, FT3, FT4, FSH, LH from early period of postoperation to preoperation and reach peak 1 years after surgery($P < 0.05$).

Endocrine Changes in Early Period of Postoperation

All of the serum hormones are decreasing in first week after surgery. For 110 cases of diabetes insipidus (58 cases didn't show polydipsia and diuresis before), 78 cases of them can return to normal urine volume by appropriate treatment last 2-4 weeks. 38.6-74.3% cases showed new endocrine disorder. HPA axis is the easiest one that became abnormal after operation, and improvement rates were 0-28.6%. For the case with abnormal HPA/HPT/GH axis pre-operation, there is no improvement case after operation, only 9 cases (12.5%) with abnormal HPG axis show improvement after operation. All of hormones showed significant decline in the early period of postoperation compare to pre-operation ($P<0.05$), indicate a pejorative and acute change of hormone in the early period of postoperation.

Endocrine Changes in Mid and Late Postoperative (Tables 2 and 3)

Patients' serum hormones were detected at 3, 6, 12 months after surgery. Most patients who were followed up showed symptoms of endocrine disorders in different degree, the long-term abnormality rates in endocrine disorders are 20.6-75.3%, and HPG axis disorder is the most common one with a incidence rate of 75.3%, disorders of HPA axis and HPT axis are followed with a rate of 61.9% and 56.7% respectively, therefore, most of postoperative patients need adrenal and thyroid hormones replacement therapy. Postoperative diabetes insipidus (DI) can be treated well using Minirin, and the incidence rate was 20.6%, has no significant statistical difference compare with the preoperative rate (p=0.412). 85 cases of patients' polydipsia, polyuria, appetite, amenorrhea, fatigue, symptoms can be relieved by single or multiple hormones replacement therapy, and are qualified to study, ordinary work, social activities, there are 8 cases of postoperative patients with completely restored to normal life, 2 cases got married and give birth to babies. The hormone replacement therapy was used in treatment of remaining 12 cases, but the curative effect is not satisfied, which 10 cases were permanent diabetes insipidus, and a long-term treatment with vasopressin tannate or minirin is needed. 127 patients (83.0%) can have a good quality of life by hormones replacement therapy after the operation.

It's worth noting that our data shows the rates of hypothyroidism and diabetes insipidus during early period of post-operation are higher than pre-operation apparently. Plasma cortisol levels significantly lower than pre-operation. The hormones level is declining continuously after operation, and shows drastic fluctuation. There are several reasons for this phenomenon; Firstly, the original hormone compensatory mechanism is damaged postoperative, and the new compensatory mechanism remains to be established. Secondly, preoperative remaining hormones maybe used up after 1 week's metabolism of the body, and intake of hormones is not fully adapted to the metabolic level of body system, therefore, there is the lowest hormones level and severe disturbance of water and electrolyte within the second weeks after operation. Beyond that, within one week post-operation is the peak period of encephaledema and intracranial infection. From the above we can come to a conclusion that correct timely treatment to maintain water and electrolyte balance and the stability of internal environment is crucial to reduce the mortality and the complications in the second week postoperative. And appropriate hormone replacement therapy can correct long-term endocrine disorders, improve the quality of life. In our data, 12 out of 146 followed-up patients can back to normal life after surgery, 6 of them even get married and have babes. 125 cases of patients who receive single or multiple hormones replacement therapy are qualified to study, ordinary work and social activities.

In conclusion, most of the craniopharyngioma patients have one or more kind of hormone deficiency in different degree, and the hormones can drop to the lowest level in the early period after the operation. An acute change in hormones can be observed within second weeks after tumor resection, and the endocrine disorder can be relieved by suitable hormon replacement therapy timely. The life quality after surgery is depended more on the tumor's growth pattern and the protection for hypothalamus and the third ventricular floor.

Table 2. Frequency characteristics of pituitary dysfunction in adult patients with craniopharyngioma.

	Pituitary Dysfunction		P
	YES(n=117)	NO(n=36)	
Gender			
Male	60	18	0.712
Female	57	18	
Tumor size			
<2cm	3	4	0.039
2~4cm	75	23	
4~6cm	27	9	
>6cm	12	0	
Tumor site			
Type Q	18	3	0.026
Type S	45	18	
Type T	54	15	
Pathological Type			
Adamantinomatous	53	12	0.357
Papillary	64	24	
Calcification			
Yes	84	15	0.256
No	33	21	
cystic			
Yes	54	17	0.562
No	63	19	
P<0.05			

Table 3. Frequency characteristics of pituitary dysfunction in different tumor type.

	Tumor type			P
	Type Q (n=21)	Type S (n=63)	Type T (n=69)	
Partial-hypopituitarism	9(42.9%)	43(68.3%)	37(53.6%)	0.006
Pan- hypopituitarism	9(42.9%)	2(3.2%)	17(24.6%)	0.000
GHD	17(81.0%)	30(47.6%)	25(36.2%)	0.000
HPG	15(71.4%)	37(58.7%)	44(63.8%)	0.047
HPT	10(47.6%)	21(33.3%)	29(42.0%)	0.038

(Table 3) contd.....

	Tumor type			P
	Type Q (n=21)	Type S (n=63)	Type T (n=69)	
HPA	12(57.1%)	18(28.6%)	18(26.1%)	0.044
DI	9(42.9%)	7(11.1%)	28(40.1%)	0.000

GROWTH FEATURES OF CHILDHOOD CRANIOPHARYNGIOMAS

The growth patterns of CPs are extremely heterogeneous [48]. Most patients have a low stature growth velocity, while others, for unknown reasons, exhibit a normal or even higher postoperative stature growth velocity that last from months to years.

These tumors were divided into two groups based on their locations according to the MRI images and/or operative findings [49, 50]: group A (infradiaphragmatic sellar tumors) and group B (suprasellar infundibulotuberal third ventricle floor [3rd VF] tumors). The origins and growth pattern of tumors are two main distinction among two groups. Tumors of intra- or infrasellar origin (group A) originate below the diaphragm and the arachnoid, in contrast, 3rd VF tumors (group B) originate in the infundibulum from back of the chiasm and in the posterior angle region between the optic tracts; growing tumors may infiltration into the third ventricle wall with or without expansion to suprasellar cisterns.

Our data showed similar results. Clinical growth failure occurred in nearly two thirds of the patients (65.9%) in Group A, while in group B, only one third patients (33.8%) showed the complication. In group A, the reduction of growth rate began in early infancy period and persisted until diagnosis, whereas in B group, the reduction began later in childhood (5– 6 years) and again, persisted till the diagnosis time Figs. (**2** and **3**). This discrepancy may result from the different tumor locations and the varying of tumor growth patterns; the tumors in group A primarily influencing the pituitary gland and distal section of the pituitary stalk (PS), whereas hypothalamus and proximal infundibulum stalk are easier damaged in group B. Therefore, we speculate that for children patients with CP, persistent growth impairment in early infancy period is consistent along their childhood.

After reviewing the patients' postoperative auxological measurements data in this study, it was found that some patients' growth patterns will be maintained after tumor removal (perhaps lasting 1– 6 years) and then experienced decelerated height velocity.

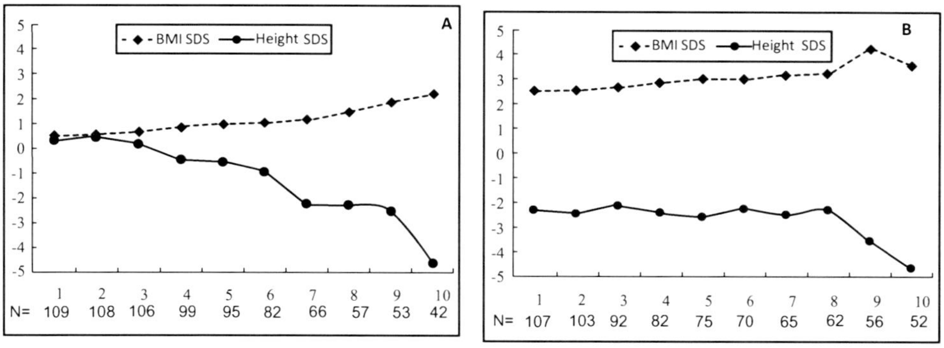

Fig. (2). The reported height and body mass index (BMI) values of patients with childhood craniopharyngioma during the 10 years before (A) and after (B) surgery. (From Ref. [57]).

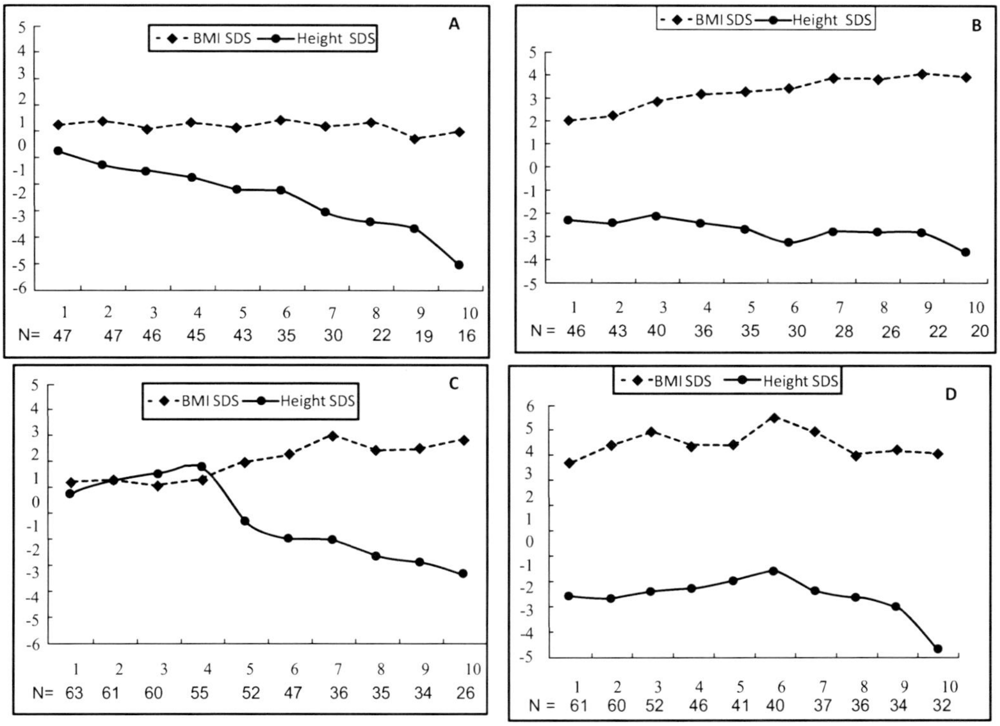

Fig. (3). Comparison of the height and body mass index (BMI) values of patients with pediatric craniopharyngioma in group A (A and B) and group B (C and D) at 10 years before (A and C) and after (B and D) surgery. (From Ref. [57]).

These findings are in accord with Blethen and Weldon's [55], which noted a substantial growth rate deceleration in patients with CP from 1.5 to 6 years after surgery. However, the fact that 18 out of 21 patients achieved a normal height indicates that these patients may grow in a relatively high rate prior to surgery.

A deeper understanding of the spontaneous growth pattern in pediatric patients with CP is essential for a properly evaluation of the effects of growth-promoting treatments among these cases. Because a delayed GH replacement treatment may result in a failure rescuing of lost height, we believe that children with CP who exhibit normal or accelerated growth after surgery should be observed at regular intervals and receive GH replacement treatment if the growth rate show an abnormal downward tendency. In our study, we observed that children with CP in group B, who were at risk for extreme postoperative obesity, had a higher body mass index (BMI) SD score (SDS) before diagnosis. These data indicate that decreased growth rates and elevated BMIs occur in patients prior to diagnosis. However, obesity arose later in the analyzed patients (i.e., shortly before the diagnosis of pediatric CP). These results are compatible with the anatomy of the sellar region. The severity of obesity significantly correlated with the tumor size among the patients in group B but not among those in group A, suggesting that the effect of the preoperative CP tumor size on the hypothalamic axis is intimately related to the tumor location.

In our study, we observed that children with CP in group B, who gained higher risk for extreme postoperative obesity, had a higher body mass index (BMI) SD score (SDS) before diagnosis. These findings indicate that decreased growth rates and elevated BMIs occur in patients prior to diagnosis. However, obesity arose later in the analyzed patients (i.e., shortly before the diagnosis of pediatric CP). These results are compatible with the anatomy of the sellar region. The severity of obesity is significantly correlated with the tumor size only among the patients in group B, suggesting that the preoperative damage of hypothalamic axis is intimately related to both the location and the size of tumors.

In our study, the fact that 19 out of 89 cases achieved normal heights after tumor resection indicated that these patients may had a relatively higher growth rate before surgery, such situation are described as "growth with GH deficiency". This phenomenon has been recognized for more than half a century in various physiological or near-physiological situations, such as the fetal period, obesity state, and in various obviously pathological states, including after the resection of suprasellar tumor [56, 57]. The reported incidences of normal or accelerated growth after CP resection in children with GH deficiency varies from 17% to 68% [58], which is consistent with our results. Interestingly, a similar tendency was observed before the surgery in our study. This rapid or normal growth was usually observed in patients with excessive weight gain and/or tumors which infiltrated into 3rd VF. Most patients with normal height in group B exhibited rapid weight gain within the first year after operation.

CONCLUSION

Despite recent advances in treatment options, craniopharyngiomas remain to be a challenging disease. Inappropriate hormone replacement therapy will lead to chronic complications, even a series of urgent, which may influence the quality of life and survival of patients. Therefore, on the basis of clinical symptoms, endocrine feedback principle and endocrine dynamic function test, it is important to standard grading evaluation of craniopharyngioma after operation. Clearly, more prospective, multi-center studies are needed to get a better sense of the long-term endocrine, psychological, and social consequences of treatment for craniopharyngioma.

CONFLICT OF INTEREST

The author (editor) declares no conflict of interest, financial or otherwise.

ACKNOWLEDGEMENTS

We should thanks Feng Zhan-peng and Zhang Shi-chao for their generous help of literature reviewing.

REFERENCES

[1] Honegger J, Buchfelder M, Fahlbusch R. Surgical treatment of craniopharyngiomas: endocrinological results. J Neurosurg 1999; 90(2): 251-7. [J]. [http://dx.doi.org/10.3171/jns.1999.90.2.0251] [PMID: 9950495]

[2] Chakrabarti I, Amar AP, Couldwell W, Weiss MH. Long-term neurological, visual, and endocrine outcomes following transnasal resection of craniopharyngioma. J Neurosurg 2005; 102(4): 650-7. [J]. [http://dx.doi.org/10.3171/jns.2005.102.4.0650] [PMID: 15871507]

[3] Sklar CA. Craniopharyngioma: endocrine abnormalities at presentation. Pediatr Neurosurg 1994; 21 (Suppl. 1): 18-20. [J]. [http://dx.doi.org/10.1159/000120856] [PMID: 7841073]

[4] Lamberts SW, de Herder WW, van der Lely AJ. Pituitary insufficiency. Lancet 1998; 352(9122): 127-34. [J]. [http://dx.doi.org/10.1016/S0140-6736(98)85043-5] [PMID: 9672293]

[5] Virk JS, Elmiyeh B, Saleh HA. Endoscopic management of cerebrospinal fluid rhinorrhea: the charing cross experience. J Neurol Surg B Skull Base 2013; 74(2): 61-7. [J]. [http://dx.doi.org/10.1055/s-0033-1333620] [PMID: 24436890]

[6] Horiguchi K, Murai H, Hasegawa Y, *et al.* Endoscopic endonasal skull base reconstruction using a nasal septal flap: surgical results and comparison with previous reconstructions. Neurosurg Rev 2010; 33(2): 235-41.

[7] Tomlinson JW, Holden N, Hills RK, *et al.* West Midlands Prospective Hypopituitary Study Group. Association between premature mortality and hypopituitarism. Lancet 2001; 357(9254): 425-31. [J]. [http://dx.doi.org/10.1016/S0140-6736(00)04006-X] [PMID: 11273062]

[8] Kassam A, Snyderman CH, Mintz A, Gardner P, Carrau RL. Expanded endonasal approach: the rostrocaudal axis. Part I. Crista galli to the sella turcica. Neurosurg Focus 2005; 19(1): E3. [J]. [PMID: 16078817]

[9] Kassam A, Snyderman CH, Mintz A, Gardner P, Carrau RL. Expanded endonasal approach: the rostrocaudal axis. Part II. Posterior clinoids to the foramen magnum. Neurosurg Focus 2005; 19(1): E4. [J].
[PMID: 16078818]

[10] Nagai AI, Minami R, Tomomatsu T. [Diagnosis and treatment of posterior pituitary insufficiency]. Saishin Igaku 1970; 25(3): 526-9. [Diagnosis and treatment of posterior pituitary insufficiency]. [J].
[PMID: 4912566]

[11] Hammer F, Arlt W. [Hypopituitarism]. Internist (Berl) 2004; 45(7): 795-811. [Hypopituitarism]. [J].
[PMID: 15241506]

[12] Erfurth EM. Endocrine aspects and sequel in patients with craniopharyngioma. J Pediatr Endocrinol Metab 2015; 28(1-2): 19-26. [J].
[http://dx.doi.org/10.1515/jpem-2014-0419] [PMID: 25514328]

[13] Lo AC, Howard AF, Nichol A, *et al.* Long-term outcomes and complications in patients with craniopharyngioma: the British Columbia Cancer Agency experience. Int J Radiat Oncol Biol Phys 2014; 88(5): 1011-8. [J].
[http://dx.doi.org/10.1016/j.ijrobp.2014.01.019] [PMID: 24661653]

[14] Tirosh A, Benbassat C, Lifshitz A, *et al.* Hypopituitarism patterns and prevalence among men with macroprolactinomas. Pituitary 2014. [J].
[PMID: 24700366]

[15] Brunner HE, Labhart A. [Coma in pituitary insufficiency. Differential diagnosis and treatment]. Internist (Berl) 1965; 6(9): 406-11. [Coma in pituitary insufficiency. Differential diagnosis and treatment]. [J].
[PMID: 5325645]

[16] Lindholm J, Kehlet H. Re-evaluation of the clinical value of the 30 min ACTH test in assessing the hypothalamic-pituitary-adrenocortical function. Clin Endocrinol (Oxf) 1987; 26(1): 53-9. [J].
[http://dx.doi.org/10.1111/j.1365-2265.1987.tb03638.x] [PMID: 3026692]

[17] Dorin RI, Qualls CR, Crapo LM. Diagnosis of adrenal insufficiency. Ann Intern Med 2003; 139(3): 194-204. [J].
[http://dx.doi.org/10.7326/0003-4819-139-3-200308050-00009] [PMID: 12899587]

[18] Agha A, Tomlinson JW, Clark PM, Holder G, Stewart PM. The long-term predictive accuracy of the short synacthen (corticotropin) stimulation test for assessment of the hypothalamic-pituitary-adrenal axis. J Clin Endocrinol Metab 2006; 91(1): 43-7. [J].
[http://dx.doi.org/10.1210/jc.2005-1131] [PMID: 16249286]

[19] Dullaart RP, Pasterkamp SH, Beentjes JA, Sluiter WJ. Evaluation of adrenal function in patients with hypothalamic and pituitary disorders: comparison of serum cortisol, urinary free cortisol and the human-corticotrophin releasing hormone test with the insulin tolerance test. Clin Endocrinol (Oxf) 1999; 50(4): 465-71. [J].
[http://dx.doi.org/10.1046/j.1365-2265.1999.00679.x] [PMID: 10468905]

[20] Robinson AG, Verbalis JG. Posterior pituitary gland. In: Larsen PR, Kroaenberg HM, Melmed S, Polonsky KS, Eds. Williams textbook of endocrinology. Philadelphia, PA: Elsevier Science 2003; pp. 281-329.

[21] Persani L, Ferretti E, Borgato S, Faglia G, Beck-Peccoz P. Circulating thyrotropin bioactivity in sporadic central hypothyroidism. J Clin Endocrinol Metab 2000; 85(10): 3631-5. [J].
[PMID: 11061514]

[22] Hartoft-Nielsen ML, Lange M, Rasmussen AK, Scherer S, Zimmermann-Belsing T, Feldt-Rasmussen U. Thyrotropin-releasing hormone stimulation test in patients with pituitary pathology. Horm Res 2004; 61(2): 53-7.
[PMID: 14646390]

[23] Ferretti E, Persani L, Jaffrain-Rea ML, Giambona S, Tamburrano G, Beck-Peccoz P. Evaluation of the adequacy of levothyroxine replacement therapy in patients with central hypothyroidism. J Clin Endocrinol Metab 1999; 84(3): 924-9. [Westwood ME, Butler GE].
[PMID: 10084572]

[24] McLellan AC, Barth JH. The combined pituitary function test in children: an evaluation of the clinical usefulness of TRH and LHRH stimulation tests through a retrospective analysis of one hundred and twenty six cases. Clin Endocrinol (Oxf) 2000; 52: 727.
[http://dx.doi.org/10.1046/j.1365-2265.2000.00996.x]

[25] Hartman ML, Crowe BJ, Biller BM, Ho KK, Clemmons DR, Chipman JJ. HyposCCS Advisory Board; U.S. HypoCCS Study Group. Which patients do not require a GH stimulation test for the diagnosis of adult GH deficiency? J Clin Endocrinol Metab 2002; 87(2): 477-85.
[http://dx.doi.org/10.1210/jcem.87.2.8216] [PMID: 11836272]

[26] Hoffman DM, Nguyen TV, O'Sullivan AJ, Baxter RC, Ho KK. Diagnosis of growth hormone deficiency in adults. Lancet 1994; 344(8920): 482-3. [J].
[http://dx.doi.org/10.1016/S0140-6736(94)91821-X] [PMID: 7914598]

[27] Consensus guidelines for the diagnosis and treatment of adults with growth hormone deficiency: summary statement of the Growth Hormone Research Society Workshop on Adult Growth Hormone Deficiency. J Clin Endocrinol Metab 1998; 83(2): 379-81.

[28] Growth Hormone Research Society; GH Research Society. Consensus guidelines for the diagnosis and treatment of growth hormone (GH) deficiency in childhood and adolescence: summary statement of the GH Research Society. J Clin Endocrinol Metab 2000; 85(11): 3990-3. [J].
[PMID: 11095419]

[29] Maghnie M, Aimaretti G, Bellone S, *et al.* Diagnosis of GH deficiency in the transition period: accuracy of insulin tolerance test and insulin-like growth factor-I measurement. Eur J Endocrinol 2005; 152(4): 589-96. [J].
[http://dx.doi.org/10.1530/eje.1.01873] [PMID: 15817915]

[30] Clayton PE, Cuneo RC, Juul A, Monson JP, Shalet SM, Tauber M. European Society of Paediatric Endocrinology. Consensus statement on the management of the GH-treated adolescent in the transition to adult care. Eur J Endocrinol 2005; 152(2): 165-70. [J].
[http://dx.doi.org/10.1530/eje.1.01829] [PMID: 15745921]

[31] Ghigo E, Aimaretti G, Gianotti L, Bellone J, Arvat E, Camanni F. New approach to the diagnosis of growth hormone deficiency in adults. Eur J Endocrinol 1996; 134(3): 352-6. [J].
[http://dx.doi.org/10.1530/eje.0.1340352] [PMID: 8616534]

[32] Bondanelli M, Ambrosio MR, Onofri A, *et al.* Predictive value of circulating insulin-like growth factor I levels in ischemic stroke outcome. J Clin Endocrinol Metab 2006; 91(10): 3928-34. [J].
[http://dx.doi.org/10.1210/jc.2006-1040] [PMID: 16882751]

[33] Aimaretti G, Corneli G, Razzore P, *et al.* Comparison between insulin-induced hypoglycemia and growth hormone (GH)-releasing hormone + arginine as provocative tests for the diagnosis of GH deficiency in adults. J Clin Endocrinol Metab 1998; 83(5): 1615-8. [J].
[PMID: 9589665]

[34] Bonert VS, Elashoff JD, Barnett P, Melmed S. Body mass index determines evoked growth hormone (GH) responsiveness in normal healthy male subjects: diagnostic caveat for adult GH deficiency. J Clin Endocrinol Metab 2004; 89(7): 3397-401. [J].
[http://dx.doi.org/10.1210/jc.2003-032213] [PMID: 15240621]

[35] Schneider HJ, Aimaretti G, Kreitschmann-Andermahr I, Stalla GK, Ghigo E. Hypopituitarism. Lancet 2007; 369(9571): 1461-70. [J].
[http://dx.doi.org/10.1016/S0140-6736(07)60673-4] [PMID: 17467517]

[36] Toogood AA, Stewart PM. Hypopituitarism: clinical features, diagnosis, and management. Endocrinol

Metab Clin North Am 2008; 37(1): 235-261, x. [J]. [http://dx.doi.org/10.1016/j.ecl.2007.10.004] [PMID: 18226739]

[37] Ascoli P, Cavagnini F. Hypopituitarism. Pituitary 2006; 9(4): 335-42. [J]. [http://dx.doi.org/10.1007/s11102-006-0416-5] [PMID: 17077946]

[38] Corneli G, Di Somma C, Baldelli R, *et al.* The cut-off limits of the GH response to GH-releasing hormone-arginine test related to body mass index. Eur J Endocrinol 2005; 153(2): 257-64. [J]. [http://dx.doi.org/10.1530/eje.1.01967] [PMID: 16061832]

[39] Popovic V, Leal A, Micic D, *et al.* GH-releasing hormone and GH-releasing peptide-6 for diagnostic testing in GH-deficient adults. Lancet 2000; 356(9236): 1137-42. [J]. [http://dx.doi.org/10.1016/S0140-6736(00)02755-0] [PMID: 11030292]

[40] Ho KK. Diagnosis of adult GH deficiency. Lancet 2000; 356(9236): 1125-6. [J]. [http://dx.doi.org/10.1016/S0140-6736(00)02748-3] [PMID: 11030286]

[41] Gómez JM, Espadero RM, Escobar-Jiménez F, *et al.* Growth hormone release after glucagon as a reliable test of growth hormone assessment in adults. Clin Endocrinol (Oxf) 2002; 56(3): 329-34. [J]. [http://dx.doi.org/10.1046/j.1365-2265.2002.01472.x] [PMID: 11940044]

[42] van Aken MO, Lamberts SW. Diagnosis and treatment of hypopituitarism: an update. Pituitary 2005; 8(3-4): 183-91. [J]. [http://dx.doi.org/10.1007/s11102-006-6039-z] [PMID: 16508719]

[43] Grunenwald S, Caron P. Central hypothyroidism in adults: better understanding for better care. Pituitary 2014. [J]. [PMID: 24554165]

[44] Shimon I, Benbassat C. Male prolactinomas presenting with normal testosterone levels. Pituitary 2014; 17(3): 246-50. [J]. [http://dx.doi.org/10.1007/s11102-013-0497-x] [PMID: 23756784]

[45] Turcu AF, Erickson BJ, Lin E, *et al.* Pituitary stalk lesions: the Mayo Clinic experience. J Clin Endocrinol Metab 2013; 98(5): 1812-8. [J]. [http://dx.doi.org/10.1210/jc.2012-4171] [PMID: 23533231]

[46] Karavitaki N, Brufani C, Warner JT, *et al.* Craniopharyngiomas in children and adults: systematic analysis of 121 cases with long-term follow-up. Clin Endocrinol (Oxf) 2005; 62(4): 397-409. [J]. [http://dx.doi.org/10.1111/j.1365-2265.2005.02231.x] [PMID: 15807869]

[47] Profka E, Giavoli C, Bergamaschi S, *et al.* Analysis of short- and long-term metabolic effects of growth hormone replacement therapy in adult patients with craniopharyngioma and non-functioning pituitary adenoma. J Endocrinol Invest 2014. [J]. [PMID: 25330765]

[48] Tiulpakov AN, Mazerkina NA, Brook CG, Hindmarsh PC, Peterkova VA, Gorelyshev SK. Growth in children with craniopharyngioma following surgery. Clin Endocrinol (Oxf) 1998; 49(6): 733-8. [J]. [http://dx.doi.org/10.1046/j.1365-2265.1998.00590.x] [PMID: 10209560]

[49] Qi S, Lu Y, Pan J, Zhang X, Long H, Fan J. Anatomic relations of the arachnoidea around the pituitary stalk: relevance for surgical removal of craniopharyngiomas. Acta Neurochir (Wien) 2011; 153(4): 785-96. [J]. [http://dx.doi.org/10.1007/s00701-010-0940-y] [PMID: 21271263]

[50] Qi S, Pan J, Lu Y, *et al.* The impact of the site of origin and rate of tumour growth on clinical outcome in children with craniopharyngiomas. Clin Endocrinol (Oxf) 2012; 76(1): 103-10. [J]. [http://dx.doi.org/10.1111/j.1365-2265.2011.04172.x] [PMID: 21752042]

[51] Koulouri O, Auldin MA, Agarwal R, *et al.* Diagnosis and treatment of hypothyroidism in TSH deficiency compared to primary thyroid disease: pituitary patients are at risk of under-replacement with levothyroxine. Clin Endocrinol (Oxf) 2011; 74(6): 744-9. [J]. [http://dx.doi.org/10.1111/j.1365-2265.2011.03984.x] [PMID: 21521256]

[52] Schmidt IL, Lahner H, Mann K, Petersenn S. Diagnosis of adrenal insufficiency: Evaluation of the corticotropin-releasing hormone test and Basal serum cortisol in comparison to the insulin tolerance test in patients with hypothalamic-pituitary-adrenal disease. J Clin Endocrinol Metab 2003; 88(9): 4193-8.
[http://dx.doi.org/10.1210/jc.2002-021897] [PMID: 12970286]

[53] Kazlauskaite R, Evans AT, Villabona CV, *et al.* Consortium for Evaluation of Corticotropin Test in Hypothalamic-Pituitary Adrenal Insufficiency. Corticotropin tests for hypothalamic-pituitary- adrenal insufficiency: a metaanalysis. J Clin Endocrinol Metab 2008; 93(11): 4245-53.
[http://dx.doi.org/10.1210/jc.2008-0710] [PMID: 18697868]

[54] Colao A, Lombardi G. Growth-hormone and prolactin excess. Lancet 1998; 352(9138): 1455-61.
[http://dx.doi.org/10.1016/S0140-6736(98)03356-X] [PMID: 9808008]

[55] Blethen SL, Weldon VV. Outcome in children with normal growth following removal of a craniopharyngioma. Am J Med Sci 1986; 292(1): 21-4. [J].
[http://dx.doi.org/10.1097/00000441-198607000-00004] [PMID: 3717202]

[56] Baskin DS, Wilson CB. Surgical management of craniopharyngiomas. A review of 74 cases. J Neurosurg 1986; 65(1): 22-7. [J].
[http://dx.doi.org/10.3171/jns.1986.65.1.0022] [PMID: 3712025]

[57] Qi S, Peng J, Pan J, *et al.* Growth and weight of children with craniopharyngiomas based on the tumour location and growth pattern. J Clin Neurosci 2013; 20(12): 1702-8.
[http://dx.doi.org/10.1016/j.jocn.2012.12.030] [PMID: 24055207]

[58] Duff J, Meyer F B, Ilstrup D M, *et al.* Long-term outcomes for surgically resected craniopharyngiomas. Neurosurgery 2000; 46(02): 291-305.

CHAPTER 17

Hypothalamus Status Evaluation

Chun-ling Ye[1,*] and **Jun-xiang Peng**[2]

[1] *College of Pharmacy, Ji'nan University, 601, Western Huangpu Avenue, Guangzhou, China*

[2] *Department of Neurosurgery, Nanfang Neurosurgery Research Institution, Nanfang Hospital, Southern Medical University, 1838 North Guangzhou Avenue, Guangzhou, China*

Abstract: Hypothalamic obesity is a condition with extremely high morbidity. Mechanisms leading to the profoundly disturbed energy homeostasis are complex. Craniopharyngioma is one of the most common pathogenesis of hypothalamic obesity, which leads to the damage of hypothalamic nucleis due to the tumor compression or/and cytokines stimulation. The purpose of the present chapter is to summarize data on the prevalence of hypothalamic obesity, discuss the clinical features and review the diagnosis and treatment of these patients. Differences tumor growth patterns and locations should be considered when comparing outcomes and survival across different treatment paradigms in patients with CP. Further studies should be conducted to better understand the mechanisms of rapid weight gain and metabolic syndrome in patients with CP and could be used to enhance effective treatments and establish prevention strategy.

Keywords: Circadian rhythm, Craniopharyngioma, Obesity.

HYPOTHALAMIC OBESITY IN CRANIOPHARYNGIOMA

Hypothalamic obesity, which was first described by Babinski [1] and Frohlich [2], is defined as significant polyphagia and weight gain and is accompany with other symptoms, such as headache, impaired vision, increased somnolence, and behavioral disturbances, especially severe hyperphagia and abnormal food-seeking behaviors. CP is one of the most common pathogenesisof hypothalamic obesity in both adults and children. Previous reports have hypothalamic obesity rates among patients with CP of 30–77% [3 - 6]. DeVile CJ [7] studied 63 patients with CP during follow-up and found that approximately 90% exhibited different degrees of obesity. This demonstrates that hypothalamic obesity in patients with CP is a common problem that deserves increased attention.

[*] **Corresponding author Chun-ling Ye**: College of Pharmacy, Ji'nan University, 601, Western Huangpu Avenue, Guangzhou, China; Tel/Fax: +8620-61641812; E-mail: yechunling2005@163.com

At our center, an analysis of growth records of children with CP was implemented and the result shows that weight and BMI gains occurred even earlier than the diagnosis of CP, meanwhile, body weight will be increased after the surgery. CP patients with tumor infiltration of hypothalamic and high BMI values had impaired accommodative response to hypoglycemia and significantly lower plasma epinephrine level.

Clinical Characteristics of CP Patients with Hypothalamic Obesity

Hyperphagia

Hyperphagia occurs immediately after CP resection, patients with hypothalamic involvement develop an incredible good and persistent appetite that is beyond control. These patients will intake much more calorie than physiological requirement and show unusual foraging behavior.

Reduced Physical Activity

CP patients with hypothalamic involvement and leptin-deficient have significantly less physically active compare to the age-matched controls or those with simple obesity

Treatment of Hypothalamic Obesity

Prevention is the best way to control the hypothalamic obesity. Surgical intervention and/or external beam radiation may be fatal to relevant nuclei in hypothalamic [8]. Treatment of hypothalamic obesity includes lifestyle intervention, pharmacotherapy, and surgery.

Lifestyle Intervention

Except the over intake of total energy result in the impaired satiety and hyperphagia which caused by the disruption of the hypothalamic nuclei,reduction of physical activity is also considered to be a major factor in the development of hypothalamic obesity in survivors of pediatric CP. In 2002 Müller and colleagues [9] reported the increase of daytime somnolence and reduction of nocturnal melatonin levels in pediatric CP patients, which might caused by some uncertain neuroendocrine mechanism, can be a strong supporting point of the hypothesis that physical activity might be decreased in pediatric CP patients.Exercise would be the next treatment approach for this reduced activity, although this often fails. Studies of physical activity programs in PWS have demonstrated benefits in terms of body fat percentage and weight loss.

Pharmacotherapy

Current drug therapies for hypothalamic obesity include dextroamphetamine, ephedrine, caffeine, sibutramine, octreotide, and triiodothyronine. Dextro-amphetamine, ephedrine, caffeine, and sibutramine are sympathomimetic. Mason PW and colleagues [10] studied five cases of treated pediatric CP with postoperative hypothalamic obesity and demonstrated that dextroamphetamine could stabilize the patients' weights and improve symptoms by targeting reduced physical activity. The incidence of side effects of dextroamphetamine such as tachycardia, hypertension, anxiety, and less sleeping can be decreased at low does. Although a large amount of hopeful therapeutic approaches had been carried out, one thing must be admitted is that there is no generally accepted pharmacological therapy for hypothalamic obesity in children and adolescents CP patients. On the other hand, obesity may be related to energy balance dysfunction, in some pathological obese mammalian models (such as a high-fat diet), researchers found that high-fat feeding in animal is sufficient to maintain cellular proliferation and neurogenesis in the median eminence, and many of the newborn cells express neuronal markers and show functional phenotypes relevant for energy-balance control. In this case however, despite the difference between the high-fat diet and hypothalamic injury, those stunning finding remind us certain new therapy for patient with CP. Further animal and cell research in molecular biological level should, of course, be performed as a part of theoretical basis of precise treatment.

Surgery

Surgical approaches to hypothalamic obesity includes vagotomy, gastric banding, and gastric bypass surgery. Animal studies have shown that vagotomy can prevent hyperinsulinemia and 326 weight loss secondary to hypothalamic injury. Müller *et al.* [11] reported four cases with reduction in both food intake and BMI after the laparoscopic adjustable gastric banding. Inge *et al.* [12] performed an Roux-en-Y gastric bypass operation on a patient who had stable but not acceptable body weight and gained a 25 kg weight loss.These results suggest that surgery can also be used as a treatment means for hypothalamic obesity. However, the efficacy and security are still ambiguous and the further research is still needed.

In conclusion, more than 100 years have passed since Babinski and Frohlich [1] first reported hypothalamic obesity. During this period, scholars have conducted much research on the etiology, pathogenesis, clinical manifestations, endocrine changing characteristics, and therapeutic strategy of CP related hypothalamic obesity and have made great progress. In particular, given the development of laboratory animal science in the past 50 years, researchers have designed animal models of hypothalamic obesity that have provided rapid developments in our understanding and studies of this disease. Despite our considerable theoretical understanding, hypothalamic obesity therapies remain ambiguous. Coinstantaneous focusing in several mechanisms is required in order to intervene this complex area. As limited number and extent of relative clinical trails, attach importance to these severe tasks is urgent needed. Multicenter combination drugs clinical trials are needed to develop an scientific accepted therapeutic schedule.

OBESITY AFTER RADICAL RESECTION OF PEDIATRIC CP: RELATIONSHIP WITH TUMOR LOCATION AND GROWTH PATTERN

CPs are sellar tumors that represent approximately 3% of all intracranial tumors and up to 10% of all pediatric brain tumors [13]. Children who underwent surgery for CP frequently suffer from severe obesity, but their growth stature is normal despite GH deficiency [14]. There are too limited studies about the relationship between growth rate and weight changes to draw a conclusive result. To investigate the features of height and weight in children treated for CP and analyze the factors that influence postoperative weights and growth rates, we explored the relationship between the growth rate and weight changes in children with CP before and after tumor resection. We included a total of 125 consecutive patients with CP who were <14 years of age and underwent surgical resection in our hospital with the aim of complete tumor removal between January 1990 and December 2010. Adjuvant radiotherapy was used in selected patients. All procedures were performed by the senior author (Qi ST). 26 recurrent cases were excluded, and the preoperative and postoperative heights and weights of remaining 89 cases before and after surgery for CP were retrospectively analyzed.

These tumors were divided into two groups based on their locations according to MRI scans and/or operative findings [15, 16]: group A (infradiaphragmatic sellar tumors) and group B (suprasellar infundibulotuberal 3rd VF tumors). The major differences between the two types lie in the tumor origins and growth patterns. Tumors of intra- or infrasellar origin (group A) originate below the diaphragm and the arachnoid. In contrast, 3rd VF tumors (group B) originate in the infundibulum from behind he chiasm and in the posterior angle region between optic tracts; growing tumors may develope into the walls of the third ventricle with or without expansion to suprasellar cisterns.

In our series, the mean BMI SDS increased from 0.71 to 2.13 during first year and to 2.62 during the second year after surgery. Children who developed hypothalamic obesity before surgery had greater increases in BMI during the first year after treatment, followed by a subsequent period of weight maintenance. An early and rapid postoperative weight gain was suggested as an apparent significant predictor of postoperative long-term severe obesity. In addition, patients who maintained a normal body weight during follow-up after receiving a diagnosis of pediatric CP had also presented with a lower BMI SDS when diagnosis. Therefore, an increased preoperative BMI in patients with CP was considered to be a powerful predictor for the development of severe obesity (Figs. **1** and **2**).

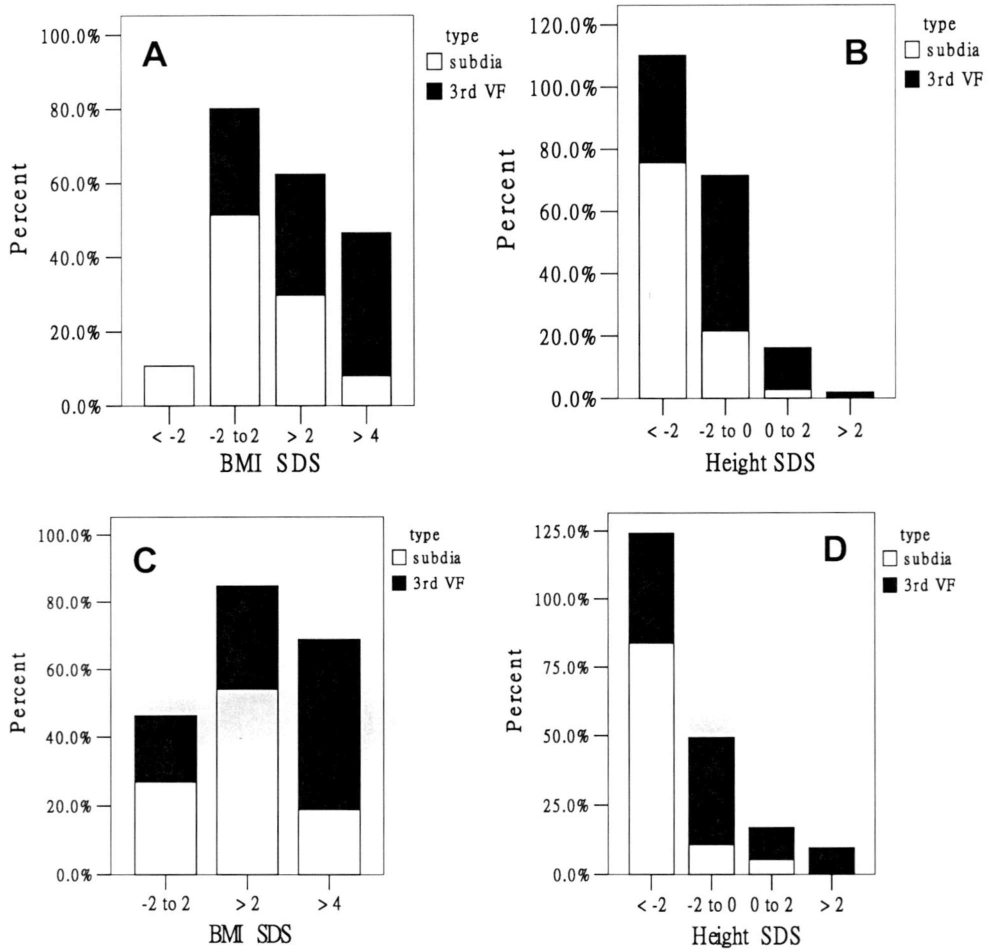

Fig. (1). Histograms summarizing the body mass index (BMI) and height SD scores (SDS) at tumor diagnosis (A, B) and at the last follow-up visit (C, D). sub-dia: Sub-diaphragm, ; 3rd VF, third ventricle floor.

A limited number of previous studies had assessed the risk factors of excessive weight gain after tumor resection had been reported in few studies. De Vile *et al.* [7] revealed a connection between the degree of hypothalamic infiltration and the severity if postoperative obesity in children with CP. Muller *et al.* [17, 18] showed that tumors infiltrate into hypothalamus can increase the risk of obesity in pediatric CP patients. Resemblance with the data from other institutions reported) [8, 16, 19 - 23], the incidence of long-term obesity in our cohort was approximately 70%. Most of our patients' BMI are normal or slightly high pre-operation, and an obviously weight gain process can be seen in one year post-operation.

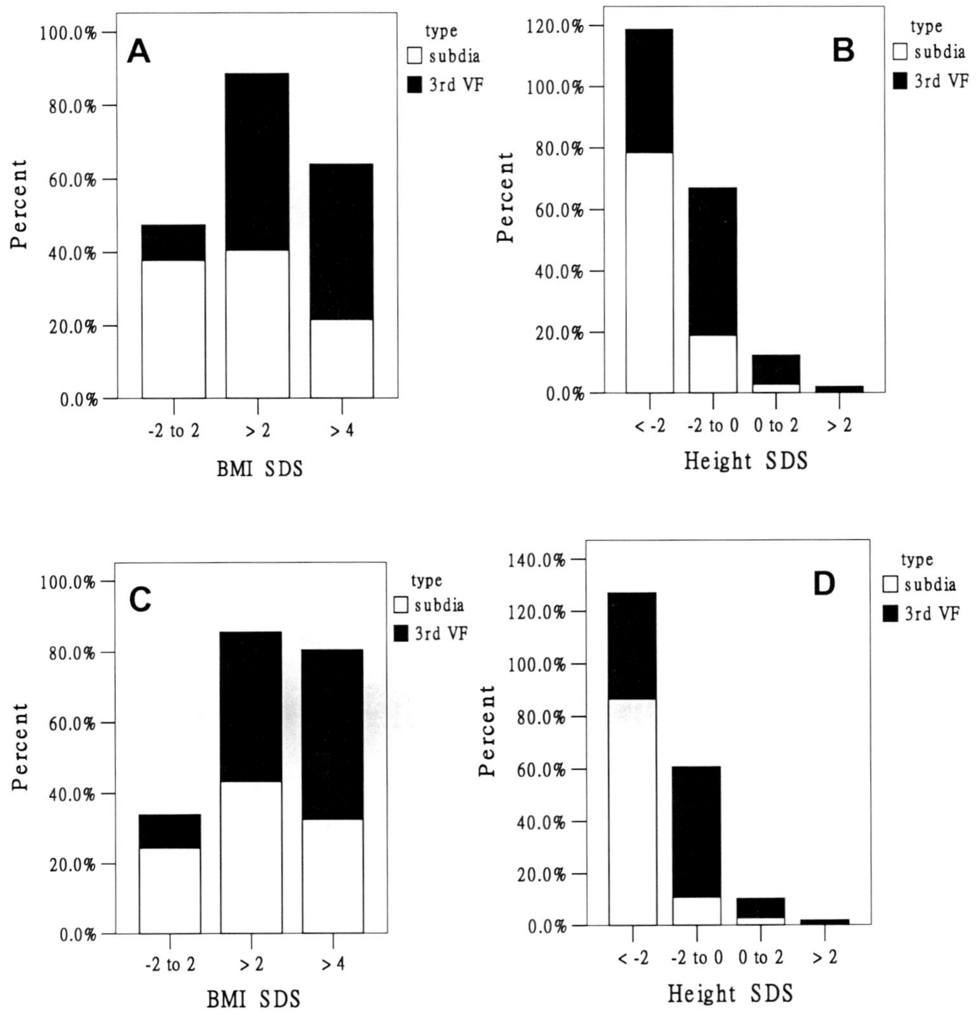

Fig. (2). Histogram summary of the body mass index (BMI) and height SD scores (SDS) during the first (A, B) and second years (C, D) after surgery. Subdia: Sub-diaphragm; 3rd VF, third ventricle floor.

The impact of obesity on surgical outcomes remains controversial. Puget *et al.* [24] found a correlation between obesity and postoperative hypothalamic lesions, whereas Villani *et al.* [25] showed no obvious correlation between obesity and the extent of tumor resection. Our data revealed no relationship between obesity at the last follow-up visit and the extent of resection; as obesity is a substantial characteristic in pediatric CP, it might be more likely related to the disease itself rather than surgery (Fig. **3**).

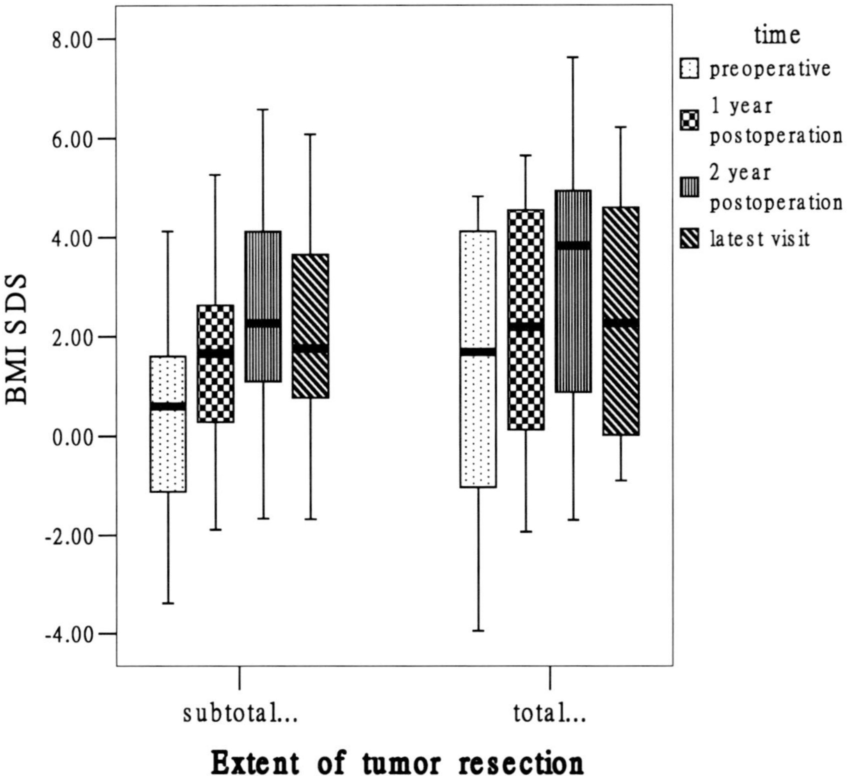

Fig. (3). Comparison of the body mass index (BMI) SD scores (SDS) in patients subjected to subtotal resection and total resection. Evolution of the BMI measured preoperatively, 1 and 2 years postoperatively, and at the last visit. None of the comparisons (Student's t test) were statistically significant.

Considerable controversy exists with regard to the relationship between the growth rate and weight changes. Some investigators [26]) have reported that patients with normal or accelerated growth rates during the post-treatment period also gained more weight than did patients with decreased growth rates. However, some authors [20] have found no relationship between the height SDS and BMI SDS or between changes in the height SDS and BMI SDS. Our observation also demonstrated that in group B, obese subjects maintained higher integrated postoperative growth rates than did non-obese subjects, although this was not true of subjects in group A. It was suggested that obese children had greater losses in height than did leaner children (Fig. **4**). There are two main reasons for this discrepancy. First, in the above studies only groups with small numbers of patients were studied for limited periods of time. Second, the relationships were not analyzed according to tumor location. Additionally, no correlation was noted between the plasma FT4 levels or hydrocortisone levels and BMI and growth rates before and after surgery, suggesting that pituitary hormone levels did not comprise the main factor influencing changes in body weight and growth rate. Therefore, the tumor location appears primary influence on growth and obesity development of obesity in pediatric CP, whereas, the degree of endocrine deficiencies or hormonal substitution hormones replacement therapy have no influence on our results.

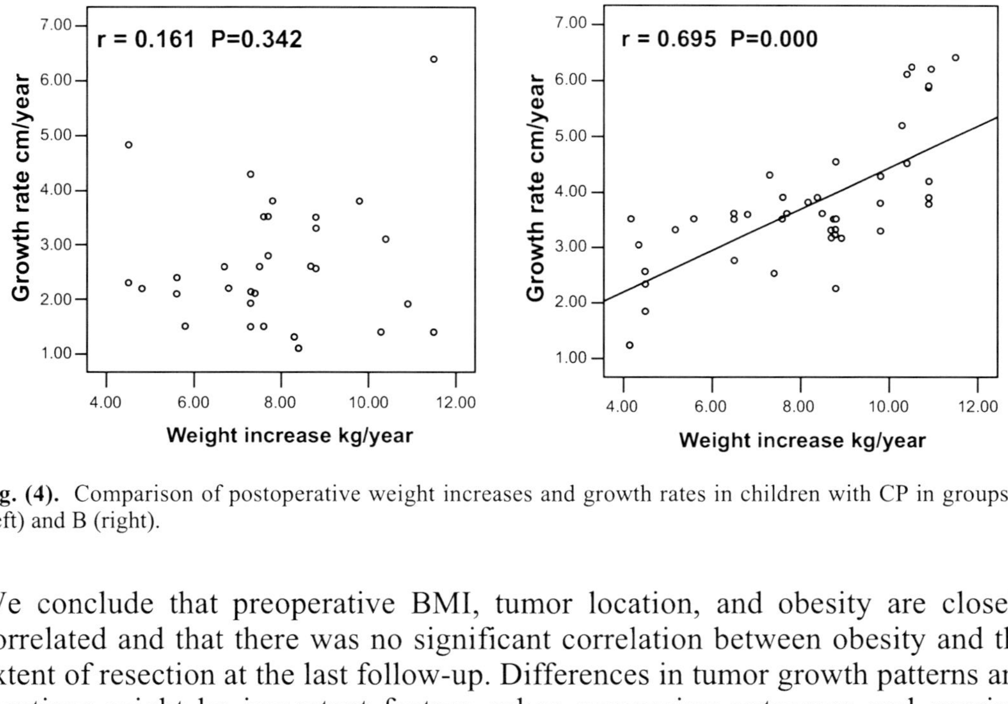

Fig. (4). Comparison of postoperative weight increases and growth rates in children with CP in groups A (left) and B (right).

We conclude that preoperative BMI, tumor location, and obesity are closely correlated and that there was no significant correlation between obesity and the extent of resection at the last follow-up. Differences in tumor growth patterns and locations might be important factors. when comparing outcomes and survival across different treatment paradigms in pediatric patients with CP. Further researches should be conducted to have a deeper view in the understanding of the mechanisms of rapid weight gain and metabolic syndrome in pediatric CP patients, as these can be used to enhance effective treatments and establish prevention programs

EMOTIONAL, MEMEORY AND CIRCADIAN RHYTHM CHANGES WITH CRANIOPHARYNGIOMA

CPs are the most common extraneural central nervous system tumors in children. Because CPs usually grow along the anatomical midline, the tumors or their related surgical excision and radiation may lead to hypopituitarism, visual field defects, obesity, sleep abnormalities, and daytime hypersomnolence (DH) frequently. DH persists despite hormone replacement or treatment of commonly associated obstructive sleep apnea (OSA). Pediatric CP patients often left sequelae after the treatment, such as severe obesity and increased daytime somnolence. Muller hypothesized that disrupted sleep patterns in patients with CP result from the stimulation or destruction of suprachiasmatic nucleus that control the hypothalamus biological rhythm.

Following CP removal, patients more often gave up their professional careers for reasons other than planned retirement. The failure in watching their diets of pediatric patients was a major problem that resulted in increasing obesity. The function of illness group with respect to social relationships, school situations, emotional control, and general vitality appeared to be disrupted disproportionately comparing to children with relatively good physical conditions and normal cognitive abilities. The postoperative occurrence and intensity of dysfunction above, as feeded back from parents, Showed no reduction as time goes on. To the contrary, as these children grow, the observed dysfunction may become even more apparent.

Despite achieving relatively good results in neuropsychological test samples, dysfunction in everyday functioning can be observed in patients after CP removal. These dysfunction are related to both cognitive and social dimensions [27 - 30]. Patients may also suffer from emotion dysfunction, To some extent, this may be caused by the irritate of the tumor to the limbic system [31]. Furthermore, social and emotional dysfunction may be secondary to endocrine hormones disruption, which cause changes in appearance such as obesity and short stature. Papazoglou and colleagues [32] noted that adaptation difficulties were more likely a general result of the tumor progression and related treatment of CP and infantile brain tumors rather than a the reduction in of intellectual ability.

Sleep/wake cycles are hypothesized to result from a balance between both circadian and homeostatic influences. Some patients with pediatric CP have complained of increased daytime somnolence. Lipton J and colleagues [33] have obtained evidence for both melatonin deficiencies and irregular circadian function in such patients, as evidenced by substantial abnormalities in 333 serially measured plasma melatonin levels. These authors speculated that a complete loss of the circadian melatonin rhythm might reflect a disruption in daytime circadian arousal mechanisms, rendering the homeostatic sleep drive unopposed and thus contributing to DH and sleep disruption in these patients. The observed absence of a nocturnal melatonin peak suggests that symptoms in these patients might respond to exogenously administered melatonin during nighttime hours. Previous studies have demonstrated low salivary melatonin levels in obese patients CP along with some improvements of self-reported DH following melatonin supplementation [9, 34].

Melatonin, a pineal indoleamine, is thought to exert a key role in both functional regulation of both hypothalamus and pituitary gland [35]. Melatonin secrete in darkness moment, as its affects on sleep patterns, it can be used to treat jet lag and other delayed sleep disorders because of its possible role as an influencer of circadian rhythms. Daily variations in melatonin levels serve as a marker of the function of this system. Low salivary melatonin levels have been documented in obese CP survivors, and melatonin supplementation has proved beneficial in some cases. Despite receiving hormonal substitution, hypothalamic injury-induced hyperphagia is difficult to manage, and severe obesity occurs postoperatively in up to 52% of affected patients; at least half of these patients experience extreme difficulty in appetite control [9].

In a previous study of patients treated for pediatric CP [34], reduced nocturnal melatonin concentrations were associated with increased daytime somnolence. The multiple sleep latency test, a standardized test of daytime somnolence, revealed severe daytime somnolence in five children who had been treated *via* hypothalamic–pituitary surgery. Accordingly, self-reported general and physical fatigue are much more in adult patients treated for CP relative to healthy controls, and the previous findings of the increase of daytime somnolence in children treated for CP were extended to and confirmed in adult patients with CP.

As CP patients often complicate with anterior pituitary dysfunction, the increased daytime somnolence may be the consequence of multiple hormones deficiency. Indeed, many interactions between the nocturnal hormones secretion of different hormones and sleep electroencephalogram parameters have been well described. Sleeping patterns changing can alter the secretion of anterior pituitary hormones. Corresponding, hormones deficiency such as primary hypothyroidism will cause the alteration of sleep pattern recorded by the multichannel sleep detector.

Muller *et al.* suggested that aggravating daytime somnolence in pediatric patients with CP was related to decreased nocturnal melatonin levels. Nocturnal melatonin levels were also found to associate with the degree of obesity (BMI) and tumor diagnosis. As hypothalamic damage is a previously reported risk factor for of severe obesity in patients with CP [34], we speculate that hypothalamic damage might be the reason of melatonin secretion disorder. in accordance with the previous literature.

In conclusion, patients with CP are more likely to gain weight and develop metabolic syndrome after treatment. Differences of tumor growth patterns and locations should be considered when comparing outcomes and survival across different treatment paradigms in patients with CP. Hypothalamic damage might have been responsible for observed disturbances in melatonin secretion. Further studies should be conducted to better understand the mechanisms of rapid weight gain and metabolic syndrome in pediatric CP and could be used to enhance effective treatments and establish prevention programs. Improvements in the prognosis and quality of life of CP survivors could be achieved through a multidisciplinary, risk-adapted neurosurgical and radiotherapeutic approach.

CONFLICT OF INTEREST

The author (editor) declares no conflict of interest, financial or otherwise.

ACKNOWLEDGEMENTS

We should thanks Feng Zhan-peng and Zhang Shi-chao for their generous help of literature reviewing.

REFERENCES

[1] Duff J, Meyer F B, Ilstrup D M, *et al.* Long-term outcomes for surgically resected craniopharyngiomas. Neurosurgery 2000; 46(2): 291-305.

[2] Virk JS, Elmiyeh B, Saleh HA. Endoscopic management of cerebrospinal fluid rhinorrhea: the charing cross experience. J Neurol Surg B Skull Base 2013; 74(2): 61-7. [http://dx.doi.org/10.1055/s-0033-1333620] [PMID: 24436890]

[3] Stahnke N, Grubel G, Lagenstein I, Willig RP. Long-term follow-up of children with craniopharyngioma. Eur J Pediatr 1984; 142(3): 179-85. [http://dx.doi.org/10.1007/BF00442445] [PMID: 6381061]

[4] Lo AC, Howard AF, Nichol A, *et al.* Long-term outcomes and complications in patients with craniopharyngioma: the British Columbia Cancer Agency experience. Int J Radiat Oncol Biol Phys 2014; 88(5): 1011-8. [http://dx.doi.org/10.1016/j.ijrobp.2014.01.019] [PMID: 24661653]

[5] Vinchon M, Weill J, Delestret I, Dhellemmes P. Craniopharyngioma and hypothalamic obesity in children. Childs Nerv Syst 2009; 25(3): 347-52. [http://dx.doi.org/10.1007/s00381-008-0754-x] [PMID: 19057910]

[6] Lustig RH. Hypothalamic obesity after craniopharyngioma: mechanisms, diagnosis, and treatment. Front Endocrinol (Lausanne) 2011; 2: 60. [http://dx.doi.org/10.3389/fendo.2011.00060] [PMID: 22654817]

[7] de Vile CJ, Grant DB, Hayward RD, Kendall BE, Neville BG, Stanhope R. Obesity in childhood craniopharyngioma: relation to post-operative hypothalamic damage shown by magnetic resonance imaging. J Clin Endocrinol Metab 1996; 81(7): 2734-7. [PMID: 8675604]

[8] Lustig RH, Post SR, Srivannaboon K, *et al.* Risk factors for the development of obesity in children surviving brain tumors. J Clin Endocrinol Metab 2003; 88(2): 611-6. [http://dx.doi.org/10.1210/jc.2002-021180] [PMID: 12574189]

[9] Müller HL, Handwerker G, Wollny B, Faldum A, Sörensen N. Melatonin secretion and increased daytime sleepiness in childhood craniopharyngioma patients. J Clin Endocrinol Metab 2002; 87(8):

3993-6.
[http://dx.doi.org/10.1210/jcem.87.8.8751] [PMID: 12161549]

[10] Mason PW, Krawiecki N, Meacham LR. The use of dextroamphetamine to treat obesity and hyperphagia in children treated for craniopharyngioma. Arch Pediatr Adolesc Med 2002; 156(9): 887-92.
[http://dx.doi.org/10.1001/archpedi.156.9.887] [PMID: 12197795]

[11] Müller HL, Gebhardt U, Maroske J, Hanisch E. Long-term follow-up of morbidly obese patients with childhood craniopharyngioma after laparoscopic adjustable gastric banding (LAGB). Klin Padiatr 2011; 223(6): 372-3.
[http://dx.doi.org/10.1055/s-0031-1284420] [PMID: 22052635]

[12] Inge TH, Pfluger P, Zeller M, *et al.* Gastric bypass surgery for treatment of hypothalamic obesity after craniopharyngioma therapy. Nat Clin Pract Endocrinol Metab 2007; 3(8): 606-9.
[http://dx.doi.org/10.1038/ncpendmet0579] [PMID: 17643131]

[13] Karavitaki N, Cudlip S, Adams CB, Wass JA. Craniopharyngiomas. Endocr Rev 2006; 27(4): 371-97.
[http://dx.doi.org/10.1210/er.2006-0002] [PMID: 16543382]

[14] Hogeveen M, Noordam C, Otten B, Wit JM, Massa G. Growth before and during growth hormone treatment in children operated for craniopharyngioma. Horm Res 1997; 48(6): 258-62.
[http://dx.doi.org/10.1159/000185531] [PMID: 9402242]

[15] Qi S, Lu Y, Pan J, Zhang X, Long H, Fan J. Anatomic relations of the arachnoidea around the pituitary stalk: relevance for surgical removal of craniopharyngiomas. Acta Neurochir (Wien) 2011; 153(4): 785-96.
[http://dx.doi.org/10.1007/s00701-010-0940-y] [PMID: 21271263]

[16] Qi S, Pan J, Lu Y, *et al.* The impact of the site of origin and rate of tumour growth on clinical outcome in children with craniopharyngiomas. Clin Endocrinol (Oxf) 2012; 76(1): 103-10.
[http://dx.doi.org/10.1111/j.1365-2265.2011.04172.x] [PMID: 21752042]

[17] Müller HL, Faldum A, Etavard-Gorris N, *et al.* Functional capacity, obesity and hypothalamic involvement: cross-sectional study on 212 patients with childhood craniopharyngioma. Klin Padiatr 2003; 215(6): 310-4.
[http://dx.doi.org/10.1055/s-2003-45499] [PMID: 14677094]

[18] Kassam A, Snyderman CH, Mintz A, Gardner P, Carrau RL. Expanded endonasal approach: the rostrocaudal axis. Part II. Posterior clinoids to the foramen magnum. Neurosurg Focus 2005; 19(1): E4.
[PMID: 16078818]

[19] Baskin DS, Wilson CB. Surgical management of craniopharyngiomas. A review of 74 cases. J Neurosurg 1986; 65(1): 22-7.
[http://dx.doi.org/10.3171/jns.1986.65.1.0022] [PMID: 3712025]

[20] Lustig RH. The neuroendocrinology of childhood obesity. Pediatr Clin North Am 2001; 48(4): 909-30.
[http://dx.doi.org/10.1016/S0031-3955(05)70348-5] [PMID: 11494643]

[21] Fiorindi A, Delitala A, Francaviglia N, Longatti P. Neuroendoscopic options in the treatment of mesencephalic expanding cysts: report of four cases and review of the literature. Clin Neurol Neurosurg 2013; 115(11): 2370-6.
[http://dx.doi.org/10.1016/j.clineuro.2013.08.025] [PMID: 24041964]

[22] Lee MH, Kim SH, Seoul HJ, *et al.* Impact of maximal safe resection on the clinical outcome of adults with craniopharyngiomas. J Clin Neurosci 2012; 19(7): 1005-8.
[http://dx.doi.org/10.1016/j.jocn.2011.09.033] [PMID: 22595354]

[23] Schöfl C, Schleth A, Berger D, Terkamp C, von zur Mühlen A, Brabant G. Sympathoadrenal counterregulation in patients with hypothalamic craniopharyngioma. J Clin Endocrinol Metab 2002; 87(2): 624-9.

[http://dx.doi.org/10.1210/jcem.87.2.8193] [PMID: 11836295]

[24] Puget S, Garnett M, Wray A, *et al.* Pediatric craniopharyngiomas: classification and treatment according to the degree of hypothalamic involvement. J Neurosurg 2007; 106(1) (Suppl.): 3-12. [PMID: 17233305]

[25] Villani RM, Tomei G, Bello L, *et al.* Long-term results of treatment for craniopharyngioma in children. Childs Nerv Syst 1997; 13(7): 397-405. [http://dx.doi.org/10.1007/s003810050108] [PMID: 9298276]

[26] Bucher H, Zapf J, Torresani T, Prader A, Froesch ER, Illig R. Insulin-like growth factors I and II, prolactin, and insulin in 19 growth hormone-deficient children with excessive, normal, or decreased longitudinal growth after operation for craniopharyngioma. N Engl J Med 1983; 309(19): 1142-6. [http://dx.doi.org/10.1056/NEJM198311103091902] [PMID: 6353237]

[27] Hadad G, Bassagasteguy L, Carrau RL, *et al.* A novel reconstructive technique after endoscopic expanded endonasal approaches: vascular pedicle nasoseptal flap. Laryngoscope 2006; 116(10): 1882-6. [http://dx.doi.org/10.1097/01.mlg.0000234933.37779.e4] [PMID: 17003708]

[28] Bawden HN, Salisbury S, Eskes G, Morehouse R. Neuropsychological functioning following craniopharyngioma removal. J Clin Exp Neuropsychol 2009; 31(1): 140-4. [http://dx.doi.org/10.1080/13803390802064599] [PMID: 18608690]

[29] Waber DP, Pomeroy SL, Chiverton AM, *et al.* Everyday cognitive function after craniopharyngioma in childhood. Pediatr Neurol 2006; 34(1): 13-9. [http://dx.doi.org/10.1016/j.pediatrneurol.2005.06.002] [PMID: 16376272]

[30] Poretti A, Grotzer MA, Ribi K, Schönle E, Boltshauser E. Outcome of craniopharyngioma in children: long-term complications and quality of life. Dev Med Child Neurol 2004; 46(4): 220-9. [http://dx.doi.org/10.1111/j.1469-8749.2004.tb00476.x] [PMID: 15077699]

[31] Ondruch A, Maryniak A, Kropiwnicki T, Roszkowski M, Daszkiewicz P. Cognitive and social functioning in children and adolescents after the removal of craniopharyngioma. Childs Nerv Syst 2011; 27(3): 391-7. [http://dx.doi.org/10.1007/s00381-010-1301-0] [PMID: 20931204]

[32] Papazoglou A, King TZ, Morris RD, Krawiecki N. Parent report of attention problems predicts later adaptive functioning in children with brain tumors. Child Neuropsychol 2009; 15(1): 40-52. [http://dx.doi.org/10.1080/09297040802036102] [PMID: 18608223]

[33] Lipton J, Megerian JT, Kothare SV, *et al.* Melatonin deficiency and disrupted circadian rhythms in pediatric survivors of craniopharyngioma. Neurology 2009; 73(4): 323-5. [http://dx.doi.org/10.1212/WNL.0b013e3181af78a5] [PMID: 19636054]

[34] Müller HL, Handwerker G, Gebhardt U, *et al.* Melatonin treatment in obese patients with childhood craniopharyngioma and increased daytime sleepiness. Cancer Causes Control 2006; 17(4): 583-9. [http://dx.doi.org/10.1007/s10552-005-9012-7] [PMID: 16596314]

[35] Brzezinski A. Melatonin in humans. N Engl J Med 1997; 336(3): 186-95. [http://dx.doi.org/10.1056/NEJM199701163360306] [PMID: 8988899]

CHAPTER 18

Clinical Manifestation and Management in Children

Jun Pan*

Department of Neurosurgery, Nanfang Neurosurgery Research Institution, Nanfang Hospital, Southern Medical University, 1838 North Guangzhou Avenue, Guangzhou, China

Abstract: In this chapter, we focused on the description of the conception, clinical manifestation, surgical treatment and prognosis of pediatric craniopharyngiomas (CP), which were extremely different from the adult patients. As most of the tumors grew with development of the pituitary gland, stalk and hypothalamic structures in pediatric patients, surgery always caused severe endocrinological and hypothalamic dysfunction. And the postrugical irradiation was also restriced for younger children, with result as big problem for the quality of life in childhooh CP. In this chapter, we proposed two types of pediatric CP: infradiaphragmatic CP and intra-third ventricular floor CP. Those two types of CP presented totally variant characteristics with aspect in clinical manifestation, surgical strategy, recurrence, and prognosis, which will also be described and discussed in details.

Keywords: Craniopharyngioma, Fuction, Obesity, Pediatric.

THE CONCEPT OF PEDIATRIC CRANIOPHARYNGIOMA

Pediatric craniopharyngioma (CP) is one of the most common pediatric tumors, accounting for 6–13% of all pediatric intracranial tumors and more than half of all sellar region tumors. Moreover, in children, CP is a common type of endocrine-related tumor [1]. Also, the actual number of CP cases among children (0–14 years) was lower than that among adults; however, in terms of the entire human lifespan, the incidence of CP was absolutely highest during childhood. Clinical trials involving CP have not used standard criteria or definitions of childhood. Most scholars consider an age of 0–16 or 0–17 years as a statistical criterion for pediatric CP. Other studies have used an age of 0–14 years as an inclusion criterion, and this range was frequently reported in studies focused on CP cases in pediatric hospitals. According to a literature review, among CP cases aged 0–16 or 0–17 years, those younger than 14 years were quite predominant. Therefore,

* **Corresponding author Jun Pan**: Department of Neurosurgery, Nanfang neurosurgery research Institution, Nanfang Hospital, Southern medical university, 1838 North Guangzhou Avenue, Guangzhou, China; Tel\Fax: +8620-61641806; E-mail: panjundu@hotmail.com

the term "pediatric CP" has been most frequently used to describe this patient population. Notably, determinations regarding whether patients belong to the pediatric CP population should be made according to the time at which diagnosis was confirmed. However, in some studies, this time point was defined as the time at which patients received treatment, which might somehow introduce bias. In our clinical series of 226 cases of CP, 96 cases belonged to the pediatric CP population and had ages ranging from 1 to 27 years. Some of these cases had long-term medical histories without treatment after diagnosis and therefore received treatment when they were older than 16 years. However, given the features of tumor origination and endocrine disorders, these cases should be classified as pediatric CP.

PRESENTING MANIFESTATION IN PEDIATRIC CP

Compared to adult CP, pediatric CP exhibits significantly different characteristics with regard to clinical manifestation, radiology, endocrinology, and hypothalamic dysfunction [2]. Therefore, we will focus on pediatric CP in this chapter. In contrast with most current studies, using the descriptions in this chapter we have subdivided childhood CPs into two types according to tumor origin: juvenile type of infradiaphragmatic CP (Id-CP) and suprasellar third ventricular floor (3rd VF) CP. The analyses of patients' clinical manifestations, radiological features, and morphological characteristics are all based on this classification.

CLINICAL MANIFESTATION

The major clinical manifestations of pediatric CPs include impaired vision, visual field defects, elevated intracranial pressure (ICP), growth retardation, and abnormal secondary sexual characters caused by endocrinological dysfunction [3]. Tumor-induced hydrocephalus can also cause an acute high ICP crisis. As a result, the patient can lapse into a coma, thus requiring emergency treatment. After analyzing a large number of clinical cases, we identified some special features associated with the clinical manifestation of pediatric CP. First, delayed diagnosis occurred more frequently in patients with pediatric CP, particularly younger patients. The major reason for this delay might be that clinical manifestations in younger patients are more easily ignored by parents. We have even met some patients with severely impaired vision that interfered with their daily lives (*e.g.*, hitting doors while walking), at which point these abnormal manifestations were noticed by their parents. Moreover, growth retardation and diabetes insipidus (DI) are not evident at early stages and are therefore easily ignored. On the other hand, elevated ICP can be easily detected. Therefore, the diagnosis might be determined by the initial presenting symptom.

Second, pediatric CPs manifest quite differently, depending on the tumor location. In general, Id-CP cases always present with impaired vision, visual field defects, growth retardation, and DI. However, hydrocephalus and elevated ICP occur less frequently with this type of tumor. Meanwhile, presurgical hypothalamic disorders are rare because of the limited hypothalamic involvement. On the other hand, suprasellar CPs that originate from the tubero-infundibulum are always accompanied by a high ICP because of tumor-induced hydrocephalus. Moreover, a small number of patients with more severe infundibular involvement may suffer from obesity, weight loss, emotional disorders, and irritation [2, 4, 5]. Epilepsy is another frequent symptom in pediatric patients and is always accompanied by the above manifestations. According to our experience, most children with CP accompanied by epilepsy have a poor prognosis. Pediatric CPs may also exhibit specific clinical manifestations and symptoms that depend on region of tumor involvement, such as rhinobyon, rhinorrhea, and protopsis caused by infrasellar CPs. Patients with cystic tumors that involve the posterior cranial fossa might suffer from hearing loss, unsteady gait, cranial nerve symptoms (abducens nerve paralysis), and hemiplegia. A huge anterior cranial fossa tumor might cause anosphrasia and mental disorders.

NEURORADIOLOGY OF PEDIATRIC CP

As described above, pediatric CPs can be divided into two types: infradiaphragmatic and suprasellar tubero-infundibular. These two types of tumors have significantly different neuroradiological features. In Id-CP cases, tumors always induce sellae turcica enlargement before involving suprasellar structures. Uniform expansion toward the suprasellar region leads to nearly all lesions having a smooth, rounded or elliptic shape without the multilobulated pattern typical of suprasellar lesions. This shape is modeled by the expansion of the mass under the diaphragm sellae. Part of the tumor originates from infrasellar structures such as the nasopharynx, sphenoid sinus, and ethmoid sinus, which might indicate an earlier occurrence and more primitive origin (such as craniopharyngeal canal migration during the fetal phase) [6 - 8]. Most tumors are large in volume; for example, the median sagittal diameter of Id-CPs in our series exceeded 4 cm. The direction of suprasellar expansion is always toward the prechiasmatic region. Therefore, in most patients the optic chiasm and anterior communicating artery complex are lifted and located above or posterosuperiorly to the tumor. The enlarged prechiasmatic space is always the main surgical space used for removal of this type of tumor.

Most pediatric suprasellar CPs originate from the tubero-infundibular part and expand toward the third ventricular cavity. In fact, this type of tumor is located inside the thin nervous tissue layer of the third ventricular walls and occupies the ventricular cavity while remaining covered by the nervous and intact ependymal layers. On radiological images, these tumors are mixed cystic-solid or purely cystic lesions that occupy part of the third ventricular cavity. Calcification is normally observed. As most such cases feature large tumors, obstructive hydrocephalus is also common. The pituitary stalk (PS) is displaced downward in most patients, as demonstrated on median sagittal or coronal MRI scans. In a small number of patients, the tumor also involves the PS, which manifests as tumor growth inside the stalk. As a result, the PS becomes thickened and is even incorporated into the tumor cystic walls.

Notably, during the development of pediatric suprasellar CP from the site of origin to the extraventricular, intracisternal space, the cystic part of the tumor can expand considerably toward the posterior cranial fossa. Although this topographic variation also occurs in a small subset of adult patients, it is predominantly observed in pediatric patients. This type of tumor still originates from the PS and expands towards the retroclivus; the posterior cranial fossa, especially the cerebellopontine angle (CPA) region, and even the upper cervical spinal canal may be involved. Normally, bilateral sites may be involved. Given the significant morphological and surgical treatment features, some scholars believe that this type of tumor should be classified as a special type of pediatric CP [9].

A few literature reports that focused on large series of cases compared the diversity of radiological images between pediatric and adult CPs. The main reason for the small number of such reports is likely that most of the literature has focused specifically on pediatric cases while ignoring differences between these and adult cases. Furthermore, many scholars have also thought the differences in radiological images from pediatric and adult cases were predominantly represented by the different pathological constitutions of these cases [10 - 12]. Nearly all squamous papillary histological variants have been observed in adult patients. Moreover, the existence of combined pathological-type CPs has further complicated the situation. Hydrocephalus has been reported in 20–38% of cases [44, 74, 86, 89, 90]; for reasons that are currently unclear, this likely occurs more frequently in pediatric populations (41–54% among children [44, 74, 90, 118] vs. 12–30% among adults [44, 74, 90]). According to our statistical analysis, apart from the influences of pathological elements, pediatric CPs are significantly larger than adult CPs. This statistical difference in tumor size remained even after analyzing only pediatric and adult adamantinomatous cases to reduce the influence of adult squamous papillary histological variants. Therefore, the more frequent incidence of hydrocephalus in pediatric cases only reflects the difference in tumor size. Notably, in a series of 45 patients, no significant differences in tumor volume was found when comparing subjects >20 and <20 years [11].

Regarding cystic tumor changes, the frequency of affected cases is considerably higher among pediatric cases than among adult cases. However, no significant difference remains if the adult squamous papillary histological variant cases are excluded. Interestingly, in a study of 91 images, there was no significant difference in tumor consistency between pediatric and adult cases [13]. In that article, skull x-ray films or computed tomography (CT) confirmed calcification incidence rates ranging from 45 to 57% [3, 14 - 17]. According to our clinical data, the incidence of calcification was higher among pediatric cases than adult cases, which agrees with previous literature reports (range: 78–100%) [3, 16 - 23]. This statistical difference remains even after excluding adult squamous papillary histological variant cases.

THE HEPOTHALAMO-PITUITARY FUNCTION AT PRESENTATION

Endocrine disorders often occur with pediatric CP, and nearly all patients present with some degree of hypopituitarism. Growth hormone (GH) axis deficiency is the most frequent manifestation. Although few clinical cases complain of growth retardation, experimental detection has indicated that GH axis deficiencies occurred in nearly 100% of patients. According to the literature, GH deficiency is present in 35–95% of evaluated patients, follicle-stimulating hormone (FSH)/luteinizing hormone (LH) deficiency in 38–82%, adrenocorticotropic hormone (ACTH) deficiency in 21–62%, thyroid-stimulating hormone (TSH) deficiency in 21–42%, and DI in 6–38%. Notably, the descriptions of hypopituitarism provided in the literature should be read more carefully, given the ununiformed nature of the evaluation criteria for endocrine disorders. In some literature reports, only the medical records of patients were analyzed according to clinical manifestations and the peripheral plasma hormone levels. This type of evaluation might harbor deviations to some extent. According to our opinion, which is based on cases from our experience, pediatric cases of Id-CP suffered more severe adenohypophyseal dysfunction. One possible reason for this difference is that the growth of juvenile Id-CP influences pituitary gland development. Another characteristic of Id-CP is the higher incidence of DI, which can reach 60%. This rate is much higher than that observed among cases of suprasellar CPs and is also higher than the rates commonly reported in the literature [2]. It is difficult to explain this phenomenon precisely. One possible reason is the influence of the tumor growth on the PS. On the other hand, the incidence of hypopituitarism was lower among cases of pediatric supradia-phragmatic CP than Id-CP. According to our data, there was a statistically significant presurgical difference between these two types of tumors. However, this difference disappeared after surgery. A few cases of childhood Id-CP exhibited obesity, mental disorders, and drowsiness. However, in most cases of this type of tumor, no significant hypothalamic disorder is evident, despite significant involvement of the 3rd VF and hypothalamus. In general, after pursuing radical tumor gross total removal, patients will suffer from different degrees of hypothalamic disorders, including obesity, mental instability, irritability, overeating, and memory dysfunction.

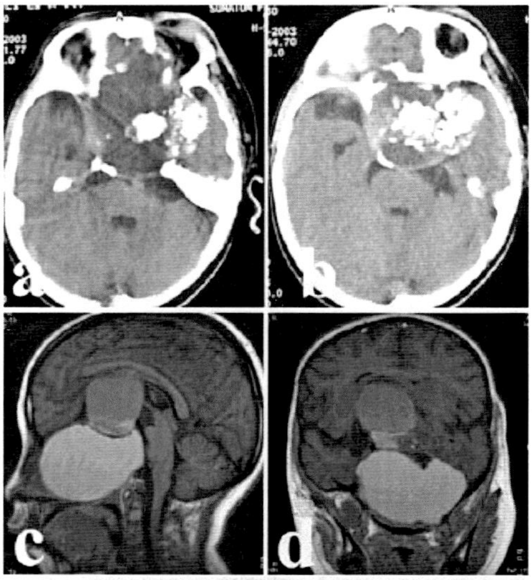

Fig. (1). CT and MRI images have an infra-sellar originating Craniopharyngioma. **A** and **B**. CT images indicated that a huge cystic and solid mixed tumor located at the infra-sellar, sellar and suprasellar region. The nasopharynx, sphenoid sinus, and ethmoidal sinus were also involved. And the big mass of calcification was inside the tumor. **C** and **D**. MRI images showed further the tumor's morphological features.

MORPHOLOGICAL FEATURES OF PEDIATRIC *VERSUS* ADULT CP

Per the description above, there are two types of pediatric CP. According to a few literature reports, Id-CP accounts for approximately 29.8–56% of all pediatric CPs. This incidence was 42% in our series [2, 24]. Pediatric Id-CP differs somewhat from adult Id-CP. In pediatric patients, these tumors are always large. Based on our data, the median sagittal maximal diameter is 4.5 ± 1.45 cm. The site of origin ranges from the nasopharynx, sphenoid sinus, and ethmoidal sinus to the pituitary fossa, with expansion along the longitudinal axis of the PS (Fig. **1**). The suprasellar expansion is similar to that of pituitary adenoma and is limited by the morphological features of the diaphragm and diaphragmatic foramen. Developmental defects in the diaphragm that lead to a large foramen remove the diaphragmatic limitations on suprasellar tumor expansion (Fig. **2**). Meanwhile, the orientation and direction of suprasellar tumors also vary. In most cases, suprasellar tumors grow toward the prechiasmatic space and lift the optic chiasm. In contrast, a few tumors expand toward the third ventricle and invaginate inside the 3rd VF (Fig. **3**). In the latter situation, the prefixed chiasm might play important role. Cavernous sinus (CS) involvement by CPs is quite rare; these tumors differ from pituitary adenomas, which more easily involve the bilateral CS (Fig. **4**). However, it is more difficult to remove CPs with true CS involvement. Given the large size of pediatric CPs, tumor development likely accompanies embryonic development of the pituitary gland. As a result, these tumors have a stronger influence on pituitary function. In our series, all patients with this type of tumor suffered from severe hypopituitarism before surgery, whereas panhypopituitarism occurred in most patients after surgery. In contrast, this phenomenon is rare among cases of adult Id-CP.

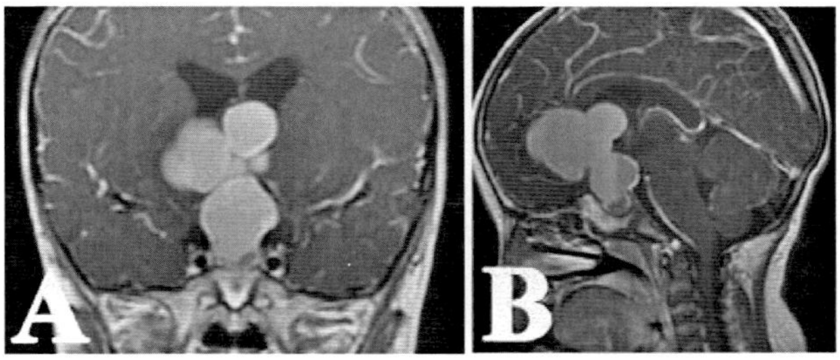

Fig. (2). MRI images indicated that the development defect of the diaphragm caused the suprasellar expansion of the CP through the diaphragmatic foramen. The tumor shaped multiple lobes.

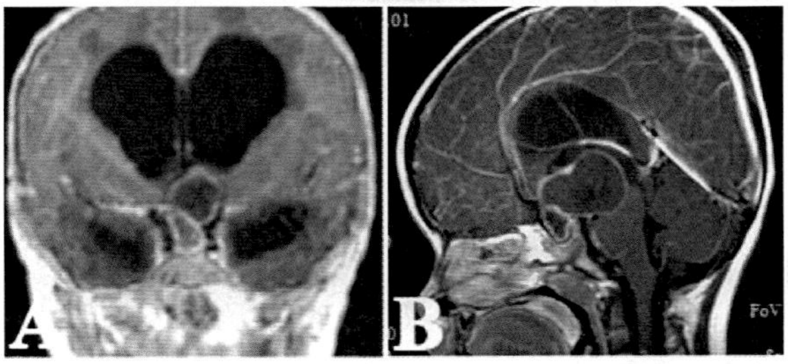

Fig. (3). A case of CP with posterior expanding, which caused a prefixed optic chiasm, invagination of the 3rd VF and occupying the third ventricular cavity.

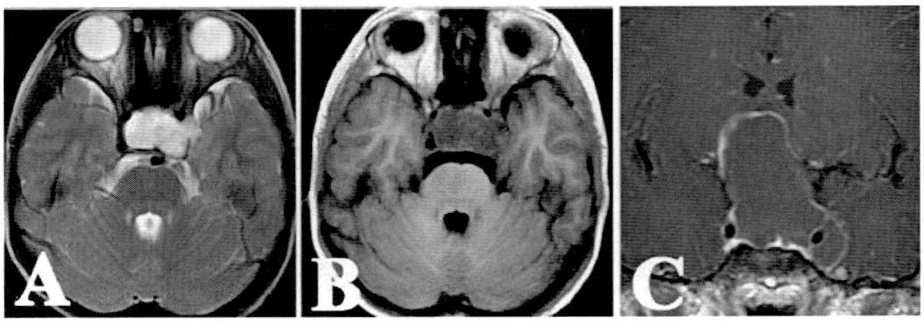

Fig. (4). MRI images indicated that a case of CP with involvement of the left side of cavernous sinus.

Adult Id-CP is very rare. In our series, this type of tumor accounted for only 10.7% of all adult CPs. Moreover, adult Id-CPs were always small-sized. The median sagittal maximal diameter of the 14 cases in our series was 2.7 ± 0.42 cm, which was significantly smaller than that of pediatric Id-CPs ($P < 0.001$). For the adult Id-CP cases, if the trans-sphenoidal surgical approach was selected, the normally compressed and distorted pituitary gland always required disruption, indicating a relatively higher site of origin. Normally, the site of adult Id-CP origin was thought to occur at the connection between the infradiaphragmatic PS to and gland near the diaphragmatic foramen. Pediatric suprasellar CPs mainly grow towards the third ventricle and occupy the third ventricular cavity; however, this type of tumor actually expands along the thin nervous tissue layer of the 3rd VF. These tumors always cause extensive enlargement of the anterior part of the third ventricle (tubero-infundibulum). Accordingly, on presurgical MRI images and during surgery, the anterior part of the third ventricle exhibits frog belly-like expansion. The suprasellar arachnoid cistern remains free of tumor (Fig. **5**). Such tumors can be considered sub-pia mater lesions. Surgical manipulation occurs inside the nervous tissue layer of the third ventricular walls. There is no significant interface between the tumor wall and the surrounding gliosis tissue of the third ventricular walls, which resulted in a difficult total tumor removal. Another morphological feature of pediatric 3rd VF CP is that these tumors are more likely to cause extensive expansion of the PS and infundibulum. The suprasellar PS expands and becomes the cystic wall of the tumor. This morphological feature renders safe tumor removal more difficult (Fig. **6**). Compared with pediatric CP, adult tubero-infundibular CPs exhibit two types of growth pattern: 1) The main body of tumor grows toward the subarachnoid cistern. More frequently, the tumor grows beneath the ventral optic chiasm and expands to the prechiasmatic space. The tumor stem is then located at the connection between the PS and tubero-infundibulum. The main tumor body is located between the ventral optic chiasm and basal membranous arachnoid around the PS. In contrast, some pediatric CPs invaginate inside the 3rd VF and expand to occupy the third ventricular cavity. Compared with pediatric tubero-infundibular CP, a higher incidence of total ventricle cavity occupation by the tumor is observed among adult cases. Although the PS is displaced downward, the stalk itself remains free of tumor involvement, which is convenient for surgical removal. Therefore, pediatric suprasellar CP is more severe than adult CP, according to the degree of tumor involvement in the third ventricular walls and hypothalamus. This difference likely contributes to underdevelopment of arachnoid structures around the PS and hypothalamus in pediatric patients. However, this point remains controversial, as some scholars believe that there might be a true difference between pediatric and adult patients with respect to the site of origin.

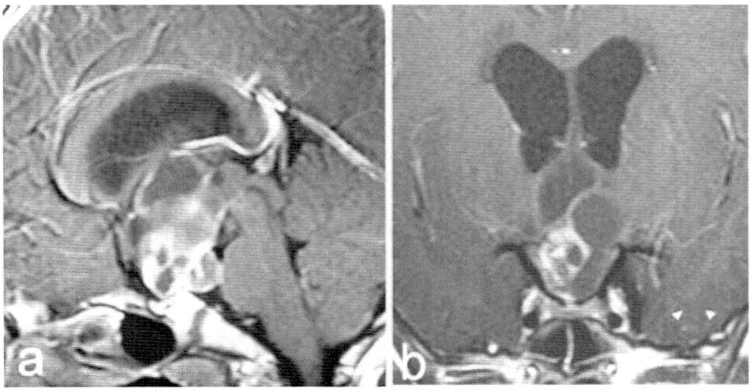

Fig. (5). MRI images of a tubero-infundibular CP. The tumor located inside the 3rd VF totally. The suprasellar cistern was free to the tumor involvement, and the pituitary stalk was intact except the frog belly expanding of the tubero-infundibulum.

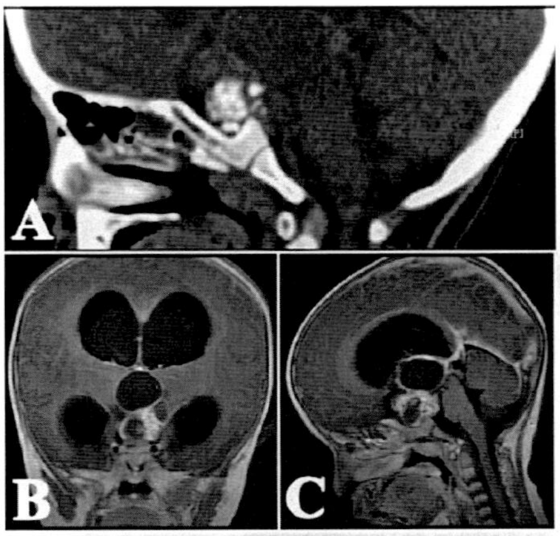

Fig. (6). CT and MRI scan of a case of 3rd VF CP. A suprasellar located cystic and solid mixed tumor caused the inflation of the full length of the pituitary stalk. The enlarged pituitary stalk became the walls of the CP, which caused big problem to remove the tumor.

In some rare cases, the cystic tumor part of suprasellar childhood CPs expands to the posterior cranial fossa Fig. (7) to form retroclivus and posterior cranial fossa CPs. Although the site of origin remains at the connection between the PS and infundibulum, the cystic tumor can expand to the interpeduncular area, retroclivus, and posterior cranial fossa. Bilateral CPA region involvement is always possible. Because of extensive expansion along the subarachnoid spaces, this type of tumor always induces cranial nerve injuries that may be accompanied by paralysis and epilepsy [25, 26]. In contrast to adult extraventricular cases with expansion toward the prechiasmatic space, pediatric extraventricular CPs with expansion to the posterior cranial fossa always adhere tightly to the 3rd VF and infundibulum, leading to considerable challenges in terms of surgical exposure and dissection.

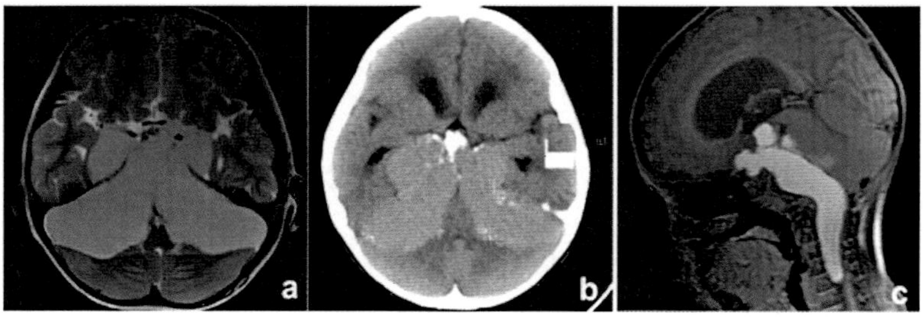

Fig. (7). A case of cystic CP with posterior expansion and involved the prepontile cistern. The low part of tumor even reached the upper cervical segment.

THERAPUTIC STRATEGY FOR PEDIATRIC CP

The therapeutic strategy for pediatric CPs remains the most controversial, which has posed significant difficulties in the establishment of an optimal therapeutic protocol. Most of the controversies focus on whether radical gross total tumor removal (GTR) or palliative surgery with irradiation therapy should be selected for pediatric CP. Most scholars believe that treatment should be individualized and should depend on the degree of tumor involvement in the hypothalamus. However, the question of how to precisely evaluate the degree of hypothalamic involvement before surgery has been quite difficult for researchers to answer. Meuric *et al.* [27], Puget S. *et al.* [28], and Sainte-Rose *et al.* [29] proposed an evaluated method for hypothalamic involvement that was based on presurgical radiological imaging (MRI), followed by surgical strategy modification according to the degree of involvement. However, distortion and compression of the 3rd VF on MRI was the only foundation for this evaluation. In our opinion, this evaluation might harbor some issues: 1) According to the tumor growth pattern, several relationships can be determined between the CP and hypothalamic structures, including compression, adherence, and even frank invasion. Presurgical MRI, however, cannot reflect tumor invasion into the nervous tissue. The current evaluation methods did not address this factor. 2) Moreover, the true relationship between the tumor and 3rd VF could not be precisely by MRI scan until recently. This point has been proven repeatedly in our clinical work; for example, based on MRI, in some cases involving CPs that were thought to grow entirely within the 3rd VF, the existence of a significant plane for surgical manipulation between the tumor and nervous tissue layer of the third ventricular walls was proven. As a result, the related intact hypothalamic–pituitary–infundibulum structure can be preserved during safe tumor removal (Fig. **8**). 3) The influences of different neurosurgeons and treatment conceptions on strategy selection were also not considered. Therefore, an evaluation method based only on hypothalamic compression and involvement on presurgical MRI scans is not suitable for use in the clinical treatment of pediatric CPs. As our opinion, because of the quite different origination site and growth pattern of infra-diaphragmatic CP (Type Q) and infundibulo-tuberal CP (Type T), it is not suitable to evaluate the hypothalamic involvement based only the images. So these two types should be subdivided when doing such evaluation.

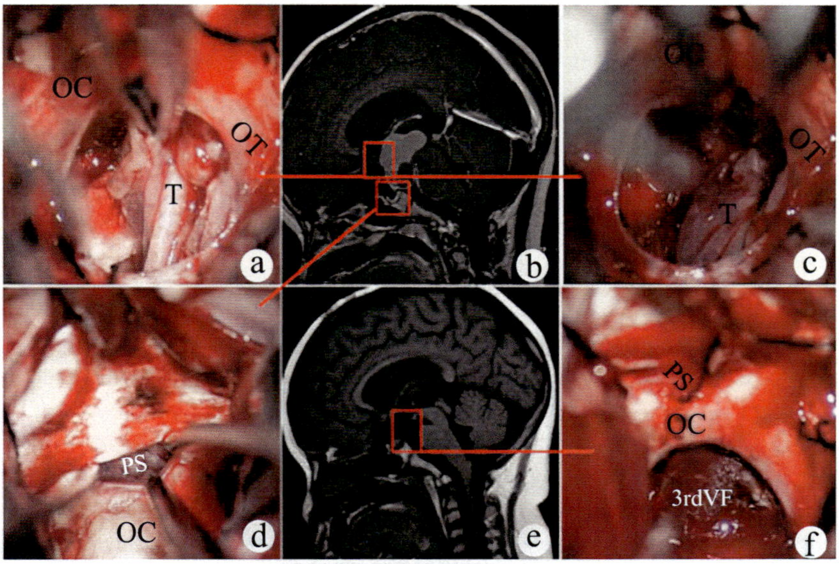

Fig. (8). The presurgical MRI and intrasurgical findings of a case of 3rd VF CP. A and C. After opening the lamina terminalis, the tumor was resected along the interface between tumor and nervous tissue layer of the 3rd VF. D. Through the 1st surgical space, the intact pituitary stalk was observed. F. After totally tumor removal, the hypothalamus-pituitary stalk-pituitary gland axis was maintained. And there was no defection observed in the 3rd VF.

There might more feasible methods for neurosurgeons to assess the hypothalamic reaction within a long-term follow-up that would be less difficult than evaluating hypothalamic involvement before surgery. In a study of 63 survivors of pediatric CP, all subjects with marked obesity after surgery exhibited evidence of significant alterations in the normal hypothalamic anatomy, with MRI data revealing either complete deficiency or extensive destruction of the 3rd VF [30]. Obesity is widely accepted to be the most significant manifestation of a long-term hypothalamic reaction. Actually, apart from the postsurgical 3rd VF morphology on MRI scans, the surgeon's judgment regarding protection of the hypothalamic structures during surgery can more precisely predict the degree of long-term hypothalamic reaction severity. We have summarized the evaluated criteria for assessing hypothalamic defects after surgery for tubero-infundibular CP (Table **1**). The method is closely related to the severity of hypothalamic dysfunction during follow-up.

Table 1. Four-grade scoring system for postoperative hypothalamic impairment in infundibulo-tuberal CPs.

Post-op scale	Criteria
GradeI	A thinned intact floor with preservation of infundibulum and stalk
GradeII	A breached floor with a small deficient at the anterior portion of the third ventricle floor with continuity of infundibulum and stalk OR the third ventricle floor occupation with tumor remnants
Grade III	A breached floor with large deficient at the posterior portion of the third ventricle floor with sacrifice of the infundibulum and stalk
Grade IV	Wholly deficient (grade V) third ventricle floor with sacrifice of the infundibulum and stalk.

PROGNOSIS OF PEDIATRIC CP

Partial or panhypopituitarism is a consistent result after surgery for pediatric CP. Similar to several previous reports [13, 31 - 35] and in contrast to anterior pituitary tumor cases, we did not observe significant relief from or restoration of preexisting hormone deficiencies after surgical CP resection. This also represents a significant difference between CPs and pituitary adenomas. As we described above, patients with pediatric Id-CP always develop severe hypopituitarism and even panhypopituitarism in most cases. Similarly, in pediatric tubero-infundibular CP cases, the incidence of postsurgical hypopituitarism also increased significantly when compared to the presurgical level [2, 13]. In our clinical cases, a few patients experienced partially restored adenohypophyseal function. In some Id-CP cases among these patients, continuity of the PS and neurohypophysis was preserved Fig. (**9**); in the other suprasellar tubero-infundibular cases, vital structures such as the 3rd VF, infundibulum and PS were protected appropriately (Fig. **10**).

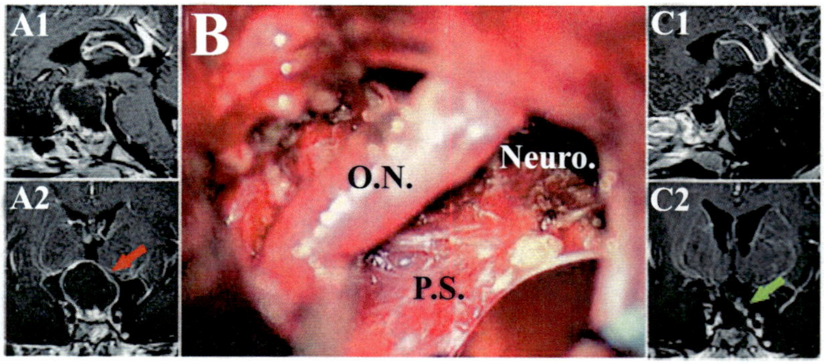

Fig. (9). A case of Id-CP with preservation of the pituitary stalk. A1 and A2. The MRI scan before surgery indicated the pituitary stalk was bias to the left side. B. In operation, along the membranous septation between neuro-hypophysis and intermediate lobe, a thin inflated pituitary stalk was maintained. C1 and C2. The MRI images after surgery showed the continuity of the hypothalamus to the pituitary stalk.

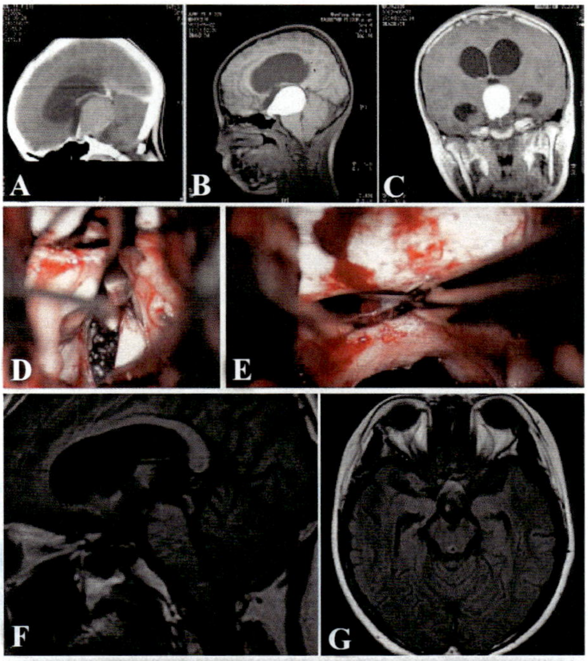

Fig. (10). A case of tubero-infundibular CP with preservation of the pituitary stalk. A~C. The CT and MRI scan before surgery indicated a cystic predominant tumor located inside the 3rd VF and occupied the 3rd ventricular cavity. D and E. Intraoperative findings showed that the tumor was totally removed through the lamina terminalis space. And the pituitary stalk was observed with intact through the 1st surgical space. F and G. The MRI after surgery indicated that the tumor was totally removed.

In pediatric patients, the phenomenon of growth without GH has been reported in some children with CP who exhibited normal or even accelerated linear growth despite harboring an untreated GH deficiency [36, 37]. Current research indicates that this phenomenon might be related to hyperinsulinemia and hyperprolactinemia, which always accompany obesity. Hyperinsulinemia and hyperprolactinemia might consequently increase IGF-1 accumulation and receptor binding, thus promoting its role in increasing the patient's height.

Hypopituitarism differs in that it can be relieved by hormone substitution, thus allowing patients to achieve a relatively good quality of life (QOL). However, hypothalamic dysfunction may severely influence a child's long-term QOL. This dysfunction can include hyperphagia and uncontrollable obesity [13, 14, 22, 38, 39]. Minor patients can also suffer from several other complications, including abnormal thirst, water and electrolyte imbalances, abnormal behaviors, mental disorders, temperature dysregulation, and daytime somnolence [14, 36, 40 - 46]. Among these manifestations, obesity is the most common complication and exists in all patients with 3rd VF tubero-infundibular CP. However, in patients with Id-

CP, significant obesity only occurs in cases with huge tumors and 3rd VF involvement or cases in which repeated recurrences and substitutive treatment cause hypothalamic injury [2]. According to current thought, obesity after CP surgery is caused by injury to the satiety center of the hypothalamus, leading to a metabolic balance disorder [47]. However, the detailed mechanism remains unknown. Possible contributing mechanisms include a lack of sensitivity to endogenous leptin. Roth *et al.* [48] demonstrated vagal mediation of hyperinsulinemia and autonomic imbalance [49], as well as reduced physical activity, which were exaggerated by neurological defects, visual failures, and somnolence [50]. Affected children who suffer from severe obesity always exhibit mental instability, solitary introversion, and irritability. Meanwhile, other dysfunctions may also occur, including DI without abnormal thirst, sleep disorders, and memory dysfunction, all of which will influence pediatric patients' QOL and learning ability. As reported by De Vile *et al.* [41] in 75 cases of pediatric CP treated *via* surgery, the IQ indices in >40% of the cases were <80. Additionally, 23% of the cases suffered from severe limb dysfunction and/or epilepsy.

Currently there are no reliable treatments for severe hypothalamic syndrome. However, our opinion is that affected children might benefit from some dietary and behavioral modifications, encouragement of regular physical activity, psychological counseling, and anti-obesity drugs; all of these can be adopted and used by parents beginning in the early postsurgical stage.

CONFLICT OF INTEREST

The author (editor) declares no conflict of interest, financial or otherwise.

ACKNOWLEDGEMENTS

Declared none.

REFERENCES

[1] Karavitaki N, Cudlip S, Adams CB, Wass JA. Craniopharyngiomas. Endocr Rev 2006; 27(4): 371-97. [http://dx.doi.org/10.1210/er.2006-0002] [PMID: 16543382]

[2] Qi S, Pan J, Lu Y, *et al.* The impact of the site of origin and rate of tumour growth on clinical outcome in children with craniopharyngiomas. Clin Endocrinol (Oxf) 2012; 76(1): 103-10. [http://dx.doi.org/10.1111/j.1365-2265.2011.04172.x] [PMID: 21752042]

[3] Van Effenterre R, Boch AL. Craniopharyngioma in adults and children: a study of 122 surgical cases. J Neurosurg 2002; 97(1): 3-11. [http://dx.doi.org/10.3171/jns.2002.97.1.0003] [PMID: 12134929]

[4] Lee YY, Wong TT, Fang YT, Chang KP, Chen YW, Niu DM. Comparison of hypothalamopituitary axis dysfunction of intrasellar and third ventricular craniopharyngiomas in children. Brain Dev 2008; 30(3): 189-94.

[http://dx.doi.org/10.1016/j.braindev.2007.07.011] [PMID: 17870266]

[5] Rath SR, Lee S, Kotecha RS, Taylor M, Junckerstorff RC, Choong CS. Childhood craniopharyngioma: 20-year institutional experience in Western Australia. J Paediatr Child Health 2013; 49(5): 403-8. [http://dx.doi.org/10.1111/jpc.12190] [PMID: 23560768]

[6] Akimura T, Kameda H, Abiko S, Aoki H, Kido T. Infrasellar craniopharyngioma. Neuroradiology 1989; 31(2): 180-3. [http://dx.doi.org/10.1007/BF00698851] [PMID: 2747897]

[7] Cooper PR, Ransohoff J. Craniopharyngioma originating in the sphenoid bone. Case report. J Neurosurg 1972; 36(1): 102-6. [http://dx.doi.org/10.3171/jns.1972.36.1.0102] [PMID: 5007266]

[8] Jiang RS, Wu CY, Jan YJ, Hsu CY. Primary ethmoid sinus craniopharyngioma: a case report. J Laryngol Otol 1998; 112(4): 403-5. [http://dx.doi.org/10.1017/S0022215100140599] [PMID: 9659511]

[9] Sarioğlu AC, Ozlen F, Hanci M, Oz B. Craniopharyngioma extended into the posterior fossa. Neurosurg Rev 1996; 19(4): 265-7. [http://dx.doi.org/10.1007/BF00314843] [PMID: 9007891]

[10] Crotty TB, Scheithauer BW, Young WF Jr, *et al.* Papillary craniopharyngioma: a clinicopathological study of 48 cases. J Neurosurg 1995; 83(2): 206-14. [http://dx.doi.org/10.3171/jns.1995.83.2.0206] [PMID: 7616262]

[11] Eldevik OP, Blaivas M, Gabrielsen TO, Hald JK, Chandler WF. Craniopharyngioma: radiologic and histologic findings and recurrence. AJNR Am J Neuroradiol 1996; 17(8): 1427-39. [PMID: 8883637]

[12] Sartoretti-Schefer S, Wichmann W, Aguzzi A, Valavanis A. MR differentiation of adamantinous and squamous-papillary craniopharyngiomas. AJNR Am J Neuroradiol 1997; 18(1): 77-87. [PMID: 9010523]

[13] Karavitaki N, Brufani C, Warner JT, *et al.* Craniopharyngiomas in children and adults: systematic analysis of 121 cases with long-term follow-up. Clin Endocrinol (Oxf) 2005; 62(4): 397-409. [http://dx.doi.org/10.1111/j.1365-2265.2005.02231.x] [PMID: 15807869]

[14] Duff J, Meyer FB, Ilstrup DM, Laws ER Jr, Schleck CD, Scheithauer BW. Long-term outcomes for surgically resected craniopharyngiomas. Neurosurgery 2000; 46(2): 291-302. [http://dx.doi.org/10.1097/00006123-200002000-00007] [PMID: 10690718]

[15] Leddy ET, Marshall TM. Roentgen therapy of pituitary adamantinomas (craniopharyngiomas). Radiology 1951; 56(3): 384-93. [http://dx.doi.org/10.1148/56.3.384] [PMID: 14834414]

[16] Banna M, Hoare RD, Stanley P, Till K. Craniopharyngioma in children. J Pediatr 1973; 83(5): 781-5. [http://dx.doi.org/10.1016/S0022-3476(73)80369-5] [PMID: 4742571]

[17] Fahlbusch R, Honegger J, Paulus W, Huk W, Buchfelder M. Surgical treatment of craniopharyngiomas: experience with 168 patients. J Neurosurg 1999; 90(2): 237-50. [http://dx.doi.org/10.3171/jns.1999.90.2.0237] [PMID: 9950494]

[18] Matson DD, Crigler JF Jr. Management of craniopharyngioma in childhood. J Neurosurg 1969; 30(4): 377-90. [http://dx.doi.org/10.3171/jns.1969.30.4.0377] [PMID: 4308176]

[19] Petito CK, DeGirolami U, Earle KM. Craniopharyngiomas: a clinical and pathological review. Cancer 1976; 37(4): 1944-52. [http://dx.doi.org/10.1002/1097-0142(197604)37:4<1944::AID-CNCR2820370446>3.0.CO;2-#] [PMID: 1260697]

[20] Zhang YQ, Wang CC, Ma ZY. Pediatric craniopharyngiomas: clinicomorphological study of 189 cases. Pediatr Neurosurg 2002; 36(2): 80-4.
[http://dx.doi.org/10.1159/000048357] [PMID: 11893889]

[21] Kahn EA, Gosch HH, Seeger JF, Hicks SP. Forty-five years experience with the craniopharyngiomas. Surg Neurol 1973; 1(1): 5-12.
[PMID: 4544703]

[22] Hoffman HJ, De Silva M, Humphreys RP, Drake JM, Smith ML, Blaser SI. Aggressive surgical management of craniopharyngiomas in children. J Neurosurg 1992; 76(1): 47-52.
[http://dx.doi.org/10.3171/jns.1992.76.1.0047] [PMID: 1727168]

[23] Hoff JT, Patterson RH Jr. Craniopharyngiomas in children and adults. J Neurosurg 1972; 36(3): 299-302.
[http://dx.doi.org/10.3171/jns.1972.36.3.0299] [PMID: 5059968]

[24] Qi S, Lu Y, Pan J, Zhang X, Long H, Fan J. Anatomic relations of the arachnoidea around the pituitary stalk: relevance for surgical removal of craniopharyngiomas. Acta Neurochir (Wien) 2011; 153(4): 785-96.
[http://dx.doi.org/10.1007/s00701-010-0940-y] [PMID: 21271263]

[25] Bashir EM, Lewis PD, Edwards MR. Posterior fast craniopharyngioma. Br J Neurosurg 1996; 10(6): 613-5.
[http://dx.doi.org/10.1080/02688699646970] [PMID: 9115662]

[26] Altinörs N, Senveli E, Erdoğan A, Arda N, Pak I. Craniopharyngioma of the cerebellopontine angle. Case report. J Neurosurg 1984; 60(4): 842-4.
[http://dx.doi.org/10.3171/jns.1984.60.4.0842] [PMID: 6608580]

[27] Meuric S, Brauner R, Trivin C, Souberbielle JC, Zerah M, Sainte-Rose C. Influence of tumor location on the presentation and evolution of craniopharyngiomas. J Neurosurg 2005; 103(5) (Suppl.): 421-6.
[PMID: 16302613]

[28] Puget S, Garnett M, Wray A, *et al.* Pediatric craniopharyngiomas: classification and treatment according to the degree of hypothalamic involvement. J Neurosurg 2007; 106(1) (Suppl.): 3-12.
[PMID: 17233305]

[29] Sainte-Rose C, Puget S, Wray A, *et al.* Craniopharyngioma: the pendulum of surgical management. Childs Nerv Syst 2005; 21(8-9): 691-5.
[http://dx.doi.org/10.1007/s00381-005-1209-2] [PMID: 16078079]

[30] de Vile CJ, Grant DB, Hayward RD, Kendall BE, Neville BG, Stanhope R. Obesity in childhood craniopharyngioma: relation to post-operative hypothalamic damage shown by magnetic resonance imaging. J Clin Endocrinol Metab 1996; 81(7): 2734-7.
[PMID: 8675604]

[31] Ahmed S, Elsheikh M, Stratton IM, Page RC, Adams CB, Wass JA. Outcome of transphenoidal surgery for acromegaly and its relationship to surgical experience. Clin Endocrinol (Oxf) 1999; 50(5): 561-7.
[http://dx.doi.org/10.1046/j.1365-2265.1999.00760.x] [PMID: 10468920]

[32] Paja M, Lucas T, García-Uría J, Salamé F, Barceló B, Estrada J. Hypothalamic-pituitary dysfunction in patients with craniopharyngioma. Clin Endocrinol (Oxf) 1995; 42(5): 467-73.
[http://dx.doi.org/10.1111/j.1365-2265.1995.tb02664.x] [PMID: 7621564]

[33] Weiss M, Sutton L, Marcial V, *et al.* The role of radiation therapy in the management of childhood craniopharyngioma. Int J Radiat Oncol Biol Phys 1989; 17(6): 1313-21.
[http://dx.doi.org/10.1016/0360-3016(89)90543-9] [PMID: 2689398]

[34] Thomsett MJ, Conte FA, Kaplan SL, Grumbach MM. Endocrine and neurologic outcome in childhood craniopharyngioma: Review of effect of treatment in 42 patients. J Pediatr 1980; 97(5): 728-35.
[http://dx.doi.org/10.1016/S0022-3476(80)80254-X] [PMID: 7431164]

[35] Honegger J, Buchfelder M, Fahlbusch R. Surgical treatment of craniopharyngiomas: endocrinological results. J Neurosurg 1999; 90(2): 251-7. [http://dx.doi.org/10.3171/jns.1999.90.2.0251] [PMID: 9950495]

[36] DeVile CJ, Grant DB, Hayward RD, Stanhope R. Growth and endocrine sequelae of craniopharyngioma. Arch Dis Child 1996; 75(2): 108-14. [http://dx.doi.org/10.1136/adc.75.2.108] [PMID: 8869189]

[37] Bucher H, Zapf J, Torresani T, Prader A, Froesch ER, Illig R. Insulin-like growth factors I and II, prolactin, and insulin in 19 growth hormone-deficient children with excessive, normal, or decreased longitudinal growth after operation for craniopharyngioma. N Engl J Med 1983; 309(19): 1142-6. [http://dx.doi.org/10.1056/NEJM198311103091902] [PMID: 6353237]

[38] Hetelekidis S, Barnes PD, Tao ML, *et al.* 20-year experience in childhood craniopharyngioma. Int J Radiat Oncol Biol Phys 1993; 27(2): 189-95. [http://dx.doi.org/10.1016/0360-3016(93)90227-M] [PMID: 8407391]

[39] Curtis J, Daneman D, Hoffman HJ, Ehrlich RM. The endocrine outcome after surgical removal of craniopharyngiomas. Pediatr Neurosurg 1994; 21 (Suppl. 1): 24-7. [http://dx.doi.org/10.1159/000120858] [PMID: 7841075]

[40] Smith D, Finucane F, Phillips J, *et al.* Abnormal regulation of thirst and vasopressin secretion following surgery for craniopharyngioma. Clin Endocrinol (Oxf) 2004; 61(2): 273-9. [http://dx.doi.org/10.1111/j.1365-2265.2004.02086.x] [PMID: 15272926]

[41] De Vile CJ, Grant DB, Kendall BE, *et al.* Management of childhood craniopharyngioma: can the morbidity of radical surgery be predicted? J Neurosurg 1996; 85(1): 73-81. [http://dx.doi.org/10.3171/jns.1996.85.1.0073] [PMID: 8683285]

[42] Griffiths AP, Henderson M, Penn ND, Tindall H. Haematological, neurological and psychiatric complications of chronic hypothermia following surgery for craniopharyngioma. Postgrad Med J 1988; 64(754): 617-20. [http://dx.doi.org/10.1136/pgmj.64.754.617] [PMID: 3249709]

[43] Lipton JM, Rosenstein J, Sklar FH. Thermoregulatory disorders after removal of a craniopharyngioma from the third cerebral ventricle. Brain Res Bull 1981; 7(4): 369-73. [http://dx.doi.org/10.1016/0361-9230(81)90031-9] [PMID: 7296306]

[44] Palm L, Nordin V, Elmqvist D, Blennow G, Persson E, Westgren U. Sleep and wakefulness after treatment for craniopharyngioma in childhood; influence on the quality and maturation of sleep. Neuropediatrics 1992; 23(1): 39-45. [http://dx.doi.org/10.1055/s-2008-1071310] [PMID: 1565216]

[45] Müller HL, Handwerker G, Wollny B, Faldum A, Sörensen N. Melatonin secretion and increased daytime sleepiness in childhood craniopharyngioma patients. J Clin Endocrinol Metab 2002; 87(8): 3993-6. [http://dx.doi.org/10.1210/jcem.87.8.8751] [PMID: 12161549]

[46] Poretti A, Grotzer MA, Ribi K, Schönle E, Boltshauser E. Outcome of craniopharyngioma in children: long-term complications and quality of life. Dev Med Child Neurol 2004; 46(4): 220-9. [http://dx.doi.org/10.1111/j.1469-8749.2004.tb00476.x] [PMID: 15077699]

[47] Daousi C, Dunn AJ, Foy PM, MacFarlane IA, Pinkney JH. Endocrine and neuroanatomic features associated with weight gain and obesity in adult patients with hypothalamic damage. Am J Med 2005; 118(1): 45-50. [http://dx.doi.org/10.1016/j.amjmed.2004.06.035] [PMID: 15639209]

[48] Roth C, Wilken B, Hanefeld F, Schröter W, Leonhardt U. Hyperphagia in children with craniopharyngioma is associated with hyperleptinaemia and a failure in the downregulation of appetite. Eur J Endocrinol 1998; 138(1): 89-91. [http://dx.doi.org/10.1530/eje.0.1380089] [PMID: 9461323]

[49] Pinkney J, Wilding J, Williams G, MacFarlane I. Hypothalamic obesity in humans: what do we know and what can be done? Obes Rev 2002; 3(1): 27-34. [http://dx.doi.org/10.1046/j.1467-789X.2002.00052.x] [PMID: 12119657]

[50] Harz KJ, Müller HL, Waldeck E, Pudel V, Roth C. Obesity in patients with craniopharyngioma: assessment of food intake and movement counts indicating physical activity. J Clin Endocrinol Metab 2003; 88(11): 5227-31. [http://dx.doi.org/10.1210/jc.2002-021797] [PMID: 14602754]

CHAPTER 19

Typical Cases of Craniopharyngioma

Jun Pan* and **Yuntao Lu**

Department of Neurosurgery, Nanfang Neurosurgery Research Institution, Nanfang Hospital, Southern Medical University, 1838 North Guangzhou Avenue, Guangzhou, China

Abstract: In this section, we have provided clinical data from 15 cases of craniopharyngioma (CP) in which the details differ with respect to growth pattern. Emphasis has been placed on performance of the presurgical analysis and determination of the surgical aims, as well as potential surgical difficulties and the selection of a proper approach to achieve satisfactory exposure for tumor removal. Along with depictions of the tumors' morphological features and schematic Fig. (**1**), we have described the surgical techniques and arachnoidal interfaces used for safe tumor removal while protecting vital neurovascular structures. Long-term follow up data have also been provided to demonstrate the patients' prognoses. These cases have been subdivided into three types: infradiaphragmatic CP (Id-CP or "Q" type), suprasellar extra-ventricular CP with expansion in the subarachnoid cistern (SeV-CP or "S" type), and suprasellar subarachnoid CP with invagination to the third ventricular walls (SiV-CP or "T" type). Because of tumor growth along the longitudinal axis of the pituitary stalk (PS), each case might display different variations. We will illustrate this in special cases.

Keywords: Craniopharyngioma, Diabetis, Infradisphargmatic, Panhypopituitarism, Subarachonidal craniopharyngioma, Third ventricular floor.

INFRADIAPHRAGMATIC CRANIOPHARYNGIOMA (TYPE "Q")

In this chapter, we describe 5 cases of Id-CP. Each case exhibited particular representative morphological features. Meanwhile, differences in the characteristics of pediatric and adult cases are also discussed.

Case 1

Medical History

This was a 6-year-old female with a 2 months' history of headache. The weight of

* **Corresponding author Jun Pan**: Department of Neurosurgery, Nanfang Neurosurgery Research Institution, Nanfang Hospital, Southern Medical University, 1838 North Guangzhou Avenue, Guangzhou, China; Tel\Fax: +8620-61641806; E-mail: panjundu@hotmail.com

Songtao Qi (Ed.)

this patient when presenting in our hospital was 24kg, and height was 125cm. So the BMI index was 15.36.

Analysis Before Surgery

The tumor was a typical Id-CP, and the patient's primary complaint was sexual hormone axis deficiency. This is also a typical presentation of adult Id-CP. The cystic CP exhibited normal tumor morphology and grew inside the pituitary fossa. A trans-nasal trans-sphenoidal approach was selected for tumor removal.

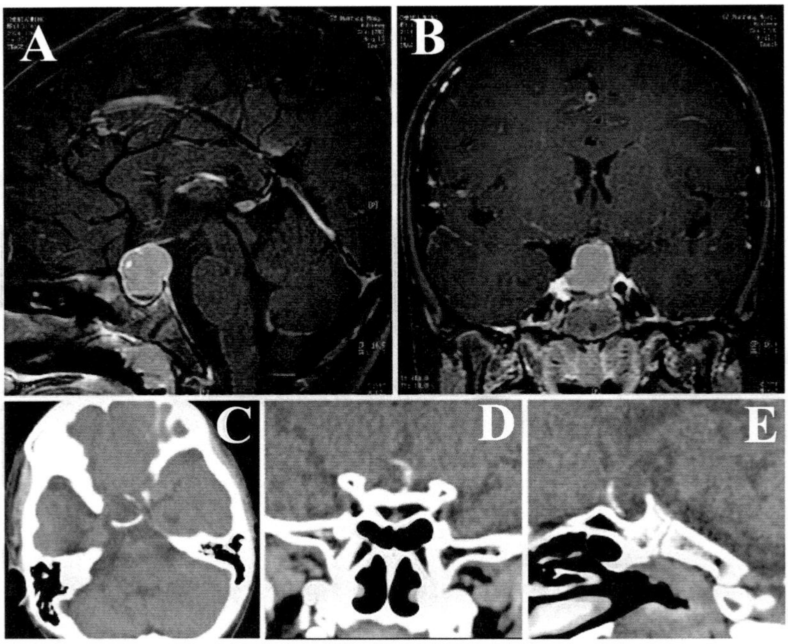

Fig. (1). Presurgical radiological images. **A-B.** Magnetic resonance imaging revealed that the cystic predominant tumor had lifted the optic chiasm and anterior communicating artery upward. The cystic wall was enhanced significantly. **C, D and E.** Computed tomography indicated eggshell-shaped calcification was observed on the tumor cystic wall.

Membranous Structures and Hierarchical Layers: (Fig. 2)

Intraoperative Findings

After opening the sellar floor dura, a thin layer of anterior lobe of pituitary gland was observed. Following by the incision of the anterior lobe, the tumor was removed along the interface of the true tumoral cystic wall. At the upper segment of pituitary stalk, the tumor fused tightly to the stalk, where was thought the originating site. The adherence was sharply dissected to remove the tumor.

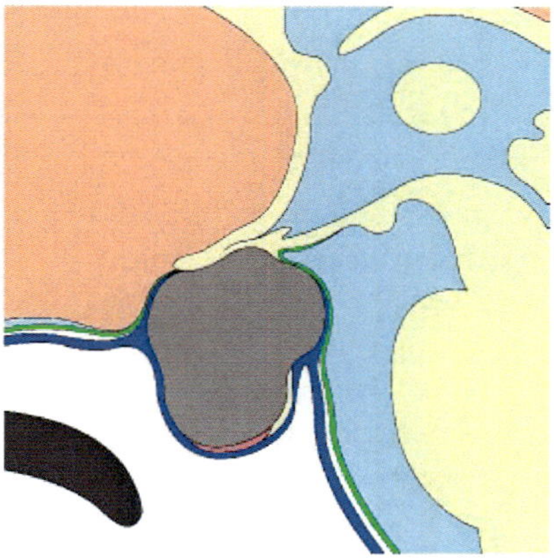

Fig. (2). Schematic Fig. (demonstrating the tumor morphology and relationships with the surrounding structures. Blue line: Dura mater (Diaphragm and sellar floor dura); Green line: Arachnoid mater.

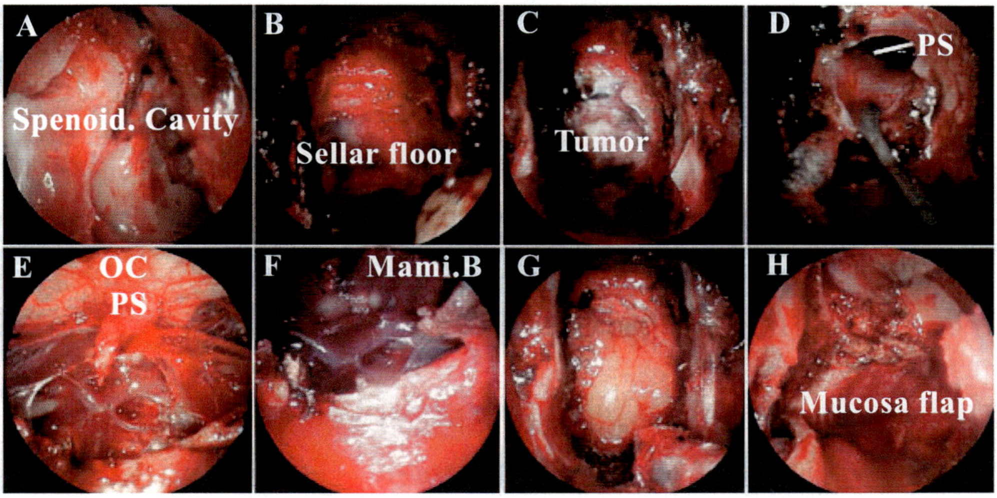

Fig. (3). Intraoperative findings. **A.** After removal of the anterior wall of sphenoidal sinus, the sinus cavity and sellar floor was exposed. **B.** After removing the bone of sellar floor and also the tuberculum sellae, the dura of sellar floor and anterior cranial floor was exposed. C. When opening the sellar floor dura, and thin layer of anterior lobe of pituitary gland was opened to expose the tumor. And a mass of calcification was observed on the anterior wall of tumor. D. At the top of tumor, the inflated pituitary stalk can be found. E. After totally tumor removal, the ventral aspect of optic chiasm and residual pituitary stalk was observed, and also the vascular structure. F. The bilateral mammillary bodies were also observed. G and H. After tumor removal, the fat, artificial dura, gelatin sponge and prepared mucosa flap were used for repairing the sellar floor.

Surgical Result

Postsurgical magnetic resonance imaging (MRI) indicated total tumor removal. His headache relieved significantly, while he suffered with significant diabetes insipidus.

Follow Up

Repeat MRI indicated intrasellar tumor recurrence during two years follow-up. And DI was significant relieved, which can be controlled by oral desmopressin. And he still suffered with pituitarism, which need to be substitute treated by prednisone and also Levothyroxine Sodium Tablets.

Clinical Pearls and Controversies

This patient is typical infra-diaphragmatic CP, which was covered by diaphragm and basal arachonidal membrane at the top of tumor. These membranous structures also separated tumor from the suprasellar structures. As concerned with the tumor's morphological features, the transsphenoidal approach was the most appropriate choice. However, it was still hard to protect the pituitary stalk in operation. Moreover, it didn't show any advantage to deal with the bilateral tumor wall in transsphenoidal approach. The recurrence of intra-sellar tumor was still the most important point within follow up period. In this case, although no recurrence happened in 2 years follow-up, it still need longer time to be followed.

Case 2

Medical History

This was an 11-year-old male patient with an 8-month history of polydipsia and polyuria and decreased vision of 2 months' duration. He had not undergone any treatment before presenting at our hospital.

Physical and Experimental Examination

At the time of admission, a neurological examination revealed no focal deficits. His daily urine volume was >4000 ml. His visual acuity was 0.08 and 0.2 in the right and left eyes, respectively, and he exhibited bitemporal hemianopia during a formal visual field examination. Endocrinological detection indicated a slightly increased prolactin (PRL) level and significantly decreased levels of several sexual hormones (testosterone, progesterone, luteinizing hormone, and estrogen).

Radiological Images Before Surgery

Presurgical MRI Fig. (**4**) studies revealed a large intra- and suprasellar, predominantly cystic mass with marked enlargement of the pituitary fossa and a rounded, symmetrical cystic suprasellar extension; on a coronal MRI scan, the intrasellar tumor region had expanded into the left-side cavernous sinus (CS). No obstructive hydrocephalus occurred, although the tumor measured 4 cm in diameter on the midsagittal plane of a preoperative MRI scan. Computed tomography revealed minor detritus calcification within the intrasellar tumor. Cortisone was administered because the patient exhibited symptoms and signs of panhypopituitarism before surgery.

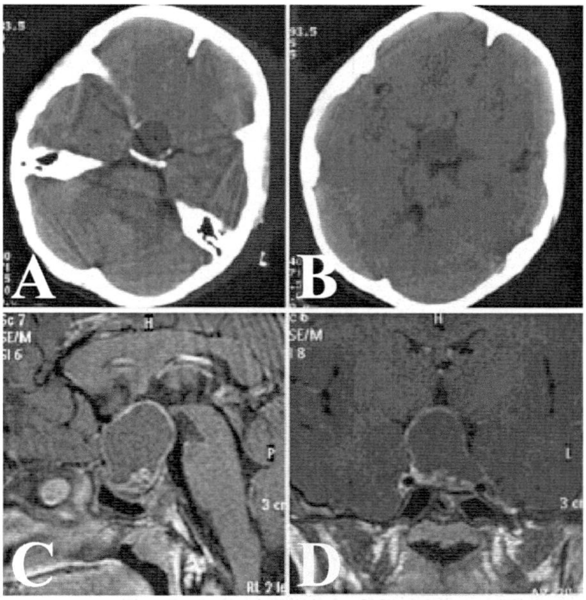

Fig. (4). Presurgical radiological images. **A-B.** Computed tomography indicated a predominantly cystic tumor in the sellar region. Punctate calcification was observed on the tumor cystic wall. **C and D.** Magnetic resonance imaging revealed that the cystic part of the tumor had lifted the optic chiasm and anterior communicating artery upward. The solid part of the tumor was located at the floor of the pituitary fossa. The cystic wall and solid tumor were enhanced significantly.

Analysis Before Surgery

This was a predominantly cystic Id-CP with solid tumor and calcification inside the pituitary fossa. The sella turcica was enlarged significantly. An interhemispheric approach was selected to attempt total tumor removal.

Membranous Structures and Hierarchical Layers: Fig. (5)

Intrasurgical Findings

After general anesthesia induction, the patient was placed in the supine position with the head fixed in a Mayfield three-pin head-holder. The head was extended slightly downward (approximately 15°), allowing the frontal lobe to spontaneously fall downward because of gravity during surgery. A standard frontobasal interhemispheric (FIH) craniotomy was performed Fig. (**6A**). A square of forehead periosteum was maintained for further frontal sinus repair. After careful dissection of the anterior interhemispheric cistern, the planum sphenoidale, optic chiasm, and cisterna lamina terminalis were exposed (black asterisks). The tumor was dissected mainly through the prechiasmatic space. The distal portion of the PS diverged and fused with the upper posterior part of the tumor capsule and elevated diaphragm sellae (DS). To preserve continuity of the PS, the diaphragm at the site of fusion between the PS and tumor should be maintained; although this site is always located behind the tumor, bias might be present in some cases. In this case, the expanded diaphragm was dissected in a circular manner through the prechiasmatic space to identify the true tumor capsule Fig. (**6C**). Next, the interface between the true capsule and diaphragm was followed to separate the adherent tumor from the normal pituitary gland. Although the tumor capsule might be extremely thin in some cases, care should be taken not to lose this interface during separation. When dissecting the posterior part of the tumor, close attention should be paid to PS continuity and the neural fibers of the stalk. Intrasellar tumors always adhere tightly to the normal neurohypophysis. The tumor capsule is easily disrupted during separation. Surgery should be more radical while maintaining a foundation of PS continuity preservation. The medial wall of the CS is always opened when dissection of the bilateral tumor part, and this causes venous bleeding. This bleeding may be significant but can be staunched using an appropriately sized gelatin sponge. After tumor removal, a smooth tumor bed should be observed.

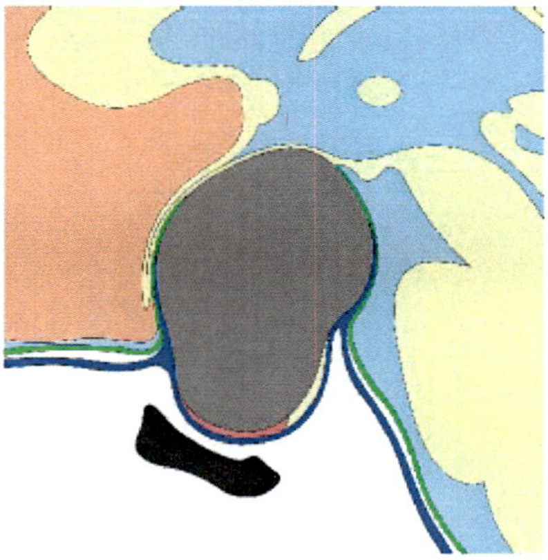

Fig. (5). Schematic Fig. (demonstrating the tumor morphology and relationships with the surrounding structures. Blue line: Dura mater (Diaphragm and sellar floor dura); Green line: Arachnoid mater.

Perioperative Treatment

Postoperative MRI obtained after 6 months revealed total tumor removal. Endocrinological detection performed 2 months after surgery indicated no new hormone deficiencies. The PRL level was normal, although the levels of several sexual hormones remained low.

Long-term Follow Up

The patient's visual symptoms had recovered by the time of the last official follow up, which was conducted at 12 months postoperatively. His diabetes insipidus (DI) recovered gradually. He was able to attend school and did not require hormone replacement therapy at the time of the last follow-up study.

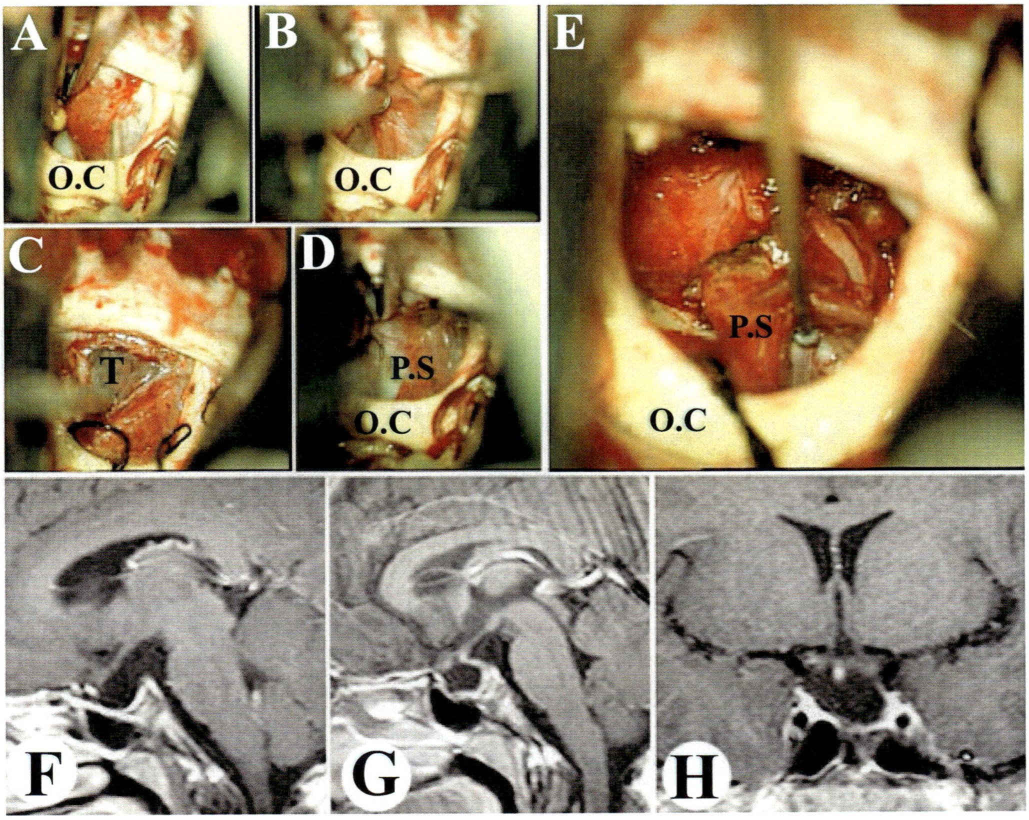

Fig. (6). Intraoperative findings and postsurgical magnetic resonance imaging (MRI). **A.** A tumor with diaphragmatic cover was exposed through the enlarged prechiasmatic space. A needle was used to reduce the cystic volume *via* decompression. **B.** The tumor was separated from surrounding neurovascular structures along the suprasellar arachnoid interface. **C.** A round incision was made to expose the true tumor wall. **D.** The intrasellar tumor part was removed. The intact proximal segment of the pituitary stalk was identified. **E.** After total tumor removal, continuity of hypothalamus–pituitary stalk axis was preserved; an extremely thin residual stalk remained at the site of tumor origin. **F-H.** Postsurgical MRI indicated total tumor removal.

Clinical Pearls and Controversies

This case is also a typical infra-diaphragmatic tumor. There was a clear interface between the tumor cystic wall and elevated diaphragm. It was very important to perform surgical manipulations along the membranous septation for safe preservation of the PS. The most important points to treat this kind of pediatric tumor was as followed: 1) The reservation of pituitary stalk or not? 2) How to remove the intra-sellar tumor totally instead of purely evacuation of cystic fluid. So the surgical pearls of this patient were 1) Showing the morphological relationship between pituitary stalk, tumor capsule, diaphragm and neuro-hypophyseal. We emphasized the dissection and separation of tumor beneath the diaphragm, which could improve the preservation of pituitary stalk. 2) The separation of tumor along the tumor's true capsule ensured the totally removed of intrasellar part of tumor.

Case 3

Medical History

This 8-year-old male patient was admitted to our neurosurgical department on August 18, 2004 with a 2-year history of intermittent headache, decreased visual acuity, and DI. His visual acuity was 0.2 in the right eye with total blindness in the left eye. He also suffered from growth retardation with a height of only 67 cm.

Physical and Experimental Examination

The patient presented with panhypopituitarism and DI. Cortisone was administered because the patient showed symptoms and signs of presurgical panhypopituitarism. Two days after his admission, the patient suffered a transient bout of unconsciousness with bilateral dilated pupils but recovered after mannitol administration.

Radiological Images Before Surgery

Presurgical MRI Fig. (7) revealed a huge, predominantly cystic intra- and suprasellar mass with marked enlargement of the pituitary fossa and a rounded and symmetrical cystic suprasellar extension. No obstructive hydrocephalus occurred although the tumor measured 8 cm in diameter on the midsagittal plane. CT revealed a rounded eggshell-like calcification around the tumor capsule wall.

Analysis Before Surgery

This patient had a huge tumor with upward expansion. Eggshell-like calcification was present on the cystic tumor walls. A predominantly right FIH was selected to remove the tumor.

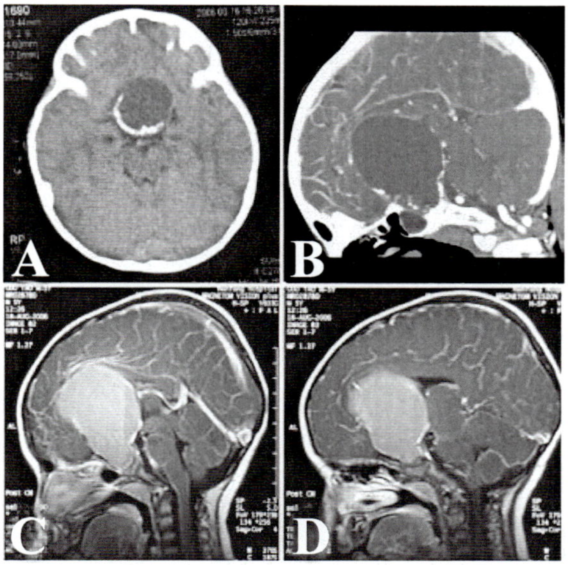

Fig. (7). Presurgical computed tomography (CT) and magnetic resonance imaging (MRI). **A-B.** CT indicated a huge cystic tumor located in the intra- and suprasellar region with significant eggshell-like calcification. **C-D.** MRI indicated that the solid part of tumor was located in the pituitary fossa. The optic chiasm and anterior communicating artery complex were displaced upward and backward.

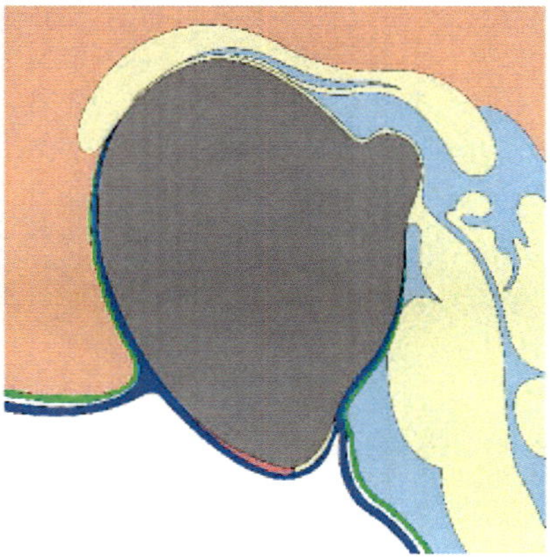

Fig. (8). Schematic Fig. (demonstrating the tumor morphology and relationships with the surrounding structures. Blue line: Dura mater (Diaphragm and sellar floor dura); Green line: Arachnoid mater.

Membranous Structures and Hierarchical Layers: Fig. (8)

Intrasurgical Findings

On August 21, 2004, 3 days after admission, complete tumor removal was performed *via* a FIH approach. A bilateral interhemispheric and predominantly right frontobasal approach was undertaken through a midline-crossing frontal craniotomy. Upon dissection of the interhemispheric fissure, the suprasellar tumor capsule was visible between two extremely prolonged optic nerves. The tumor capsule surfaces were continuous with the elevated diaphragm sellae and dura mater of the skull base Fig. (**9**). First, a piece of tumor capsule was cut through the wide space between the two optic nerves for pathological study. After tumor capsule decompression, the suprasellar tumor capsule could be easily dissected from the chiasm, AcoA, and 3rd VF. However, the tumor had adhered to the upper infundibulum around the tuber cinereum, where the PS connected, and acute dissection was required to free the adhesions while avoiding the hypothalamic structures. After manipulating the suprasellar portion, the diaphragm or the cystic tumor wall was dissected in a circular manner around the tuberculum sellae, interclinoid ligament, and dorsum sellae, and the intrasellar portion of the tumor was removed *via* erasion through the enlarged sellae. A gelatin sponge was used to stop bilateral venous bleeding from the CS. A routine watertight dural closure and bone flap replacement was performed.

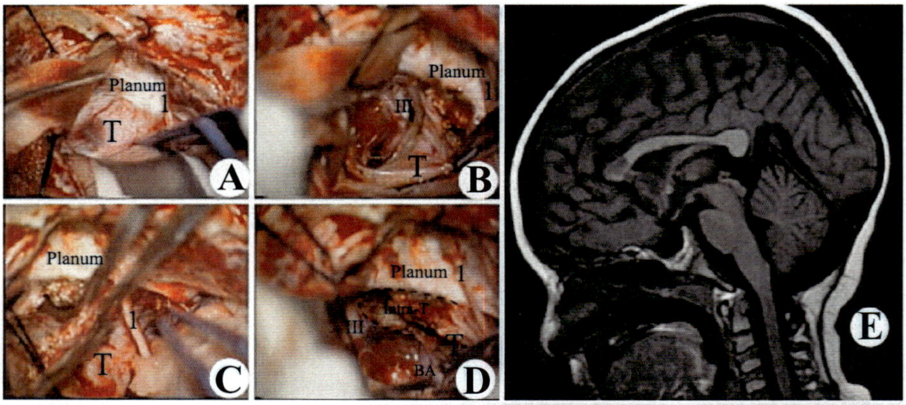

Fig. (9). Intraoperative findings. **A.** The diaphragm-covered tumor was exposed through the enlarged prechiasmatic space. The bilateral optic nerves were distorted and thinned following long-term compression by the tumor. **B-D.** After separating the tumor from the surrounding neurovascular structures along the arachnoidal interface, the diaphragm was cut in a circular manner (dotted line) to display the true tumor wall. **E.** After total tumor removal, sagittal magnetic resonance imaging indicated preservation of the third ventricle floor.

A pathological study revealed a typical adamantinomatous CP. Postoperatively, the patient exhibited DI and required hormone replacement for a few months. He was discharged on September 17, 2004. Six months after surgery, his health was well maintained without hormone replacement except for antidiuretic hormone (ADH) therapy (1–deamino–8–D–arginine vasopressin [DDAVP], 0.05 mg twice daily). His right eye vision improved markedly after surgery. No tumor recurrence was observed during the most recent MRI study Fig. (**10**) on April 8, 2006. Despite poor left eye vision, he had resumed independent performance of daily activities.

Perioperative Treatment

After surgery, the patient's water and electrolyte levels were monitored carefully. DI and hyponatremia were the main perioperative complications and were relieved after treatment.

Long-term Follow Up

No tumor recurrence was detected during a 6-year follow-up period. The patient suffered from growth retardation and panhypopituitarism. Hormone substitutive therapy was continued.

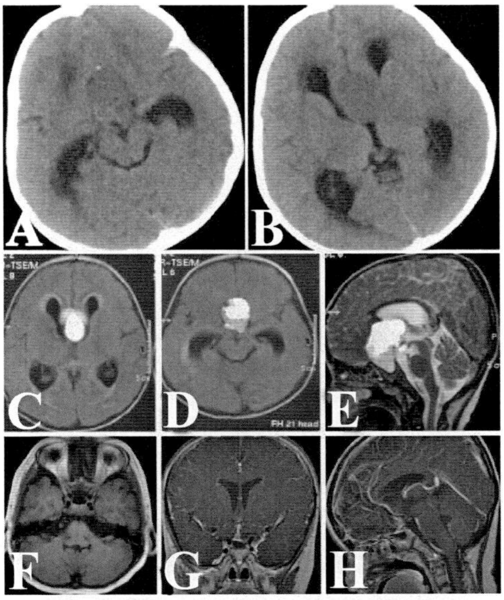

Fig. (10). Presurgical and postsurgical radiological images. **A-B.** Presurgical computed tomography data. **C-E.** Presurgical magnetic resonance imaging (MRI) data. **F-H.** Postsurgical MRI data.

Clinical Pearls and Controversies

This case indicated the therapeutic dilemma of huge infra-diaphragmatic CP. It was common that the nervous fibers of pituitary stalk inflated and attenuated when extremely supra-sellar expanding. As the result, the residual nervous fibers of stalk was difficult to identified and not to mention the reservation.

Case 4

Medical History

A 3-year-old male patient presented at our hospital with a 1-month history of headache, polyuria, and intermittent epilepsy.

Physical and Experimental Examination

The patient exhibited strabismus and abducens nerve paralysis in the left eye. Endocrinological detection indicated hypopituitarism. His levels of sexual hormones and GH were significantly decreased, and his PRL level was slightly increased.

Radiological Images Before Surgery

Presurgical CT indicated a quasi-circular cystic tumor located in the intra- and suprasellar region. Small punctate calcification was distributed inside the pituitary fossa. Enhanced CT revealedthe cystic wall enhanced roundly. MRI indicated a mixed cystic-solid tumor that occupied the anterior part of the third ventricular cavity along with slightly hydrocephalus. The optic chiasm and AcoA were lifted upward, thus enlarging the first surgical space. The cystic fluid was slightly hyperintense on T1 and hyperintense on T2-weighted MRI.

Membranous Structures and Hierarchical Layers: Fig. (11)

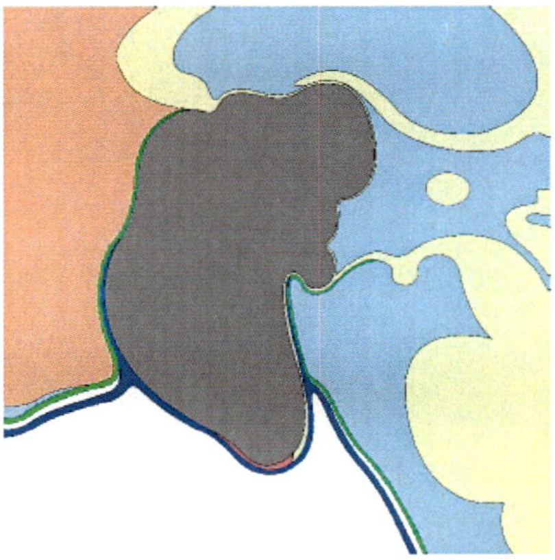

Fig. (11). Schematic Fig. (demonstrating the tumor morphology and relationships with the surrounding structures. Blue line: Dura mater (Diaphragm and sellar floor dura); Green line: Arachnoid mater.

<u>*Intrasurgical Findings*</u>

The sellar region was exposed by dissection of the interhemispheric fissure. The diaphragm-covered tumor and basal membranous arachnoid were observed. The tumor was separated from the surrounding structures along the arachnoidal interface. The PS, which had been inflated by the tumor, was umbrella-shaped. The diaphragm was cut in a circular manner to reveal the true tumor capsule. Along the interface, the neurohypophysis had a clear membranous border that could be freed from the tumor. The PS was ruptured to facilitate total tumor removal.

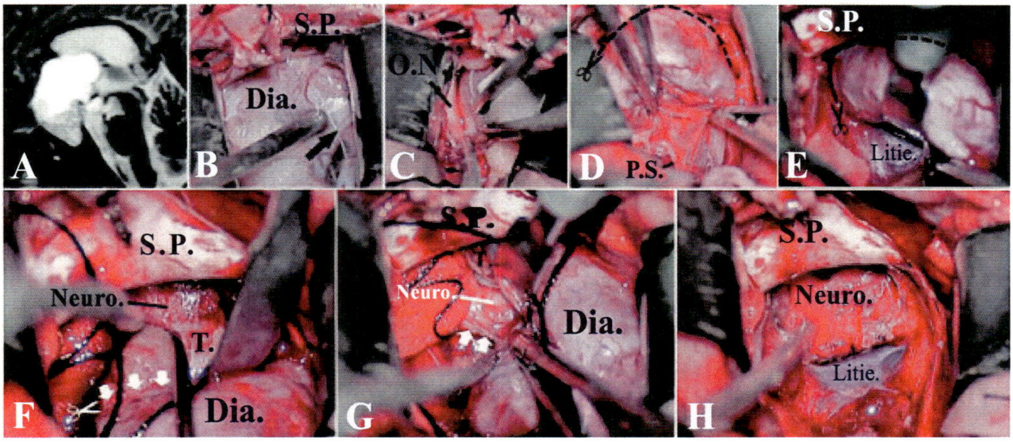

Fig. (12). Intrasurgical findings. **A.** Presurgical MRI showed an intra- and suprasellar infradiaphragmatic craniopharyngioma that occupied the anterior part of the third ventricle and caused minor hydrocephalus. **B.** The diaphragm-covered tumor and overlaid basal membranous arachnoid layer (**black arrow**) were exposed *via* a frontobasal interhemispheric approach. **C.** The bilateral optic nerves were bluntly dissected from the tumor because of the diaphragmatic and arachnoid separation. **D.** At the top of the tumor, the pituitary stalk was inflated into a frog belly shape. The dotted lines (**scissor**) indicate the round incision that opened the diaphragm. **E.** The tumor was found to be completely covered by diaphragm on exposure at the dorsum sellae. The Liliequist membrane could also be identified. **F.** After making a round diaphragmatic incision (**white scissor and arrows**), the true tumor was observed. It was not difficult to bluntly separate the tumor from the neurohypophysis using a microdissector. The neurohypophyseal surface was smooth with an apparent cover of membranous septation. **G.** The incision (**White arrows**) and smooth neurohypophysis were also identified bilaterally. **H.** The neurohypophysis was preserved after total tumor removal. The anterior sphenoidal planum and posterior Liliequist membrane were also observed. **Dia.**, Diaphragm; **S.P.**, Sphenoidal planum; **O.N.**, Optic nerve; **P.S.**, Pituitary stalk; **Lilie.**, Liliequist; **Neuro.**, Neurohypophysis; **T.**, Tumor.

Perioperative Treatment

Pathological analysis confirmed the diagnosis of adamantinomatous craniopharyngioma. MRI confirmed total tumor removal. Postsurgical endocrinological detection indicated panhypopituitarism.

Long-term Follow Up

No recurrence was detected during a 3-year follow-up. The patient continued to exhibit growth retardation and panhypopituitarism, which necessitated hormone supplementation.

Clinical Pearls and Controversies

The expanding way of this huge infra-diaphragmatic tumor indicated the developmental defection of diaphragmatic foramen. The tumor extruded towards the 3rd ventricular floor through enlarged foramen. So although it was infra-diaphragmatic tumor, the total tumor removal will inevitably cause the injury of the hypothalamic structures located at the anterior part of 3rd ventricular floor. In spite of the continuity of pituitary stalk cannot be preserved, the reservation of the residual neuro-hypophyseal structures when dissection of tumor hinted that the membranous structure between adeno- and neuro-hypophyseal might provide a separating interface for safely dissecting.

Case 5

Medical History

A 7-year-old male patient presented with a 2-year history of intermittent headache and decreased visual acuity. He also exhibited growth failure, emaciation, and partial hypopituitarism as well as visual deterioration (right eye: 0.1, left eye: 0.3) and bitemporal hemianopsia.

Physical and Experimental Examination

The routine blood and urine analysis results were normal; however, the patient exhibited low levels of plasma sexual hormones (testosterone, progesterone, follicle-stimulating hormone, luteinizing hormone, and estrogen). An insulin stimulation test for cortisol and GH revealed subnormal responses.

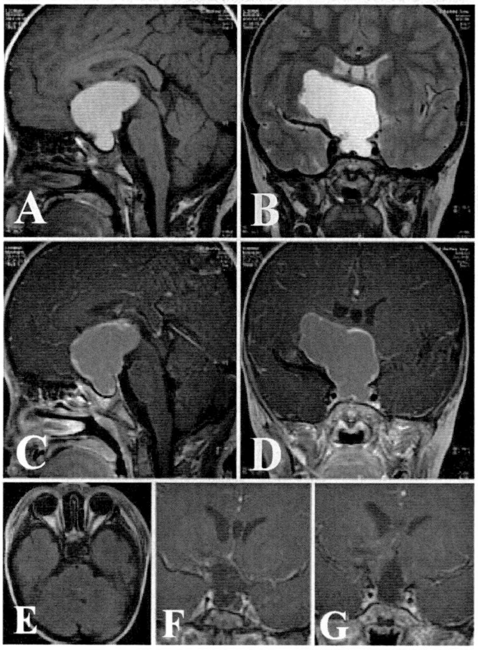

Fig. (13). Presurgical and postsurgical magnetic resonance imaging data.

Radiological Images Before Surgery

An intra- and supra-sellar, predominantly cystic mass was identified Fig. (**13**). CT revealed no significant calcification. The location of the optic chiasm was determined by the AcoA and ACA and was displaced anteriorly and upward. Enhanced MRI revealed enhancement of the cystic tumor wall in a circular area. On a coronal scan, extreme rightward expansion of the cystic tumor was observed. No obstructive hydrocephalus was observed consequent to the tumor growth pattern and direction of expansion.

Analysis Before Surgery

1. Surgical and topographic tumor classification: intra- and suprasellar Id-CP (Type "Q").
2. Relationship with the AcoA: The AcoA complex was displaced anteriorly and upward.
3. Tumor growth initiated below the diaphragm and arachnoid. The suprasellar tumor was covered by the diaphragma sellae and arachnoid above the diaphragm.
4. Surgical excision should be the first-line therapy. The FIH approach was ultimately selected to reach the lesion.

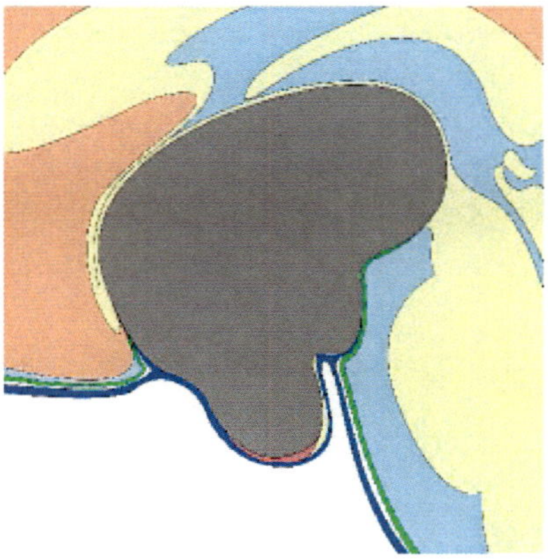

Fig. (14). Schematic Fig. (demonstrating the tumor morphology and relationships with the surrounding structures. Blue line: Dura mater (Diaphragm and sellar floor dura); Green line: Arachnoid mater.

Intrasurgical Findings

A standard frontobasal interhemispheric craniotomy was performed Fig. (**15**). The bone flap extended beyond the median line with the lowest margin as near as possible to the floor of the anterior cranial fossa. The mucosa inside the frontal sinus was removed carefully after opening the bone window. The bone of the posterior sinus wall was removed and drilled to provide additional exposure. The sinus cavity was completely filled with bone wax and antibiotic powder to reduce the risk of intracranial infection. A curved incision was made near the skull base to open the bilateral dura mater beside the superior sagittal sinus. The anterior part of the superior sagittal sinus was subsequently ligated, followed by removal of the cerebral falx. The dural flap was turned rearward.

Postoperative Course

Postoperatively, the patient suffered severe transient DI. Hyponatremia was the major presentation of electrolyte imbalances. The symptoms were relieved by fluid and electrolyte replacement. Endocrinological detection revealed evidence of panhypopituitarism. The patient's visual function recovered significantly. A postsurgical MRI study after 1 year confirmed total tumor removal and preservation of the 3rd VF (Fig. 42 E-G).

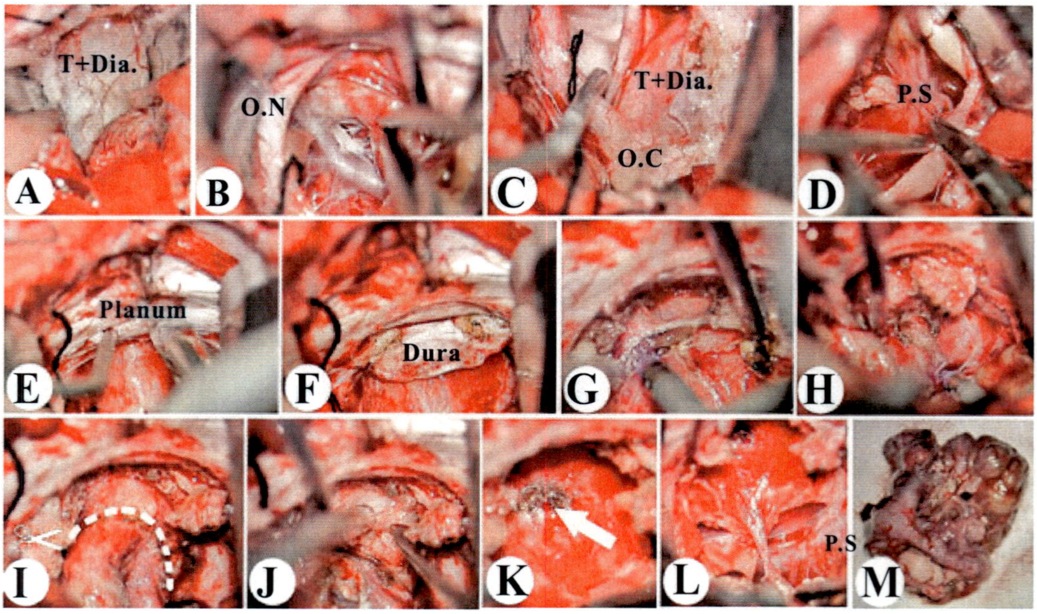

Fig. (15). Intraoperative findings. **A-C.** The diaphragm-covered tumor was exposed after dissecting the interhemispheric fissure. The surrounding neurovascular structures were separated from the tumor along the diaphragm. The bilateral optic nerves and chiasm were separated. **D.** The pituitary stalk exhibited severe tumor involvement. **E-H.** The dura mater was cut at the tuberculum sellae, and the bone was drilled to increase exposure of the intrasellar region. **I.** The surface diaphragm was incised in a circular manner to expose the true tumor wall. **J.** The intrasellar tumor was separated along the tumor wall. **K.** At the floor of pituitary fossa, a membranous ligament that connected the tumor was also dissected. **L.** The severely involved pituitary stalk was ruptured to avoid tumor recurrence. **M.** The tumor was totally removed.

Long-term Follow Up

After 3 years of follow-up, the patient still required oral prednisone and Euthyrox to treat panhypopituitarism. Although his DI was relieved, he still required desmopressin therapy. His BMI increased from a presurgical value of 15.6 to 18.3.

Clinical Pearls and Controversies

This patient was similar with the case 4. However, we drilled off the tuberculum sellae to enlarge the direct exposure of intrasellar part of tumor, which also provided the possibility to remove the tumor along the true boundary.

CISTERNAL CRANIOPHARYGIOMA (TYPE "S")

Case 1

Medical History

A 51-year-old female with headache and decreased visual accuracy of bilateral eyes for 4 months. She didn't suffer with nausea and vomiting.

Physical and Experimental Examination: Fig. (16)

Physical examination revealed no significant positive results except for temporal hemianopia of right eye and decreased vision in bilateral eyes. And the endocrinological detection before surgery indicated normal hormone level.

Radiological Images Before Surgery

Computed tomography (CT) indicated a suprasellar lesion with round enhancement but without significant calcification. Magnetic resonance imaging (MRI) revealed a suprasellar cystic tumor (2.6 x 3cm) located beneath the optic chiasm. The tumor expanded from the optic chiasmatic cistern to the prepontile cistern. The prechiasmatic space was enlarged. A normal PS was identified to be displaced towards left side.

Analysis Before Surgery

The tumor originated from the subarachnoid segment of the PS, as indicated by the intracisternal location of the tumor on MRI. Inflated growth caused the tumor to occupy the suprasellar arachnoidal cistern instead of further involving the 3rd VF, and also expanded backwards with occupying the prepontile cistern. The tumor generally grew in an extra-axial pattern. Therefore, a right eyebrow keyhole approach was selected for tumor dissection. And purely endoscopic surgery was selected because the less invasion to the 3rd VF. Preservation of the pituitary stalk and 3rd VF neural structures was attempted.

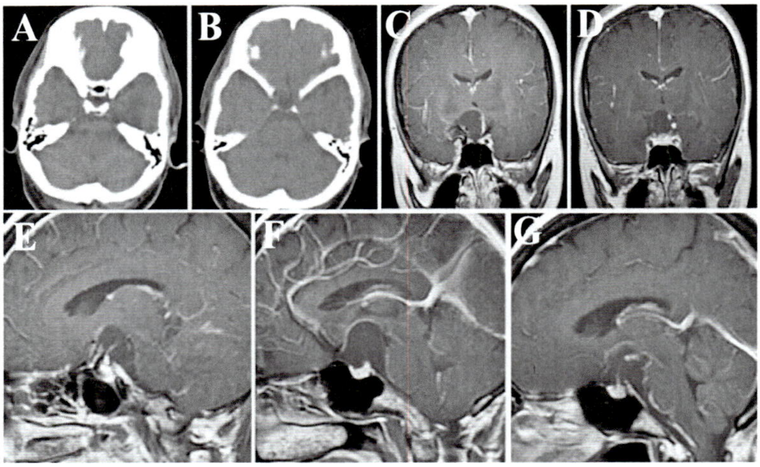

Fig. (16). Presurgical radiological images of the present case. **A-B.** CT scan before surgery indicated a suprasellar lesion without significant calcification. **C-G.** Sagittal and coronal MRI scans showed that the tumor mainly occupied the prechiasmatic subarachnoid cistern space, and expanded backwards to the prepontile cistern. The site of tumor origin was located in the middle segment of the pituitary stalk. The normal pituitary stalk was displaced to the left side of the tumor.

Membranous Structures and Hierarchical Layers: Fig. (17)

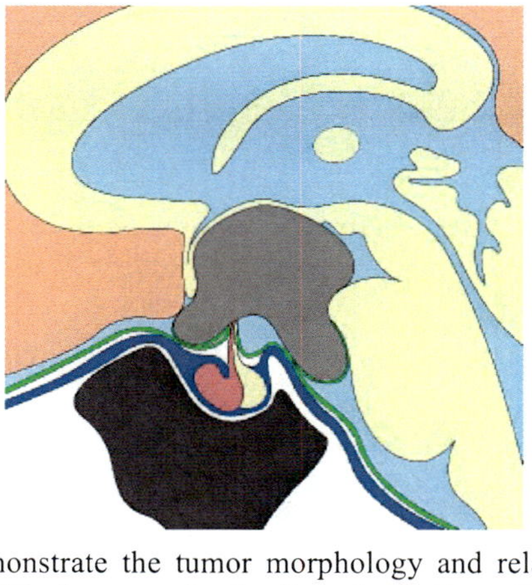

Fig. (17). Schematic Fig. (demonstrate the tumor morphology and relationships with the surrounding structures. Blue line: Dura mater (Diaphragm and sellar floor dura); Green line: Arachnoid mater.

Intrasurgical Findings

A right-eyebrow keyhole approach was used. After dissection of the lateral fissure to release the CSF, the second surgical space was predominantly use to expose the tumor. The prechiasmatic space was enlarged by the tumor, which originated from the tubero-infundibular part of the PS with suprasellar growth. The tumor located within the suprasellar arachnoid cistern was covered by arachnoid trabeculae. The arachnoid separated the tumor from surrounding neurovascular structures. Especially the Liliequist membrane separated the posterior part of tumor to the branches of the basilar artery. The tumor stem, which grew outside of the 3rd VF and was considered to have originated from the upper PS segment, could be observed clearly. The continuity of the hypothalamus–PS was preserved.

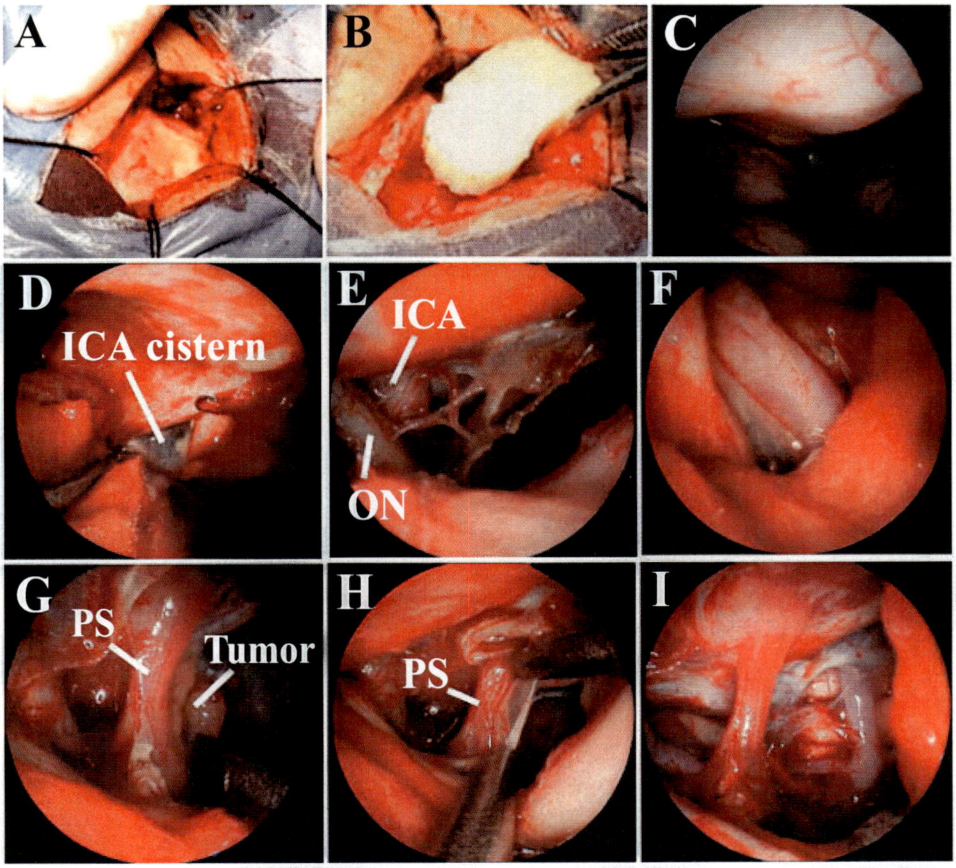

Fig. (18). Intraoperative findings. **A-B.** Right eyebrow keyhole approach and the bone flap. **C~E.** The lateral fissure was dissected and released the CSF. After opening the ICA cistern, the ICA and the right side optical nerve was observed. F~H. Through the second surgical space (ICA-chiasmatic space), the observed tumor was entirely located outside the ventricular cavity and which was separated from the suprasellar region *via* arachnoidal trabeculae. At the ventral optic chiasm, the tumor adhered tightly to the tubero-infundibular part of the pituitary stalk, which was thought to be the site of origin. **I.** After total tumor removal, the pituitary stalk and third ventricular floor were preserved anatomically. A defect was observed on the pituitary stalk at the tumor origin.

Paraoperative Treatment and Occurrence of Complications

MRI after surgery showed the tumor was totally removed and the pituitary stalk was preserved. Although the patient continued to suffer from hypopituitarism and transient DI, the symptom was gradually resolved and controlled well.

Long-term Follow Up

No tumor recurrence was observed during a 2-year follow-up period. The endocrinological evaluation indicated near-normal hormone levels. The patient had a good QOL, could perform activities of daily living, and resumed his presurgical employment.

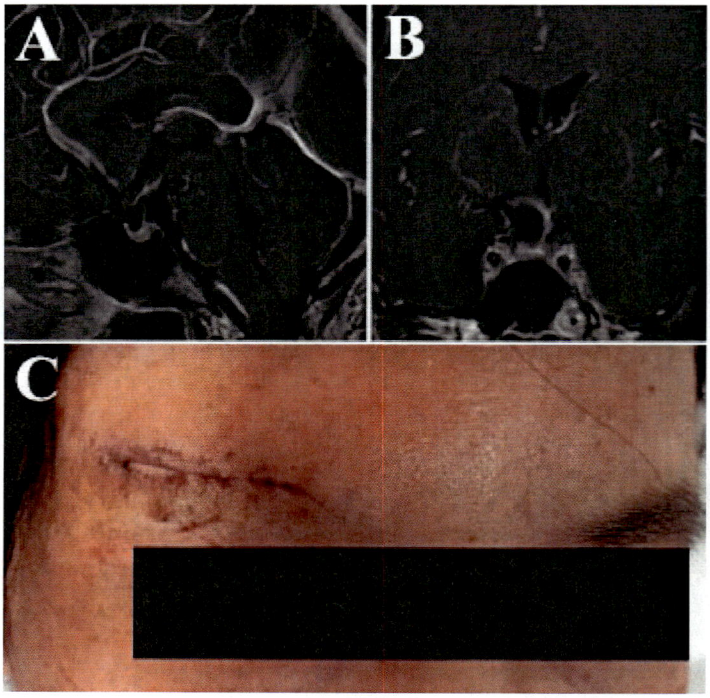

Fig. (19). The radiological image after surgery. A~B MRI scan indicated the tumor was totally removed and the pituitary stalk was preserved well. C. Photo of the present patient indicated the incision.

Pearls and Controversies

The tumor of this patient was purely suprasellar extra-ventricular location. The approaches for selection included extra-axial corridor (Sub-frontal and pterional approaches), extended transsphenoidal endoscopic approach. Here, we provided a trans-eyebrow sub-frontal keyhole approach to surgical removal of CP with the aid of endoscopy. Multiple surgical view of endoscopy can provide better exposure for identification of the interface between tumor and surrounding optical chiasm, pituitary stalk, *et al.* As the result, the retraction of these vital structures by the traditional microscopic sub-frontal approach will be avoided.

Case 2

Medical History

This was a 24-year-old female patient with a 2-year history of menstrual disorders and a 2-month history of amenorrhea. She experienced repeated headaches, decreased visual accuracy, and olfactory dysfunction for 1 month without nausea or vomiting.

Physical and Experimental Examination

The patient exhibited normal consciousness, and no significant positive results were detected during physical examination. Endocrinological detection indicated only a slightly increased prolactin (PRL) level. A growth hormone (GH) releasing test *via* insulin application indicated no other hypophyseal axis hormone deficits besides GH.

Radiological Images Before Surgery

Presurgical MRI indicated a suprasellar cystic lesion. The normal PS was presented clearly with the posterior of the tumor. The cystic walls were significantly enhanced on enhanced MRI. The main tumor body had grown externally through the enlarged prechiasmatic space. The optic chiasm and anterior communicating artery (AcoA) were displaced upward. On transverse MRI, the cystic lesion was found to have expanded bilaterally to reach the sylvian fissure on the left side.

Analysis Before Surgery

1. Patient's General Condition: No positive signs other than decreased vision, visual field defects, and dysosmia were detected during physical examination. Regarding endocrinological disorders, the patient had suffered from menstrual disorders for 2 years and amenorrhea for 2 months. The decreased GH level indicated hypopituitarism of the GH axis.
2. Surgical Challenges: The cystic tumor involved several subarachnoid spaces, including the chiasmatic cistern, exterior and interior carotid artery cisterns (left side), and olfactory cistern. Part of the cystic wall intruded into the ventral aspect of the frontal lobe. The left-side internal carotid artery (ICA) and its branches as well as cranial nerve III were surrounded by the tumor, which required sharp surgical dissection. Coarse calcification had tightly adhered to the PS and possible to the left carotid artery Fig. (**21**).

3. Surgical Aim: Total tumor removal while attempting to anatomically preserve hypothalamus–infundibulum–pituitary axis continuity.
4. Surgical Strategy: The presented external CP growth in this case was typical. This subarachnoid intracistern CP originated from the subarachnoid segment of the PS. The main cystic tumor body grew through the enlarged first space to the anterior cranial fossa and might have caused olfactory dysfunction. Following extreme elevation of the bilateral optic nerves, the tumor expanded bilaterally through the enlarged second space. Despite this extensive expansion, the tumor surface remained covered by the arachnoid membrane, which separated the tumor from the surrounding neurovascular structures. An extra-axial approach and manipulations should be selected to avoid invasion of vital neural tissues.

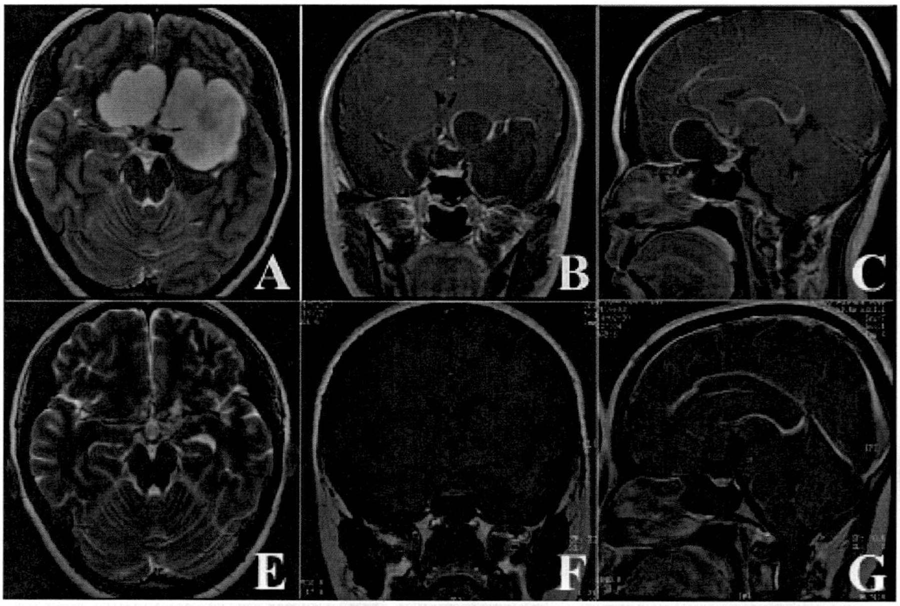

Fig. (20). Presurgical and postsurgical magnetic resonance imaging (MRI). **A-C.** Presurgical MRI indicated a cystic tumor mainly located at the optic chiasmatic cistern with extensive expansion to the anterior cranial fossa and right-side middle fossa through the enlarged first space. The pituitary stalk is located at the right posterior side of the tumor. **D-E.** Postsurgical MRI indicated total tumor removal with preservation of the pituitary stalk and third ventricle floor.

Membranous Structures and Hierarchical Layers: Fig. (21)

Intrasurgical Findings

For tumor removal, a right-side frontotemporal approach with a relatively large bone flap was selected to expose both the anterior fossa tumor capsule and lateral temporalis part of the tumor.

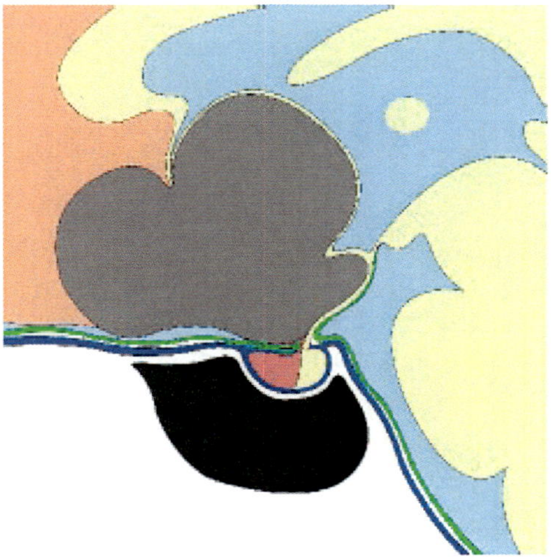

Fig. (21). Schematic Fig. (demonstrating the tumor morphology and relationships with the surrounding structures. Blue line: Dura mater (Diaphragm and sellar floor dura); Green line: Arachnoid mater.

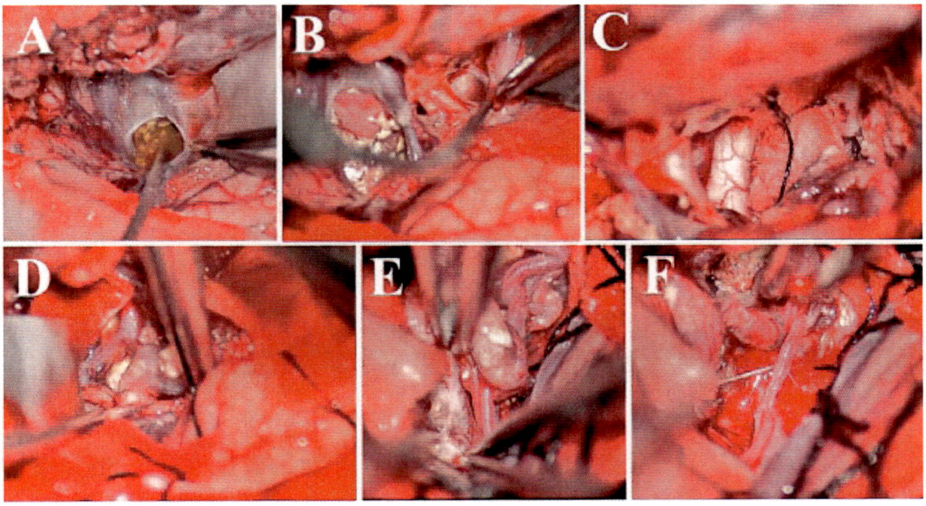

Fig. (22). Intraoperative findings. **A:** After craniotomy, the lateral fissure was dissected to expose the tumor. The huge cystic tumor was located beneath the arachnoid membrane. Therefore, the tumor had expanded along the potential space between the frontal lobe and arachnoid, causing tight adhesion between the tumor cystic wall and nervous tissue that required sharp dissection. Punctate calcification was observed on the tumor wall. **B-C** After sharp dissection, the bilateral optical nerves were exposed. **D.** The calcified tumor had adhered tightly to the left side of the internal carotid artery (ICA) and its branches, thus presenting significant challenges to surgical removal. **E-F.** The ICA branches were separated from the tumor and preserved well.

Perioperative Treatment

Endocrinological detection indicated significant decreases in the free T3 and thyroid-stimulating hormone (TSH) levels. Disordered water and electrolyte balances were detected and treated as usual; however, this patient experienced these symptoms over the long term because of the longer time required to separate the PS from the tumor calcification.

Long-term Follow Up

Total tumor removal was proven during a 2.5-year follow-up period. After surgery, the patient suffered from transient oculomotor nerve palsy, which recovered during follow-up. However, regarding the endocrinological evaluation, the menstrual disorder and low thyroxine level persisted. Prednisone and levothyroxine tablets were administered as substitutive treatment. Her weight increased slightly without other hypothalamic dysfunction such as obesity.

Pearls and Controversies

The presentation of this case showed the expanding of craniopharyngioma from intra-cisternal (optical chiasmatic cistern) to surrounding cisterns. This case of tumor expanded predominantly to the anterior cranial fossa, sub-frontal base and signle lateral temporal lobe. As the extremely expanding, the transsphenoidal approach couldn't selected in this case. As the result, we selected enlarged fronto-temporal approach. Through extra-axial corridor, the tumor was removed along the boundary. The anterior part of hypothalamic structures was proved to be without involved by tumor. The pituitary stalk was preserved. Fortunately, this female patient was pregnant at two years after surgery, which indicated the best outcome of this type of tumor.

Case 3

Medical History

This was an 18-year-old female patient. She had a 5-year history of headache with progressive deterioration and a 6-month history of decreased visual accuracy. She also reported a 2-year history of menstrual disorder with amenorrhea of 6 months' duration.

Physical and Experimental Examination

Ophthalmic evaluation indicated no significant abnormalities in her vision or visual field. Presurgical endocrinological detection indicated only slight increases in PRL and progesterone (PRGE).

Radiological Images Before Surgery

Presurgical CT scans indicated a solid lesion with coarse calcification located in the suprasellar region. MRI revealed a mixed solid-cystic tumor in the suprasellar region. The cystic part of the lesion expanded and grew towards the clivus and displaced the pones and left side of the peduncle backward. The solid part of the tumor was located superiorly with significant enhancement; this might have been the site of origin and calcification. The optic chiasm was displaced upward, although the first space was not enlarged.

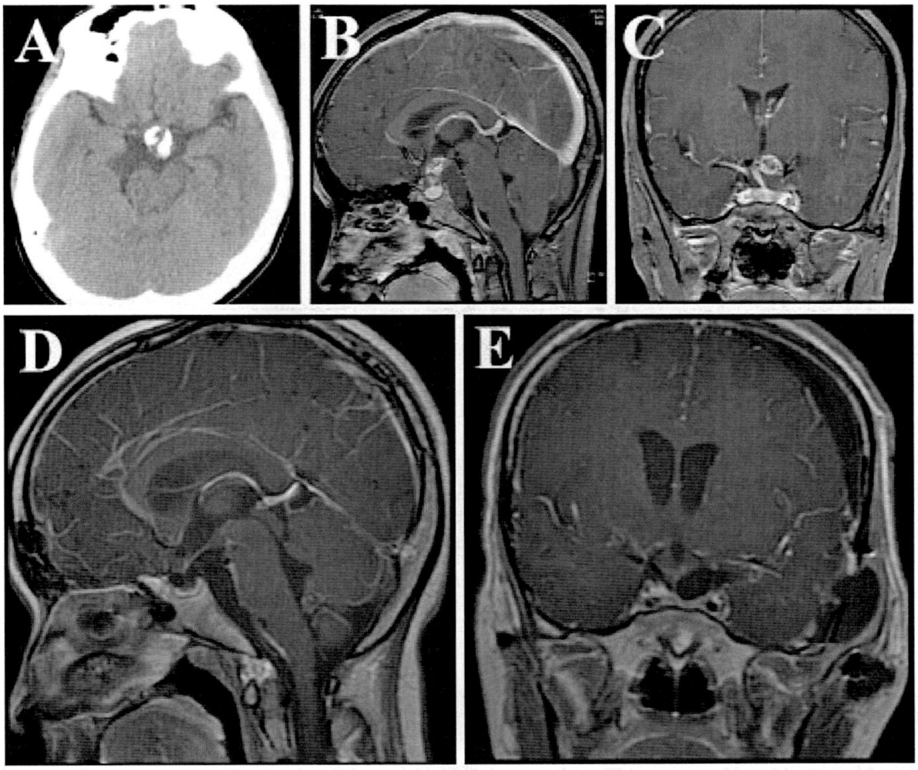

Fig. (23). Presurgical and postsurgical radiological images. **A.** Presurgical computed tomography indicated a solid tumor with coarse calcification located in the suprasellar arachnoid cistern. **B-C.** Presurgical magnetic resonance imaging (MRI) suggested a relationship between tumor and the pituitary stalk and third ventricle floor (3rd VF). On a sagittal scan (**B**), the solid part of the tumor appears to be located at the tubero-infundibulum, whereas the cystic tumor has expanded to the retroclivus region and is located between the 3rd VF and Liliequist's membrane. A coronal scan indicated rightward displacement of the pituitary stalk, suggesting that the tumor origin is located on the left side of the tubero-infundibulum. **D-E.** Postsurgical MRI after 1 year indicated total tumor removed and good 3rd VF preservation.

Analysis Before Surgery

1. Patient's General Condition: The physical examination revealed no positive signs other than headache and amenorrhea.
2. Surgical Aim: The tumor grew outside the ventricle, and the arachnoid membrane separated the tumor wall from the nervous tissue of the 3rd VF except at the infundibular site of tumor origin. Therefore, gross total tumor

removal should be pursued and the anatomical continuity of the 3rd VF-infundibulum-PS should be preserved.

3. Surgical Difficulty: Two points of difficulty were observed in this case. 1) The anatomical tumor location. As the majority of the tumor had expanded to the retro-clivus, the usual skull base approach could not expose the site of tumor origin. Furthermore, the patient's vision and visual field were normal, so optic nerves or chiasm retraction should be avoided if possible. 2) The huge calcification mass presented the greatest challenge to preservation of PS continuity. In this case, the huge calcification might cause severe tumor adherence to the PS and posterior circulation vessels, which would present significant challenges to surgical safety.
4. Surgical Strategy: This is a typical case of a tumor with subarachnoid origination and extensive posterior growth. The site of origin might have been located in the middle and upper segments of the PS with a bias toward the right side. Although the main direction of growth was backward and the tumor even reached the middle clivus, Liliequist's membrane and the basilar artery and its branches remained separate from the tumor and thus protected. The PS was distorted and displaced to the left side. As the first space was not enlarged, the second and third spaces represented the most potentially important corridors for manipulation in the suprasellar region. The tentorium required dissection to expose the tumor located at the posterior cranial fossa. Endoscopy should be used to assist with direct exposure of the relationship between the tumor and neurovascular structures to enhance safety during tumor separation. Despite extensive expansion, the extra-axial approach should be selected because of the extra-ventricular growth.

Membranous Structures and Hierarchical Layers: Fig. (24)

Intrasurgical Findings

A Left-Side Frontotemporal Trans-Tentorium Approach was Selected

Surgical Result

The tumor was totally removed with PS preservation. Transient oculomotor nerve palsy occurred and diabetes insipidus (DI) occurred.

Perioperative Treatment

For this patient, perioperative treatment included close monitoring of the intake and output volumes and electrolyte levels. Intramuscular or oral ADH (desmopressin) was used according to the urine volume and blood sodium level to help the patient transition through the period of profuse urination.

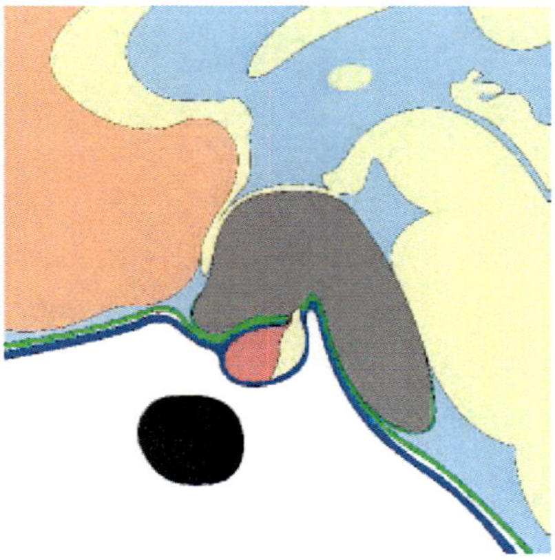

Fig. (24). Schematic Fig. (demonstrating the tumor morphology and relationships with the surrounding structures. Blue line: Dura mater (Diaphragm and sellar floor dura); Green line: Arachnoid mater.

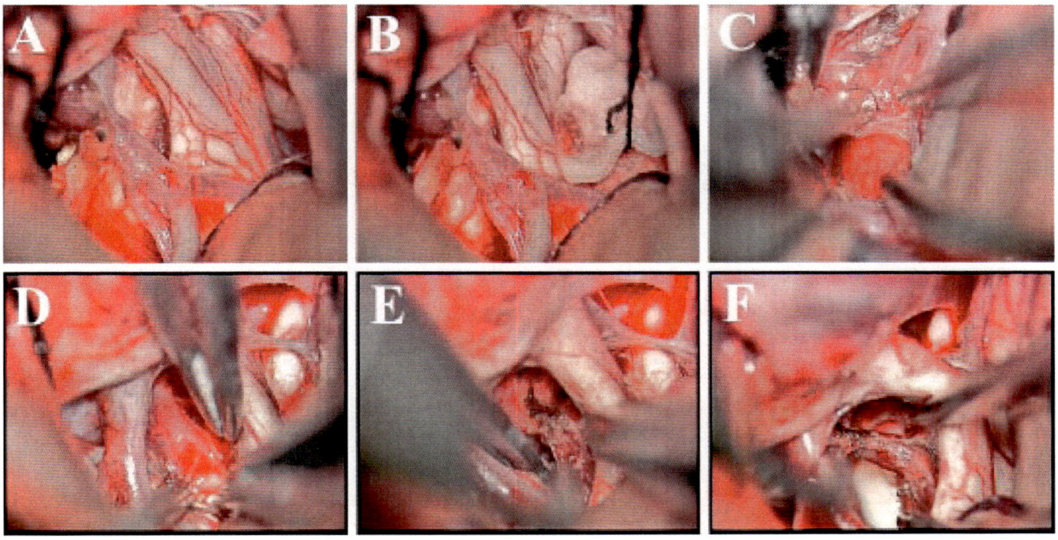

Fig. (25). Intra-operative findings. **A.** After dissecting the lateral fissure, the optic chiasm and the left side of the internal carotid artery (ICA) and its branches were exposed. The ICA lateral space was the main corridor used for manipulation. The subfrontal and terminalis lateral arachnoid were sufficiently dissected to observe the bulging lamina terminalis space. **B.** Above the lamina terminalis, a piece of cotton was used to push the tumor downward, after which the ICA-optic space and ICA lateral space could be used to remove the tumor directly. **C.** The tumor cystic wall surrounded the main branches of the ICA. During surgery, the arachnoidal interface was followed strictly to avoid injuring the vessel and cranial nerves. Notably, given the extensive expanding, blind tumor retraction should be avoided if the tumor cystic wall cannot be observed directly. **D.** Through the ICA-optic space, the pituitary stalk was observed. There was no arachnoidal interface at the infundibular site of tumor origin, necessitating sharp dissection. Anatomical preservation of the pituitary stalk was pursued. **E-F.** After tumor removal, the site of tumor origin was exposed. The pituitary stalk and third ventricle floor were preserved intact.

Long-term Follow Up

No tumor recurrence occurred during a 4-year follow-up period. Vision accuracy decreased slightly in the left eye. The right eye remained normal. DI recovered gradually beyond 1 year after surgery. The patient still suffered from hypopituitarism and menstrual disorders. She took prednisone and euthyrox tablets. Her weight increased slightly (body mass index [BMI] from 23.8 before surgery to 26.2 kg/m^2 at the last follow-up examination) without other manifestations of hypothalamic injury.

Pearls and Controversies

This case indicated another kind of expanding of suprasellar extra-ventricular CP, which expanded predominantly to the dorsum sella and clivus. As the result, it will be quite difficult to expose the posterior cranial tumor by the approaches of anterior or lateral corridor. So we selected temporal modification of pterional approach. The tumor was totally removed by combined usage of pterional and sub-temporal corridor, and the pituitary stalk was preserved in the meantime.

Case 4

Medical History

This patient was a girl aged 5 years and 7 months. The hearing in her left ear had decreased significantly and progressively for 3 months; the hearing in her right ear had decreased, leading to hearing loss, along with an unstable gait for 2 months.

Physical and Experimental Examination

No significant positive symptoms were detected except slight dysphagia and an unsteady gait. As in other patients with extra-arachnoid CP, the patient only presented with sexual hormone deficiencies according to endocrinological detection.

Radiological Images Before Surgery

Presurgical CT indicated a huge cystic tumor located in the sellar region, bilateral ambiens cistern, and interpeduncular cistern. Significant calcification was identified in the sellar region. As the tumor occupied the third ventricular cavity, the patient suffered from hydrocephalus. MRI indicated that a huge cystic tumor had originated from the posterior PS with extensive backward expansion to the prepone cistern that reached the C4 level. The tumor occupied the bilateral ambiens cistern. A normal PS was identified at the front of the tumor.

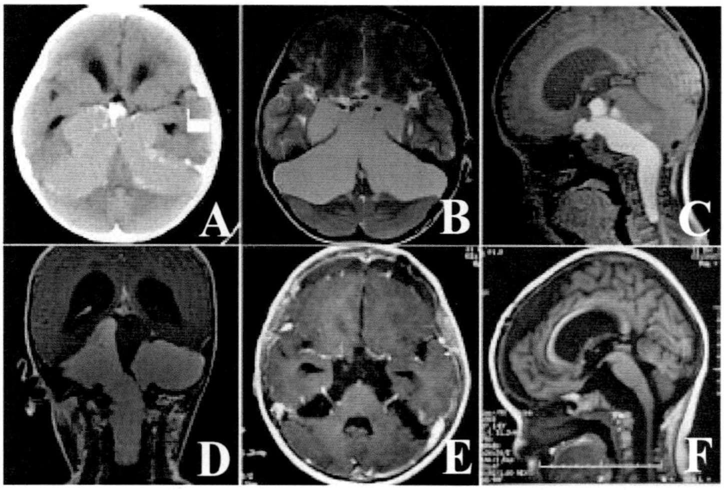

Fig. (26). Presurgical and postsurgical radiological images. **A.** Presurgical computed tomography indicated coarse calcification in the sellar region and significant punctate calcification distributed over the cystic walls. **B-D.** Presurgical magnetic resonance imaging revealed a huge cystic tumor that originated from the sellar region and expanded extensively, reaching the bilateral CPA region and upper cervical canal. **E and F.** Following surgery, total tumor removal was confirmed.

Analysis Before Surgery

1. Patient's General Condition: This was a 5-year-old patient with a huge tumor. There were many positive signs of cranial nerve and brain stem involvement. This patient also suffered from hypopituitarism and growth retardation.
2. Surgical Aim: Despite the huge size, the main tumor body remained inside the subarachnoid space. Therefore, following the selection of an appropriate approach to provide sufficient tumoral exposure, total tumor removal was the aim of surgery for this patient. As usual, preservation of the anatomical 3rd VF–infundibulum–PS continuity was attempted.
3. Surgical Difficulty: 1) This was a young child with a huge tumor and extensive, bilateral involvement. It was difficult to provide sufficient exposure. Sharp dissection was needed to separate the tumor from the cranial nerves and vessels. 2) The higher location of the 3rd VF, caused by tumor involvement in the interpeduncular cistern, rendered it difficult to provide direct exposure during surgery. 3) A huge calcification was detected at the tubero-infundibular part of the PS, which is generally considered the site of tumor origin.

Membranous Structures and Hierarchical Layers

The main tumor body was located at the subarachnoid cistern; more precisely, the tumor was extra-pia mater and subarachnoid (see the schematic Fig. **27**).

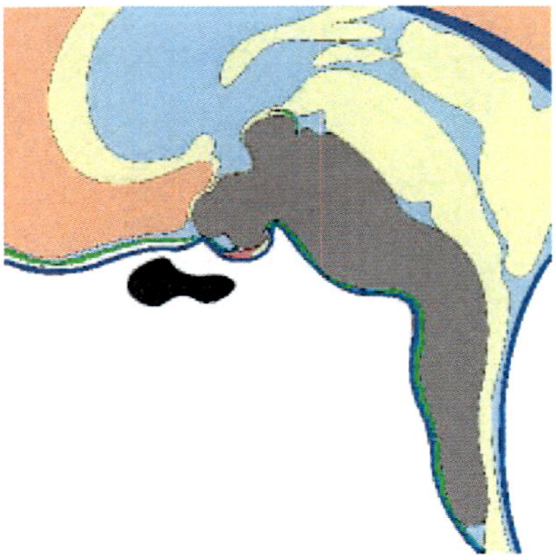

Fig. (27). Schematic Fig. (demonstrating the tumor morphology and relationships with the surrounding structures. Blue line: Dura mater (Diaphragm and sellar floor dura); Green line: Arachnoid mater.

Intra-surgical Findings

A right-side frontotemporal trans-tentorium approach was selected. The bone flap was modified and enlarged toward the temporal squama. During surgery, the tentorium was incised to provide greater exposure of the tumor with posterior cranial fossa involvement.

Perioperative Treatment

Endocrinological detection indicated no new hormone disorders relative to the presurgical results. Levels of several sexual hormones remained low. The unstable gait was relieved. The patient's hearing increased significantly within 6 months after surgery. She continued to suffer from hypopituitarism and minor DI, which was well controlled by low-dose desmopressin. Long-term prednisone use was needed as substitutive hormone deficiency therapy.

Long-term Follow Up

No tumor recurrence was observed *via* MRI during a 2.5-year follow-up period. The patient's weight increased slightly, and DI recovered. However, long-term prednisone and euthyrox treatment were required for hormone deficiency treatment.

Pearls and Controversies

The expanding mode of this extra-ventricular CP was also common, which was subdivided to a special subtype called as posterior cranial CP by some scholars. This case is a typical one with extremely posterior expanding. Except that the tumor was huge with involved multiple anatomical areas, the difficulties of surgery also presented at the encasement of the tumor to the surrounding cranial nerves. As the result, the protection of the related cranial nerves should be paid more attention to. It was important for pursuing the totally tumor removal that dissecting along the interface of tumoral cystic wall. If the interface was missing, the tumor will be residual easier.

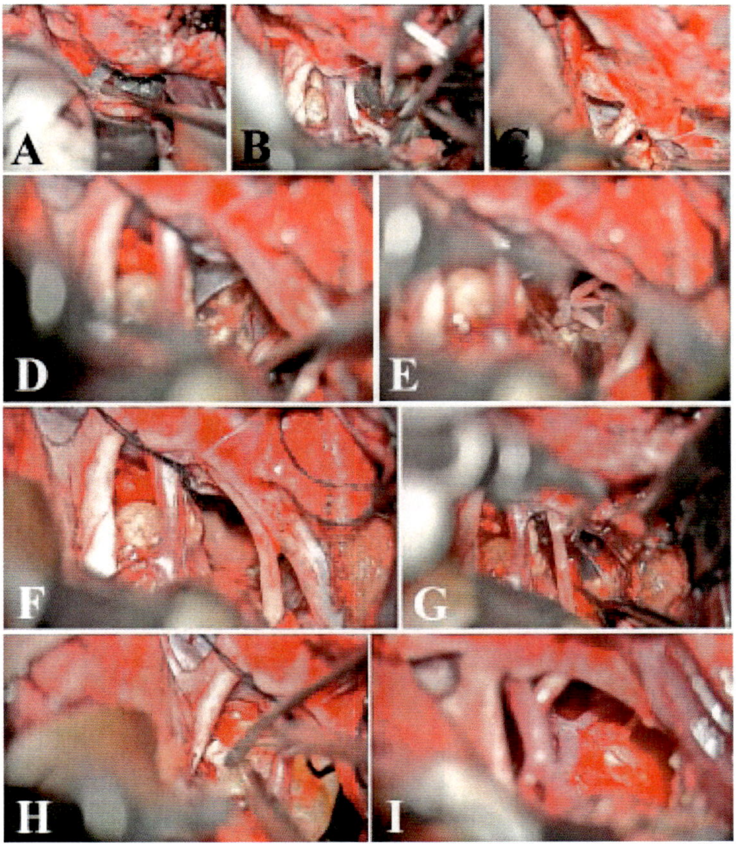

Fig. (28). Intraoperative findings. **A.** After dissecting the sylvian fissure, the relationship between the basal arachnoid membrane and tumor was displayed. The cystic tumor was located inside the subarachnoid cistern. **B.** Further exposure of the tumor with expansion to the right-side temporal lobe. The tumor cystic wall surrounded the oculomotor nerve, which was dissected after intratumor decompression. **C.** The solid tumor was dissected through the internal carotid artery (ICA)-optic space. Significant adherent calcification (black asterisk) distorted the pituitary stalk significantly. **D.** Through the enlarged ICA-III nerve space, the posterior cranial fossa tumor was exposed. The tumor was located between the third ventricle floor and diencephalon lobe of the Liliequist membrane. **E.** An arachnoid interface remained between the tumor and cranial nerves. **F.** The tumor was exposed mainly through the median and lateral ICA spaces and the lateral III nerve space. **G.** A tentorial incision was made to enlarge the exposure. **H.** The site of tumor origin remained at the tubero-infundibular pituitary stalk, necessitating sharp dissection. **I.** After total tumor removal, the brain stem, basilar artery, and bilateral vertebral arteries were exposed.

Case 5

Medical History

This case was a 51-year-old female patient. She presented with a 2-month history of progressively decreasing visual accuracy and vomiting.

Physical and Experimental Examination

No significant positive physical results were observed. Endocrinological detection indicated slight abnormalities, such as low secretion levels of several sexual hormones. An insulin stimulation test indicated normal cortisol axis and thyroxine axis function and a GH hormone axis deficiency.

Radiological Images Before Surgery

Presurgical CT revealed an intra- and suprasellar mixed cystic-solid tumor. No significant calcification was observed inside the tumor. Sagittal MRI indicated a mixed cystic-solid tumor in the intra- and suprasellar region with extensive extension towards the third ventricular cavity and interpeduncular cistern. The normal pituitary gland and stalk could not be identified *via* MRI. The optic chiasm and AcoA were displaced upward and anteriorly, leading to a small first surgical space. On coronal MRI, the cystic tumor had a lobular shape because of arterial restriction (A1 and A2 segment of the anterior carotid artery [ACA]).

Analysis Before Surgery

1. Patient's General Condition: This was a 51-year-old female with amenorrhea. The major complaint was decreased vision. Partial hypopituitarism was observed before surgery.
2. Surgical Aims: To recover vision accuracy and achieve total tumor removal. Preservation of the intact 3rd VF and PS was attempted.
3. Surgical Difficulty: The tumor predominantly involved the retro-stalk and interpeduncular region and was quite difficult to expose. There was no significant abnormal pituitary function or hypothalamic dysfunction before surgery. Therefore, it was important to protect the anatomical continuity of the 3rd VF–infundibulum–PS to provide a good quality of life (QOL) for the patient. The site of tumor origin remained beneath the pia mater of the PS. The tumor predominantly grew externally, as indicated by the cystic extension. As the upper and posterior tumor margins upwardly compressed the 3rd VF, a piece of cotton was inserted into the lamina terminalis cistern to push the tumor into direct vision and facilitate tumor dissection from the 3rd ventricle infundibulum area through the second and third spaces. Septation of the suprasellar arachnoid

membranes allowed preservation of the vital neurovascular structures. Protection of the perforating branches required additional attention. The normal pituitary gland and diaphragm were displaced downward.

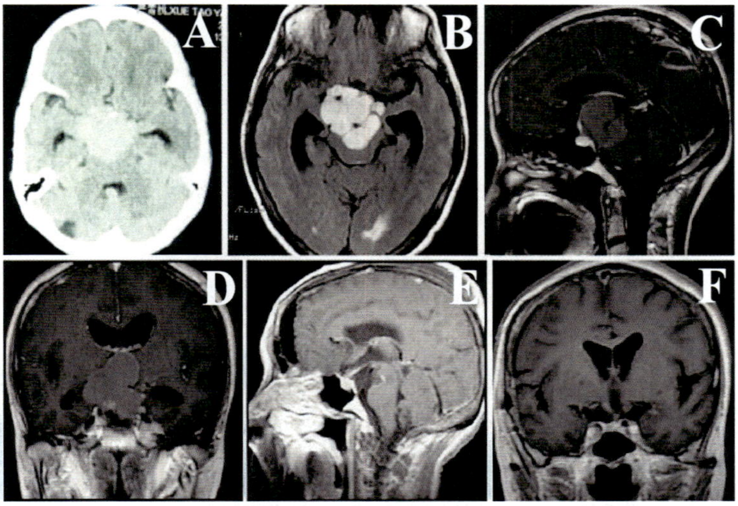

Fig. (29). Presurgical and postsurgical radiological images. **A.** Presurgical CT showed a mixed cystic-solid tumor in the suprasellar region with punctate calcification. **B-D.** Presurgical MRI revealed a tumor with extensive expansion to the interpeduncular cistern and clivus region. The pituitary stalk was displaced to the anterior of the tumor. On a transverse scan, the vessels were surrounded by the cystic tumor. **E-F.** Postsurgical MRI confirmed total tumor removal. The pituitary stalk and third ventricle floor remained intact.

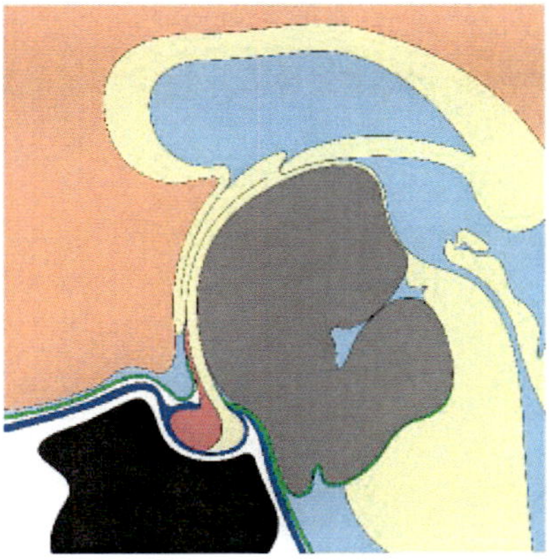

Fig. (30). Schematic Fig. (demonstrating the tumor morphology and relationships with the surrounding structures. Blue line: Dura mater (Diaphragm and sellar floor dura); Green line: Arachnoid mater.

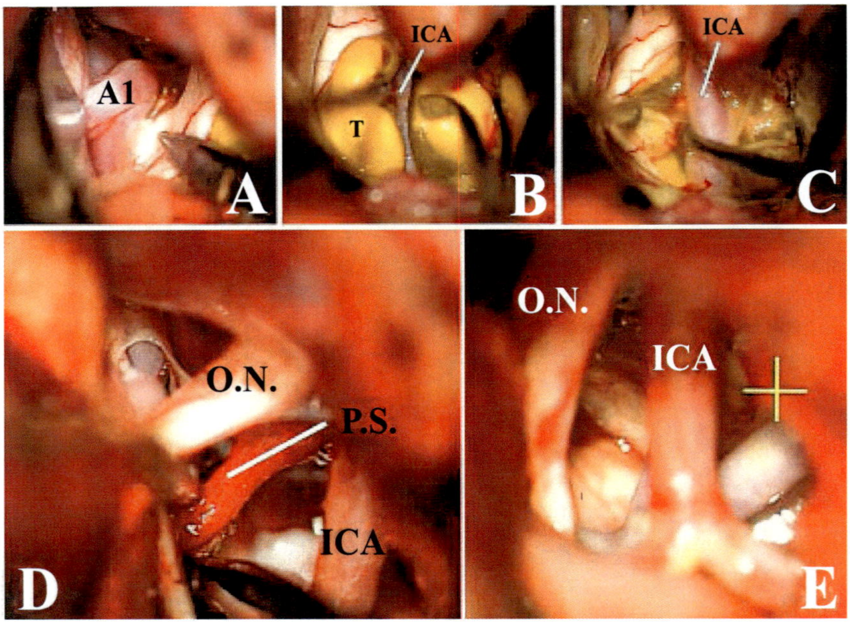

Fig. (31). Intraoperative findings. **A-C.** After dissecting the right-side lateral fissure, a cystic tumor with yellow cystic fluid was exposed. **D-E.** Through the second and third surgical spaces, the tumor was observed to envelop the ICA with a relative clear arachnoid interface. This interface was followed to separate the tumor from vital neurovascular structures. **F-H.** The site of tumor origin was located at the posterior aspect of the upper PS segment. **I-K.** The site of tumor origin was dissected for total tumor removal. **L-M.** After tumor removal, the neurovascular structures of the sellar region were preserved, including continuity of the hypothalamus–pituitary stalk.

Intrasurgical Findings

A right side frontotemporal approach with an enlarged temporal bone flap was used. After dissecting the right lateral fissure, a cystic tumor was observed to occupy the second and third surgical spaces. The ICA was enveloped by the tumor. Blunt dissection revealed a remaining membranous septation between the tumor and vital neurovascular structures such as the ICA and ventral aspect of the optic chiasm. Total tumor separation from the surrounding structure revealed the site of origin at the posterior aspect of the PS. After total tumor removal, hypothalamus–PS continuity was preserved.

Perioperative Treatment

The patient continued to exhibit hypopituitarism and minor DI, which was well controlled by low-dose desmopressin.

Long-term Follow Up

No tumor recurrence occurred within a 3-year follow-up period. The patient's weight increased to a BMI of 26.4. Her optical vision also increased. Oral prednisone was needed to treat a hormone deficiency. The desmopressin was not needed for long-term period, as the DI was relieved significantly.

Pearls and Controversies

This is another typical case of CP withretro-chiasmatic expanding. Pre-fix of optical chiasm might play an important role for tumor extension. As concerned of the origination, the tumor located between diencephalon leaf of Liliequist membrane and the pia mater of third ventricular floor. Understanding such morphological features could maximize the protection of the nervous structures. On the other hand, the transsphenoidal approach might play more important role in surgical treatment of such CP with this special growth mode.

CISTERNAL CRANIOPHARYGIOMA (TYPE "S")

Case 1

Medical History

A 59-year-old male patient presented with a 3-month history of headache and dizziness and progressive aggravation and vomiting of 1 week's duration. The patient had not undergone any treatment before presenting at our hospital.

Physical and Experimental Examination

The patient exhibited normal consciousness as well as normal visual acuity and vision field with no significant defects; his bilateral pupil sizes and reflections were normal. Endocrinological detection indicated normal hormone levels.

Radiological Images Before Surgery

Computed tomography (CT) indicated a mixed cystic-solid lesion occupying the intrasellar and suprasellar region along with a small amount of punctate calcification on the cystic wall. Magnetic resonance imaging (MRI) revealed a typical tubero-infundibular type craniopharyngioma (CP) with a protruding cystic lesion that had occupied the third ventricular cavity and caused hydrocephalus. According to our classifications, the tumor type was "subarachnoidal" and "T". The solid tumor was located at the median and left side of the infundibulum with anterior extension through the first space. The lower segment of the pituitary stalk (PS) was normal as indicated by the red arrow in Fig. (**32**).

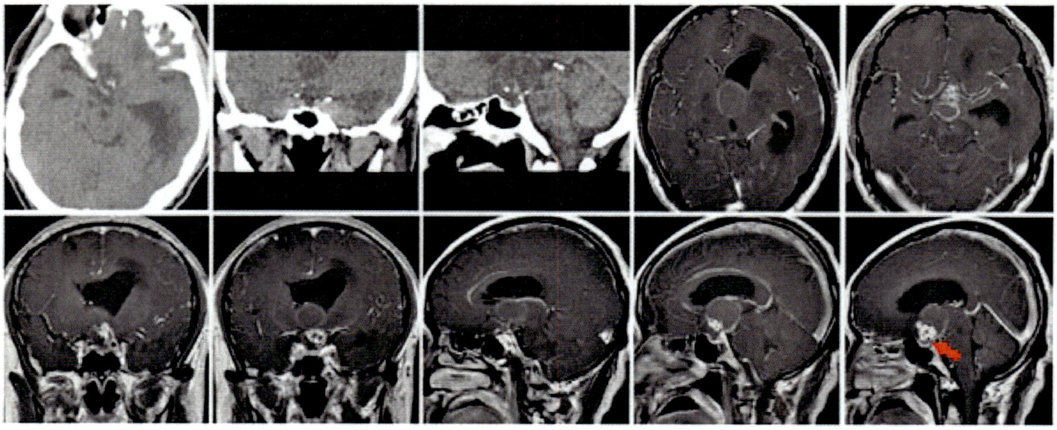

Fig. (32). Clinical presurgical images from the typical Case 1. The red arrow indicates the intact lower segment of the pituitary stalk.

Analysis Before Surgery

This tumor was a typical adult tubero-infundibular CP. Regarding its origin, according to pioneering histological findings published by Erdheim, the nests of epithelial cell remnants that give rise to CPs (following his embryological theory concerning the origin of CP from an incompletely involuted craniopharyngeal duct) are mainly found in two areas: (1) at the anterior-superior surface of the pituitary gland–PS junction and (2) at the interface between the pars tuberalis and infundibulum. In this case, the site of origin was the latter location. As shown in the schematic drawing, the main tumor body was tumor located inside the arachnoid sleeve of the PS (ASPS). As a result, there was no significant interface between the tumor and tubero-infundibulum. However, part of the tumor extended to the subarachnoid cistern through the prechiasmatic space (first space) and the arachnoidal sleeve still covered the surface of this part of the tumor, providing a surgical interface between the surrounding structures.

Regarding surgical approach selection, the posterior tumor border was located behind the anterior communicating artery (AcoA) complex and reached the anterior commissure. Therefore, a frontobasal interhemispheric (FIH) approach was selected. The lamina terminalis space was opened to dissect the tubero-infundibular part of the tumor. Extra-axial spaces (*e.g*., first and second spaces) were used to remove the external part of tumor, and cotton pads were needed to push the tumor upward inside the third ventricle floor (3rd VF) to facilitate dissection through the lamina terminalis. In such cases, if the AcoA complex obstructs exposure of the terminalis space and good development of the bilateral A1 and A2 segments, the AcoA artery can be dissected to provide sufficient exposure.

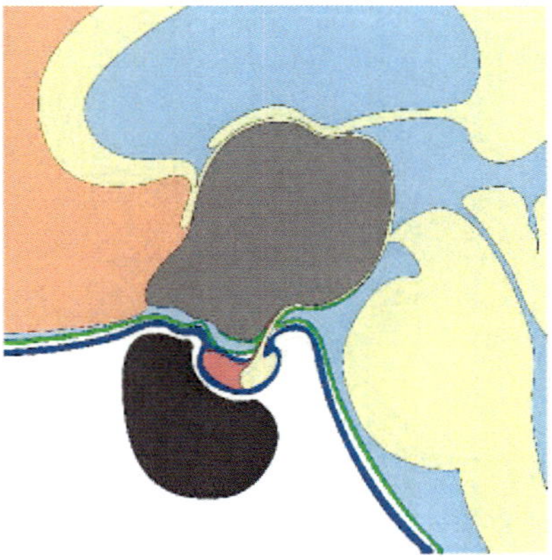

Fig. (33). Schematic Fig. (demonstrating the tumor morphology and relationships with the surrounding structures.

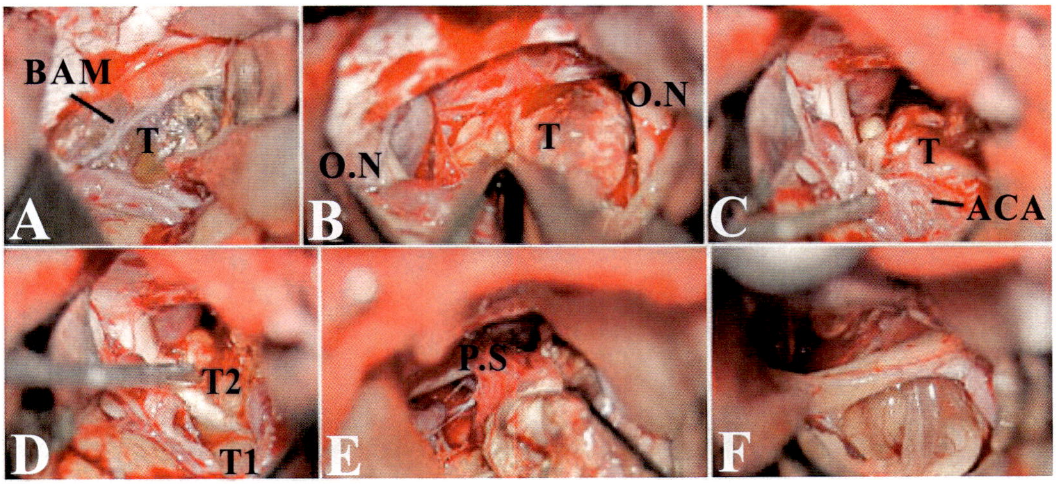

Fig. (34). Intraoperative findings. **A.** After dissecting the anterior interhemispheric fissure, the basement arachnoid membrane-covered suprasellar tumor was exposed. **B.** Through the enlarged prechiasmatic space, the tumor located inside the suprasellar arachnoid cistern was dissected. **C.** Relationship of the tumor and anterior communicating artery complex. **D.** The tumor originated from the hypothalamic infundibulum and expanded posteriorly toward the third ventricle floor (3rd VF; T1 in Fig. () and also anteriorly to the arachnoidal cistern (T2 in Fig. (). **E.** Relationship of tumor with the pituitary stalk. **F.** After removing the tumor inside the 3rd VF, the third ventricular cavity was entered by opening the lamina terminalis.

Intrasurgical Findings

A FIH approach was used to remove the tumor. Through an enlarged prechiasmatic approach, the basement arachnoid membrane (BAM)-covered tumor was exposed. The relationship between the tumor and PS was observed after dissecting the suprasellar tumor that had protruded from the infundibulum. The tumor had originated from the infundibulum, with expansion backward toward the 3rd VF and also forward to the subarachnoid cistern. The lamina terminalis was opened to remove the tumor located inside the nervous tissue layer of the 3rd VF.

Perioperative Treatment

The postsurgical recovery was uneventful except for minor diabetes insipidus (DI), a water-electrolyte imbalance disorder, and partial hypopituitarism. The patient's fluid input and output volume and plasma sodium levels were monitored.

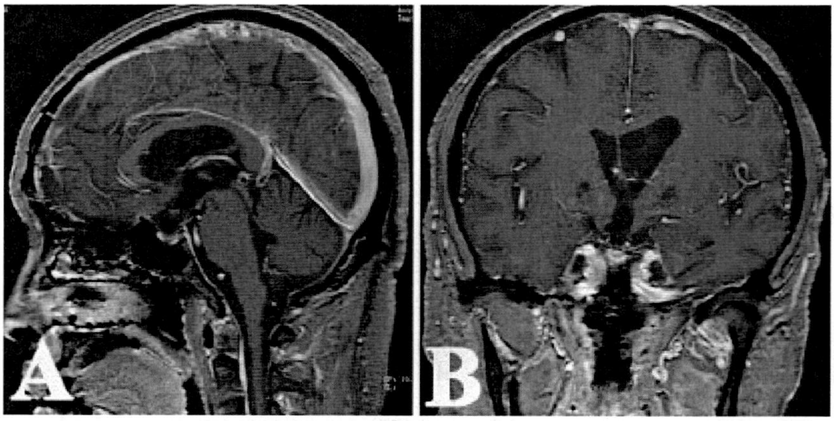

Fig. (35). Postsurgical magnetic resonance imaging confirmed total tumor removal.

Long-term Follow Up

No tumor recurrence was detected after 8 years of follow-up. The patient's pituitary function partially recovered. He required supplemental oral prednisone therapy to treat hormone insufficiency. His thyroxine axis function recovered, and he did not require euthyrox substitution. His body mass index (BMI) increased slightly from 20.3 before surgery to 22.4. His visual acuity was completely recovered.

Pearls and Controversies

There always existed controversies about the relationship between tumor and 3rd ventricular floor. If the nervous tissue of 3rd ventricular floor located at the top of the tumor or displaced to the ventral of the tumor? In this case, the intraoperative Fig. (s clearly indicated that the tumor penetrated the third ventricular floor and displayed as an intra- and extra-ventricular morphology. The result provided great understanding and helps for dealing with this key point within the surgery of craniopharyngioma.

Case 2

Medical History

A 7-year-old male patient presented with a 6-month history of headache, decreased visual acuity, polyuria, and polydipsia. He had not undergone any surgical treatment at other hospitals.

Physical and Experimental Examination

The patient exhibited normal consciousness with visual acuity of 0.5 and 0.3 in the right and left eyes, respectively. Endocrinological detection indicated a slight increase in T4 and slight decrease in progesterone (PRGE).

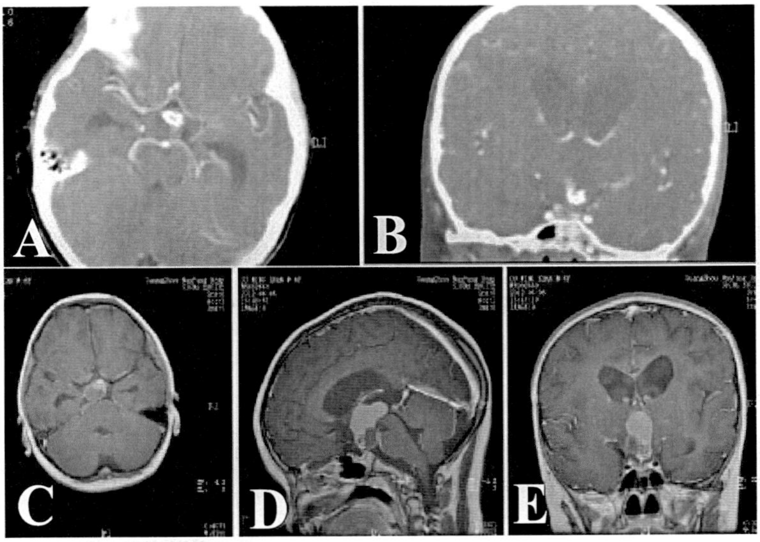

Fig. (36). Presurgical computed tomography (CT) and magnetic resonance imaging (MRI) of Case 5. **A-B.** Presurgical CT indicated a predominantly cystic tumor in the suprasellar region without significant calcification. **C-E.** MRI indicated a tumor that had originated from the infundibular part with invagination into the third ventricular floor and occupation of the third ventricular cavity.

Radiological Images Before Surgery

CT indicated a mixed cystic-solid suprasellar lesion with a small calcification mass in the infundibulum. The cystic tumor occupied the third ventricular cavity and had caused hydrocephalus. MRI revealed a typical infundibulotuberal CP. The solid tumor was located at the infundibulum, a possible site of origin. The cystic tumor extended backwards to occupy most of the third ventricular cavity and obstruct the foramen of Monro. The lower segment of the PS was normal, as indicated by the red arrow in Fig. (**37**).

Analysis Before Surgery

This was a typical 3rd VF CP. On presurgical MRI, the relationship of tumor to the nervous tissue of the 3rd VF could not be clearly identified. During surgery, however, there was a clearly identifiable interface between the tumor and hypothalamus. The intact 3rd VF and pituitary stalk were preserved.

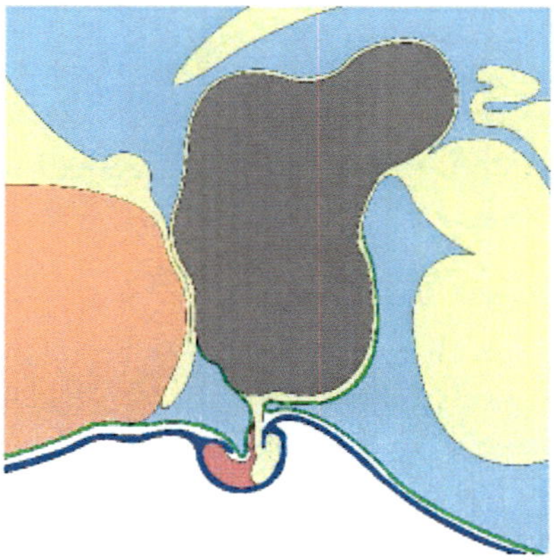

Fig. (37). Schematic Fig. (demonstrating the tumor morphology and relationships with the surrounding structures.

Intra-Surgical Findings

A FIH approach was used to remove the tumor.

Paraoperative Treatment and Occurrence of Complications

The patient's postsurgical recovery was uneventful except for transient DI and a minor water-electrolyte disorder.

Long-term Follow Up

No tumor recurrence was detected after 3 years of follow-up. The patient had not significant dysfunction except for a slight increase in weight. He did not require long-term hormone substitution. His BMI increased slightly from 24.6 before surgery to 25.9.

Pearls and Controversies

The tumor of this patients was seemed as locating purely inside the third ventricular cavity. By presurgical images, the 3rd ventricular floor was involved severely, which was belong to the Grade 2 of the hypothalamic involvement classification. However, in operation, the nervous tissue of third ventricular floor could be maintained intact. Moreover, the tumor boundary was clear, which could be clearly identified and separated. So it should be a valuable project being worthy to be investigated for neurosurgeon that how to confirm if a infundibulo-tuberal CP could be radical total removed by presurgical images.

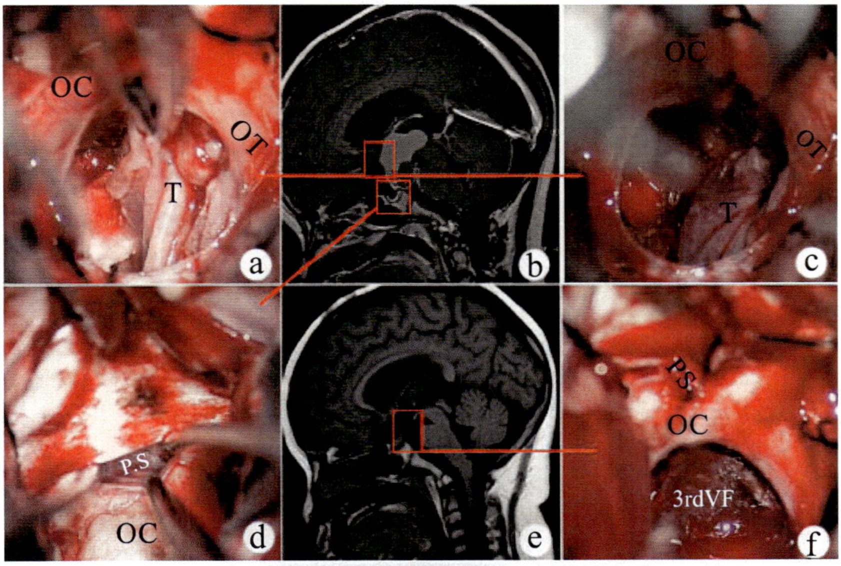

Fig. (38). Intraoperative findings. **A.** The lamina terminalis was opened to expose the tumor. The tumor was dissected along the interface between the tumor and nervous tissue layer of the third ventricular floor (3rd VF). **B.** Presurgical sagittal magnetic resonance imaging (MRI). **C.** The site of tumor origin remained at the infundibular part of the pituitary stalk, where the tumor was sharply dissected while attempting to preserve the hypothalamus–pituitary stalk axial continuity. **D.** A small prechiasmatic space was observed. **E.** Postsurgical sagittal MRI. **F.** The 3rd VF was well preserved after total tumor removal.

Case 3

Medical History

A 54-year-old male patient presented with a 2-mont history of progressive nausea, vomiting, and decreased visual acuity. The patient had not undergone any surgical treatment at other hospitals.

Physical and Experimental Examination

The patient exhibited normal consciousness. Endocrinological detection indicated slight increases in fT4, FSH, and PRL.

Radiological Images Before Surgery

CT indicated a solid suprasellar tumor without significant calcification. MRI showed the lesion originating from the tubero-infundibulum without excessive extension. The tumor was significant enhanced on the T1-weighted enhanced MRI. According to our classification, the tumor type was "subarachnoidal" and "T". The lower segment of the PS was normal.

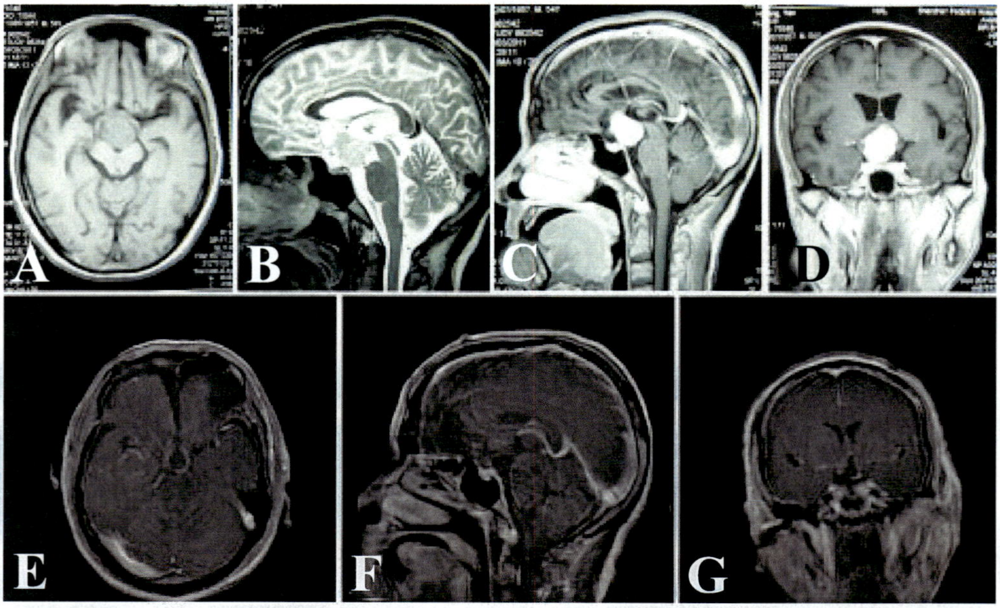

Fig. (39). Presurgical and postsurgical magnetic resonance imaging (MRI) of Case 6. **A-D.** Presurgical MRI. **E-G.** Postsurgical MRI indicated total tumor removal.

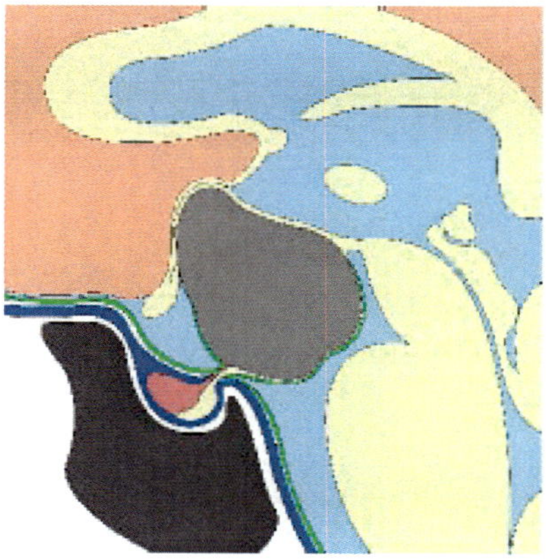

Fig. (40). Schematic Fig. (demonstrating the tumor morphology and relationships with the surrounding structures).

Intrasurgical Findings

A FIH approach was used to remove the tumor.

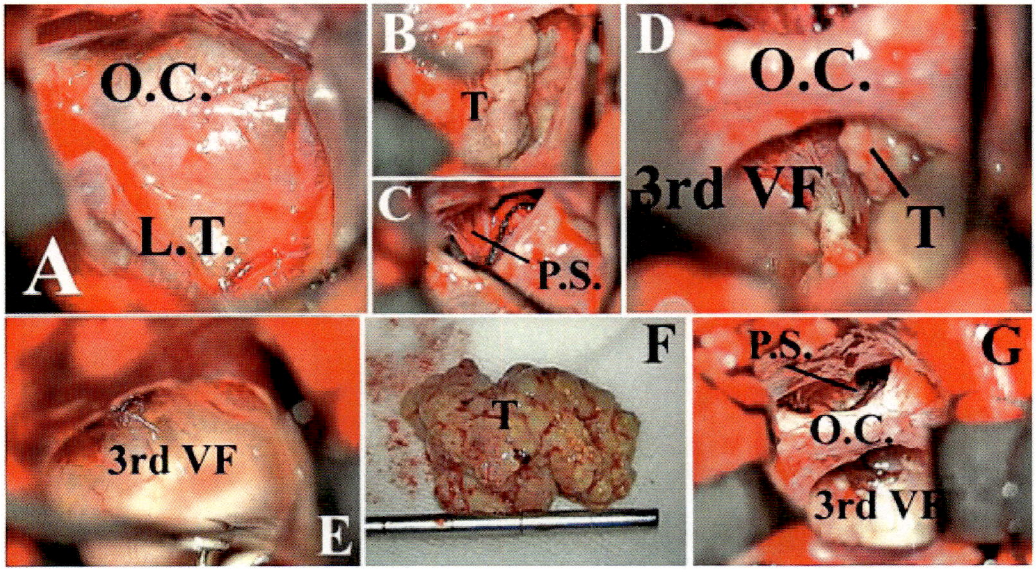

Fig. (41). Intraoperative findings. **A.** After dissecting the interhemispheric fissure, the optic chiasm and bulged lamina terminalis were exposed. **B-C.** The tumor was exposed and separated after opening the terminalis. The intact lower segment of the pituitary stalk was observed through the first surgical space. **D.** Site of tumor origin at the upper segment of the pituitary stalk. **E.** The third ventricle floor (3rd VF) remained intact except at the site of origin. **F.** The tumor was totally removed. **G.** After tumor removal, a defect existed in the anterior part of the 3rd VF (site of origin).

Perioperative Treatment

The patient's postsurgical recovery was uneventful except for moderate DI and a water-electrolyte disorder. After active fluid substitution treatment and sodium level adjustments, the patient's condition was relieved.

Long-term Follow Up

A recurrent tumor was identified after 2 years of follow-up. External beam radiation therapy was used to treat the recurrent tumor. The tumor subsequently remained stable during an additional 2 years of follow-up. The patient exhibited significant weight gain and a increase in BMI from 21.4 to 26.3.

Pearls and Controversies

This case was a typical Squamous papillary CP. So we indicated the typical growth pattern and surgical manipulation of this kind of tumor in this case. The most part of the nervous tissue of 3rd ventricular floor can be reserved.

Case 4

Medical History

A 35-year-old male patient presented with a 6-month history of sexual disorder, memory loss, polydipsia, and polyuria. The patient had not undergone any surgical treatment at other hospitals.

Physical and Experimental Examination

The patient exhibited normal consciousness. Endocrinological detection indicated slightly increased FSH and PRL levels.

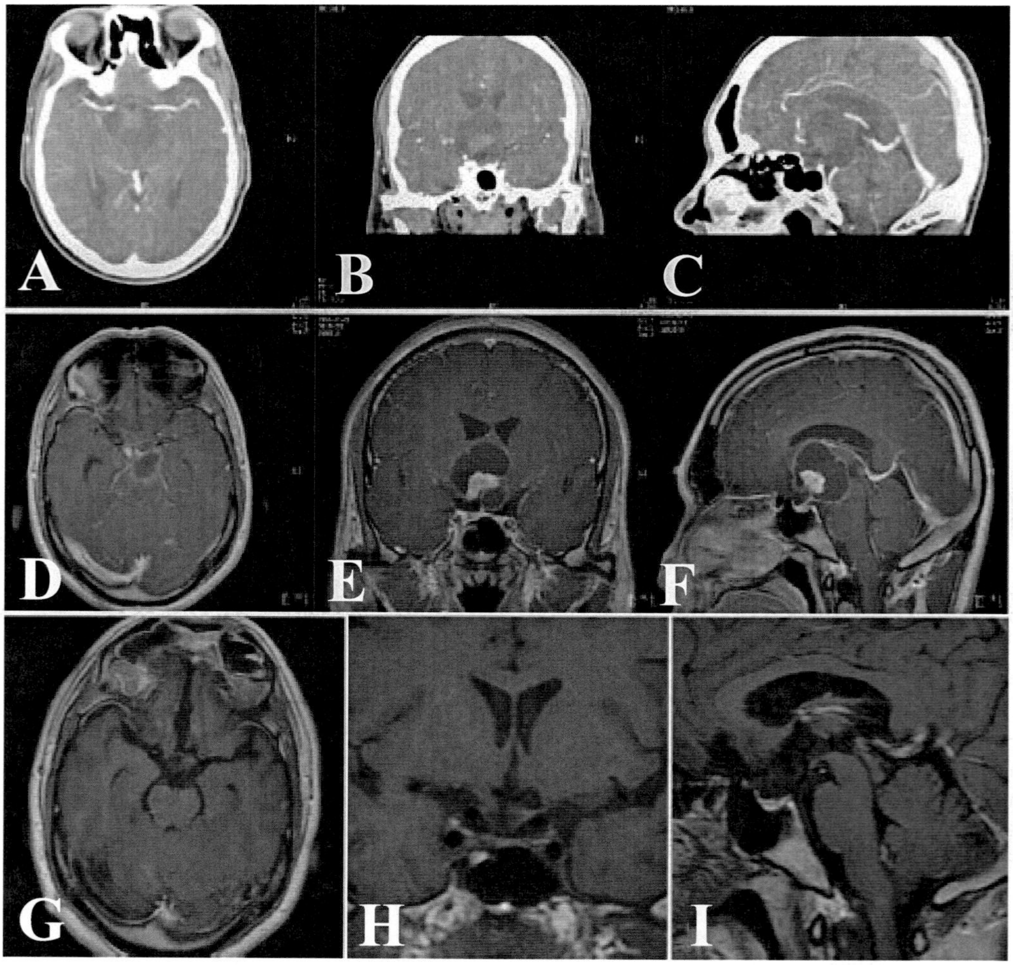

Fig. (42). Presurgical and postsurgical computed tomography and magnetic resonance imaging.

Radiological Images Before Surgery

This was a typical admantinomatous tumor located in the third ventricular walls. An interhemispheric approach was indicated in combination with opening of the lamina terminalis to remove the tumor.

Analysis Before Surgery

A FIH approach was selected to remove the tumor. The prefixed chiasm limited exposure of the lamina terminalis. The AcoA could be dissected to provide greater exposure after evaluating the bilateral A1 and A2 segments of the ACA.

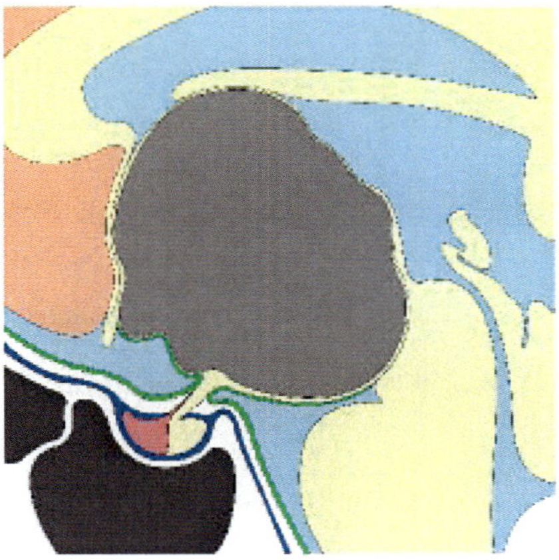

Fig. (43). Schematic Fig. (demonstrating the tumor morphology and relationships with the surrounding structures.

Intrasurgical Findings

After dissecting the interhemispheric fissure, the sellar region structure was exposed. The prefixed chiasmatic space restricted the use of the first surgical space. Following sufficient exposure of the lamina terminalis, the AcoA complex was visible. The AcoA itself was short and small with Hubner recurrent artery origination. Through the small first space, the intact lower segment of the PS was observed. Because the bilateral A1 and A2 segments of the ACA were well developed, the AcoA was dissected at the right side of the Hubner recurrence artery. The entire lamina terminalis was subsequently exposed. Next, the bilateral ICA was separated from the enlarged 3rd VF. After opening the terminalis, the tumor inside the 3rd VF was separated from the nervous tissue layer of the 3rd VF. The 3rd VF remained intact after total tumor removal.

Perioperative Treatment

The patient's postsurgical recovery was uneventful except for moderate DI and a water-electrolyte disorder. These conditions were relieved after active fluid substitution treatment and sodium level adjustments.

Long-term Follow Up

Tumor regrowth was identified after a 1-year follow-up. Gamma-knife radiotherapy was used to treat the recurrent tumor. The tumor remained stable during a subsequent 3-year follow-up study. The patient exhibited significant weight gain, with a slight increase in BMI from 22.8 to 26.3.

Pearls and Controversies

The reason for choosing this case was because that it provided the typical morphological features of the cystic degeneration in squamous papillary CP. In the meantime, tumor residual at the lateral wall of third ventricle recurred during follow-up period, which was controlled well by Gamma knife. So the conclusion of poor therapeutic value of Gamma knife to CP could be revised. It needed further evaluation of Gamma knife for small tumor residual.

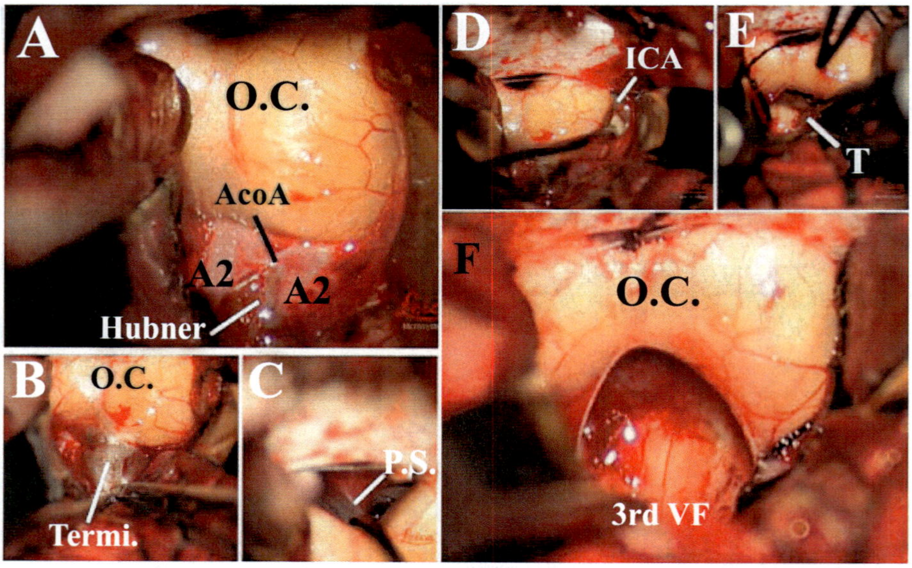

Fig. (44). Intraoperative findings. **A.** After dissecting the interhemispheric fissure, the bulged terminalis and small first surgical space (due to the prefixed optic chiasm) were observed. The anterior communicating artery (AcoA) complex and Hubner recurrence branch were exposed. **B.** Because the A1 and A2 segments of the anterior carotid artery were well developed, the AcoA was dissected at the right side of the Hubner branch, which was kept intact. **C.** The lower segment of the pituitary stalk was observed through the first surgical space. **D.** The right side of the internal carotid artery was separated from the third ventricle floor (3rd VF) along the arachnoidal interface. **E.** Following sufficient exposure, the lamina terminalis was opened to reveal the tumor. . The tumor was located inside the nervous tissue layer of the 3rd VF. The intact 3rd VF was preserved after total tumor removal.

Case 5

Medical History

A 21-year old male patient presented with a 6-month history of severe headache and memory disorder.

Physical and Experimental Examination

No significant positive physical signs were observed. Endocrinological detection indicated panhypopituitarism. The PRL level was increased slightly.

Radiological Images Before Surgery

CT indicated a suprasellar tumor with calcification in the third ventricular cavity. MRI indicated a predominantly cystic tumor that had originated from the tubero-infundibular part of the PS. The tumor had expanded towards the 3rd VF. The lower segment of the PS was intact, whereas the upper segment was severely inflated. The cystic wall was significantly enhanced on T1-weighted enhanced MRI.

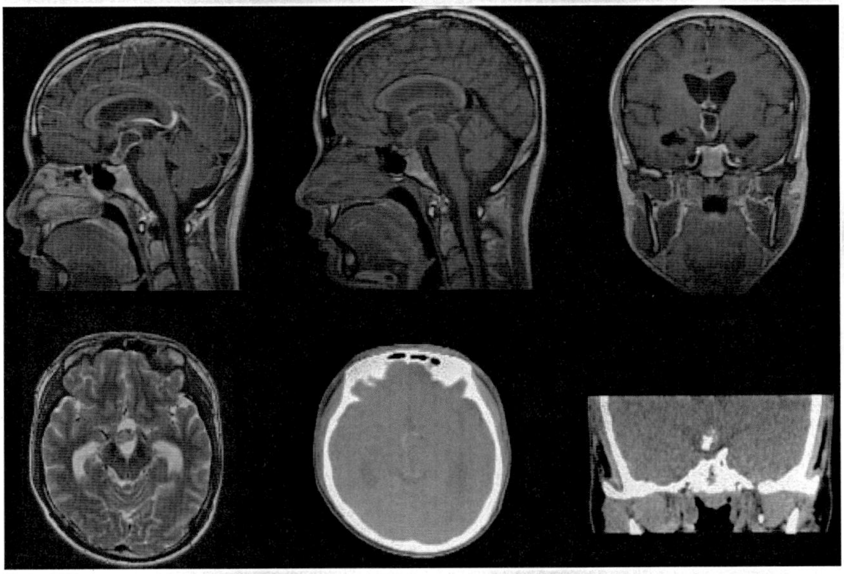

Fig. (45). Presurgical computed tomography and magnetic resonance imaging.

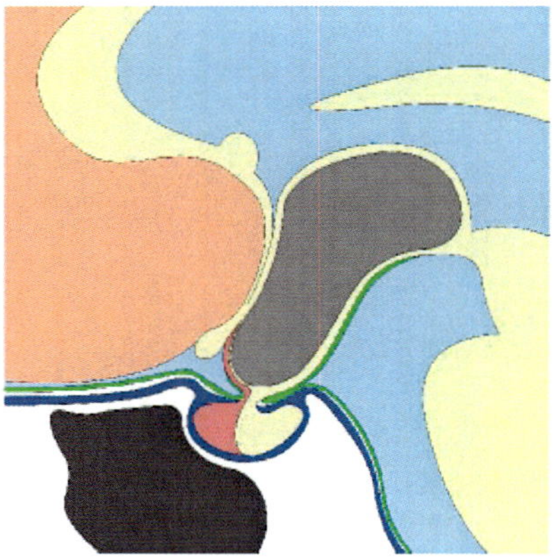

Fig. (46). Schematic Fig. (demonstrating the tumor morphology and relationships with the surrounding structures.

Intra-Surgical Findings

A FIH approach was used to remove the tumor. The arachnoid sleeve-covered lower segment of the PS was observed through the small prechiasmatic space. The lamina terminalis was opened. The nervous tissue layer of the 3rd VF was opened to expose the true tumor. The tumor was separated while attempting to protect the 3rd VF.

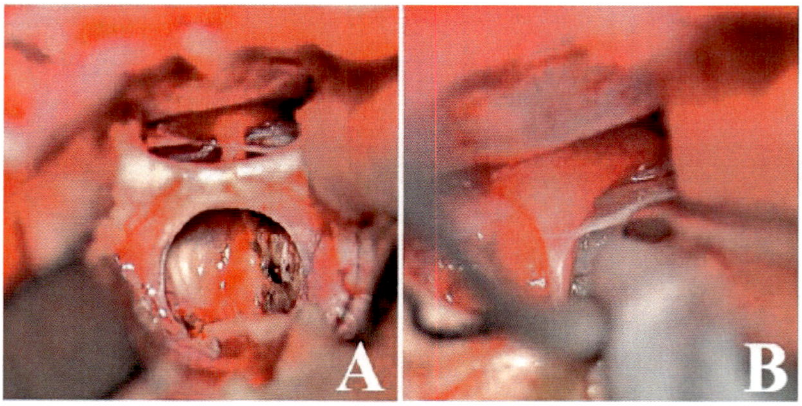

Fig. (47). Intraoperative findings. After tumor removal, the intact 3rd ventricular nervous tissue was observed. And the continuity of pituitary stalk to the infundibulo-tuberalis was maintained.

Perioperative Treatment

Pathological analysis confirmed the diagnosis of adamantinomatous CP. Postsurgical endocrinological detection indicated panhypopituitarism.

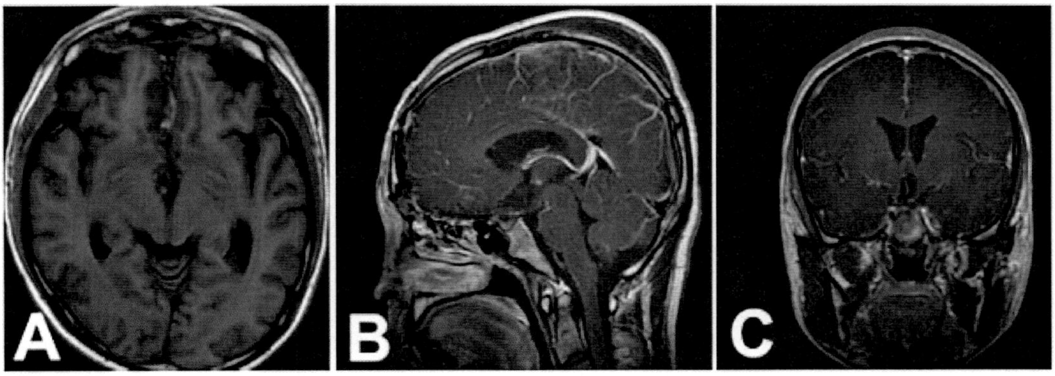

Fig. (48). Postsurgical magnetic resonance imaging indicated total tumor removal.

Long-term Follow Up

No tumor recurrence was detected after 2 years of follow-up. The patient's sexual function remained deficient. He suffered from growth retardation and required oral prednisone and euthyrox as substitution therapy for hypopituitarism. The patient also exhibited significant weight gain. His BMI increased slightly from 25.2 to 28.2.

Pearls and Controversies

This case showed a craniopharyngioma with the special growth pattern in presurgical images. But as matter of fact, this is a common morphological feature of the trans-infundibular type of CP. As this tumor's volume was small, the relationship of tumor to pituitary stalk and infundibulo-tuberalis can be displayed more clearly. The rounded enhancement of tumor's boundary indicated the severe involvement of surrounding nervous tissue. So even a small tumor, the patient suffered severe hypothalamic reaction after surgery.

CONFLICT OF INTEREST

The authors (editor) declares no conflict of interest, financial or otherwise.

ACKNOWLEDGEMENTS

Declared none.

Afterword

Many days have passed; it has been 4 years since we began writing this book. Although most of our time was spent on clinical analyses and investigations in order to remain synchronous with new trends, research related to craniopharyngioma continued to shift rapidly worldwide with each passing day. The clinical data and experiences have progressed remarkably, despite our concerns with our own changes. The annual number of craniopharyngioma patients increased from 20–30 to 60–70 cases. Moreover, recurrent tumors also increased significantly in different areas of China, suggesting a different therapeutic trend. Despite that this book is now fully completed after careful, critical research, it becomes obvious that many dilemmas, controversies, and questions about craniopharyngioma remain and will require further investigation and follow-up.

First, we admit that craniopharyngioma should no longer be classified as a rare intracranial lesion. Rather, it should be considered one of the most common congenital benign tumors, especially in pediatric patients. Second, extremely urgent fields that require further evaluation include surgical treatment with the aim of gross total tumoral removal, endoscopic transsphenoidal surgery, and a comparison of the curative effects of these treatments. Third, the impact of endocrine-related diseases on the long-term quality of life of craniopharyngioma patients should be further investigated to improve surgical safety. Fourth, radiotherapy and stereotactic radiosurgery (SRS) remain in common use for the treatment of craniopharyngioma. Notably, many centers utilize SRS as a routine treatment. Our opinion, based on the results from our single center, is that radiotherapy and SRS seriously affect the patient's quality of life, as well as secondary surgery manipulation. Therefore, it is critical to conduct a correct evaluation of the role and efficacy of SRS. Fifth, the influence of craniopharyngioma on endocrinology is more severe than that of other lesions that occur in a similar location, such as adenomas. The achievement of more accurate endocrinological monitoring and more effective treatment substitutions remains challenging with respect to the long-term survival of some patients worldwide. Finally, the difficulty of craniopharyngioma surgery is undeniable, leading to study requirements and a long learning curve. Meanwhile, it is fairly difficult to correct endocrine disorders. Therefore, Cushing's description from the last century, "Craniopharyngioma is a problem making neurosurgeon so depressed and difficult", largely remains true nowadays. It is foreseeable that in the era of big data and accurate medical treatment, the above-described challenging issues will eventually be resolved properly. This process requires not only the superb surgical techniques of neurosurgeons and a deeper understanding of the growth patterns of this disease, but also multidisciplinary collaborations with endocrinologists and radiosurgeons. In addition, the new developments from basic research on the mechanism of this disease are also anticipated.

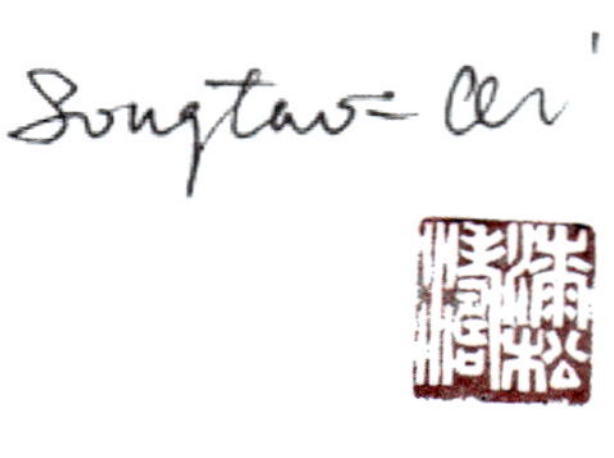

SUBJECT INDEX

A

B

C

D

E

F

G

H

I

O

P

R

S

T

U

V

W

Made in United States
North Haven, CT
04 November 2026

21727486R00241